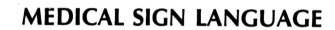

MEDICAL SIGN LANGUAGE

MEDICAL SIGN LANGUAGE

Easily Understood Definitions of Commonly Used Medical, Dental and First Aid Terms

By

W. JOSEPH GARCIA

Director
Silent Environment Educational Kamp
Ellensburg, Washington

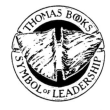

CHARLES C THOMAS • PUBLISHER
Springfield • Illinois • U.S.A.

Published and Distributed Throughout the World by

CHARLES C THOMAS • PUBLISHER
2600 South First Street
Springfield, Illinois, 62717, U.S.A.

© *1983 by* CHARLES C THOMAS • PUBLISHER
ISBN 0-398-04805-3 (cloth)
ISBN 0-398-04806-1 (paper)
Library of Congress Catalog Card Number: 82-40446

With THOMAS BOOKS *careful attention is given to all details of
manufacturing and design. It is the Publisher's desire to present books
that are satisfactory as to their physical qualities and artistic possibilities
and appropriate for their particular use.* THOMAS BOOKS *will be true
to those laws of quality that assure a good name and good will.*

Printed in the United States of America
R-1

**Project Creator
and Director**
W. Joseph Garcia

Illustrators
Kay Meacham
Camille Cole Buch
Victoria Yarbrough

Anatomical Drawings By
Lynn McCowin
Victoria Yarbrough
Kay Meacham

Written By
Lynn Carlson
Marsha Nash
W. Joseph Garcia

Cover Designed By
Camille Cole Buch

**Technical Assistance
Sign Language**
Jer Loudenback
Sheryl Kool
Theresa Smith
Frank Caccamise, Ph.D.

Medical
Patrick Smith, M.D.
Jud Weaver, D.D.S.
William R. Meyer, O.D., P.S.

Edited By
Joseph Zwaniziger
David Canzler, Ph.D.
W. Joseph Garcia
Jer Loudenback
Marsha Nash
Sheryl Kool
LuAnn Newton

Special Assistance By
Terry Stratton
Susan Nagamine
Lucinda Sorensen
Joseph Zwaniziger
Susan Barto
Mary Northrup
Kathy Peters
Karen Stevens

Production and Photographics By
Kay Meacham
Victoria Yarbrough
Marsha Nash
W. Joseph Garcia

This manual is dedicated to
my Mother and Father
and Mr. Felix and Mrs. Barbra McGinnis
who made the entire project possible.

INTRODUCTION

To the Medical Facility:

It is suggested at least one person on staff per working shift be enrolled in an American Sign Language (ASL) class. This manual will greatly assist one in communicating medical information to the deaf once understanding of ASL is acquired. A medical facility may wish to keep this manual on hand for reference when an interpreter or individual with signing experience is not available. This manual may assist in communicating medical information to the deaf under these circumstances.

To the Deaf Individual:

This manual was designed to provide the reader with clear, easily understood definitions of commonly used medical, dental, and first aid terms.

To the Interpreter for the Deaf:

This manual offers suggestions for interpreting medical terms. In cases where we were unable to equate a sign for some terms, the interpreter may sign the accompanying definitions, which were written in a manner to facilitate interpreting English into American Sign Language.

For terms with a common sign variation used widely by the deaf, a second or third suggested sign will be included.

A different face and the letters a, b, c, or d are used to show the sign's variations. Dotted lines show the beginning positions of the hands. (DM) = double movement, (SM) = single movement, and (MM) = multiple movement.

There are several hand shapes referred to throughout the manual. They are as follows:

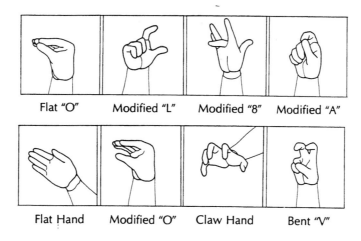

Flat "O"   Modified "L"   Modified "8"   Modified "A"

Flat Hand   Modified "O"   Claw Hand   Bent "V"

To the Beginning Signer:

Take classes in American Sign Language (ASL). Learn the syntax and morphology of ASL in addition to the cultural aspects of the deaf society, and then this manual will be valuable to you. Any text that only provides vocabulary lists should be avoided until understanding of the ASL language structure is obtained.

It would be inappropriate to try to include in this Introduction the principles of American Sign Language. I believe more would be gained by the beginner learning this information through the instructor of an ASL class.

An important point to make is that giving a deaf person a written note is not an accurate way to achieve communication. English is a second language to the deaf and not their native language. Lou Fant wrote in the Introduction to his text, *An Introduction to Ameslam,* "Imagine yourself in a glass sound proof booth with a pencil and paper. Outside is a person trying to teach you to read, write and speak the Japanese language." How well would you master the language? How long would it take? How comfortable would you be trying to communicate your medical problems and needs, especially in written form, through this language?

ACKNOWLEDGMENTS

A special thanks to the Leonardt Foundation for giving birth to the SEEK program.

The following individuals and organizations helped open communication between the deaf and medical services by supporting this project.

Sunnen Foundation
E.K. and Lillian F. Bishop Foundation
M.J. Murdock Foundation
Unigard Insurance Company
Charis Fund
Seattle First National Bank
William Randolph Hearst Foundation
Joseph Wharton Foundation
Boeing Company Charitable Trust
Scott B. and Annie P. Appleby Trust
Grover Hermann Foundation
Norman Archibald Charitable Fund
Safeco Insurance
Jennie S. Baker Foundation
Rainier National Bank
Wausau Insurance Company
Forest Foundation
Washington National Insurance
General Mills Foundation
Pacific Northwest Bell
Record Printing
NuArc Company, Inc.
Kalart Victor Corporation
M.P. Goodkin Company
Dale Meredith
Valley Cafe
Koh-I-Noor Rapidograph, Inc.
Grange Insurance
Safeway Company, Inc.
Ellensburg Junior Womens Club
Kreonite, Inc.
Amos-Hill Veneer & Lumber Company
Dietrich-Post Company
Elmo Corporation
North American Van Lines, Inc.
J.C. Penney Co., Inc.
Richard Photo Products
Mrs. Joan K. Snyder
Mr. Arnold Thorsen
Widex Hearing Aid Company
Dr. R.P. Whittaker
Vivitar Corporation

CONTENTS

Introduction

MEDICAL SIGN LANGUAGE

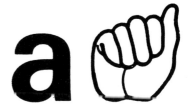

ABDOMEN

The belly; the part of the body below the chest and above the legs. It includes the stomach, intestines, gallbladder, spleen, liver, pancreas and bladder. *See Figure 1*

(1) The fingertips of the right "flat" hand make a circle on the lower stomach.(SM)

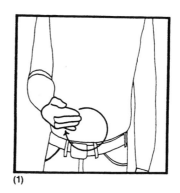

ABDOMINAL CRAMP

A tightening of the muscles in the abdomen which is very painful and dangerous.

*An **abdominal cramp** may be a warning of a severe problem.*

(1) The fingertips of the right "flat" hand make a circle on the lower stomach.(SM)

(2) Sign CRAMP — both "claw" hands are at stomach level with palms facing in. Move both hands into "S" hands and twist in opposite directions as if wringing out a cloth. (SM)

* *The facial expression should show pain.*

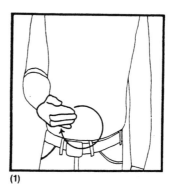
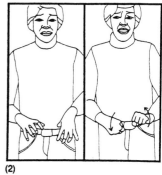

ABERRATION

An error in the way the lens of the eye focuses light.

*Due to an **aberration**, her vision was blurred.*

(1) Sign SEE — the right "V" hand faces in at eye level. Move the hand out forward.(SM)

(2) Both "five" hands face each other at eye level, with the right hand on the inside. Move both hands alternately from right to left a few times.(MM)

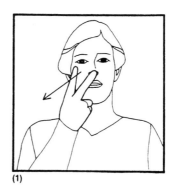
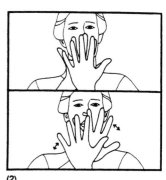

3

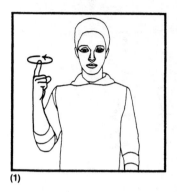
(1)

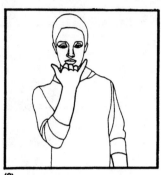
(2)

ABNORMAL

Not right, not normal, irregular or unusual.

Being sick for a long time is abnormal.

(1) Sign SOMETHING — the right "one" hand faces left at chest level and makes a small circle, keeping the wrist stiff.(SM)
(2) Sign WRONG — the right "Y" hand faces in under the chin.(SM)

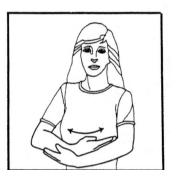
a.(1)

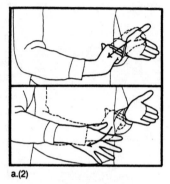
a.(2)

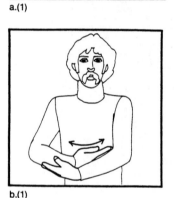
b.(1)

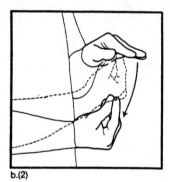
b.(2)

ABORTION

A natural or medically caused removal of a baby from the uterus before it is ready to be born.

It is important to watch for infection following an abortion.

a. (1) Sign BABY — the right hand and forearm face up, resting on the left hand and forearm which also face upward. Both are then rocked back and forth as if holding a baby.(MM)
(2) The left "flat" hand faces right at stomach level. The right "claw" hand moves down the left palm into an "A" hand then opens into a "five" hand as it is thrown down.(SM)
b. (1) Sign BABY — the right hand and forearm face up, resting on the left hand and forearm which also face upward. Both are then rocked back and forth as if holding a baby.(MM)
(2) The left cupped hand faces down at stomach level. The fingertips of the right "flat-O" hand touch the left palm. Move the right hand down towards the floor.(SM)

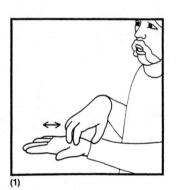
(1)

ABRASION

A wound caused by the scraping away of the skin with something rough.

It is important to thoroughly clean an abrasion to prevent infection.

(1) The left "flat" hand faces up at chest level. The right "claw" hand scratches back and forth on the left palm.(MM)

* *The right "flat" hand could rub the exact injured area following this sign.*

4

ABSCESS

A collection of pus in an infected area of the body, usually near an opening in the skin or a wound.

A doctor should be seen when an abscess is present because it may spread and infect the entire body.

ABSORB

To soak up.

One reason bandages are used is to absorb blood and fluids from wounds.

(1) Both "five" hands face in at waist level. Move both hands up to chest level, ending in "flat-O" hands.(SM)

* The mouth movement should imitate sucking in the air.

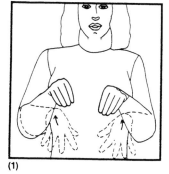

(1)

ABSTINENCE

Going without sexual activity. Abstinence can also be used to mean going without anything, as alcohol, food or drugs.

A doctor may advise abstinence after a woman has a baby to prevent infection in her vagina and to allow any damage done during labor to be repaired.

a. (1) Sign SEX — the right "X" hand faces out and touches at the temple and then the upper jaw. (SM)
(2) The left "one" hand faces down at waist level. The right "X" hand faces down and hooks over the left index finger. Move both hands up to chest level. (SM)
b. (1) Sign SEX — the right "X" hand faces out and touches at the temple and then the upper jaw. (SM)
(2) Sign NONE — both "flat-O" hands face down at shoulder level. Move both hands out forward and to the sides.(SM)

* If food, drugs, or alcohol is meant, the sign for "food", "drugs", or "alcohol" should be signed followed by the NONE sign.

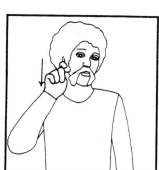

a.(1)

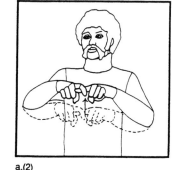

a.(2)

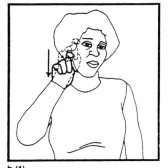

b.(1)

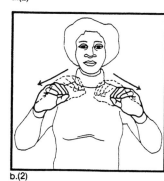

b.(2)

ABUSE

Wrong or improper use of something or someone, resulting in injury.

Drug and alcohol abuse are problems in today's society.

(1) Sign WRONG — the right "Y" hand faces in at the chin (SM)
(2) Sign USE — the left "S" hand faces down at chest level. The right "U" hand faces out and makes a small circle then touches the left hand.(SM)

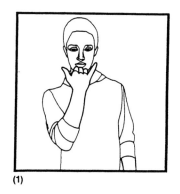

(1)

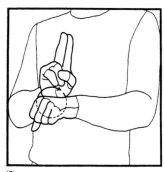

(2)

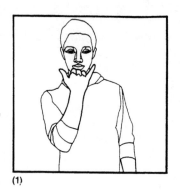 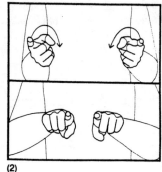

ACCIDENT

An undesirable, unexpected event resulting in damage.

The best way to avoid an accident is by being careful all of the time.

(1) Sign WRONG — the right "Y" hand faces in at the chin (SM)

(2) Sign HAPPEN — both "one" hands face up at chest level. Move both hands in and down, ending with palms facing down.(SM)

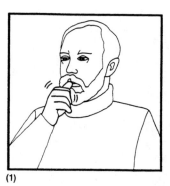 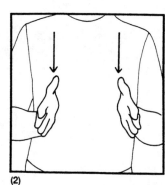

ACCIDENT VICTIM

A person involved in an accident.

An accident victim should get quick medical help.

(1) Sign SUFFER — the back of the thumb of the right "A" hand touches the chin. Pivot the hand slightly from left to right a few times.(MM)

* *The facial expression should show suffering.*

(2) Sign PERSON — both "flat" hands face each other at chest level. Move both hands down to waist level.(SM)

ACCOMMODATION

In optometry, the changes in the eye which allow us to see things that are different distances from us.

In accommodation, the muscles in the ciliary body help change the shape of the lens, allowing images at different distances to be focused on the retina.

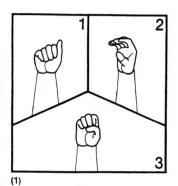 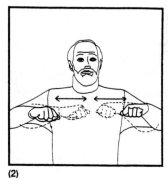

ACE BANDAGE®

The name under which a kind of bandage is sold. An ace bandage has elastic in it to make it stretchy.

An ace bandage is often used to apply firm constant pressure on a part of the body.

(1) Fingerspell "A-C-E".

(2) Both "A" hands face down at chest level. Move both hands out to the sides and then in a few times as if imitating something stretching. (MM)

(Continued on next page)

(3) Sign BANDAGE — the left "B" hand faces in at chest level. The right "B" hand also faces in. Circle the right hand out and around the left hand a few times as if imitating wrapping a bandage. (MM)

* This should be signed at the area where the bandage is being applied.

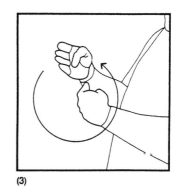

(3)

ACETYLSALICYLIC ACID
The chemical name for aspirin.

> *Acetylsalicylic acid is mixed with other chemicals to make common pain relievers.*

ACHE
A dull, persistent pain; the pain itself.

> *A continuous ache anywhere in the body is usually a sign that something is not right, and a doctor should be seen.*

(1) Sign PAIN — both "one" hands face each other with palms facing in. Twist both hands in opposite directions a few times.

*This can be signed at the area of an ache. Facial expression should show pain.

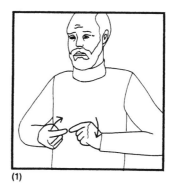

(1)

ACHILLES TENDON
The connecting tissue between the muscles in the calf and the heel. *See Figure 5*
(1) The right index finger points to the tendon.

ACID
A chemical that has a sour taste and will cause burns; in chemistry, a substance which can give up a proton or a hydrogen ion; the common slang name for L.S.D. (lysergic acid diethylamide).

> *All acids should be labeled and handled with great care.*

a. (1) Fingerspell "A-C-I-D" if referring to the chemical.

b. (1) Fingerspell "L-S-D" if referring to the drug.

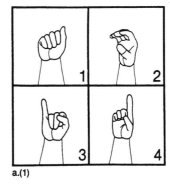

a.(1)

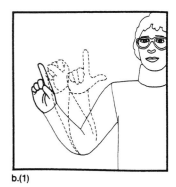

b.(1)

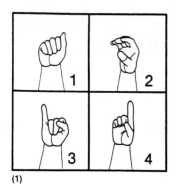
(1)

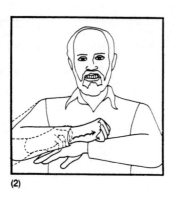
(2)

ACID BURNS

Those burns on the skin caused by contact with an acid.

*After washing an **acid burn** for 20 minutes, pain may still be present.*

(1) Fingerspell "A-C-I-D".
(2) The left "flat" hand faces down at chest level. The fingertips of the right "claw" hand climb up the left hand as if imitating eating away. (MM)

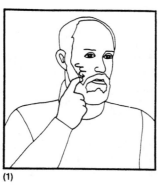
(1)

ACNE

A disease of the skin which results in small red bumps caused by an inflammation in the gland at the bottom of a hair in the skin. Acne, which usually occurs during adolescence, may be made worse by a poor diet, allergies, nervousness or not enough of a vitamin.

***Acne** can be treated by keeping the skin clean, not eating oily foods, using things on the skin which dry it out, and using antibiotics.*

(1) The index finger of the right "one" hand taps the face a few times.(MM)

ACOUSTIC

In audiology, having to do with sound or hearing.

*A room with flat walls does not have the same **acoustic** quality as a room with rough surfaces.*

ACRID

Harsh or strong smelling or tasting.

*An infected wound may have an **acrid** smell.*

(1) Sign SMELL — the fingertips of the right "flat" hand brush against the nose a few times.(MM)
(2) Sign TASTE — the middle finger of the right "eight" hand touches the tongue or lower lip.
(3) Sign STRONG — both "S" hands face in at chest level. Move both hands down slightly. (SM)
* The facial expression should reflect strong smelling or tasting.

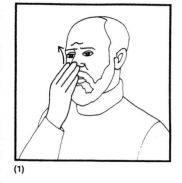
(1)

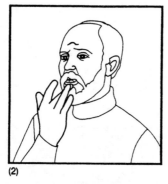
(2)

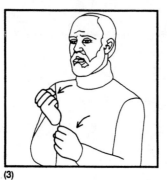
(3)

8

ACROPHOBIA

The fear of being in high places.

Acrophobia may be treated with therapy and counseling.

(1) Sign LOOK DOWN — the right "V" hand faces down at eye level and moves down.(SM)

* *The eyes should follow the movement of the right hand.*

(2) Sign FAR — the left "A" hand with the thumb extended, is at shoulder level facing in. The right "A" hand with the thumb extended, faces in at shoulder level and moves down and out.(SM)

* *The eyes should follow the movement of the right hand.*

(3) Sign FEAR — both "A" hands face each other at shoulder level. Move both hands in towards the body, ending in "five" hands, palms facing in.(SM)

* *The facial expression should show fear.*

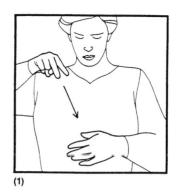
(1)

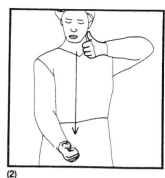
(2)

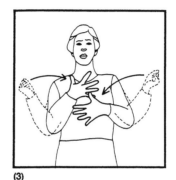
(3)

ACUITY

In optometry, clearness or sharpness of vision.

The chart used by optometrists measures your visual acuity.

(1) Sign SEE — the right "V" hand faces in at eye level. Move the hand out forward.(SM)

(2) Sign CLEAR — both "flat-O" hands face out at shoulder level. Move both hands out into "five" hands.(SM)

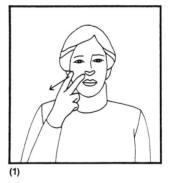
(1)

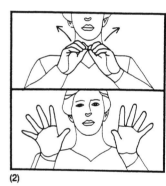
(2)

ACUPUNCTURE

A procedure used to treat a problem, relieve pain or to make an area unable to feel things. Acupuncture has been used in the Far East for centuries to treat disorders and as an anesthetic. In the early 1970's, acupuncture started to be used more in the United States as an anesthetic. In acupuncture, long, thin needles are placed in the skin in certain places and moved around, or a small electric charge is put through them.

Head, neck, chest and abdominal surgery have been done using acupuncture to stop the pain while the person is awake.

(Continued on next page)

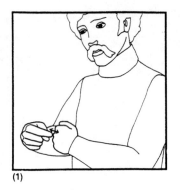

(1)

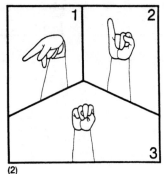

(2)

ACUPUNCTURE, *continued*

(1) The left "A" hand faces in at chest level. The index finger of the right "one" hand taps the back of the left hand a few times.(MM)

* *This can be signed at the area of acupuncture.*

(2) Fingerspell "P-I-N".

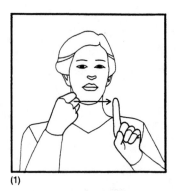

(1)

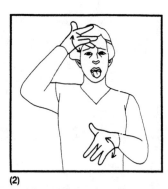

(2)

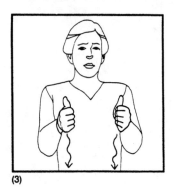

(3)

ACUTE

Happening quickly and severely.

> *An acute illness is one that starts suddenly and becomes worse very rapidly.*

(1) The left "one" hand faces out at shoulder level. The right "S" hand faces in at shoulder level. The right hand sharply hits the index finger of the left hand.(SM)

(2) Sign SICK — the middle finger of the right "eight" hand touches the forehead. The middle finger of the left "eight" hand touches the stomach. Twist both hands slightly.(SM)

* *The facial expression should show sickness or pain.*

(3) Both "A" hands with thumbs extended, face each other at chest level. Move both hands down in a wiggling movement to waist level.(SM)

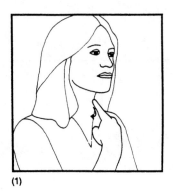

(1)

ADAM'S APPLE

The piece of cartilage at the front of the neck, part of the trachea. *See Figure 4*

(1) The right index finger points to the area of the Adam's Apple and imitates it's shape.(SM)

ADAPT

To change and live comfortably in a different environment.

In order to adapt to cold climates, one must wear the proper clothing.

(1) Sign CHANGE — the right "A" hand is on top of the left "A" hand. Twist both hands so that the left hand ends up on top of the right hand. (SM)

(2) Sign BECOME — the right "flat" hand is on top of the left "flat" hand. Twist both hands so that the left hand ends up on top of the right hand. (SM)

(3) Sign HABIT — both "five" hands cross at the wrists at chest level, palms facing down. Move both hands down to waist level, ending in "S" hands. (SM)

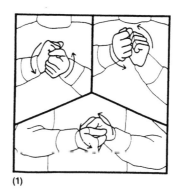
(1)

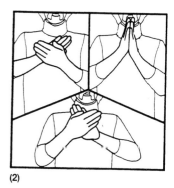
(2)

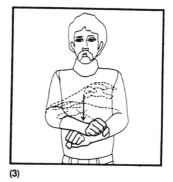
(3)

ADDICT

A person who has a habit or need for a drug.

It is difficult for an addict to quit taking drugs he is addicted to on his own.

(1) Sign PERSON — both "flat" hands face each other at chest level. Move both hands down to waist level.(SM)

(2) The index finger of the right "one" hand hooks the corner of the mouth and moves back slightly.(SM)

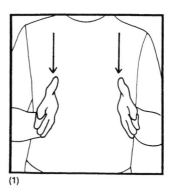
(1)

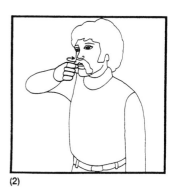
(2)

ADDICTED

Referring to a person who must take certain drugs because it has become a physical or mental habit, and discomfort would result if the drugs were not taken.

The slang word "junkie" is meant when referring to a person who is addicted to heroin or other narcotic drugs.

(1) Sign BECOME — the right "flat" hand is on top of the left "flat" hand. Twist both hands so that the left hand ends up on top of the right hand.(SM)

(2) Sign HABIT — both "five" hands cross at the wrists at chest level, palms facing down. Move both hands down to waist level, ending in "S" hands.(SM)

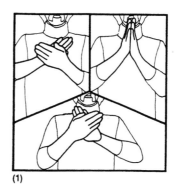
(1)

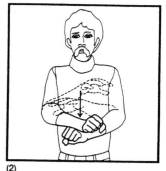
(2)

11

ADENECTOMY

The surgical removal of a gland or adenoid growth.

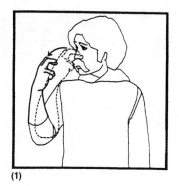

If a person has adenomatosis, (tissue growths over the glands) an adenectomy may be done.

(1) The right bent "V" hand moves from eye level down.(SM)

ADENOID

A collection of soft tissue in the upper throat.

When the adenoid becomes infected and swells, ear infection and deafness may result.

ADHESION

The abnormal joining together of two structures because of inflammation.

The intestines may be blocked if an adhesion forms after an abdominal injury.

ADHESIVE

A substance that sticks to another substance.

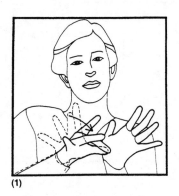

Adhesive bandages should not be put on serious burns.

(1) The left "flat" hand faces right at chest level. The right "flat" hand faces left at chest level. Move the right hand towards the left, ending in an "eight" hand with the thumb and index finger touching the left palm.(SM)

ADHESIVE STRIP

A small piece of tape with gauze attached, sealed in a sterile wrapper for use on small wounds.

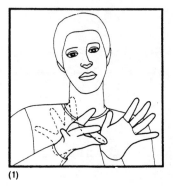
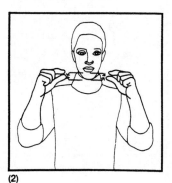

A "Band-Aid® " is a common type of adhesive strip.

(1) The left "flat" hand faces right at chest level. The right "flat" hand faces left at chest level. Move the right hand towards the left, ending in an "eight" hand with the thumb and index finger touching the left palm.(SM)

(2) Both "G" hands face each other at chest level and move out toward the sides.(SM)

12

ADHESIVE TAPE

Sticky tape commonly used in medicine and first-aid to hold dressings in place.

Adhesive tape is a very important part of a first-aid kit.

(1) The left "flat" hand faces right at chest level. The right "flat" hand faces left at chest level. Move the right hand towards the left, ending in an "eight" hand with the thumb and index finger touching the left palm.(SM)

(2) The left "flat" hand faces down at waist level. The fingertips of the right "H" hand move across the back of the left hand.(SM)

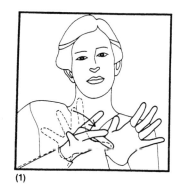 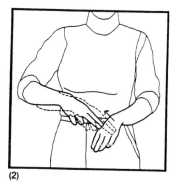

(1) (2)

ADMINISTER

To give or apply a remedy or medicine to a patient.

When you administer any drugs to children, be sure to follow directions.

ADMIT

To allow someone or something to enter.

Before a nurse can admit you to a hospital, you must fill out forms.

(1) The left "flat" hand faces down at chest level. The right "flat" hand faces down at shoulder level. Move the right hand down under the left hand and out forward.(SM)

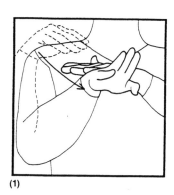

(1)

ADOLESCENCE

The period of life between childhood and adulthood.

The common age of adolescence is usually between 12 and 17 years of age.

(1) The right "S" hand touches the chin and moves down a few times.(MM)

(2) Sign TWELVE — the right "two" hand faces in at chest level. The fingertips of the index finger and middle finger close to tap the thumb twice. (DM)

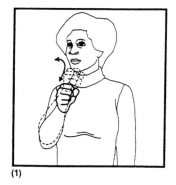 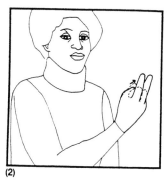

(1) (2)

(Continued on next page)

13

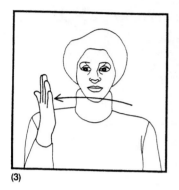

(3)

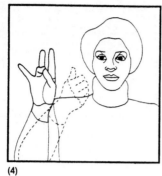

(4)

ADOLESCENCE, *continued*

(3) The right "flat" hand faces left and moves from left to the right.(SM)

(4) Sign SEVENTEEN — the right "A" hand faces left and then makes a "seven" facing out.(SM)

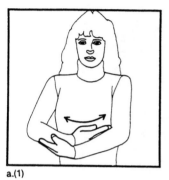

a.(1)

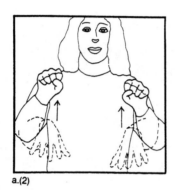

a.(2)

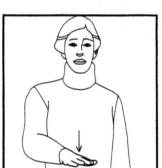

b.(1)

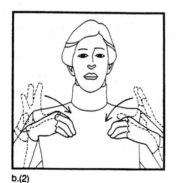

b.(2)

ADOPT

To make something or someone part of one's life or family.

Many families adopt children when they can't have children of their own.

a. (1) Sign BABY — the right hand and forearm face up, resting on the left hand and forearm which also face upward. Both are then rocked back and forth as if holding a baby.(MM)

(2) Both "five" hands face in at waist level. Move both hands up to chest level, ending in "S" hands.(SM)

b. (1) Sign CHILD — the right "flat" hand faces down at waist level and moves as if patting the head of an imaginary child.(SM)

(2) Sign ACCEPT — the thumbs of both "five" hands touch the chest, palms facing each other. Move both hands into the body, ending in "flat-O" hands, with the fingertips touching the chest.(SM)

ADRENAL GLANDS

Two glands above the kidneys that make adrenaline and other hormones and compounds. *See Figure 11*

ADRENALINE

A hormone that acts as a stimulant when a person is excited, afraid, or in threat of danger; also called epinephrine. In these situations its release causes activity in the body, such as faster heartbeat, and more blood going to muscles.

Doctors sometimes give adrenaline to people with asthma.

ADVISE

To give someone else ideas about solving a problem.

Doctors advise pregnant women to stop smoking, drinking and taking unnecessary drugs.

(1) The left "flat" hand faces down at chest level. The right "flat-O" hand rests on top of the left hand. Move the right hand up and forward into a "five" hand.(MM)

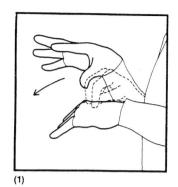

(1)

AFFECT

To influence or to cause change in something.

Some antibiotics affect the growth of bacteria by stopping them from spreading.

(1) The left "flat" hand faces down at chest level. The right "flat-O" hand rests on top of the left hand. Move the right hand up and forward into a "five" hand.(SM)

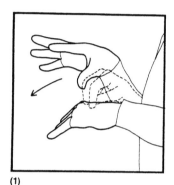

(1)

AFTERBIRTH

The material that comes out of the mother's vagina immediately following the birth of a child.

The afterbirth includes the placenta, umbilical cord, and the membranes that surround the baby while in the womb.

(1) The left "flat" hand faces down at chest level. The right "flat" hand faces left on top of the left hand. Move the right hand out forward over the top of the left hand.(SM)

(2) Sign BIRTH — the left "flat" hand faces in at chest level. The right "flat" hand moves down under the left hand and then out forward.(SM)

(3) Both "five" hands face up at chest level. Move both hands to the sides then up, with the palms ending facing each other.(SM)

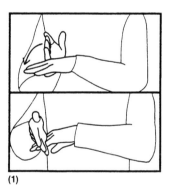

(1)

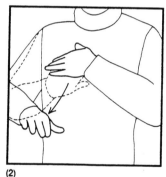

(2)

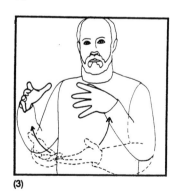

(3)

AGE

The amount of time a person has been alive. It is usually counted in years.

The amount of a drug a doctor gives may depend on the age of a patient.

(Continued on next page)

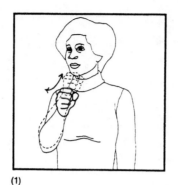
(1)

(1) The right "S" hand touches the chin and moves down a few times.(MM)

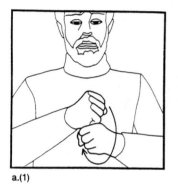
a.(1)

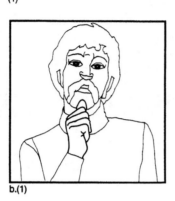
b.(1)

AGONY

Great mental or physical pain. Extreme suffering.

> *Doctors give medicines to help stop the **agony** of badly burned patients.*

a. (1) The right "S" hand is on top of the left "S" hand at chest level. Both hands face in. Slowly move the right hand out and around the left hand.(SM)

* *The facial expression should show agony. The movement should be done slowly.*

b. (1) Sign SUFFER — the back of the thumb of the right "A" hand touches the chin. Pivot the hand slightly from left to right a few times.(MM)

* *The facial expression should show suffering.*

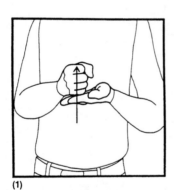
(1)

AID

To give assistance or help.

> *To give the right **aid** to an injured person, you must have correct training.*

(1) Sign HELP — the left "flat" hand faces up at waist level. The right "S" hand faces left on top of the left palm. Move both hands up to chest level.(SM)

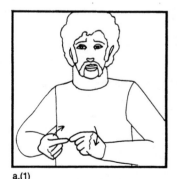
a.(1)

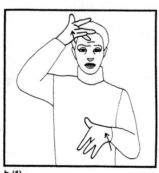
b.(1)

AILMENT

Any illness, injury, disease, or sickness.

> *If an **ailment** becomes worse, a doctor should be seen.*

a. (1) Sign PAIN — both "one" hands face each other with palms facing in. Twist both hands in opposite directions a few times.

* *This can be signed at the area of an ailment. The facial expression should show pain.*

b. (1) Sign SICK — the middle finger of the right "eight" hand touches the forehead. The middle finger of the left "eight" hand touches the stomach. Twist both hands slightly.(SM)

* *The facial expression should show sickness or pain.*

AIRSICK

Upset stomach and vomiting caused by the motion of an airplane.

Sometimes drinking soft drinks helps prevent a person from becoming airsick.

(1) The right thumb, index and pinky fingers are extended at shoulder level, the palm faces down. Shake the hand slightly forward and back a few times.(MM)
(2) Sign SICK — the middle finger of the right "eight" hand touches the forehead and the middle finger of the left "eight" hand touches the stomach. Twist both hands slightly.(SM)

* The facial expression should show sickness or pain.

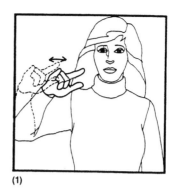
(1)

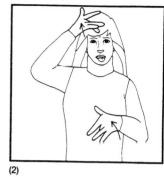
(2)

AIRSPLINT

A device that can be inflated with air and used to hold broken bones still until they can be put in a cast by a doctor.

The Ski Patrol uses airsplints because they are light and easy to carry around.

(1) The thumbs and index fingers of both "G" hands make a rectangle.(SM)
(2) Both "S" hands face down at the mouth, the left hand on the outside. Move both hands slightly to the sides, ending in open "five" hands as if blowing something up.(SM)
(3) The left "flat" hand faces down with the arm bent at the elbow. The right arm is also bent at the elbow. Place the right "flat" hand on the left arm then under the left arm as if imitating a splint.(SM)

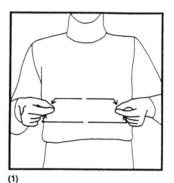
(1)

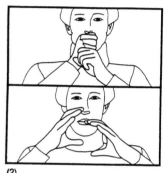
(2)

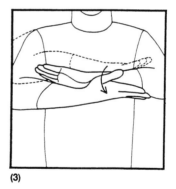
(3)

AIRWAY

Any of the tubes or passages that lead from outside the body into the lungs.

The larynx is the beginning of the airway.

(1) The index finger of the right "one" hand moves from the nose down the right side of the throat.(SM)

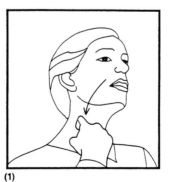
(1)

17

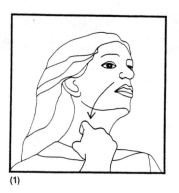
(1)

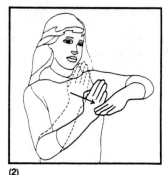
(2)

AIRWAY OBSTRUCTION

Something that blocks the flow of air in the airway.

The most common type of airway obstruction is meat that is not chewed enough.

(1) The index finger of the right "one" hand moves from the nose down the right side of the throat.(SM)

(2) Sign BLOCK — the left "flat" hand faces down at chest level. The right "flat" hand faces left at shoulder level. Move the right hand down to touch the left hand.(SM)

ALBUMIN

A protein found in animals and vegetables. It mixes well with liquids and is the main protein in the blood.

Albumin helps keep water in the bloodstream so it flows easily.

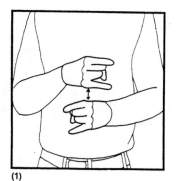
(1)

ALCOHOL

The common term for a liquid containing the chemical ethyl alcohol, such as wine, beer, or whiskey.

There are also many different kinds of alcohol used for different medical and industrial purposes.

(1) The right fist with the index and pinky fingers extended is on top of the left fist with the index and pinky fingers extended at chest level, palms facing in. Tap the hands together a few times.(MM)

* *Fingerspell if referring to rubbing alcohol.*

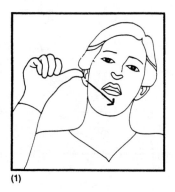
(1)

ALCOHOLIC

A person addicted to alcohol.

An alcoholic usually has mental, physical and emotional problems that affect his health.

(1) The right "A" hand with the thumb extended faces out at shoulder level. Move the hand down several times.(MM)

ALCOHOLISM

The disease of being addicted to alcohol.

The cause of alcoholism is unknown, however, it is a disease and should be treated as a disease.

ALCOHOLICS ANONYMOUS

An organization whose members are alcoholics, concerned with helping people with alcoholism; commonly known as "A.A." Alcoholics Anonymous is located in almost all major cities.

People with drinking problems or family members of problem drinkers can receive help from Alcoholics Anonymous.

(1) Fingerspell "A·A"

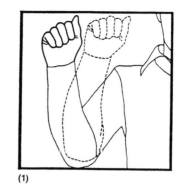

(1)

ALERT

Mentally aware, prepared or able to pay attention to things going on.

Some drugs, such as stimulants, will make a person more alert and others, such as narcotics and depressants, will make them less alert.

(1) Both "G" hands are at the sides of the head, facing out. Flick the fingers of both hands open wide and at the same time open the eyes wide.(SM)

* This may also be a repeated motion.

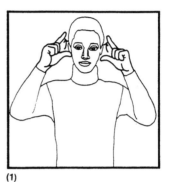

(1)

ALIMENTARY CANAL or TRACT

The tubes and structures that food moves through while being digested.

The alimentary canal, starting at the mouth and ending at the anus, includes the pharynx, esophagus, stomach, small and large intestines, and the rectum.

ALLERGEN

A substance or thing, usually a protein, that is the cause of a person's allergy.

Allergens can be things that are inhaled, such as pollen or dust, foods and drugs, or things that are touched.

ALLERGIC REACTION

The abnormal activities that go on in a person's body when that person is exposed to something he is allergic to (an allergen).

There are many different allergic reactions a person can have, some of which are cold-like symptoms, such as sneezing and runny eyes and nose, swelling or a rash.

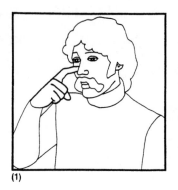
(1)
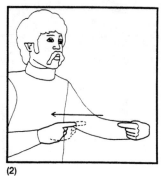
(2)

ALLERGY

An abnormal reaction of the body to certain substances (allergens) which bother only some people.

Eczema, asthma, hay fever, rashes, hives, or cold-like symptoms may all be signs of an allergy to something.

(1) The index finger of the right "one" hand touches the nose.(SM)
(2) Both "one" hands face each other at chest level. Move the right hand away from the left hand.(SM)

ALVEOLUS

In dentistry, the space in the bone of the jaws that a tooth sits in. A tooth is held in place in its alveolus by a material called cementum. *See Figure 25*

AMALGAM

In dentistry, a combination of powdered metals, including silver, which are mixed with mercury and used to make fillings for teeth.

Amalgam is an inexpensive way to fill teeth and lasts 5-15 years.

AMBLYOPIA

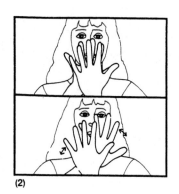
(1)
(2)

Blurred or poor vision when there is no disease of the eye present and nothing wrong with the shape of the eye.

Amblyopia may be caused by alcohol, diabetes, drugs, tobacco, some toxic substance, or most commonly, the abnormal balance of the muscles that move the eyes.

(1) Sign SEE — the right "V" hand faces in at eye level. Move the hand out forward.(SM)
(2) Both "five" hands face each other at eye level, with the right hand on the inside. Move both hands alternately from right to left a few times.(MM)

AMBULANCE

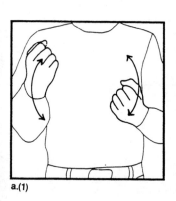
a.(1)
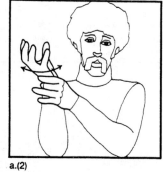
a.(2)

A special car or truck used to carry sick or injured people to clinics or hospitals.

Ambulances have special equipment in them to treat people while they are being moved.

a. (1) Sign CAR — both "S" hands face in at chest level. Move the hands up and down alternately as if holding on to a steering wheel of a car.(MM)
(2) The right "claw" hand faces up at shoulder level and twists from left to right a few times as if imitating the flashing light of an ambulance. (MM)

(Continued on next page)

b. (1) Sign CAR — both "S" hands face in at chest level. Move the hands up and down alternately as if holding on to a steering wheel of a car.(MM) (2) Both "claw" hands face up at shoulder level. Twist both hands from left to right a few times as imitating the flashing light of an ambulance. (MM)

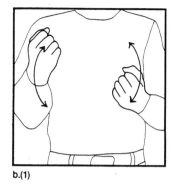
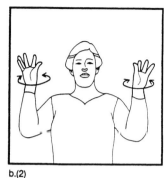

b.(1)   b.(2)

AMBULATORY

Being able to walk; not confined to bed.

Ambulatory patients may recover faster because they can exercise.

(1) Sign CAN — both "A" hands face out at shoulder level. Move both hands down forward, ending at chest level with the palms facing down. (SM)
(2) Sign WALK — both "flat" hands face down at chest level. Move both hands alternately forward and back a few times as if imitating walking. (MM)

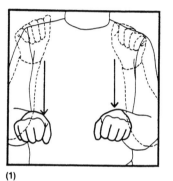
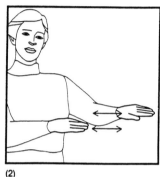

(1)   (2)

AMINO ACIDS

A group of substances made up of carbon, hydrogen, oxygen and nitrogen which when connected in certain ways form proteins.

Proteins in food we eat are broken down in the stomach into amino acids and then used to make other proteins we need for normal growth.

AMITRIPTYLINE

A drug used to make a person feel less depressed; sold under the name of Elavil®

Besides acting to lessen depression, amitriptyline also acts as a sedative and may make a person feel tired.

AMNESIA

The inability to remember things that have happened in the past. A partial or complete loss of memory.

Some causes of amnesia are an injury to the head, old age, alcoholism, mental disease and epilepsy.

(1) The fingertips of the right "five" hand touch the forehead. Move the hand out into a "S" hand. (SM)
(2) The middle finger of the right "eight" hand moves across the forehead from left to right. (SM)

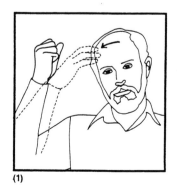
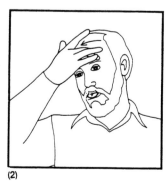

(1)   (2)

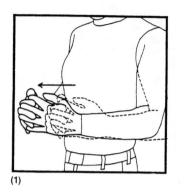
(1)

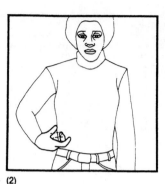
(2)

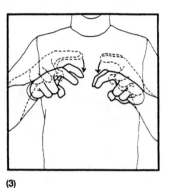
(3)

AMNIOCENTESIS

The process of inserting a needle into the uterus, removing a sample of fluid which the fetus floats in, and checking the fluid to see if anything is wrong.

The fluid removed during an amniocentesis is studied to see if a baby is healthy and normal.

(1) Sign PREGNANT — the fingers of both "five" hands are together at the stomach. Move both hands out forward as is showing the stomach growing. (SM)

(2) The right "K" hand is placed at the right side of the stomach. Move the thumb out from the hand as if drawing liquid out of the stomach. (SM)

(3) Sign ANALYZE — both "V" hands face down at chest level. Drop both hands down at the wrists a few times. (MM)

AMNIONIC FLUID

Colorless, transparent liquid which protects the fetus from injury and helps control the temperature in the sac; also called "waters" or "bag of waters." Each hour, about one third of the amnionic fluid is absorbed and new fluid is made to replace it.
See Figure 14

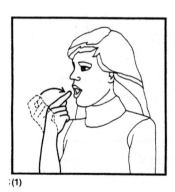
:(1)

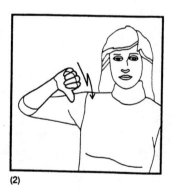
(2)

AMOBARBITAL

A barbiturate drug which acts as a depressant or sedative and slows down the body's activities, causing relaxation and sleep. The slang name for amobarbital is "blue devils."

Amobarbital, like other depressants, should not be taken with alcohol.

(1) Sign PILL — the thumb and index finger of the right hand touch, the palm faces the mouth. Flick the index finger towards the mouth as if popping a pill into the mouth. (SM)

(2) Sign DOWNER — the right fist with thumb pointing down, moves down at should level twice. (DM)
* This is a general sign for depressants ("downers"). The specific type of drug should also be fingerspelled and all side effects explained.

22

AMPHETAMINE

A type of mildly addictive drug which acts as a stimulant. Benzedrine® is one name that amphetamine is sold under.

Amphetamines are used by doctors to control narcolepsy.

(1) Sign PILL — the thumb and index finger of the right hand touch, the palm faces the mouth. Flick the index finger towards the mouth as if popping a pill into the mouth. (SM)

(2) Sign UPPER — the right fist with thumb pointing up, moves up at shoulder level twice. (DM)

* *This is a general sign for stimulants ("uppers"). The specific type of drug should also be fingerspelled and all side effects explained.*

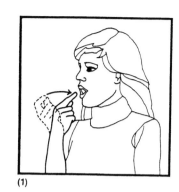
(1)

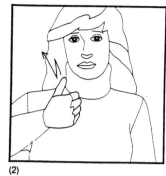
(2)

AMPICILLIN

An antibiotic used for infections caused by certain kinds of bacteria. Ampicillin is made from penicillin.

Ampicillin is used on some infections of the bladder and some infections of the intestine.

AMPUTATION

Surgical removal of a limb or other body part because of disease or injury.

Amputations may be done on breasts because of cancer or fingers or toes because of frostbite.

(1) The right "flat" hand faces in and moves down past the left bent arm as if cutting it off. (SM)

This can be signed on any body part that is being amputated.

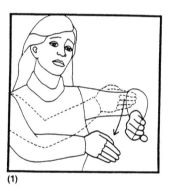
(1)

AMPUTEE

A person who has had a limb removed by amputation.

An amputee may be fitted with an artificial limb called a prosthesis.

AMYL NITRATE

A clear, quickly evaporating liquid used to make blood vessels larger.

People who have angina pectoris attacks carry amyl nitrate capsules and break them under their noses to relieve pain.

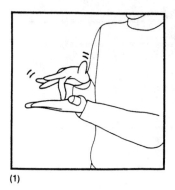
(1)

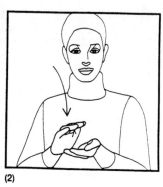
(2)

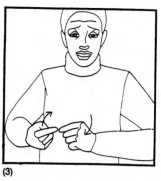
(3)

ANALGESIC

A medicine which lessens or relieves pain.

*Aspirin is a commonly used **analgesic** which can be bought without a prescription.*

(1) Sign MEDICINE — the left "flat" hand faces up at chest level. The middle finger of the right "eight" hand touches the left palm and the hand pivots slightly from left to right. (MM)

(2) Sign REDUCE — the left "flat" hand faces up at chest level. The right "flat" hand faces down at shoulder level. Move the right hand down to the left hand. (SM)

(3) Sign PAIN — both "one" hands face each other with palms facing in. Twist both hands in opposite directions a few times. (MM)
*The facial expression should show pain.

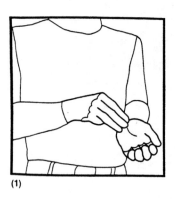
(1)

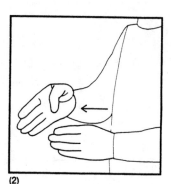
(2)

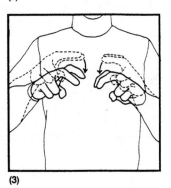
(3)

ANALYST

A doctor who investigates the mental processes of someone.

*An **analyst** will talk with a person about past experiences and feelings to help him see why a current mental problem exists.*

(1) Sign DOCTOR — the right "M" hand touches the left inside wrist. (DM)

(2) Sign SPECIALIZE — the left "B" hand faces right at chest level. The right "B" hand faces left on top of the left hand. Move the right hand straight out on the left index finger. (SM)

(3) Sign ANALYZE — both "V" hands face down at chest level. Drop both hands down at the wrists a few times. (MM)

ANALYZE

To look at something closely and examine its parts to see how it works, what it is made of or what is wrong with it.

(Continued on next page)

ANALYZE, *continued*

Doctors often **analyze** the blood from sick people to find out what is wrong.

(1) Both "V" hands face down at chest level. Drop both hands down at the wrists a few times. (MM)

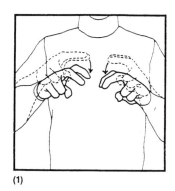
(1)

ANAPHYLAXIS

A severe allergic reaction to a substance, usually a protein, which causes shock. It usually happens when a person has been exposed to the substance before. The symptoms of anaphylaxis come on fast and may include breathing problems, weakness, paleness, chest pain, unconsciousness and perhaps death.

Anaphylaxis may be caused in some people by a bee sting, eating a certain food, or the injection of a drug.

ANATOMICAL OBSTRUCTION

The blocking of a tube or passage by a part of the body or by swelling because of injury or infection.

The term anatomical obstruction is commonly used when talking about something that blocks breathing, such as the tongue dropping and blocking the throat or swelling which closes air passages.

ANATOMY

The study of the body's structure and parts.

Anatomy is one of the first things a person learns when preparing to become a doctor.

(1) Sign BODY — the fingertips of both "flat" hands touch first the chest area and then the stomach area. (SM)
(2) Sign STUDY — the left "flat" hand faces up at waist level. The right "S" hand faces down at chest level. Move the right hand down towards the left hand, ending in a "five" hand. (SM)

May also wiggle the fingers of the right hand after the movement.

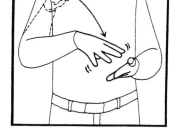
(1)   (2)

ANCESTORS

A person's parents, grandparents, great grandparents and so on.

Many features that make us the way we are come from our ancestors.

(Continued on next page)

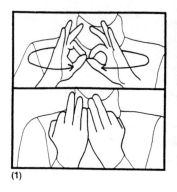

(1)

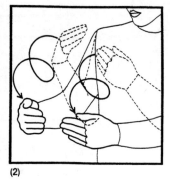

(2)

ANCESTORS, *continued*

(1) Sign FAMILY — both "F" hands face out at chest level with the thumbs and index fingers touching. Move both hands slightly out and around, ending with the pinky fingers touching and the hands facing in. (SM)

(2) Sign GENERATION — both cupped "flat" hands face in at the right shoulder. Move both hands alternately in forward circular movements to waist level. (SM)

ANEMIA

An abnormal condition caused by a shortage of red blood cells in the body or not enough hemoglobin inside the red blood cells. Symptoms of anemia are paleness, weakness and shortness of breath.

Anemia is commonly caused by a lot of bleeding after an injury, a poor diet, or if red blood cells are abnormal and are not replaced fast enough.

ANESTHESIA

A state in which a person cannot feel all or a part of his body; a loss of sensation.

Anesthesia causes a person to not feel pain during an operation.

ANESTHETIC

A substance which causes a person not to feel pain or touch; something which causes anesthesia.

An anesthetic can be a drug or a gas and is usually given before an operation.

(1) The right "five" hand covers the nose and mouth and taps a few times. (MM)

Substitute "injection", "drink" or "pill" instead of gas, depending on the way the anesthetic is being given.

(2) Sign BODY — the fingertips of both "flat" hands touch the chest area and then the stomach area. (SM)

(3) Sign FREEZE — both "five" hands face down at chest level. Move both hands up slightly ending in "claw" hands. (SM)

* *If a local anesthetic is referred to, point to the area that is to be frozen then sign FREEZE, instead of signing BODY.*

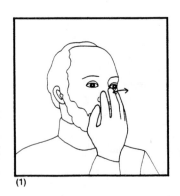

(1)

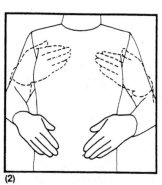

(2)

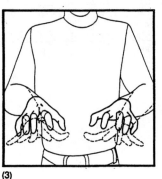

(3)

ANEURYSM

An enlargement in one spot of a blood vessel, usually the aorta, caused by a weakness in the vessel's wall.

Aneurysms are dangerous because the vessel balloons out and may rupture.

ANGEL DUST

See PCP

ANGINA PECTORIS

A sharp, severe pain in the chest, usually around the heart, which may spread to the arms, neck or jaw. The person will have a feeling of pressure around the heart, will not move, may be sweating and very afraid.

Angina pectoris is caused by the heart not getting enough blood because of heart disease or physical exercise.

ANIMAL

A living thing which is not a plant.

All animals have certain characteristics such as being able to move, having a nervous system, and needing certain foods for growth and activity.

(1) The fingertips of both "five" hands touch the chest. While keeping the fingertips in place, pivot both hands in and out a few times, bending at the knuckles. (MM)

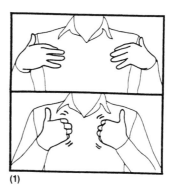

ANIMAL BITE

A break in the skin caused by the teeth of an animal.

Animal bites, especially those caused by wild animals, should be cleaned well and a doctor should be seen.

(1) Sign ANIMAL — the fingertips of both "five" hands touch the chest. While keeping the fingertips in place, pivot both hands in and out a few times, bending at the knuckles. (MM)
(2) Sign BITE — the left "flat" hand faces in at chest level. The right "C" hand moves up to bite the pinky finger side of the left hand. (SM)

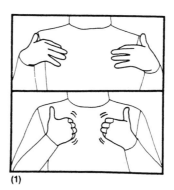
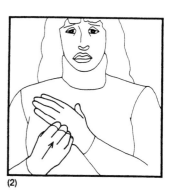

27

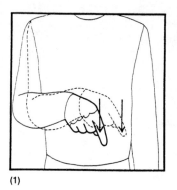 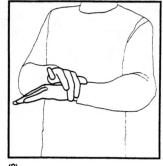

(1)   (2)

ANKLE

The joint between the lower leg and foot and the area around that joint. *See Figure 1*

(1) The right "one" hand points down to the feet. (DM)
(2) The right hand grabs the left wrist. (SM)

* *It may be necessary to fingerspell the word ANKLE.*

ANOMALY

An organ, structure, or other thing which is not normal, not right, irregular or unusual.

> *A birth defect would be an anomaly.*

ANOREXIA NERVOSA

The symptom of a mental illness causing loss of appetite. Anorexia nervosa occurs usually in young girls between the ages of 12 and 21 and sometimes in older men and women. It causes loss of weight, amenorrhea in women (menstruation stops) and impotence in men. This is one of the few psychiatric disorders in children that can cause death if not treated.

> *A woman with anorexia nervosa may need psychiatric therapy in a hospital if she will not eat.*

ANTACID

Something that will make an acid less strong.

> *An antacid is often eaten to make gastric juices less strong.*

ANTERIOR

Referring to a structure or thing at the front or in front of something. The face is on the anterior part of the head. *See Figure 1*

ANTERIOR TIBIAL ARTERY

A major blood vessel in the front of the lower leg which supplies blood to the front of the lower leg, ankle and foot. *See Figure 6*

ANTHRAX

A severe infectious disease caused by a bacteria which usually affects cattle and sheep. People can get anthrax by being around the hide, hair, or wastes of an infected animal.

Anthrax may attack the lungs, the intestinal tract or more commonly, the skin where it causes ulcers and sores.

ANTIBIOTIC

A natural or man-made substance used on or in the body to kill or stop the growth of bacteria.

Antibiotics should be taken for as long as the doctor tells you to take them — not just until you feel better.

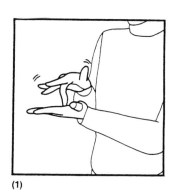
(1)

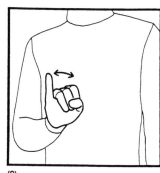
(2)

(1) Sign MEDICINE — the left "flat" hand faces up at chest level. The middle finger of the right "eight" hand touches the left palm and pivots slightly from left to right a few times. (MM)

(2) Sign INFECTION — the right "I" hand faces out and shakes slightly from left to right a few times. (MM)

* *Mouth the word "infection" while signing.*

(3) Both "flat-O" hands face up at chest level. While moving the hands down sideways, brush the thumbs across the other fingers, ending in "A" hands. (SM)

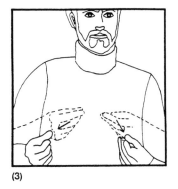
(3)

ANTIBODY

A type of protein made by special cells in the body because something has gotten into the body that is not supposed to be there.

Antibodies travel around the body and attack and help destroy the materials that are not supposed to be in the body.

ANTIDOTE

A substance which, when given to a person, will stop a poison or lessen its effects.

The antidote is often given on the label of a bottle of something that is poisonous to people or animals.

ANTIGEN

A substance which, when it gets into the body in some way, causes antibodies to be made.

Examples of antigens are bacteria, poisons made by bacteria, or organs and blood donated by another person.

ANTIHISTAMINE

A substance made by the body and released when there is injury to cells to lessen the effects of histamine.

Antihistamines lessen swelling, make blood vessels smaller and stop fluids from collecting where they should not.

ANTISEPTIC

Something that prevents the growth of and may destroy harmful bacteria.

Antiseptics are used in hospitals and by doctors to control many kinds of dangerous bacteria.

ANTISOCIAL

The condition of not wanting to be around other people, of wanting to do things that most people don't think are right, or to do things that hurt a society or community.

People with antisocial feelings may be able to get help from a psychologist.

ANTITOXIN

A man-made antibody used by doctors which makes the poisons made by some kinds of bacteria not work.

If you step on a rusty nail and haven't had a tetanus shot for a long time, a doctor may want to give you a tetatanus antitoxin injection to protect you.

ANTIVENIN

A substance given to people who have been bitten by poisonous insects or snakes to stop the poison from working.

Antivenin is made by giving animals the venom of a poisonous insect or snake, letting them make a substance in their body to stop the poison, and then taking out part of the blood which has that substance.

ANTIVENOM

A substance given to people who have been bitten by poisonous snakes, to stop the poison from working.

Antivenom is a common name for antivenin.

ANUS

The circular, muscular opening between the folds of the buttocks. The anus is the end of the digestive tract which lets wastes pass out of the body. *See Figure 12 or 13*

a. (1) The palm of the left "F" hand faces outward at chest level. The finger of the right "one" hand makes a small circle indicating the anus. (SM)

b. (1) The right "one" hand points in the direction of the buttocks.

* These are two variations to the sign anus. They could be used together to clarify the meaning.

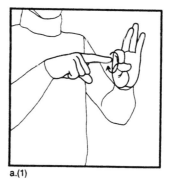
a.(1)

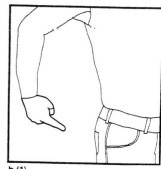
b.(1)

ANVIL

The common name for the incus, one of the tiny bones in the middle ear, which helps transmit sound waves from the eardrum to the inner ear. *See Figure 20*

ANXIETY

Worry, uneasiness, or fear about the future.

Many people show great anxiety when at a doctor's or dentist's office.

(1) Both "B" hands face out at head level. Both hands move in an alternating circular motion in front of the face, as if brushing the nose with the backs of the fingertips. (MM)

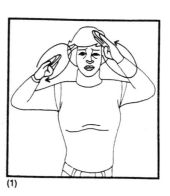
(1)

AORTA

The large, major artery which leaves the heart and then branches into smaller arteries and takes blood to all parts of the body. *See Figure 15 or 16*

APEX

The end, highest point or tip of something.

The apex of a tooth would be the end of the root.

APHAKIA

In optometry, when the crystalline lens of the eye is gone.

> *When aphakia is present, one can still see, although it is difficult to focus on objects.*

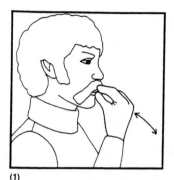
(1)

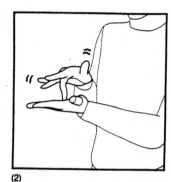
(2)

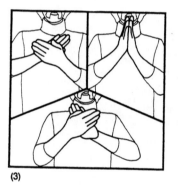
(3)

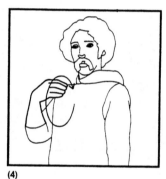
(4)

APHRODISIAC

A drug or food which increases the desire of a person to have sexual intercourse.

> *People sometimes use an aphrodisiac to try to cure sexual problems caused by age or psychological problems.*

(1) Sign EAT — the fingertips of the right "flat-O" hand tap the mouth a few times. (MM)

(2) Sign MEDICINE — the left "flat" hand faces up at chest level. The middle finger of the right "eight" hand touches the left palm and the hand pivots slightly from left to right. (MM)

(3) Sign BECOME — the right "flat" hand is on top of the left "flat" hand. Twist both hands so that the left hand ends up on top of the right hand. (SM)

(4) Sign DESIRE — the fingertips of the right "C" hand brush down the chest then out and around in a circular movement. (MM)

APOPLEXY

The condition in which a person becomes unconscious, falls to the ground and becomes paralyzed, usually on one side of the body, because of a broken blood vessel or a plugged artery in the brain.

> *Apoplexy is another word for a stroke.*

APICOECTOMY

Removal of the end of a tooth's root. Apicoectomy is also called a root resection.

> *An apicoectomy is usually done so a dentist can get at the tissue around the root of a tooth to remove diseased tissue.*

APPENDECTOMY

Removal of the appendix by surgery.

> *If a person has extremely bad pain on the right side due to an infected appendix, an appendectomy would probably be done.*

(Continued on next page)

(1) Fingerspell "A-P-P-E-N-D-I-X"
(2) Sign OPERATE — the thumb of the right "A" hand moves across the right lower stomach.(SM)
(3) The right fist with the thumb tucked inside, faces in at the right lower stomach. Flick the thumb out of the fist. (SM)

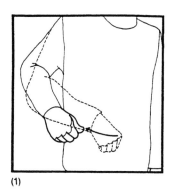

(1)

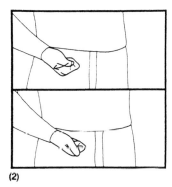

(2)

APPENDICITIS

An inflammation of the appendix.

*Symptoms of **appendicitis** may include very severe pain in the lower right hand side of the abdomen, vomiting and a high temperature.*

APPENDIX

The worm-like tube 3 inches in length which is closed at the end and is attached to the start of the large intestine (colon). *See Figure 9*

(1) Fingerspell "A-P-P-E-N-D-I-X"

APPETITE

A person's desire for food.

*When people get sick, they often lose their **appetite**.*

(1) Sign HUNGRY — the right "C" hand brushes down the chest in a slow, long movement. (SM)

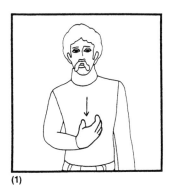

(1)

APPLY

To put something on something else or to bring into contact with something.

*After you stop a wound from bleeding, you should **apply** a clean dry bandage.*

(1) The left "S" hand faces down at chest level. The right "U" hand faces out and makes a small circular movement then touches the left wrist. (SM)

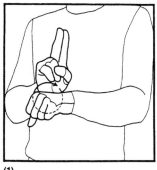

(1)

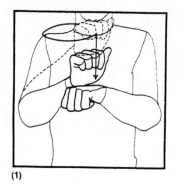
(1)

APPOINTMENT

Plans made to do something or meet someone at a certain time and place.

*You should make an **appointment** to see a doctor or a dentist when you first are aware of a problem.*

(1) The left "S" hand faces down at chest level. The right "A" hand makes a horizontal circle above the left hand then moves down to rest on top of the left hand. (SM)

AQUEOUS

Having water in it or being like water.

*Most things which are injected are **aqueous** substances.*

AQUEOUS HUMOR

The watery, clear liquid found between the cornea and the lens in the front part of the eye. *See Figure 22*

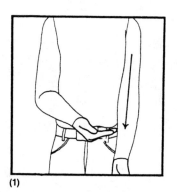
(1)

ARM

The limb which goes from the shoulder to the wrist. The part of the limb that goes from the elbow to the wrist is referred to as the forearm. *See Figure 2*

(1) The right "cupped" hand brushes down the left arm. (SM)

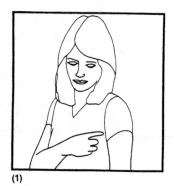
(1)

ARMPIT

The rounded space under the upper arm. *See Figure 1*

(1) The right index finger points to the left armpit. (SM)

AROMATIC

Having a sweet, spicy or good smell.

*Many medicines which must be drunk or swallowed are **aromatic** to make them easier to take.*

(Continued on next page)

(1) Sign SMELL — the fingertips of the right "flat" hand brush against the nose a few times. (MM)

(2) Sign GOOD — the fingertips of the right "flat" hand touch the mouth then move the hand down, ending facing up at chest level. (SM)

* *The facial expression should reflect good smelling.*

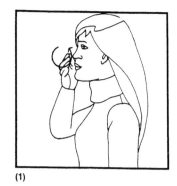
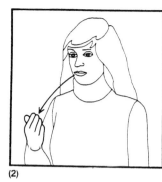

(1) (2)

ARSENIC

A very poisonous substance used to make insecticides, weed killers and some medicines.

> *Someone poisoned by **arsenic** will have a smell of garlic on the breath, pain throughout the digestive tract, vomiting, diarrhea, dehydration, coma, and convulsions and may die.*

(1) Sign MEDICINE — the left "flat" hand faces up at chest level. The middle finger of the right "eight" hand touches the left palm and the hand pivots slightly from left to right. (MM)

(2) Sign POISON — both bent "V" hands cross at the wrists and face in at chest level. (SM)

* *This is just a general sign and the specific type of poison should be fingerspelled.*

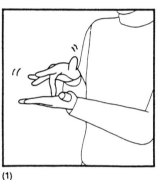
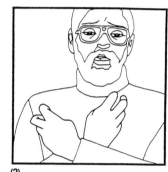

(1) (2)

ARTERIOSCLEROSIS

Thickening and hardening of the walls of blood vessels, especially the arteries, which make blood flow more difficult and may cause high blood pressure.

> *The cause of **arteriosclerosis** is unknown, but exercise, not eating a lot of fatty foods, not smoking, and avoiding stress help to prevent it.*

ARTERY

A kind of blood vessel which carries blood from the heart to other parts of the body.

> *An **artery** carries blood which has a lot of oxygen in it to the capillaries in the tissues where the oxygen is released and waste is picked up.*

(Continued on next page)

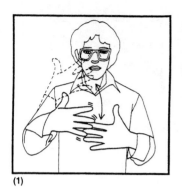
(1)

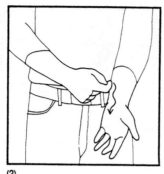
(2)

ARTERY, *continued*

(1) Sign BLOOD — the left "five" hand is at chest level with the palm toward the body. The palm of the right "five" hand is toward the body with the middle fingertips touching the mouth. Move the right hand down the back of the left hand. Wiggle the fingers of the right hand as it moves. (MM)

* This movement should be short, repeated and somewhat restrained.

(2) The right index finger moves in a squiggling line down the inside of the left lower arm. (SM)

* "A-R-T-E-R-Y" should be fingerspelled and it's functions explained to distinguish it from veins.

ARTHRITIS

A general term for inflammation of a joint which causes pain, swelling, stiffness and often changes the shape of the joint.

> *Among the many causes of arthritis, some are infec-tions, such as tuberculosis or gonorrhea, and damage to a joint.*

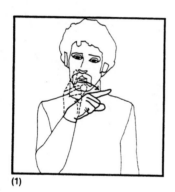
(1)

ARTIFICIAL

Man-made, not natural; an object or action.

> *Artificial legs have knee joints that work almost as well as real joints.*

(1) Sign FALSE — the right "L" hand faces left and brushes to the left past the nose. (SM)

ARTIFICIAL INSEMINATION

A procedure in which a doctor places live sperm in a woman's vagina so the woman may become preg-nant without having sexual intercourse.

> *Artificial insemination is used when a couple can't have a baby because something is wrong with the man's sperm, and a donor's sperm must be used.*

ARTIFICIAL LIMB

See PROSTHESIS

ARTIFICIAL PACEMAKER

See PACEMAKER

ARTIFICIAL RESPIRATION

Breathing done with the help of a machine or another person.

Artificial respiration can be done by a machine or, in emergencies, by people doing mouth to mouth breathing.

* Also see MOUTH TO MOUTH.

ASCARID

A kind of large, white, round worm which is a parasite of man and pigs. A person is infected with ascarids by swallowing food or water which has the eggs in it. The worm hatches in the intestine and then travels around the body, goes to the lungs, moves up the trachea and is swallowed so it ends up back at the intestines. Symptoms of having ascarids are damage and infection in the lungs, loss of weight, stomach pains, rashes, restlessness and perhaps blockage of the intestine.

An ascarid infection can be treated with drugs.

ASCORBIC ACID

See VITAMIN C

ASEPTIC

Sterile or free from germs.

Keeping equipment, rooms, hands, floors and anything else in a hospital or doctor's office as aseptic as possible will help prevent the spread of diseases.

(1) Sign CLEAN — the left "flat" hand faces up at chest level. The right "flat" hand brushes down the left palm. (SM)

The facial expression and sharpness of movement will emphasize the sterile aspect of the sign CLEAN.

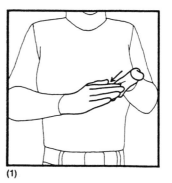
(1)

ASLEEP

Sleeping or referring to something which is numb.

When someone has sat on their leg wrong and cut off the blood flow it will tingle and feel numb and the person may say that his leg is "asleep".

(1) Sign FREEZE — both "five" hands face down at chest level. Move both hands up slightly ending in "claw" hands. (SM)

* This sign means the numbing of a body part and not the act of sleeping.

* The sign meaning the act of sleeping is under the term SLEEP.

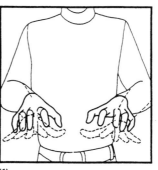
(1)

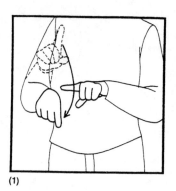

(1)

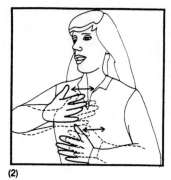

(2)

ASPHYXIA

Stopping or interferring with breathing so that air cannot get to the lungs. As a result, there is less oxygen in the body and an increase in carbon dioxide. The symptoms of asphyxia are difficulty in breathing, a bluish color to the skin and perhaps convulsions, unconsciousness and death.

Asphyxia can be caused by choking, too much of a depressant or anesthetic, a crushing injury of the chest, a lessening in the amount of oxygen in the air or something being stuck in the throat.

(1) Sign CAN'T — the left "one" hand faces down at chest level. The index finger of the right "one" hand moves down and strikes the left index finger. (SM)
(2) Sign BREATHE — both "five" hands move in and out from the chest with quick, short, repeated movements. (MM)

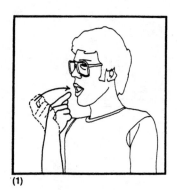

(1)

ASPIRIN

A very common drug containing acetylsalicylic acid, used for relieving pain and lowering fevers.

Because aspirin is so easy to get, many people take it too often.

(1) Fingerspell "A-S-P-I-R-I-N".
(2) Sign PILL — the thumb and index finger of the right hand touch, the palm faces the mouth. Flick the index finger towards the mouth as if popping a pill into the mouth. (SM)

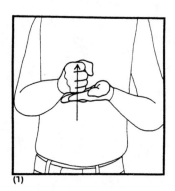

(1)

ASSIST

To help or give aid.

A person trained to give first-aid will assist injured people before they can be taken to a doctor.

(1) Sign HELP — the "flat" left hand is facing up at waist level. The right "S" hand faces left on top of the left palm. Move both hands up to chest level.(SM)

ASSISTANT

A person who helps or aids another person in doing something.

Nurses often act as a doctor's assistant.
(1) The right "L" hand faces left at waist level. The left "A" hand is on top of the right thumb and faces right. Move both hands up to chest level.(SM)

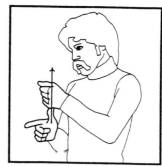

(1)

ASTHMA

A condition in which a person coughs a great deal and has trouble breathing because the tubes taking air from the trachea to the lungs tighten or swell.

Asthma is often caused by an allergy.

ASTIGMATISM

A vision defect caused by a cornea which is not curved smoothly and which doesn't focus images on the retina correctly, causing blurred vision.

If astigmatism is not corrected with glasses or contact lenses, a person may have headaches or the eyes may get tired.

ATHLETE'S FOOT

A contagious skin infection caused by a fungus which grows on feet. Symptoms of athlete's foot are redness, itching, cracking of the skin, blistering and scaling.

Athlete's foot can be prevented by keeping feet clean and dry, wearing clean socks and exposing the feet to air when possible.

ATRIAL FIBRILLATION

Quick and irregular beating of the atria of the heart, so the heart doesn't pump blood well.

A person with atrial fibrillation is not having a heart attack and it will not cause death, but the person may be very uncomfortable.

ATRIUM, ATRIA

The two chambers of the heart which sit on top of the ventricles. The right atrium receives the blood from all of the body except the lungs through the vena cava and when it is full, contracts and forces blood into the right ventricle. The left atrium receives blood which has oxygen in it from the lungs through the pulmonary veins and, when it is full, contracts and forces blood into the left ventricle. *See Figure 15 or 16*

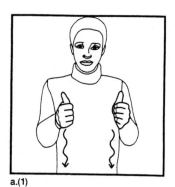
a.(1)

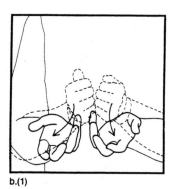
b.(1)

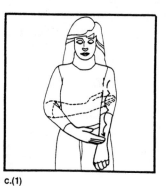
c.(1)

ATROPHY

The becoming smaller or wasting away of an organ or a tissue. Atrophy can be caused by not using the part, disease or damage to the nerve or blood supply to the area.

When an arm or leg is in a cast, there is some atrophy of the muscles because the part is not used.

a. (1) Both "A" hands with thumbs extended, face each other at chest level. Move both hands down in a wiggling movement to waist level. (SM)

b. (1) Both "A" hands face each other at chest level. Move both hands out forward slightly, opening into "five" hands. (SM)

c. (1) The right "flat" hand faces in and moves down the left arm several times. (MM)

ATROPINE

A drug made from the belladonna or deadly nightshade plant. Atrophine is used as a heart or breathing stimulant, to relax muscles and to dry up parts of the body and prevent secretions.

Atropine is often given to people before they have an anesthetic.

ATTACK

The sudden coming on of a disease or a symptom.

A person who is allergic to pollen may have an attack of hay fever.

(1) The left "one" hand faces out at shoulder level. The right "S" hand faces in at shoulder level. The right hand sharply hits the left index finger. (SM)

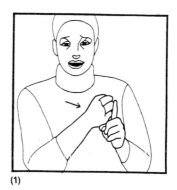

(1)

ATTITUDE

A person's behavior about feelings or his state of mind about something or somone.

Sometimes a person's positive attitude about getting over a disease or injury will help them get better.

(1) The right "A" hand makes a circle over the left chest.(SM)

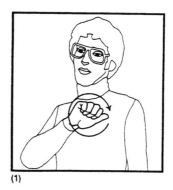

(1)

AUDIOGRAM

The picture, visual record, or chart which comes from an audiometer that shows how well a person hears.

All children should have an audiogram in their school file that is updated regularly.

AUDIOLOGIST

One who specializes in diagnosing and treating hearing defects.

An audiologist uses an audiometer to test a person's hearing.

(1) Sign DOCTOR — the right "M" hand touches the left inside wrist.(DM)

(Continued on next page)

(1)

41

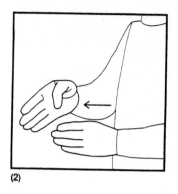
(2)

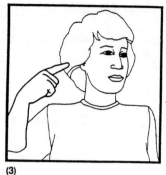
(3)

AUDIOLOGIST, *continued*

(2) Sign SPECIALIZE — the left "B" hand faces right at chest level. The right "B" hand faces left on top of the left hand. Move the right hand straight out on the left index finger. (SM)

(3) Sign EAR — the right index finger points to the right ear.(SM)

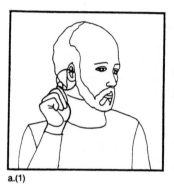
a.(1)

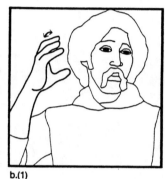
b.(1)

AUDIOLOGY

The science which deals with hearing.

Audiology deals with hearing defects and the treatment of those defects.

a. (1) The right "A" hand faces out and makes a small circle at the right ear. (SM)

b. (1) The right "claw" hand twists slightly from left to right a few times at the right ear. (MM)

* *This is a newer sign. The full word AUDIOLOGY should be fingerspelled and explained before the sign is used.*

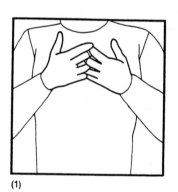
(1)

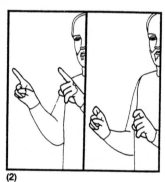
(2)

AUDIOMETER

An instrument which tests how well we hear.

An audiometer produces a wide range of sounds and measures the amount of sound we hear.

(1) Sign MACHINE — both "five" hands mesh together at chest level and bounce up and down a few times. (MM)

(2) Sign TEST — both "one" hands face out at shoulder level with the index fingers pointing up. Move both hands down slightly, at the same time bending and straightening the index fingers. Repeat this movement three times until the hands end at waist level. (MM)

(3) Sign HEAR — the index finger of the right "one" hand points to the right ear. (SM)

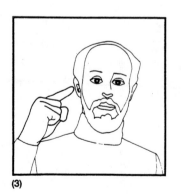
(3)

AUDITORY

Referring to hearing or the organs which help us hear.

> *The auditory health of a person means the condition of the ears or how well a person hears.*

(1) The index finger of the right "one" hand points to the right ear. (SM)

* This is a general sign for ear or hear. The full word "A-U-D-I-T-O-R-Y" should be fingerspelled and explained before the sign is used.

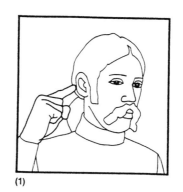
(1)

AUDITORY NERVE

The nerve which connects the ear with the brain, having one part which carries information to the brain, allowing us to hear, and another part which helps us keep our balance. The auditory nerve is also called the acoustic nerve. *See Figure 20*

AURA

The symptoms or warning signs a person feels which let him know he is about to have an attack, convulsions or seizure, as with epilepsy.

> *The aura may be a feeling or may involve the senses as sight, where one would see flashes of light.*

AURISCOPE

An instrument used to examine the ear.

> *An auriscope usually has a little light and a magnifying lens so the inside of the ear can be seen.*

AUTISM

A mental disorder in which a person's interest or attention is totally on himself, leaving him out of touch with the real world.

> *A child with autism feels alone and wants to stay that way, so he will withdraw from people, his movements will repeat again and again, and he will often have speech problems.*

43

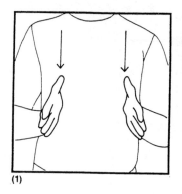
(1)

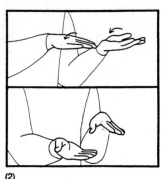
(2)

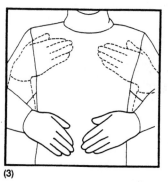
(3)

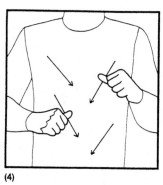
(4)

AUTOPSY

Examination of a dead person's body and organs to see what the cause of death was or to see if there was any disease.

An autopsy may be done on a person that died of unknown causes.

(1) Sign PERSON — both "flat" hands face each other at chest level. Move both hands down to waist level. (SM)

(2) Sign DEAD — the left "flat" hand faces up at chest level. The right "flat" hand faces down at chest level. Turn both hands to the right so that the left hand ends facing down and the right hand ends facing up. (SM)

(3) Sign BODY — the fingertips of both "flat" hands touch first the chest area and then the stomach area. (SM)

(4) The extended thumbs of both "A" hands brush down the chest in short, repeated movements. (MM)

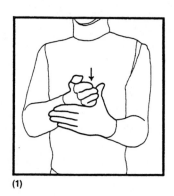
(1)

AVERAGE

Something which is in the middle and not extreme.

A normal, healthy person's temperature may be anywhere between 98° F and 99° F but the average is 98.6°.

(1) The left "flat" hand faces in at chest level with the thumb extended. The right "flat" hand faces left and moves down to tap the left hand between the thumb and index finger. (SM)

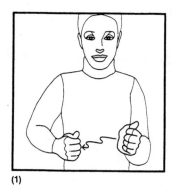
(1)

AVOID

To stay away from something.

Dentists tell people who have a lot of cavities to avoid things with a lot of sugar in them.

(1) Both "A" hands are together at chest level. Move the right hand toward the body in a left and right wavy motion.(SM)

AVULSION

The tearing or ripping away of a part of the body.

When there is an avulsion of a finger, toe or even a whole limb, it may be reattached to the body by a surgeon if the part is sent along with the victim to the hospital.

(1) Sign TEAR — both "A" hands face down at chest level and move slightly to the sides as if tearing something. (SM)

* This is a general sign for tear. It is recommended that "skin", "ligament", or "muscle" be fingerspelled following the sign TEAR as necessary.

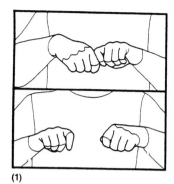
(1)

AWKWARD

Clumsy, hard to handle or difficult.

Young people, growing quickly, are often awkward.

(1) The right "three" hand faces down at waist level and the left "three" hand faces down at chest level. Alternately change the levels of both hands a few times. (MM)

* The facial expression should look awkward.

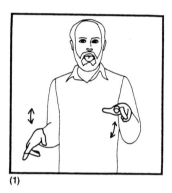
(1)

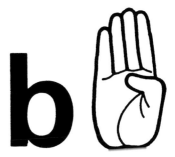

b

BABY

A very young child, one just born or an infant.

*There are several vaccines that **babies** should have to help keep them from getting certain diseases.*

(1) The right hand and forearm face up, resting on the left hand and forearm which also face up. Both are then rocked back and forth as if holding a baby.(MM)

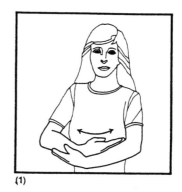
(1)

BACITRACIN

An antibiotic made by a bacteria which will stop an infection caused by other kinds of bacteria.

***Bacitracin** is most commonly used on wounds or infections on the skin.*

BACK

The posterior or rear part of the body from the neck down to the buttocks. *See Figure 3*

(1) The right "flat" hand pats the back a few times. (MM)

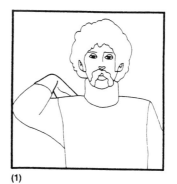
(1)

BACKACHE

A common problem of pain and tenderness in the muscles or the places they attach to in the lower back.

*A **backache** can result from infection, problems with the backbone, disorders with ligaments attached to the spinal column, muscle injury or a problem in another part of the body.*

(Continued on next page)

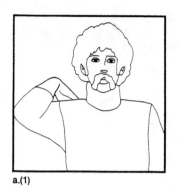
a.(1)

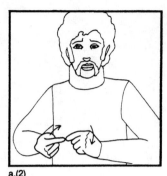
a.(2)

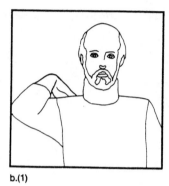
b.(1)

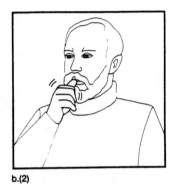
b.(2)

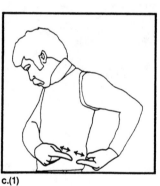
c.(1)

BACKACHE, *continued*

a. (1) Sign BACK — the right "flat" hand pats the back a few times. (MM)

(2) Sign PAIN — both "one" hands face each other with palms facing in. Twist both hands in opposite directions a few times. (MM)

This can be signed at the area of pain. The facial expression should show pain.

b. (1) Sign BACK — the right "flat" hand pats the back a few times. (MM)

(2) Sign SUFFER — the back of the thumb of the right "A" hand touches the mouth and pivots slightly from left to right a few times. (SM)

* *The facial expression should show pain or suffering.*

c. (1) Both "one" hands face each other at the lower back area. Move both hands in and out from each other a few times. (MM)

The facial expression should show pain. This can also be signed by twisting both "one" hands slightly in opposite directions a few times. (MM)

BACKBOARD

A board which is used to hold a person's neck and spine still while he is being moved from the place of an accident to medical help.

If a person has a neck or back injury, a backboard should be used.

BACKBONE

The series of bones which go from the base of the skull to the pelvis. The backbone is also called the spinal column or vertebral column. The backbone supports the trunk, head, neck and arms.

See Figure 26

(Continued on next page)

(1) Sign BACK — the right "flat" hand pats the back a few times. (MM)
(2) Both "F" hands face down at waist level, the right hand slightly above the left hand. Move the right hand up to chest level as if imitating the shape of the backbone.

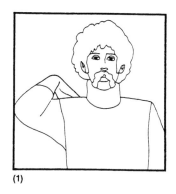
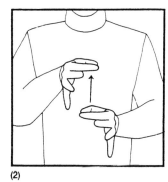

(1)   (2)

BACKFLOW

Moving or flowing in a direction opposite the normal direction.

*When someone vomits, there is a **backflow** of stomach contents through the esophagus.*

BACKRUB

The rubbing or massaging of a person's back to relax them, relieve pain or help blood circulate.

*People who must lie in bed for long periods of time are given **backrubs** to prevent bed sores.*

(1) Sign BACK — the right "flat" hand pats the back a few times. (MM)
(2) Both "flat" hands, with thumbs extended, move into "flat-O" hands. The movement imitates giving a backrub. (MM)

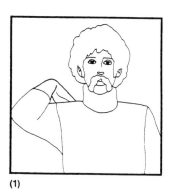
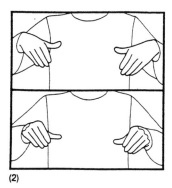

(1)   (2)

BACTERIA

Very tiny plant-like one celled living things which are found everywhere and cannot be seen with the naked eye. Some kinds of bacteria can reproduce very quickly and build up large numbers. Some kinds of bacteria live with us and cause no harm, some we use to help us, and others can cause infections and disease.

Bacteria are very important in nature for breaking down dead things and freeing materials found in them for use in living things.

BAG OF WATERS

The bag of fluid which surrounds a baby while it is in the uterus. The bag of waters usually pushes open the lower end of the uterus and it may be seen surrounding the baby's head. The bag of waters is also called the amnion and the fluid in it is called the amnionic fluid.

(Continued on next page)

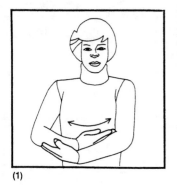
(1)

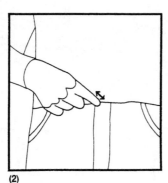
(2)

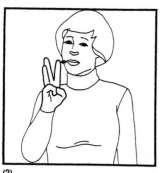
(3)

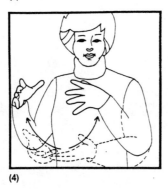
(4)

BAG OF WATERS, *continued*

*The **bag of waters** usually bursts and releases the fluid it contains before the baby's head comes out but if it hasn't, it should be torn so the fluid is released and the baby can't inhale it.*

(1) Sign BABY — the right hand and forearm face up, resting on the left hand and forearm which also face upward. Both are then rocked back and forth as if holding a baby. (MM)

(2) The index finger of the right "one" hand points to the stomach a few times. (MM)

(3) Sign WATER — the index finger of the right "W" hand taps the mouth a few times. (MM)

(4) Both "five" hands face up at waist level. Move both hands out and up as if imitating the shape of a sac or bag. At the same time, the cheeks should puff out a little.

BALANCE

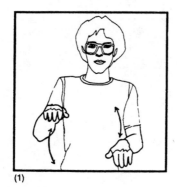
(1)

A condition in which the levels of the different components of the body (fluid, protein, etc.) stay the same.

*The kidneys help control the fluid **balance** of the body by making sure there is the correct amount of water in the fluids in and around the cells.*

(1) The left "flat" hand faces down at chest level. The right "flat" hand faces down at waist level. Alternately move both hands up and down, changing the level of the hands. (MM)

BALD

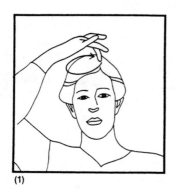
(1)

No hair or areas without hair on a part of the body which usually has it, especially the head.

*Being **bald** may be a natural part of aging for some people or may be caused by illness, having a fever for a long time, drugs, emotions or a poor diet.*

(1) The middle finger of the right "eight" hand makes a small circle on top of the head as if showing a bald spot. (SM)

*This can also be signed at the area of baldness.

BANDAGE

A piece of cloth or other material that is placed on a part of the body to hold dressings or splints in place, apply pressure to an area, hold something still, stop bleeding or cover an injury to keep it clean.

A bandage can be made of cotton, gauze, muslin, rubber, paper, elastic or materials which are sticky.

(1) The left "B" hand faces in at chest level. The right "B" hand also faces in and circles out and around the left hand as if imitating wrapping a bandage. (MM)

* This sign can be made at the location of the wound or where the bandage is intended to be placed.

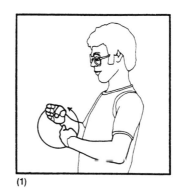

(1)

BAND-AID®

The brand name for small bandages or adhesive strips used for small or minor injuries.

Band-Aids® are sterile and wrapped in paper and come in many different sizes.

(1) The fingertips of the right "H" hand move up across the left "flat" hand. (SM)

* This sign could also be placed at the location of the injury.

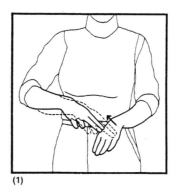

(1)

BARBITURATE

Any of a group of substances used as sedatives or depressants and which act on the nervous system causing relaxation and sleep. If barbiturates are used for a long time they can cause addiction. Examples of barbiturates are seconal, amytal, pentothal and phenobarbital.

The effects of a barbiturate are stronger when it is taken with alcohol, however, the combination may cause death.

(1) Sign PILL — the thumb and index finger of the right hand touch, the palm faces the mouth. Flick the index finger towards the mouth as if popping a pill into the mouth. (SM)

(2) Sign DOWNER — the right "A" hand with the thumb pointing down, moves down at shoulder level twice. (DM)

* This is a general sign for depressants ("downers"). The specific type of drug should also be fingerspelled and all side effects explained.

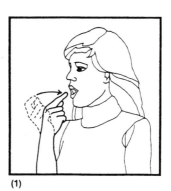

(1)

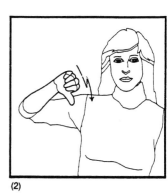

(2)

51

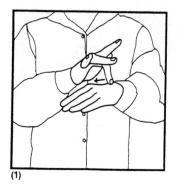
(1)

BARE

Being open to view, naked or not covered.

*An open wound shouldn't be left **bare** or infection may get in it.*

(1) The left "flat" hand is at waist level with the palm down. The middle finger of the right "eight" hand touches the left wrist and moves outward along the fingers.(SM)

BASAL METABOLIC RATE

The rate at which the body uses energy in order to support life-sustaining processes. It is determined by measuring how much oxygen a person uses while he is awake but resting completely.

*When a person is sick, his **basal metabolic rate** should be higher because he is fighting a disease.*

BASAL METABOLISM

The smallest amount of energy a person needs to stay alive.

***Basal metabolism** includes the energy needed for the heart to beat, to move the muscles which help us breathe, and to keep the kidneys working and the nervous system active.*

BASILIC VEIN

An important large vein on the inner side of the biceps.

*The **basilic vein** is usually used for blood drawing and intravenous injections.*

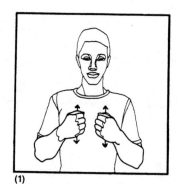
(1)

BATH

A tub or basin with water and perhaps other things in it which a person sits in to clean himself or to treat a problem.

*The **bath** water can be hot or cold and can have things such as carbon dioxide, herbs, salt or other medicines added to it to help a sick person.*

(1) Both "A" hands rub up and down on the chest a few times. (MM)

* This is a short, repeated and restrained movement.

52

BATHE

To take a bath, or to wash and clean the body or a part of the body by dipping it in or covering it with water.

Doctors sometimes tell people with wounds to bathe around the injury so it will not get wet.

(1) Both "A" hands rub in a circular movements on the chest as if bathing. (MM)

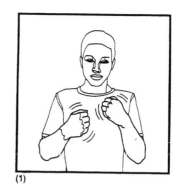
(1)

BATHROBE

A comfortable, loose-fitting piece of clothing worn over pajamas or to cover up the body.

When someone is going to stay in a hospital for a while, he should bring along a bathrobe and slippers.

(1) Sign BATH — both "A" hands rub up and down on the chest a few times. (MM)
(2) Both "A" hands face out at the shoulders. Move both hands forward with the hands facing in as if imitating putting on a bathrobe. (SM)

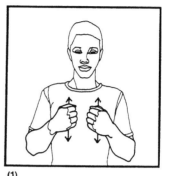
(1)

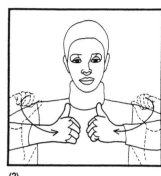
(2)

BED

A piece of furniture for sleeping or resting on.

A hospital bed can be moved up or down for the comfort of a patient.

(1) The head rests in the palm of the right hand.(SM)

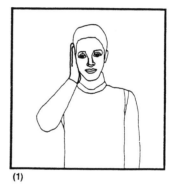
(1)

BEDPAN

A pan or bowl that a person goes to the toilet into when they cannot get out of bed.

A bedpan should be cleaned out after each use.

(1) Both "cupped" hands face up at waist level. Move both hands out and up as if imitating the shape of a bedpan. (SM)

(Continued on next page)

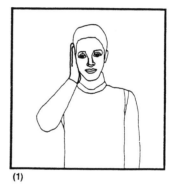
(1)

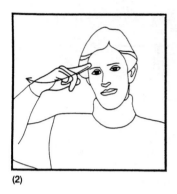
(2)

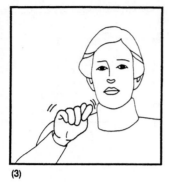
(3)

BEDPAN, *continued*

(2) Sign FOR — the index finger of the right "one" hand touches the forehead, the palm faces in. Turn the hand out so that the palm faces out. (SM)
(3) The right "T" hand faces out and shakes slightly from left to right. (MM)

BEDRAIL

A rail or device which is attached to the side of a bed to keep a person from falling or getting out of bed.

*Most hospitals require a **bedrail** to be put up for children and older people.*

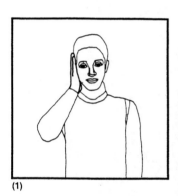
(1)

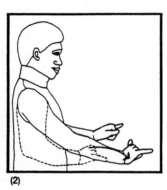
(2)

BEDREST

The act of staying in bed to rest and recover from an injury or disease.

*When a person has a serious operation, **bedrest** is important for quick healing.*

(1) Sign BED — the head rests on the palm of the right "flat" hand. (SM)
(2) Both "Y" hands face down at waist level. Move the right hand slightly forward. (SM)

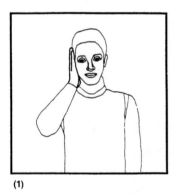
(1)

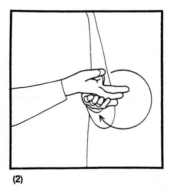
(2)

BEDRIDDEN

Being confined to bed because of an injury or disease.

*It is important to move a **bedridden** patient often and keep their sheets clean and dry to prevent bedsores.*

(1) Sign BED — the head rests on the palm of the right "flat" hand. (SM)
(2) The right "H" hand faces up on the palm of the left "flat" hand. Move both hands out forward in a circular motion. (MM)

BEDSIDE MANNER

The way a doctor acts around his patients.

*A doctor's **bedside manner** is important to keep a patient confident.*

(Continued on next page)

(1) Sign DOCTOR — the right "M" hand touches the left inside wrist. (MM)

(2) Sign ATTITUDE — the right "A" hand with the thumb extended makes a small circle from left to right then touches the left chest. (SM)

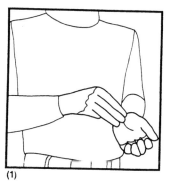
(1)

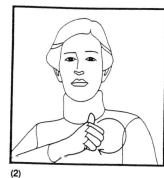
(2)

BEDSORE

A sore or ulcer on a person caused by lying in one position for a long time. Bedsores are caused by a person's weight pushing on the skin for a long time and stopping circulation of blood in the area. They are most common on the buttocks, elbows, shoulderblades, and end of the spine.

*A **bedsore** can be prevented by moving a person often, rubbing the skin with alcohol, dusting with powder and keeping the sheets and pajamas clean and dry.*

(1) Sign BED — the head rests on the palm of the left "flat" hand. (SM)

(2) The right "H" hand faces up on the palm of the left "flat" hand. Move both hands out forward in a circular motion. (MM)

(3) The right "F" hand faces out at the location of the bedsore. (SM)

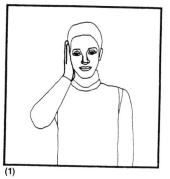
(1)

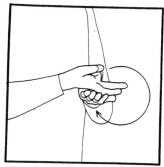
(2)

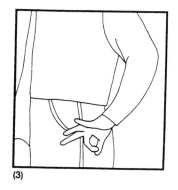
(3)

BEDWETTING

Urinating in bed at night while sleeping.

*Not drinking anything for a few hours before going to bed and waking up a couple times during the night to go to the bathroom may stop **bedwetting**.*

(1) The right "five" hand faces in at face level. Move the hand down slightly into "flat-O" hand, at the same time the eyes close as if sleeping. (SM)

(2) Both "flat-O" hands face in at waist level. Move both hands down the legs into "five" hands, as if imitating wetting the pants. (MM)

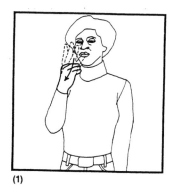
(1)

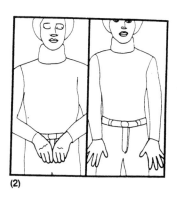
(2)

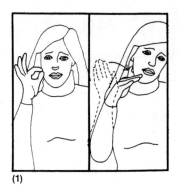

(1)

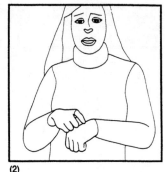

(2)

BEE STING

A sore caused by a bee putting its sharp stinger into the skin and injecting a small amount of poison. Most people experience only pain, itching, redness and swelling in the area. A small number of people may have a severe allergic reaction or an anaphylactic reaction (a reaction causing convulsions, unconsciousness, and sometimes death) from a bee sting.

A bee sting may be treated by putting ice or baking soda paste on it; taking an antihistamine may help.

(1) The right "F" hand faces out and the index finger and thumb touch the right cheek. The right "flat" hand then faces left and brushes past the right cheek. (SM)

(2) The right index finger taps the top of the left hand. (SM)

This can be signed at the area of the sting.

BEHAVIOR

The way someone acts or conducts himself.

People showing anti-social behavior usually do not have many friends.

(1) Both "C" hands face out at chest level. Move both hands alternately towards the center in circular movements. (MM)

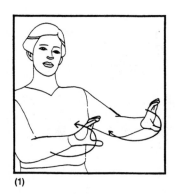

(1)

BELCH

To let air out noisily through the mouth from the stomach.

People may belch because they swallowed air when they ate, because gas was formed in the stomach from the food or because the food contained gas.

BELLADONNA POISONING

Poisoning caused by eating the shiny black berries of the belladonna or deadly nightshade plant. Symptoms of belladonna poisoning are a dry mouth, sore throat, thirst, hot dry skin, a very high temperature, confusion and excitement.

Belladonna poisoning is also called atropine poisoning.

BELLY

The abdomen or stomach area. *See Figure 1*

(Continued on next page)

(1) The fingertips of the right "cupped" hand pat the stomach a few times. (MM)

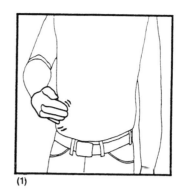
(1)

BELLYACHE

A pain in the stomach or abdomen.

A bellyache can be caused by the flu, eating too much, eating spicy foods or cramps.

(1) The fingertips of the right "cupped" hand pat the stomach a few times. (MM)
(2) Sign PAIN — both "one" hands face each other with palms facing in. Twist both hands in opposite directions a few times. (MM)
The facial expression should show pain.

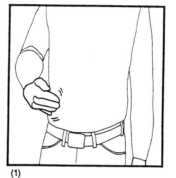
(1)

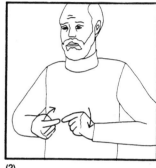
(2)

BELLYBUTTON

The common name for navel. The small hole or scar in the center of our abdomens where the umbilical cord entered our bodies when we were inside our mother's womb. See Figure *1*

(1) The right "F" hand faces in at the bellybutton. (SM)

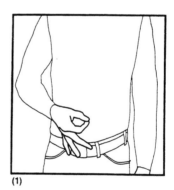
(1)

BENIGN TUMOR

A tumor or growth on the body which is not getting worse, not growing and not dangerous to the health.

A benign tumor is a tumor which is not cancerous.

BENNIES

The slang name for Benzedrine.

Some people refer to bennies as speed.

(1) Sign PILL — the thumb and index finger of the right hand touch, the palm faces the mouth. Flick the index finger towards the mouth as if popping a pill into the mouth. (SM)
(2) Sign UPPER — the right "A" hand with the thumb pointing up, moves up at shoulder level twice. (DM)
* This is a general sign for stimulants ("uppers"). The specific type of drug should also be fingerspelled and all side effects explained.

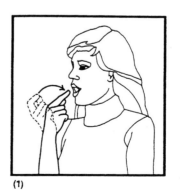
(1)

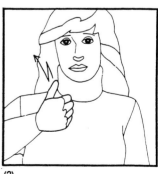
(2)

BENZEDRINE®

The trade name which the drug amphetamine is sold under. Amphetamine acts as a stimulant, making a person more alert.

Benzedrine may be used to treat narcolepsy or help people lose weight.

* Sign Bennies or speed followed by fingerspelling B-E-N-Z-E-D-R-I-N-E.

BETTER

A good change or improvement of a past condition.

*A person with an infection will feel **better** as antibodies made by the body start killing the infection.*

(1) Sign IMPROVE — the right "flat" hand moves up the arm touching several times on the way up.(MM)

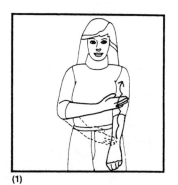
(1)

BEVERAGE

A general word for a drink, usually not used when talking about water.

*Examples of **beverages** are milk, beer, coffee, and soda pop.*

(1) Sign DRINK — the right "C" hand moves towards the mouth as if imitating taking a drink. (SM)

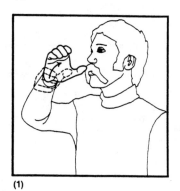
(1)

BICEPS

The large muscle in the front part of the upper arm between the elbow and shoulder, or the muscle on the back of the thigh. The biceps muscle in the arm (the biceps brachii) and the biceps muscle in the leg (the biceps femoris) are used to bend the arm or leg. *See Figure 4*

BICUSPIDS

The name for a kind of tooth. There are a total of eight bicuspids in an adult's mouth, four on the top and four on the bottom. Bicuspids are the first two teeth behind the canine or cuspid tooth. They have two bumps on the crown and are used for crushing or grinding food. The biscuspids are also called premolars. *See Figure 24*

* Point to teeth and fingerspell B-I-C-U-S-P-I-D-S.

BIFOCAL GLASSES

Glasses whose lenses are divided into two halves so a person who is both nearsighted and farsighted can see clearly at all distances.

The upper lens of bifocal glasses is made so that a person can see things far away clearly and the lower lens is made so the person can see things close to him clearly.

(1) Sign GLASSES — both "G" hands face each other and move across the eyes. (SM)
(2) The index fingers of both "one" hands draw a line across the eyes as if dividing the imaginary lenses. (SM)

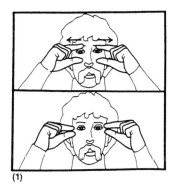
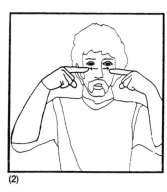
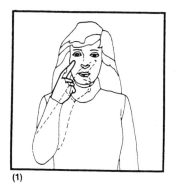
(1)   (2)

BILE

A substance made in the liver and then moved to the gallbladder where it is stored until it is secreted into the upper part of the small intestine to help in digestion.

Bile helps break down fats and contains parts of red blood cells which have been destroyed.

BINDER

A broad bandage usually wrapped firmly or snugly around the chest or abdomen to hold a dressing in place, to provide support or to cover a large wound. (In emergencies, towels make good binders.)

Care must be taken not to tie a binder so tightly that it makes breathing difficult.

BINOCULAR VISION

A term used in optometry for the process in normal vision in which the images formed by the two eyes appear to be one image.

Binocular vision gives us depth perception, that is, it enables us to judge how far away objects are.

(1) Sign EYES — the right index finger points to both eyes. (DM)
(2) Both "F" hands face out at the sides of the head. Move both hands towards each other until they overlap. (SM)

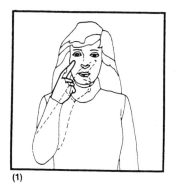
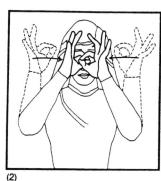
(1)   (2)

BIOFEEDBACK

A procedure or system in which a person is taught to control certain body activities that he normally has no control over.

Using biofeedback, a person may be able to more consciously control heart rate, blood pressure, muscle activity or brain activity.

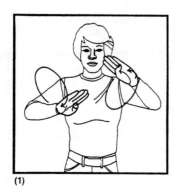
(1)

BIOLOGY

The study of life and living things.

Biology includes the study of plants and animals, how they are put together and how they work.

(1) Both "B" hands face out at chest level. Move both hands alternately in circles up and inward a few times. (MM)

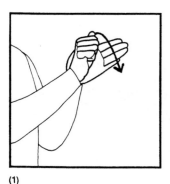
(1)

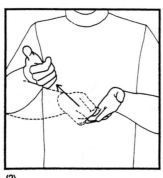
(2)

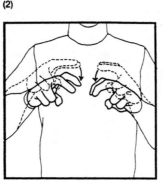
(3)

BIOPSY

The examination of a small piece of tissue taken from a living person to see if there is something wrong or if there is a disease present.

A microscope is often used to examine the tissue taken in a biopsy.

(1) The thumb of the right "A" hand moves down the fingers of the left "flat" hand as if cutting. (SM)
(2) The left "flat" hand faces up at chest level. The right fist, with the thumb tucked inside, faces up on the left palm. Move the right hand up and at the same time, flick the thumb out. (SM)
(3) Sign ANALYZE — both "V" hands face down at chest level. Drop both hands down into bent "V" hands a few times. (MM)

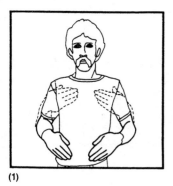
(1)

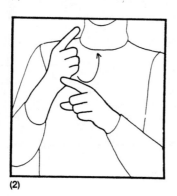
(2)

BIORHYTHMS

The regularly repeated activities or processes that go on in the body.

Some of the activities of the body which involve biorhythms are menstruation in women, temperature changes in the body during the day, and the alternation of sleeping and being awake.

(1) Sign BODY — both "flat" hands face in. The fingertips of both hands touch the chest and then the stomach. (SM)
(2) Sign REGULAR — the left "one" hand points out, the palm facing right and the right "one" hand points out, the palm facing left on top of the left hand. Tap the hands in a circular movement, at the same time, both hands move across the body from left to right. (MM)

BIOTIN

A vitamin found in many foods, especially liver, kidney, yeast, milk and egg yolks; also called Vitamin H. Biotin is widely needed in the body to help many enzymes work normally.

BIRTH

The movement of a baby from the uterus through the vagina to the outside; the act of delivering a baby.

*The **birth** of a child occurs around nine months after fertilization of the egg.*

(1) Sign BORN — the left "flat" hand faces up at waist level. The right "flat" hand faces in. Move the hand out and down on the left palm. (SM)

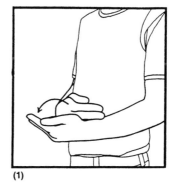
(1)

BIRTH CANAL

The vagina and the part of the uterus a baby moves through when it is being born.

*The **birth canal** is normally smaller in diameter than a baby but during late pregnancy and during labor it expands enough to let the baby through.*

BIRTH CERTIFICATE

An official record of a person's birth.

*A **birth certificate** is filled out by the attending doctor; it has the names of the baby's parents, the date and time of birth, and the place of birth on it.*

(1) Sign BORN — the left "flat" hand faces up at waist level. The right "flat" hand faces in. Move the hand out and down on the left palm. (SM)
(2) The thumbs of both "C" hands tap a few times, the palms face out at chest level. (MM)

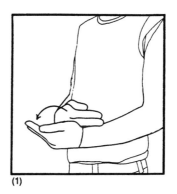
(1)
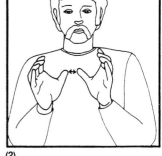
(2)

BIRTH CONTROL

The methods or procedures a man and woman use to control pregnancy, limiting the number of children they have or allowing them to choose when they will have children. Birth control is also called "contraception".

*Examples of **birth control** are the IUD, diaphragm, the contraceptive pill, the rhythm method, abortion and sterilization.*

a. (1) Fingerspell "B-C".

* It may be necessary to fingerspell "B-I-R-T-H C-O-N-T-R-O-L" first and then use the abbreviation "B-C".

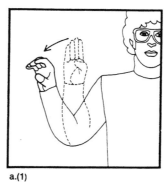
a.(1)

(Continued on next page)

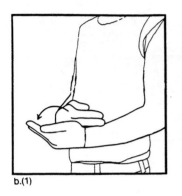
b.(1)

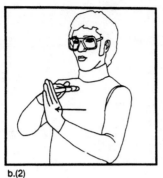
b.(2)

BIRTH CONTROL, *continued*

b. (1) Sign BORN — the left "flat" hand faces up at waist level. The right "flat" hand faces in. Move the hand out and down on the left palm. (SM)
(2) Sign PREVENT — both "flat" hands cross at chest level and move out forward slightly. (SM)

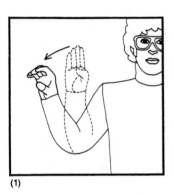
(1)

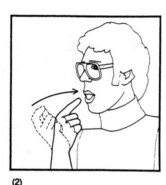
(2)

BIRTH CONTROL PILL

Pills which contain one or two chemicals which are like the hormones made by a woman. Birth control pills are taken in 28 day cycles. The hormone-like substances imitate pregnancy, so no eggs are released from the ovaries. (With no egg in the fallopian tubes or uterus, pregnancy cannot occur.) Birth control pills are also called "contraceptive pills" or just "The Pill".

*When taken as directed, **birth control pills** are almost 100% effective but they may also cause side effects like nausea, weight gain, depression, high blood pressure, vaginal infections and perhaps liver tumors or other kinds of cancer.*

(1) Fingerspell "B-C".
(2) Sign PILL — the thumb and index finger of the right hand touch, the palm faces the mouth. Flick the index finger towards the mouth as if popping a pill into the mouth. (SM)

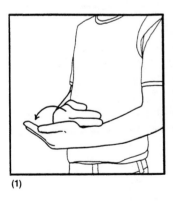
(1)

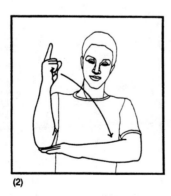
(2)

BIRTHDAY

The day of someone's birth.

*A person's **birthday** is usually celebrated each year on that date.*

(1) Sign BORN — the left "flat" hand faces up at waist level. The right "flat" hand faces in. Move the hand out and down on the left palm. (SM)
(2) Sign DAY — the left "flat" hand faces down at chest level, with the arm bent. The right "one" hand points up, with the elbow resting on the fingers of the left hand. Move the right hand down to rest on the left arm. (SM)

BIRTH DEFECT

A bodily part missing, misshapen or unable to function properly at birth.

Birth defects can be inherited (as in mongolism), caused by infections of the mother during pregnancy, or by the mother's use of certain drugs.

(1) Sign BORN — the left "flat" hand faces up at waist level. The right "flat" hand faces in. Move the hand out and down on the left palm. (SM)
(2) Sign SOMETHING — the right "one" hand points up at chest level and makes a small circle, keeping the wrist stiff. (SM)
(3) Sign WRONG - the right "Y" hand faces in under the chin. (SM)

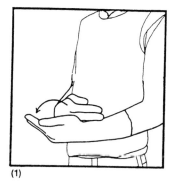

(1)

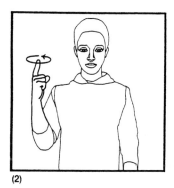

(2)

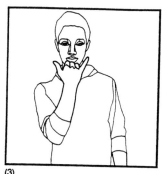

(3)

BIRTHMARK

A mark or discolored area on the body present at birth.

Birthmarks may be caused by a collection of blood vessels under the skin or an abnormal collection of substances responsible for skin color.

(1) Sign BORN — the left "flat" hand faces up at waist level. The right "flat" hand faces in. Move the hand out and down on the left palm. (SM)
(2) The right "F" hand faces out on the face. (SM)

* *This should be signed at the area of the birthmark.*

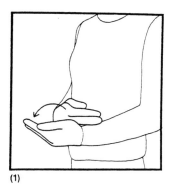

(1)

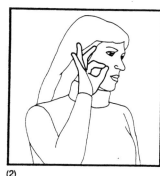

(2)

BIRTHPLACE

The place where one was born; also the place where something originally started.

It is important to know your birthplace because it is a commonly asked question on health forms.

(1) Sign BORN — the left "flat" hand faces up at waist level. The right "flat" hand faces in. Move the hand out and down on the left palm. (SM)
(2) Sign WHERE — both "five" hands face up at chest level and move slightly from left to right. (MM)

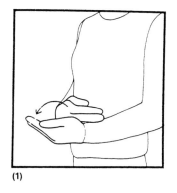

(1)

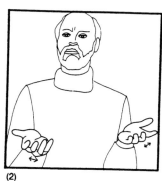

(2)

63

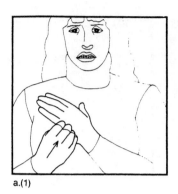

a.(1)

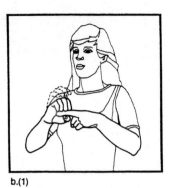

b.(1)

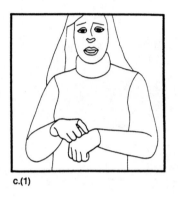

c.(1)

BITE

Puncturing or tearing of the skin and underlying tissue by an animal's teeth or an insect's stinger. In dentistry, the term means the fit of the teeth when brought together; also called occlusion.

Animal bites may cause redness and swelling, pain, itching or throbbing and should be treated so that they don't become infected.

a. (1) Sign BITE — the left "flat" hand faces in at chest level. The right "C" hand bites the pinky finger side of the left hand. (SM)

* *This should be signed if referring to a large bite.*

b. (1) Sign BITE — the left "one" hand points out at chest level. The right "C" hand bites the left index finger. (SM)

* *This should be signed if referring to a small bite.*

c. (1) Sign BITE — the left "S" hand faces down at chest level. The index finger of the right "one" hand taps the back of the left hand a few times. (MM)

* *This should be signed if referring to an insect bite.*

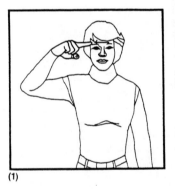

(1)

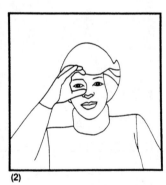

(2)

BLACK EYE

The discoloration of the eye or the area around the eye resulting from bumps or injury, caused by blood leaking into the area. There will be pain, swelling and a change in the color of the skin to red or purple and then to green or yellow.

Applying cold towels to a black eye will help prevent swelling.

(1) Sign BLACK — the index finger of the right "one" hand moves across the forehead from left to right. (SM)

(2) The right "C" hand faces left over the right eye. (SM)

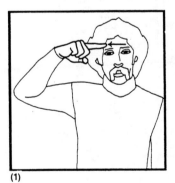

(1)

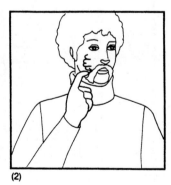

(2)

BLACKHEAD

A kind of pimple on the skin with a dark center in it.

A blackhead is caused by a plug forming in the opening of a skin gland and then turning dark color when exposed to air.

(1) Sign BLACK — the index finger of the right "one" hand moves across the forehead from left to right. (SM)

(2) The index finger of the right "one" hand taps the right cheek a few times as if imitating pimples. (MM)

* *This can be signed at the area of the blackhead.*

BLACKOUT

A short period of unconsciousness.

A blackout is caused by not enough blood being circulated to the brain.

(1) The right "K" hand moves slightly down from chest level into an "O" hand. (SM)

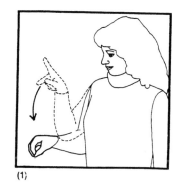

(1)

BLADDER

The expandable, bag-like organ at the front of the lower abdomen. The bladder is connected to the kidneys by the ureters and receives urine made by the kidneys. *See Figure 9*

BLAND DIET

A diet mild in flavor and texture; free of irritation.

A bland diet consists of foods that are low in fiber and have small amounts of spices, acids and fats in them.

BLANKET

A piece of material (wool, cotton, or synthetic) used as a covering to hold in body heat.

A blanket is used to prevent shock by helping keep the body temperature at 98.6°.

(1) Both "five" hands face in at waist level. Move both hands up to shoulder level, ending in "flat-O" hands as if imitating pulling a blanket up. (SM)

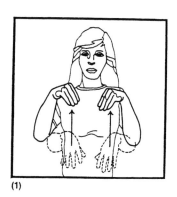

(1)

BLEED

The act of losing blood. (See BLOOD)
(1) Sign RED — the index finger of the right "one" hand brushes down the chin a few times. (MM)
(2) The left "five" hand is at chest level with the palm towards the body. The palm of the right "five" hand is towards the body with the middle fingertips touching the mouth. Move the right hand down the back of the left hand. Wiggle the fingers of the right hand as it moves. (SM)

*This movement should be longer and slower.

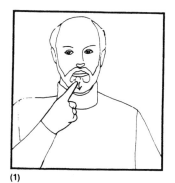

(1)

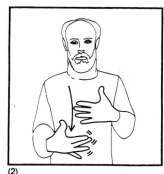

(2)

BLEEDER'S DISEASE
See HEMOPHILIA

BLEEDING SICKNESS
See HEMOPHILIA

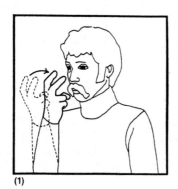
(1)

BLIND
A temporary or permanent loss of sight.

Blindness can be caused by damage or disease in the brain, looking at too bright a light (sun), emotional or mental problems, or damage or disease in the eye.

(1) The right bent "V" hand faces in at eye level and moves in slightly towards the eyes. (SM)

BLIND SPOT
The place on the retina where the optic nerve leaves the eye. There are no cones or rods in this area so no vision can occur.

The blind spot is another name for "optic disk".

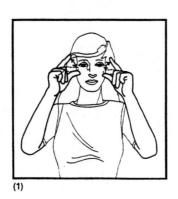
(1)

BLINK
To quickly close and open the eyelid.

Blinking helps spread tears over the eye, which keeps the eye from drying out, and it brushes away dust which may have landed on the eye.

(1) The thumbs and index fingers of both "G" hands touch, the palms face out at the sides of the eyes. Flick the fingers open as if imitating the eyes blinking, and at the same time, the eyes should blink. (SM)

*This can be signed with only the right hand to mean one eye blinking.

BLISTER
A small bump on the skin caused by a fluid, usually serum, blood, or pus collecting between the layers of skin.

Blisters are usually caused by something rubbing or pinching the skin or by minor burns.

BLOOD

The red fluid that the heart pumps through the arteries, veins and capillaries of the body. The blood is made up of red blood cells, white blood cells, platelets and the plasma in which they float.

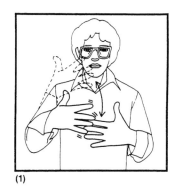
(1)

Blood carries nutrients, hormones, antibodies and oxygen to the body's cells and takes away carbon dioxide and wastes.

(1) The left "five" hand is at chest level with the palm toward the body. The palm of the right "five" hand is toward the body with the middle fingertips touching the mouth. Move the right hand down the back of the left hand. Wiggle the fingers of the right hand as it moves. (MM)
This movement should be short, repeated and somewhat restrained.

BLOOD BANK

A place where blood or plasma is stored until it is needed by someone.

When someone donates blood to a blood bank, the blood is checked for any abnormalities or disease.

BLOOD CLOTTING

The process in which blood changes into a jelly-like mass which doesn't flow normally. When we are bleeding, a clot will form over the hole in the blood vessel and act like a plug to stop the blood from flowing out.

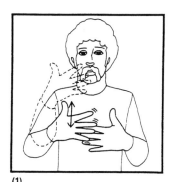
(1)

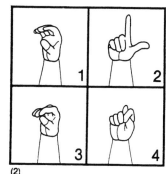
(2)

Blood clotting or coagulation is caused by certain substances in the plasma coming together to form a net which blood cells become trapped in.

(1) Sign BLOOD — the left "five" hand is at chest level with the palm toward the body. The palm of the right "five" hand is toward the body with the middle fingertips touching the mouth. Move the right hand down the back of the left hand. Wiggle the fingers of the right hand as it moves. (MM)
This movement should be short, repeated and somewhat restrained.

(2) Fingerspell "C-L-O-T".

BLOOD COUNT

The number of red blood cells or white blood cells in a certain amount of blood.

A blood count is done using a microscope so the cells can be seen.

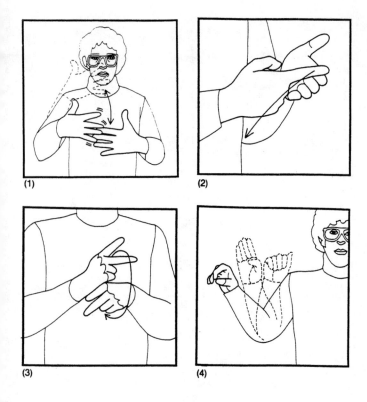

(1)

(2)

(3)

(4)

BLOOD GROUP

An inherited characteristic of the blood divided into four groups (A, B, AB and O) depending on the kind of protein (antigen) on the surface of the red blood cells.

In transfusions it is important that the blood donor and the receiver of blood belong to the same blood group because blood of one group reacts to blood of another group.

(1) Sign BLOOD — the left "five" hand is at chest level with the palm toward the body. The palm of the right "five" hand is toward the body with the middle fingertips touching the mouth. Move the right hand down the back of the left hand. Wiggle the fingers of the right hand as it moves. (MM)
This movement should be short, repeated and somewhat restrained.

(2) Sign WHAT — the left "flat" hand faces right at chest level. The index finger of the right "one" hand moves down the fingers of the left hand. (SM)

(3) Sign KIND — the right "K" hand faces left on top of the left "K" hand which faces right. Move both hands out forward in a circular movement. (SM)

(4) Fingerspell "A-B-O", indicating the types of blood.
The facial expression should indicate questioning when signing.

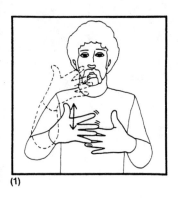

(1)

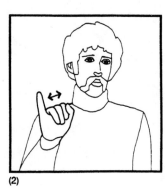

(2)

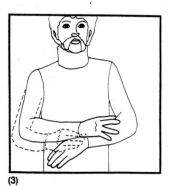

(3)

BLOOD POISONING

A general term for an infection of the blood caused by the presence of different bacteria, germs or poisons and wastes in the blood.

The symptoms of blood poisoning are fever and chills, abscesses, and red patches on the skin.

(1) Sign BLOOD — the left "five" hand is at chest level with the palm toward the body. The palm of the right "five" hand is toward the body with the middle fingertips touching the mouth. Move the right hand down the back of the left hand. Wiggle the fingers of the right hand as it moves. (MM)
This movement should be short, repeated and somewhat restrained.

(2) Sign INFECTION — the right "I" hand faces out and shakes slightly from left to right. (MM)
* Mouth the word "infection" while signing.

(3) The left arm is bent and faces down. The right "flat-O" hand faces down on the back of the left hand and moves up the left arm into a "five" hand. (SM)

BLOOD PRESSURE

A measurement of how hard the blood is pushing on the walls of the blood vessels. The measurement varies depending on whether the heart is contracting or relaxed. The blood pressure is measured with a cuff or band which is wrapped around the arm and inflated with air. The person taking the blood pressure listens with a stethoscope to the movements of blood in the vessels.

Blood pressure is usually written with one number over another number, the top number is the blood pressure when the heart contracts and the bottom number is the pressure when the heart is relaxed.

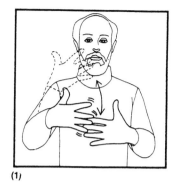 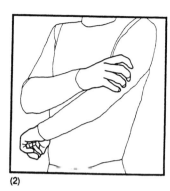

(1) Sign BLOOD — the left "five" hand is at chest level with the palm toward the body. The palm of the right "five" hand is toward the body with the middle fingertips touching the mouth. Move the right hand down the back of the left hand. Wiggle the fingers of the right hand as it moves. (MM)
This movement should be short, repeated and somewhat restrained.
(2) The right "claw" hand grabs the left upper arm. (SM)

BLOODSHOT

A term describing the discoloration caused by blood collected in the blood vessels in an area.

The eyes are said to be bloodshot when the tiny blood vessels in the conjunctiva fill with blood and make the white of the eyes look red.

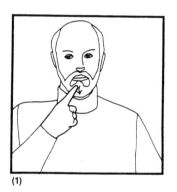 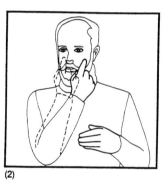

(1) Sign RED — the index finger of the right "one" hand brushes down the chin a few times. (MM)
(2) The right index finger points to both eyes. (DM)

BLOODSTREAM

The flow of blood through the circulatory system.

The heart, veins and arteries provide a travel system for the bloodstream.

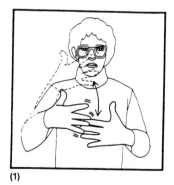 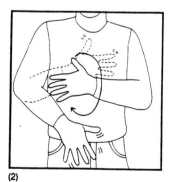

(1) Sign BLOOD — the left "five" hand is at chest level with the palm toward the body. The palm of the right "five" hand is toward the body with the middle fingertips touching the mouth. Move the right hand down the back of the left hand. Wiggle the fingers of the right hand as it moves. (SM)
This movement should be short, repeated and somewhat restrained.
(2) The left "five" hand faces in at chest level. The right "five" hand faces in and moves out and around the left hand in a circular movement, with the fingers wiggling at the same time. (MM)

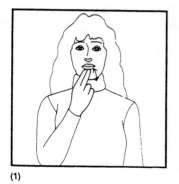
(1)

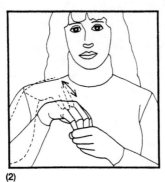
(2)

BLOOD SUGAR

Sugar in the form of glucose which is carried in the blood to the cells where it is used for energy.

Blood sugar levels will rise after a person eats because glucose is removed from the food.

(1) Sign SUGAR — the fingertips of the right "H" hand brush down the chin a few times. (MM)
*This can also be signed by brushing the fingertips of the right "flat" hand down the chin a few times. (MM)

(2) Sign IN — the fingertips of the right "flat-O" hand move into the fist of the left "O" hand, both at chest level. (MM)

(3) Sign BLOOD — the left "five" hand is at chest level with the palm toward the body. The palm of the right "five" hand is toward the body with the middle fingertips touching the mouth. Move the right hand down the back of the left hand. Wiggle the fingers of the right hand as it moves. (MM)
*This movement should be short, repeated and somewhat restrained.

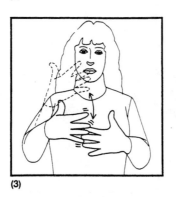
(3)

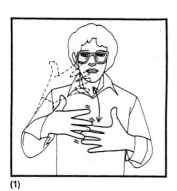
(1)

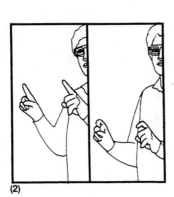
(2)

BLOOD TEST

A laboratory examination of blood taken from a person to see what sort of chemicals or substances are in it, how much of a substance is in it, and to see if the cells are normal.

There are many different kinds of blood tests which can be done and a doctor will ask to do tests which may help him find out what is wrong with someone.

(1) Sign BLOOD — the left "five" hand is at chest level with the palm toward the body. The palm of the right "five" hand is toward the body with the middle fingertips touching the mouth. Move the right hand down the back of the left hand. Wiggle the fingers of the right hand as it moves. (MM)
*This movement should be short, repeated and somewhat restrained.

(2) Sign TEST — both "one" hands point up at shoulder level with the palms facing out. Move both hands down slightly and at the same time bend the index fingers. Repeat this movement three times, with the hands ending at waist level. (MM)

BLOOD VESSELS

The veins, arteries and capillaries which carry blood. *See Figures 6 and 7*

BLUE DEVILS
See AMOBARBITAL

BLUNT INJURY
See CONTUSION

BLUR
A haziness or fuzziness of sight.

*A person's vision usually becomes **blurred** just before passing out.*

(1) The right "five" hand faces out at eye level. The left "five" hand faces in, in front of the right hand. Move the hands in opposite directions from left to right as if the fingers are imitating blurring. (MM)

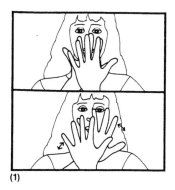
(1)

BODY
The whole structure of a person or animal.

*A clean, healthy, well-cared-for **body** helps one feel good about oneself.*

(1) Both "flat" hands face in. The fingertips of both hands touch the chest and then the stomach. (DM)

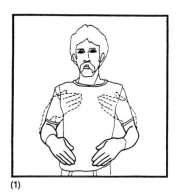
(1)

BOIL
A round area of inflammation in the skin caused by bacteria infecting a gland or the base of a hair.

Boils can be very painful and should be treated by a doctor.

(1) Fingerspell "B-O-I-L".
(2) The left "flat" hand faces right at chest level. The fingertips of the right "claw" hand touch the left palm. Open the right hand slightly, leaving the fingertips on the left palm, as if imitating a boil. At the same time, the cheeks should puff out a little. (SM)

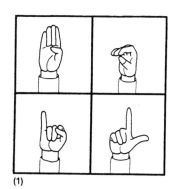
(1)
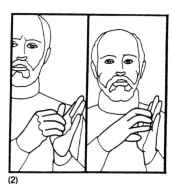
(2)

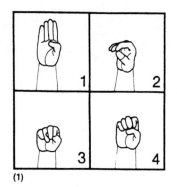
(1)

BONE

The hard, white substance that makes up the skeleton of the body. Bone contains minerals such as calcium and phosphorus which make it hard. The bones act as a frame and support the body and also protect certain organs. They also store minerals and the center of some bones (the marrow) make blood cells.

Bone is not just minerals, but is a special tissue with its own blood supply, alive and constantly changing.

(1) Fingerspell "B-O-N-E".

BONE FRAGMENT

A small piece of bone that has been broken off by an injury.

Bone fragments can cut and damage tissue around the site of an injury.

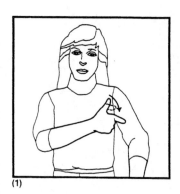
(1)

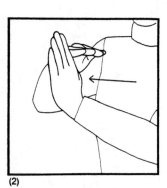
(2)

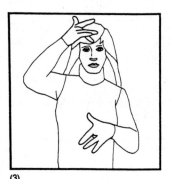
(3)

BOOSTER SHOT

A later dose of a vaccine given to help increase the protection provided by earlier doses.

A booster shot is usually given a couple of weeks or more after the first shot.

(1) Sign INJECTION — the right "L" hand faces in with the index finger touching the upper arm. Move the thumb of the right hand in as if injecting something into the left arm. (SM)
(2) Sign PREVENT — both "flat" hands cross at chest level and move out forward slightly. (SM)
(3) Sign DISEASE — the middle finger of the right "eight" hand touches the forehead and the middle finger of the left "eight" hand touches the stomach. (SM)

BOTULISM

A severe type of food poisoning caused by eating food which has a certain kind of toxin bacteria (Clostridium botulinum) growing in it. Not much food has to be eaten to make someone sick because the bacteria is very poisonous. Symptoms are dizziness, weakness, vomiting, and in severe cases, paralysis of the heart, respiratory and central nervous systems, causing death.

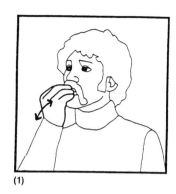 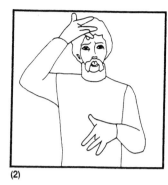

(1)　　　　(2)

Botulism can be prevented by cooking all foods completely, especially meats, correctly boiling containers when home canning and by always cleaning surfaces after preparing foods.

(1) Sign EAT — the fingertips of the right "flat-O" hand touch the mouth. (SM)
(2) Sign SICK — the middle finger of the right "eight" hand touches the forehead and the middle finger of the left "eight" hand touches the stomach. (SM)

* This is a general sign for food poisoning. The word "B-O-T-U-L-I-S-M" should also be fingerspelled to specify the specific type of poisoning.

BOWEL

The part of the digestive tract beyond the stomach, consisting of the small bowel and the large bowel, or colon. *See Figure 9*

BOWEL MOVEMENT

The release of solid wastes or feces from the rectum through the anus.

People vary in how often they have bowel movements; it is not necessary to have one a day to stay healthy.

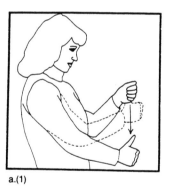 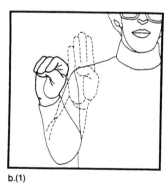

a.(1)　　　　b.(1)

a. (1) Sign FECES — the left "A" hand faces right at chest level. The thumb of the right "A" hand is inside the left fist. Move the right hand down, keeping the left hand in place. (SM)
b. (1) Fingerspell "B-M".

BRACE

A device which is attached to a structure or part and used to steady or hold it in a certain position.

When a person's spine or teeth are not straight, braces can be worn to straighten them.

BRACHIAL

Referring to the arm.

(Continued on next page)

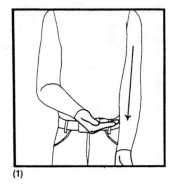
(1)

One would apply pressure to the artery in the brachial to control the bleeding of a victim's hand.

(1) Sign ARM — the fingertips of the right "cupped" hand brush down the left arm. (SM)

BRACHIAL ARTERY

The main artery supplying fresh blood to the arm. When pressure is applied to the brachial artery in the inner upper arm between the elbow and shoulder, severe bleeding in the arm can be slowed. *See Figure 6*

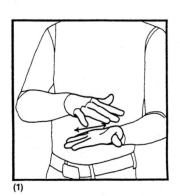
(1)

BRAILLE

A system or form of reading and writing that allows the blind to "see" by touch or feeling.

The Braille system uses small, raised dots in different patterns to form numbers and letters.

(1) The left "flat" hand faces up at waist level. The right "five" hand faces down and moves across the left palm as if reading braille. (MM)

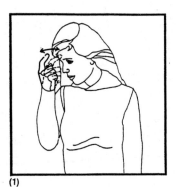
(1)

BRAIN

The large, soft organ made up of nerve tissue found inside the cranium. The brain is made up of five parts — the cerebrum, cerebellum, pons, medulla oblongota, and midbrain, and extends down the vertebral canal as the spinal cord. The brain receives nerve impulses or messages from all over the body, controls the body's activities and is responsible for thought, memory, reasoning and emotions. *See Figure 17 or 18*

(1) The index finger of the right "one" hand taps the forehead. (MM)

BRAIN DAMAGE

A general word for some injury to the brain. The injury could be caused by many things like abnormal development, poisoning by drugs or chemicals, not enough oxygen getting to the brain, a stroke or an accident.

With treatment, therapy, training and education many people with brain damage can learn skills and lead full, normal lives.

(1) Sign BRAIN — the index finger of the right "one" hand taps the forehead. (MM)

(2) Sign DAMAGE — the left "five" hand faces up at chest level. The right "five" hand faces down at chest level. Move both hands towards the center, into "A" hands facing each other. Continue through until the arms cross. Then move both hands back to their beginning positions, with the right "five" hand facing down and the left "A" hand facing up.

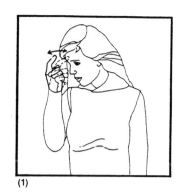

(1)

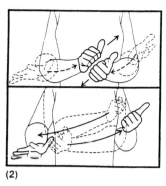

(2)

BRAIN FEVER

A disease caused by an infection of the brain. Symptoms are a severe headache, temperature and vomiting.

Brain fever is another name for meningitis or encephalitis.

BRAIN WAVES

The regular changes in the electrical activity of the brain. There are several different kinds of brain waves which occur in the brain depending on whether the person is sleeping, awake, concentrating, or has epilepsy.

Brain waves are recorded by an electronic encephalograph.

BREAK

A fracture of a bone or other material.

It is important to splint a break so the joints above and below the broken bone will not move.

(1) Both "S" hands are together at chest level with the palms facing down. Turn both hands up as if breaking something. (SM)

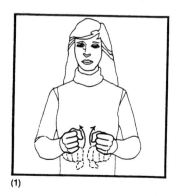

(1)

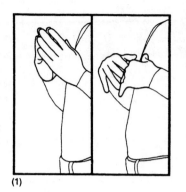

(1)

BREAKDOWN

A general term for various types of mental illness that come from not being able to cope with daily problems.

It is important to seek help in times of high stress to avoid mental breakdown.

(1) Both "flat" hands touch at the fingertips to form a peak. The fingers point up. Bend the fingers down as if the peak collapsed.(SM)

BREAKING WIND

See FLATULENCE

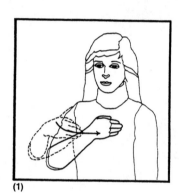

(1)

BREAST

Referring to the upper, front part of the chest or for one of the mammary glands, the enlarged fatty glands on the chest of a woman which produce milk after she has had a baby.

The breasts of a woman are actually a collection of glands surrounded by fat which, when certain hor- mones are made by the body, produce milk.

(1) The fingertips of the right "cupped" hand touch the right and then the left chest. (DM)

BREASTBONE

The flat bone at the front of the chest which the clavicles or collar bones and the front part of the ribs attach to. Breastbone is another name for ster- num. *See Figure 26*

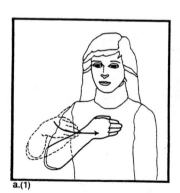

a.(1)

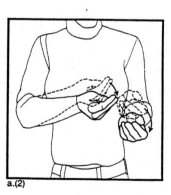

a.(2)

BREASTFEED

Feeding a baby with mother's milk from the breast.

Breastfeeding an infant is a good way to help build up antibodies in his system.

a. (1) Sign BREAST — the fingertips of the right "cupped" hand touch the right and then the left chest. (DM)

(2) Both "flat-O" hands face up at the left chest. Drop both hands down slightly. (SM)

(Continued on next page)

BREASTFEED, *continued*

b. (1) Sign BABY — the right hand and forearm face up, resting on the left hand and forearm which also face upwards. Both are then rocked back and forth as if holding a baby. (MM)
(2) The left "cupped" hand faces up at the left chest. The right "cupped" hand faces up slightly above the left hand. Open and close the fingers of the right hand, forming a "flat-O" hand. (MM)

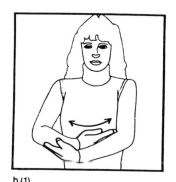

b.(1)

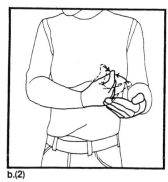

b.(2)

BREAST SELF-EXAMINATION

The procedure in which a woman checks her breast for any abnormality, lump or hardness which may be a sign of breast cancer. Breast self examinations should be done once a month, just after the menstrual period and also once a month in women who have gone through menopause. To examine her breasts, a woman lies down and puts one hand behind her head. With the flattened fingers of the other hand she gently examines the breast on the side with the arm behind her head. To examine the breast, she starts at the outer edge of the breast and checks an area with tiny circular motions. She then works her way around the outer edge of the breast in a circle, staying the same distance away from the nipple, checking each small area with the tiny circular motions. After finishing the circle, she moves her fingers in closer to the nipple and makes another circle, examining her breast in the same way. She does this until she has examined the whole breast. The other breast is checked in the same way. This whole procedure is repeated sitting up, with the hand still behind the head. Each nipple should then be gently squeezed to check for any discharge. At this time, the woman should also stand in front of a mirror (with her hands raised above her head) and check each breast for any change in shape or size or any puckering. If there is anything abnormal discovered or any lump a doctor should be seen immediately.

*Breast cancer, which is the most common type of cancer and the leading cause of cancer deaths in women, can be found earlier and treated with more success if a woman does regular **breast self-examinations**.*

(Continued on next page)

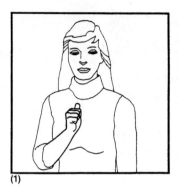
(1)

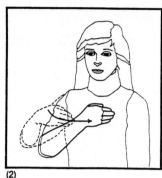
(2)

(1) Sign MYSELF — the right "A" hand faces left with the back of the thumb touching the chest. (SM)
(2) Sign BREAST — the fingertips of the right "cupped" hand touch the right and then the left chest. (DM)
(3) The fingertips of the right "flat" hand circle the left chest as if imitating examining the breast. (MM)

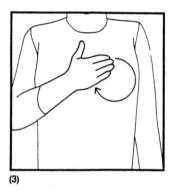
(3)

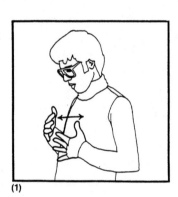
(1)

BREATH

The air which is taken into or inhaled and let out of or exhaled from the lungs during respiration.

The way someone's breath smells or the sounds it makes when moving in the airways may help a doctor tell if something is wrong.

(1) Both "five" hands move in and out from the chest as if imitating breathing. (MM)

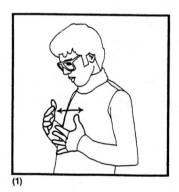
(1)

BREATHING

The act or process of taking in or inhaling and letting out or exhaling air.

The normal rate of breathing, about 16 breaths per minute, can be increased by certain diseases or exercise and decreased by some drugs and unconsciousness.

(1) Both "five" hands move in and out from the chest as if imitating breathing. (MM)

78

BRIDGE

In dentistry, a set of artificial teeth which are used to replace missing teeth and are held in place by being attached to a person's natural teeth. (This can also be the connection between two things; a narrow band of tissue.)

Most bridges are permanently attached but some can be made to be temporarily attached so that they can be removed.

(1) The index finger of the right "one" hand points to the teeth. (SM)
(2) Sign FALSE — the right "L" hand faces left and brushes past the nose. (SM)
(3) The index finger and thumb of the right hand imitate putting a bridge in the mouth. (SM)

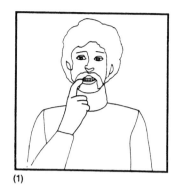

(1)

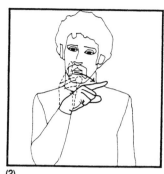

(2)

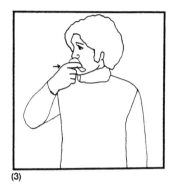

(3)

BROMIDE®

A group of drugs made by combining the substance bromine with another substance which acts as a depressant.

Bromides used to be used as sedatives but because of bad side effects and the discovery of new drugs, they aren't used much any more.

BRONCHI

The two main branches off the bottom of the trachea which go to the lungs. One bronchus goes into each lung, where it branches into smaller passages leading to the air sacs. *See Figure 10*

BRONCHITIS

An inflammation of the lining of the tubes which take air into the lungs, the bronchi. Symptoms of bronchitis are pain in the chest, a cough and fever.

Bronchitis can be caused by air pollution, smoking, a virus or bacteria infecting the airways, or allergies.

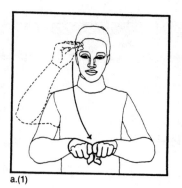

a.(1)

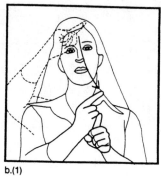

b.(1)

BROTHER

A term used to describe relationship between children. A brother is a male child with the same mother and father as another child.

When only one parent is in common, the term half-brother is used.

a. (1) The fingertips of the right "flat-O" hand touch the forehead. The left "one" hand is facing down, pointing out at waist level. Move the right hand down next to the left hand, ending in an "one" hand, pointing out. (SM)

b. (1) The index finger of the right "one" hand touches the forehead. The left "one" hand is facing down, pointing out at waist level. Move the right hand down into a "one" hand and then tap the left hand once. (SM)

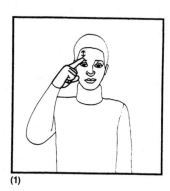

(1)

BROW

The part of the face from the eyes to the hairline, the forehead. *See Figure 1*

(1) The index finger of the right "one" hand moves from the right eyebrow to the hairline. (DM)

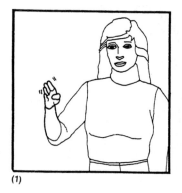

(1)

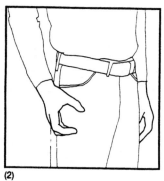

(2)

BRUISE

An injury in which the skin is not cut, but the small blood vessels beneath the skin are damaged allowing blood to leak out and causing the skin to change color to purple.

Bruises can be treated by applying cold to the area after the injury.

(1) Sign BLUE — the right "B" hand faces out at chest level. Pivot the hand slightly from left to right a few times. (MM)

(2) The right "C" hand faces in on the area of the bruise. (SM)

BRUSHING TEETH

The act of removing food particles from the surface and between the teeth.

Flossing and brushing teeth regularly will help keep plaque and tartar from building up and causing tooth decay.

(Continued on next page)

(1) The index finger of the right "one" hand imitates brushing the teeth. (MM)

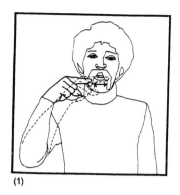

(1)

BUNION

Inflammation of the joint of the big toe causing pain and swelling.

Bunions, most common in women, are caused by wearing shoes that are too tight for many years.

BUR

Any of differently shaped small attachments for a dental drill. Burs are made out of a very hard, rough material.

The head of the drill turns very quickly and the dentist, by using different burs, can grind, smooth, cut, or drill into the teeth.

BURN

Skin or deeper tissue injury caused by being exposed to heat, chemicals, electricity or radiation for too long a time. The effects of a burn vary depending on what caused it, its strength and how long it lasted. The most common type of burn is the burn caused by heat, the thermal burn. These burns are grouped into first, second and third degree burns, depending on how badly the skin is damaged.

One must never put lotions or ointments on a severe burn, only a clean dry bandage.

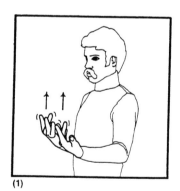

(1)

(1) Sign FIRE — both "five" hands face in with the fingers pointing up at chest level. Wiggle the fingers and move both hands up slightly. (MM)

* *This can be signed with one hand under the area of the burn.*

BURNPADS

Large, thick pads which can be quickly applied to an area.

Burnpads are so-called because they are often used on burns.

BURSA

A sac found around joints and over bones near the skin which contains a fluid that reduces the friction between two structures.

A bunion is caused by irritation of the bursa around the joint of the big toe.

BURSITIS

The inflammation of a bursa caused by overuse or injuries, causing pain and swelling in the area. Locations often affected by bursitis are the shoulder, elbow, knee and big toe.

Bursitis is treated with rest, pain relievers, heat and sometimes cortisone injections.

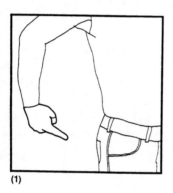

(1)

BUTTOCKS

The fleshy part of the body on the lower back side of the hips. The buttocks are formed by the gluteus maximus muscles. *See Figure 3*

(1) The right index finger points to the buttocks. (SM)

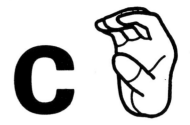

C

CADAVER

A dead human body; a corpse.

Medical schools use cadavers to train their students in anatomy.

(1) Sign BODY — both "flat" hands face in. The fingertips of both hands touch the chest and then the stomach. (SM)

(2) Sign DEAD — the left "flat" hand faces up at chest level. The right "flat" hand fces down at chest level. Turn both hands to the right so that the left hand ends facing down and the right hand ends facing up. (SM)

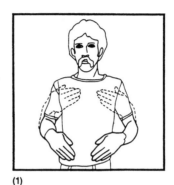

(1)

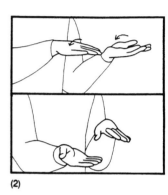

(2)

CAFFEINE

A drug that acts as a stimulant and makes a person urinate. It will make a person feel temporarily more alert and less tired. It is found in coffee, tea and some soft drinks and is added to some pain relievers.

Taking in too much caffeine can cause poisoning with symptoms of irregular heartbeat, trembling, nervousness and difficulty in sleeping.

a. (1) Sign COFFEE — the left "S" hand faces in at chest level. The right "S" hand moves in counterclockwise circles above the left hand as if imitating a coffee grinder. (MM)

b. (1) Sign TEA — the left "O" hand faces in at chest level. The right "F" hand moves in counterclockwise circles above the left hand. (MM)

(2) Sign DRINK — the right "C" hand faces left and moves towards the mouth as if imitating taking a drink. (SM)

(3) Both "A" hands face out at the sides of the eyes. Open both hands, and at the same time, open the eyes wide. (SM)

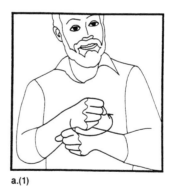

a.(1)

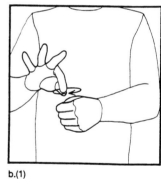

b.(1)

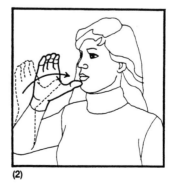

(2)

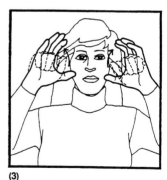

(3)

* There is no sign for caffeine. To explain the idea of caffeine, fingerspell "C-A-F-F-E-I-N-E" and sign COFFEE or TEA, then DRINK, WIDE AWAKE. Further explanation may be necesary.

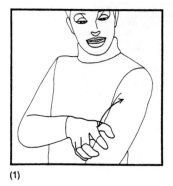
(1)

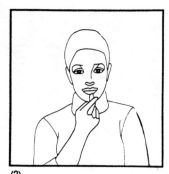
(2)

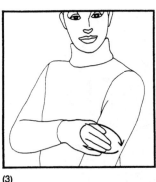
(3)

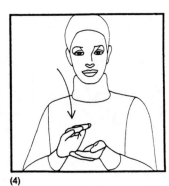
(4)

CALAMINE

A pink powder mostly of zinc oxide used to make a soothing lotion that relieves skin irritations.

Calamine lotion is used on minor skin irritations like poison ivy and sunburn.

(1) The right "claw" hand itches up and down the left upper arm a few times. (MM)

(2) Sign PINK — the middle finger of the right "P" hand brushes down the chin a few times. (MM)

(3) The fingertips of the right "flat" hand rub in a circular movement on the left arm.

* This could be signed where the calamine is being applied.

(4) Sign REDUCE — the left "cupped" hand faces up at chest level. The right "cupped" hand faces down at shoulder level and moves down to the left hand. (SM)

CALCIUM

A substance which is important in the body for making bones and teeth, helping the blood clot and for making the muscles and nerves work. Good sources of calcium are beans, cheese, milk and egg yolk.

Pregnant women need a lot more calcium than other people for normal development of bones and other structures in the baby's body.

CALCULUS

An abnormal formation of hard objects in body passages or cavities. A calculus, commonly called a stone, is usually made up of minerals.

The kidneys, ureters, bladder, urethra, gallbladder and bile duct are places where a calculus may form or be found.

CALF

The rear, fleshy part of the lower leg. The calf is made up of the soleus and gastrocnemius muscles. *See Figure 3*

(1) The right index finger points to the calf of the leg.

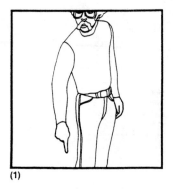
(1)

CALLUS

A hard, thickening of skin caused by pressure or friction; also the hard tissue that forms on the ends of broken bones.

A callus is commonly seen on the hand or the foot.

a. (1) Fingerspell "F-O-O-T".

b. (1) Sign HANDS — the left "flat" hand brushes up the back of the right hand, then the right "flat" hand brushes up the back of the left hand. (SM)

(2) Sign SKIN — the index finger and thumb of the right hand pinch the right cheek. (SM)

(3) Sign HARD — the left "bent-V" hand faces down at chest level. The knuckles of the right "bent-V" hand tap the back of the left hand a few times. (MM)

(4) The right "F" hand faces down on top of the left palm. (SM)

* Fingerspell "F-O-O-T" or sign HANDS, whichever applies, then sign (2), (3), and (4).

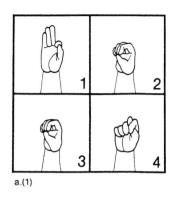

a.(1)

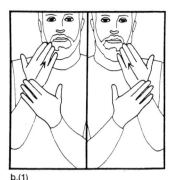

b.(1)

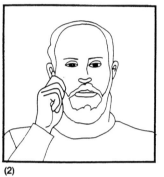

(2)

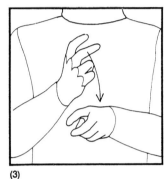

(3)

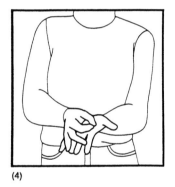

(4)

CALM

A feeling of peace, quiet or relaxation.

People are often given a drug to calm them before they have an operation.

(1) Both "flat" hands cross at the lips. Move both hands down and out, ending with both hands facing down. (SM)

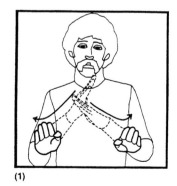

(1)

85

CALORIE

A unit of heat. The amount of energy a food provides is measured in calories. The calorie used in nutrition is the amount of heat needed to raise the temperature of a kilogram of water 1° C.

Fats provide more calories than proteins or carbohydrates.

CANAL

In medicine, a narrow tube, duct or passage through bone or tissues.

Bone contains small canals with blood vessels which carry nutrients through the bone.

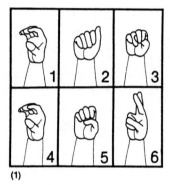

(1)

CANCER

An uncontrolled, disorganized and abnormal cell growth. Cancer cells don't work correctly, use up the body's energy and replace the normal cells in an organ so the organ doesn't work. A cancer can grow by spreading directly to tissue next to the affected area or by cells being carried from the original site by the blood or lymph system. This is why finding the disease early is important. Since cancer can affect many organs or parts of the body, there are many different symptoms. Some symptoms are a lump or thickening in an area, a sore that won't heal, a cough, problems swallowing, difficulty in digesting food, sudden weight loss, a change in the size or appearance of a wart or mole or bleeding or discharge from an area. The exact cause of cancer is unknown but exposure to some substances (carcinogens) and constant irritation will make it more likely that a person will get a certain form of cancer. Surgery, chemotherapy and radiation are used to treat cancer.

Malignancy, malignant tumor, malignant growth, neoplasm and carcinoma are all words for cancer.

(1) Fingerspell "C-A-N-C-E-R".

86

CANDIDIASIS

An infection of the respiratory tract, the mouth and digestive tract or more often, of the female vagina which is caused by a yeast. The yeast lives in these places normally but under some conditions, they may increase in number and cause an infection. When they infect the vagina, there is irritation in the area, itching and a discharge from the vagina. Candidiasis is also called Moniliasis or yeast infection.

A woman who is diabetic, pregnant, taking birth control pills, or taking antibiotics is more likely to get candidiasis; it can be treated with medicines placed in the vagina.

CANINE TEETH

See CUSPIDS

CANKER SORE

A small sore or ulcer on the inside of the mouth.

The cause of many canker sores is unknown but some may be caused by a food allergy.

(1) Fingerspell "S-O-R-E".
(2) The right index finger points to the corner of the mouth or the spot of the canker sore. (SM)

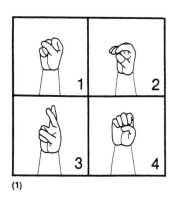
(1)

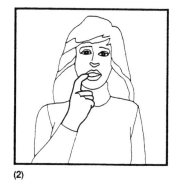
(2)

CANNABIS

See MARIJUANA

CAP

An artificial tooth made of gold, silver or porcelain used to replace a tooth that has been badly chipped, decayed or has died.

A cap is another name for "crown."

(1) The right index finger points to a tooth.

(2) The right "claw" hand faces down on top of the left fist. (SM)

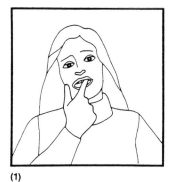
(1)

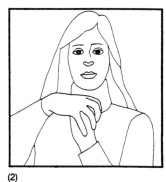
(2)

CAPILLARY

A very small blood vessel that connects the smallest arteries to the smallest veins.

Capillaries have very thin walls so the blood is very close to the tissues, allowing the exchange of materials.

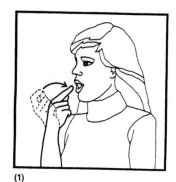

(1)

CAPSULE

A small container made of gelatin containing a dose of medicine.

A capsule enables someone to swallow a medicine without tasting it.

(1) Sign PILL — the thumb and index finger of the right hand touch, the palm faces the mouth. Flick the index finger towards the mouth as if popping a pill into the mouth. (SM)

CARBOHYDRATES

Substances made up of only carbon, hydrogen and oxygen arranged in different ways. Carbohydrates are an important source of energy in our diets.

Examples of carbohydrates are sugars, such as glucose and fructose, and starches.

CARBON

An element; a basic substance found in all living things and organic compounds. Carbon makes life possible when it combines with hydrogen, oxygen and nitrogen. In food, carbon acts as a source of energy.

Common forms of pure carbon are coal and diamonds.

CARBON DIOXIDE

A gas that cannot be seen or smelled and is made up of carbon and oxygen (CO_2).

Carbon dioxide is made when things rot or burn, and is found in the air exhaled from animals.

CARBON MONOXIDE

A very poisonous, odorless, colorless gas (CO) made up of carbon and oxygen.

Carbon monoxide is formed by the incomplete burning of organic material, and may be found in automobile exhaust, coal and wood fire smoke and in mines and sewers.

CARBUNCLE

An infection of the tissue under the skin, caused by bacteria. A carbuncle is a large, inflammed area with several openings that allow pus to escape.

A carbuncle, worse than a boil, is very painful and can make a person very sick.

CARCINOGEN

A substance that causes cancer.

Examples of carcinogens are some types of radiation, certain chemicals, such as cigarette tar, and some viruses.

(1) Sign SOMETHING — the right "one" hand points up at chest level and makes a small circle, keeping the wrist stiff. (SM)
(2) Sign CAUSE — both "A" hands face up at chest level. Move both hands down and towards the left, ending in "five" hands at waist level. (SM)
(3) Fingerspell "C-A-N-C-E-R".

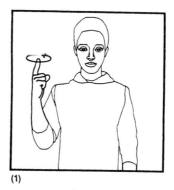
(1)

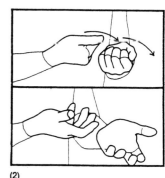
(2)

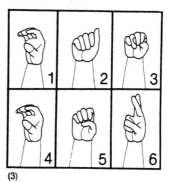
(3)

CARCINOMA

See CANCER

CARDIAC

Referring to the heart.

Cardiac muscle found in the heart is different from muscle found in other parts of the body.

(1) Sign HEART — the middle finger of the right "eight" hand taps the chest a few times.

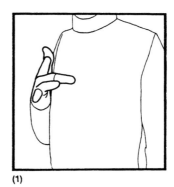
(1)

CARDIAC ARREST
See HEART ATTACK

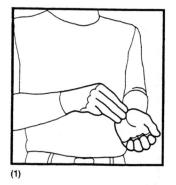
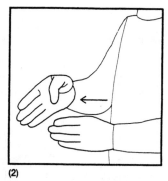
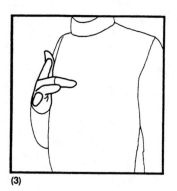

CARDIOLOGIST

A doctor who specializes in treating heart diseases.

A person who has had a heart attack or some sort of heart damage may be seen by a cardiologist.

(1) Sign DOCTOR — the right "M" hand touches the left inside wrist. (DM)
(2) Sign SPECIALIZE — the left "B" hand faces right at chest level. The right "B" hand faces left on top of the left hand. Move the right hand straight out on the left index finger. (SM)
(3) Sign HEART — the middle finger of the right "eight" hand taps the chest a few times.

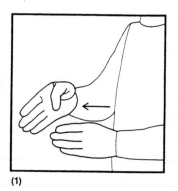
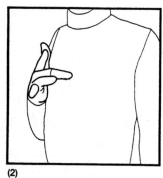

CARDIOLOGY

The branch of medicine that deals with the heart, how it works and its diseases.

Cardiosclerosis (hardening of the cardiac tissues and arteries) is one disease that is studied in cardiology.

(1) Sign SPECIALIZE — the left "B" hand faces right at chest level. The right "B" hand faces left on top of the left hand. Move the right hand straight out on the left index finger. (SM)
(2) Sign HEART — the middle finger of the right "eight" hand taps the chest a few times.

CARDIOPULMONARY RESUSCITATION

A combination of artificial respiration and artificial blood circulation. Cardiopulmonary resuscitation, also called CPR, will get oxygen to the lungs of a person who has stopped breathing and get the blood to circulate in a person whose heart has stopped beating.

A person needs special training to be able to do car-diopulmonary resuscitation.

(1) Fingerspell "C-P-R".

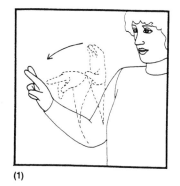
(1)

CARIES

In dentistry, the decay or rotting of a tooth caused by the wastes of bacteria.

The number of dental caries a person gets can be reduced by drinking water which has fluoride in it.

(1) The right index finger points to a tooth. (SM)
(2) Both "A" hands, with thumbs extended, face in at chest level. Move both hands down the sides in a wavy motion. (SM)

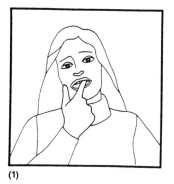
(1)

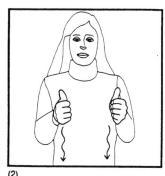
(2)

CAROTID ARTERIES

The major arteries supplying blood to the head.
See Figure 6

CARPAL BONES

The eight bones which make up the wrist. All eight bones together are called the carpus. *See Figure 26*

(1) Fingerspell "B-O-N-E".
(2) The right hand grabs the left wrist.

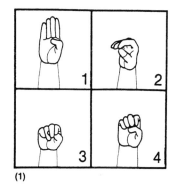
(1)

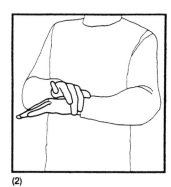
(2)

CARRIER

A healthy person who has a disease-causing germ but doesn't have the symptoms or signs of the disease.

A carrier of a disease can spread the disease to other people without knowing it.

CARTILAGE

A firm and strong tissue that can stand a lot of pulling and pressure. Cartilage provides support, covers the ends of bones in joints so they move smoothly against each other and connects bones to each other. Cartilage is also called gristle.

Cartilage is found in the trachea and bronchi, and helps keep these airways open.

CAST

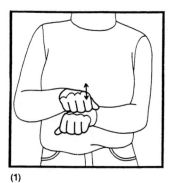
(1)

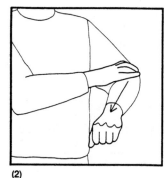
(2)

A stiff, hard wrapping made up of plaster of paris and gauze placed around a broken bone. The word "cast" is also used in dentistry for a mold taken of the teeth and gums, usually out of wax, plastic or plaster of paris.

A cast is placed on a bone to hold it still so it will heal faster and correctly.

(1) The left "A" hand faces down at chest level. The knuckles of the right "A" hand tap the back of the left hand a few times. (MM)
(2) The right "C" hand faces down and moves down the left arm as if imitating a cast on the arm. (SM)

* This should be signed at the location of the cast.

* These signs refer to a cast on broken bones.

CASTOR OIL

An oil made from the seeds of the castor oil plant, which acts as a laxative.

In the digestive tract, castor oil is made into an irritating substance that causes the entire tract to be emptied.

CASTRATE or CASTRATION

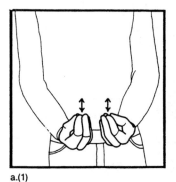
a.(1)

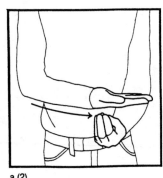
a.(2)

To remove the testicles or ovaries; removal of the sex glands.

Gelding is the castration of a male animal and spaying is the castration of a female animal.

a. (1) Sign TESTICLES — both "flat-O" hands are near each other at waist level with the fingers pointing up. Move both hands down.
(2) Sign REMOVE — the left "flat-O" hand is at waist level with the fingers pointing up. The left "flat" hand faces up and moves across the fingertips of the left hand.(SM)

(Continued on next page)

b. (1) Sign OVARIES — place both "F" hands on the lower abdomen, facing in.

(2) Both fists face out with the thumbs tucked inside, the hands face out at the sides of the lower abdomen area. Flick the thumbs out of both fists. (SM)

* For MALE: Sign a.(1) and (2). For FEMALE: Sign b.(1) and (2).

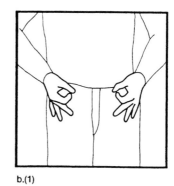

b.(1)

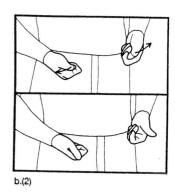

b.(2)

CASUALTY

A person who is injured or killed in an accident.

When a casualty dies, he is generally called a fatality.

(1) The right "A" hand with the thumb extended faces left at chest level and bounces slightly forward a few times. (MM)

(2) Sign HURT — both "one" hands point to each other and twist in opposite directions a few times. (MM)

* The facial expression should reflect pain.

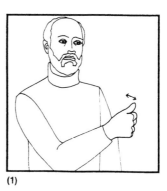

(1)

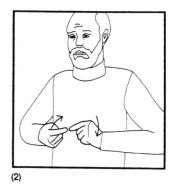

(2)

CATARACT

A clouding of the crystalline lens of the eye so that light rays can't pass through, causing poor vision and perhaps blindness. Cataracts may occur in older people as a part of aging and in younger people because of disease. Cataracts can be treated in most people by an operation in which the lens is removed and replaced by special glasses or contact lenses.

Cataracts are a common cause of poor vision and blindness in older people.

(1) Sign EYE — the right index finger points to the right eye. (SM)

(2) Sign WHITE — the right "five" hand touches the chest and moves out ending in a "flat-O" hand. (SM)

(3) The left "S" hand faces in at chest level. The right "cupped" hand moves over the left fist as if imitating covering something. (SM)

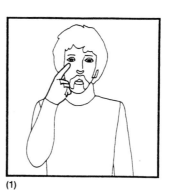

(1)

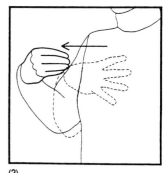

(2)

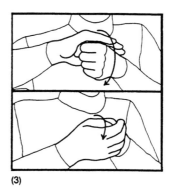

(3)

CATARRH

An old term for inflammation of a mucus membrane causing a lot of mucus to be produced.

When a person has a cold or an infection of the respiratory tract, there is often catarrh in the nose and throat.

CATHETER, CATHETERIZATION

A thin, hollow tube made of plastic, metal or rubber inserted into a passage or tube of the body to remove fluid from an area, keep a passage open or to remove a blockage.

The most common type of catheterization is that of the bladder, in which the catheter is passed through the urethra to the bladder to drain out urine.

CAT SCANNER

A highly developed machine used for taking X ray photographs of tissues and organs; also called "cat scan."

A cat scanner is widely used for finding tumors in the body.

(1) Fingerspell "X-R-A-Y".
(2) Sign MACHINE — both "five" hands mesh together at chest level and bounce up and down a few times. (MM)

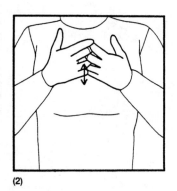

(1)

(2)

CAUDAL

Referring to a tail-like structure or the buttocks or end of an animal.

The caudal vertebrae in humans are less developed than those in most animals.

CAUSE

Something that produces or is responsible for an effect or result.

Viruses and bacteria are the causes of many diseases.

(1) Both "A" hands face up at chest level. Move both hands down and towards the left, ending in "five" hands at waist level. (SM)

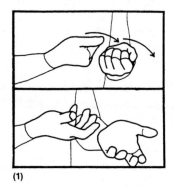

(1)

CAUSTIC

Referring to things that can burn, dissolve or eat something away.

Caustic substances, such as strong acids or alkalis, can destroy or damage living tissue.

(1) Sign CHEMICAL — both "C" hands face out at shoulder level. Move both hands in alternate circular movements towards the center, then down and out to the sides. (MM)

(2) The left "flat" hand faces down at chest level. The fingers of the right "claw" hand climb up the back of the left hand as if imitating the hand eating away at something. (MM)

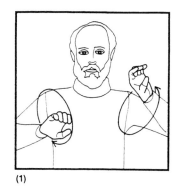

(1)

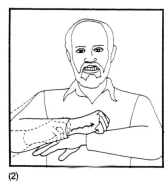

(2)

CAUTERIZE

To destroy body tissue by burning with heat, chemicals or electricity.

A part of the body may be cauterized to stop or prevent bleeding, to destroy tumors or to destroy excess tissue around a wound.

CAVITY

In medicine, a hollow space or area in the body.

Examples of a cavity are the chest cavity or the abdominal cavity.

(1) The left "C" hand faces right at chest level. The middle finger of the right "eight" hand is inside the left hand.

(2) Move the right hand up slightly into a "S" hand. (SM)

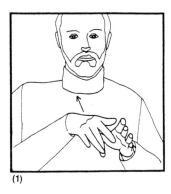

(1)

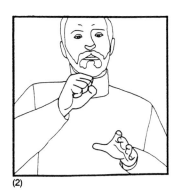

(2)

CAVITY, dental

In dentistry, a hole in the tooth.

A deep cavity may allow infection into the pulp of a tooth if not treated.

(1) Fingerspell "C-A-V-I-T-Y".

(Continued on next page)

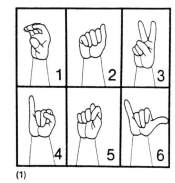

(1)

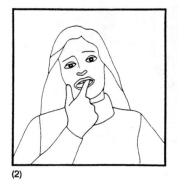
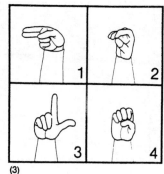

(2) The index finger of the right "one" hand points to a tooth. (SM)

(3) Fingerspell "H-O-L-E".

CECUM

A pouch at the start of the large intestine. The appendix is connected to the bottom of the cecum. *See Figure 9*

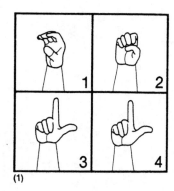

CELL

The tiny structure which makes up plants and animals and carries on all the processes that make life possible. There are cells of many different types, depending on what they do and where they are located. New cells are made when the old cells divide. The cell is made up of a nucleus, which directs the cell's activities, and is surrounded by the cytoplasm, which holds special structures and substances that carry out the chemical activities of the cell.

> *The nucleus and cytoplasm are surrounded by a cell membrane which holds everything together and allows materials into and out of the cell.*

(1) Fingerspell "C-E-L-L".

* This may need to be explained before fingerspelling "C-E-L-L".

CELLULOSE

A carbohydrate made up of glucose molecules connected in a certain way. Cellulose makes up the outer wall of plant cells and provides support. Although humans cannot digest cellulose, it provides bulk and helps with the movement of materials through the intestines.

> *Cellulose is also called plant fiber or roughage.*

CEMENTUM

A thin layer of a bone-like substance found on the root of a tooth which holds a tooth in its socket.

> *The cementum acts like a glue which attaches the dentin of the root of the tooth to the bone of the jaw.*

CENTER FOR DISEASE CONTROL

An organization in Atlanta, Georgia, which investigates, studies and tries to control diseases.

If there is a possible epidemic of a disease, the Center for Disease Control will investigate possible causes of the disease.

(1) Fingerspell "C-D-C".

* *An explanation should follow as fingerspelling is not clear enough.*

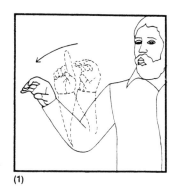

(1)

CENTIGRADE

A system of measurement which has one hundred divisions in it. Centigrade is most often used when referring to a thermometer which has one hundred degrees in it.

0° on the centigrade scale is the temperature at which water freezes and 100° is the temperature at which water boils.

(1) The left "one" hand points up and faces right at chest level. The right "one" hand points left and faces down. Move the right index finger up and down the left index finger a few times. (MM)
(2) The right "C" hand shakes slightly from left to right a few times. (MM)

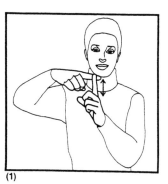

(1)

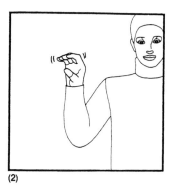

(2)

CENTRAL NERVOUS SYSTEM

That part of the nervous system which is made up of the brain and spinal cord. *See Figure 8*

(1) Fingerspell "C-N-S".

* *An explanation should follow as fingerspelling is not clear enough.*

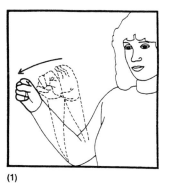

(1)

CENTRAL VISUAL ACUITY

In optometry, the higher sensitivity of the eye to see an object in the center of the field of vision.

Central visual acuity is caused because there are more rods and cones at the center of the retina than at the side.

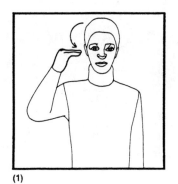
(1)

CEPHALIC
Referring to the head.

Cephalic version is the turning of a fetus' head during labor to make the delivery easier.

(1) The fingers of the right "cupped" hand touch the top part of the head and then move down slightly to touch the lower part. (SM)

CERATOMETER
An instrument used by an optometrist to measure the cornea of the eye.

The ceratometer measures the curvature of the cornea so contact lenses can be made to fit.

CEREBELLUM
The back part of the brain, underneath the cerebrum and in back of the pons and medulla oblongata. The major activities of the cerebellum are coordination of muscle movement and control of posture. *See Figure 17 or 18*

CEREBRAL HEMORRHAGE
Bleeding in the cerebrum of the brain from a broken blood vessel. Cerebral hemorrhage is often caused by high blood pressure. Symptoms of a cerebral hemorrhage are sudden unconsciousness, noisy breathing, a red face, and paralysis on one side of the body.

Cerebral hemorrhage is also called a stroke or apoplexy.

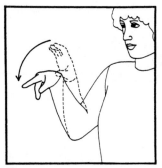
(1)

CEREBRAL PALSY
Abnormal development of the nervous system because of damage to the brain at birth. The symptoms appear in infancy and include poor muscle control and coordination.

Children with cerebral palsy can't be cured but are treated with training, therapy and surgery to correct physical problems.

(1) Fingerspell "C-P".

* *This should be explained or completely fingerspelled before using only "C-P".*

CEREBROSPINAL FLUID

The clear fluid found in the hollow center of the spinal cord, in the ventricles of the brain and around the brain and spinal cord. The fluid acts as a cushion, protecting the brain and spinal cord from injury.

The cerebrospinal fluid is examined when a person is suspected of having certain diseases, such as meningitis, a brain abscess, encephalitis or polio.

CEREBROVASCULAR ACCIDENT

The breaking or plugging of a blood vessel in the brain, causing a sudden, severe attack. During a cerebrovascular accident, one suddenly becomes unconscious, has a red face, noisy breathing and paralysis on one side of the body.

A cerebrovascular accident (CVA) is also called a stroke or apoplexy.

CEREBRUM

The largest part of the brain, divided into two halves and found in the upper part of the skull. The cerebrum takes in information from all parts of the body, helps control muscle movement and is the part of the brain responsible for memory, learning, reasoning, intelligence and emotions. *See Figure 18*

CERTIFY

To make sure, confirm as true or to guarantee.

All doctors must certify their training by hanging college diplomas and medical school certificates in their offices for all patients to see.

(1) The left "flat" hand faces up at waist level. The right "S" hand faces left and moves down to touch the left palm, then up. (SM)

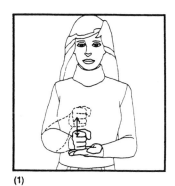
(1)

CERVICAL

Referring to the neck or a neck-like structure.

Damage to the cervical region can be very dangerous because there are many large blood vessels in the area, and the spinal cord and trachea also run through the area and may be injured.

(1) The fingers of the right "cupped" hand touch the top of the neck and then move down slightly to touch the bottom of the neck. (SM)

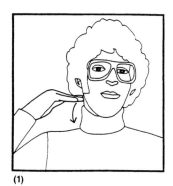
(1)

CERVICAL VERTEBRAE

The seven vertebrae in the neck region.
See Figure 26

CERVIX

The lower, narrow part of the uterus. Part of the cervix extends into the vagina. *See Figure 12*

CESAREAN SECTION

An operation in which a baby is delivered from the uterus by cutting through the abdomen into the uterus. This means of giving birth is used when giving birth naturally would endanger the mother or the baby.

A cesarean section is commonly done if the baby is too large to pass through the pelvic opening.

a. (1) Sign PREGNANT — The fingers of both "five" hands mesh together at stomach level. Move both hands out slightly forward as if showing the stomach growing. (SM)

(2) Sign OPERATE — the right "A" hand faces in at the left stomach area. Move the hand from left to right across the stomach as if the thumb is imitating cutting the stomach. (SM)

(3) The left "flat" hand faces in at chest level. The right "cupped" hand faces down behind the left hand. Move the right hand down and under the left hand then out forward. (SM)

b. (1) The right "C" hand shakes slightly from left to right a few times. (MM)

(2) Sign OPERATE — the right "A" hand faces in at the left stomach area. Move the hand from left to right across the stomach as if the thumb is imitating cutting the stomach. (SM)

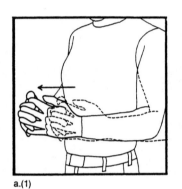
a.(1)

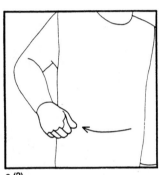
a.(2)

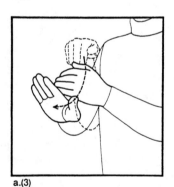
a.(3)

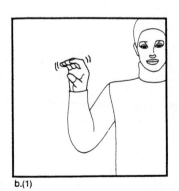
b.(1)

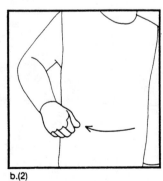
b.(2)

CESSATION OF BREATHING

The stopping of breathing.

A cessation of breathing can be caused by drowning, electrocution, shock, poisoning by drugs such as alcohol or narcotics or a blockage of an airway.

(1) Sign BREATHE — both "flat" hands move in and out from the body a few times as if imitating breathing. (MM)
*This movement should be short and repeated.

(2) Sign STOP — The left "flat" hand faces up at chest level. The right "flat" hand faces left and moves down to sharply hit the left palm. (SM)

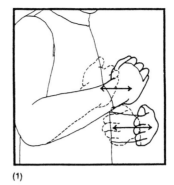 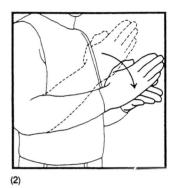

(1)   (2)

CHAFING

Inflammation of the skin caused by irritations from clothing or irritations on other parts of the skin.

Chafing usually occurs in the groin or anal regions, between fingers or toes, the wrists and the neck area.

(1) Sign SKIN — the index finger and thumb of the right fist grab the right cheek. (SM)
(2) The left "flat" hand faces up at chest level. The right "flat" hand faces down on top of the left palm and rubs back and forth on the left palm a few times. (MM)

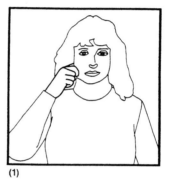 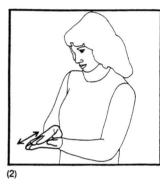

(1)   (2)

CHAIR CARRY

A way of carrying someone by putting them on a chair and then having two people pick up the chair.

The chair carry should not be used with people who may have a neck, back or leg injury.

CHANCRE

A hard ulcer or sore which is the first symptom of syphilis and may appear anywhere, especially on the mouth, penis, urethra, eyelid or vulva. The chancre will appear 2-4 weeks after the person was infected and will heal without leaving a scar.

When a person has a chancre, the disease is highly contagious and the chancre itself has many of the disease-causing germs in it.

CHANGE OF LIFE

See MENOPAUSE

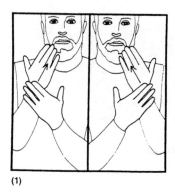
(1)

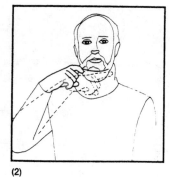
(2)

CHAPPED HANDS or LIPS

The cracking, roughening or reddening of the skin of the hands or lips because of wind, cold or moisture. Using strong detergents or soaps can also cause chapped hands.

Drying hands well after washing, using hand lotions and protecting the hands in cold weather and when doing rough work can help prevent chapped hands.

(1) Sign HANDS — the left "flat" hand brushes up the back of the right "flat" hand and then the right "flat" hand brushes up the back of the left "flat" hand. (SM)

(2) Sign DRY — the index finger of the right "one" hand points to the left and moves across the mouth from left to right .(SM)

* *If chapped lips are referred to, point to the lips then sign DRY.*

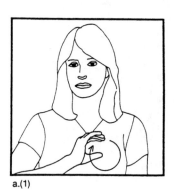
a.(1)

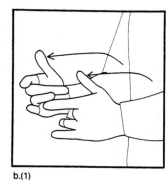
b.(1)

CHARACTER, CHARACTERISTIC

The usual or typical traits, features or qualities of someone or something.

When a doctor is diagnosing a disease he will examine the person for certain characteristics of the disease.

a. (1) The right "C" hand faces left at the left chest. The right hand makes one small circle from left down and around, then touches the left chest. (SM)

b. (1) Both middle fingers of both "eight" hands touch the chest, then move out forward. (SM)

* *The lips should make a "PA" movement.*

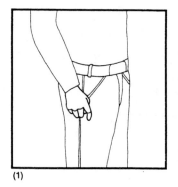
(1)

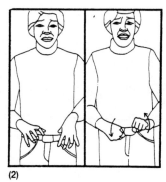
(2)

CHARLEY HORSE

Soreness, a spasm, pain or stiffness in a muscle caused by injury or overworking the muscle.

Charley horse is usually used to describe pain occurring in the muscle of the leg.

(1) The index finger of the right "one" hand points to the area of the charleyhorse.(SM)

(2) Sign CRAMP — both "claw" hands face in at the area of the cramp. At the same time, close the hands into "S" hands and twist both hands in opposite directions. (MM)

* *The facial expression should show pain.*

CHART

A record of a person's illness.

A chart contains personal information about a person and also medical information such as medications given, temperature, pulse, respiratory rate, blood pressure and doctor's and nurses' notes.

(1) The left "five" hand faces right at chest level. The fingertips of the right "five" hand brush down the left palm, then the backs of the fingertips brush out across the palm and fingers of the left hand. (SM)

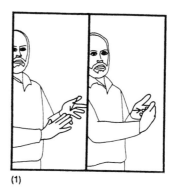

(1)

CHEEK

The side of the face or the buttocks.

Cheek is often used as a slang term for the buttocks.

a. (1) The index finger of the right "one" hand points to the right cheek. (SM)
* *Use this sign if referring to the side of the face.*
b. (1) The index finger of the right "one" hand points to the right buttock. (SM)
* *Use this sign if referring to the buttocks.*

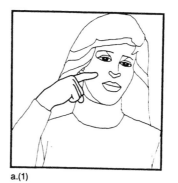

a.(1)

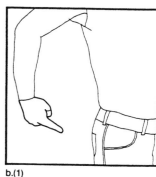

b.(1)

CHEMICAL

A combination of pure substances which are put together in certain amounts and in certain ways. Examples of chemicals are water, which is made up of the pure substances hydrogen and oxygen, and salt, which is made up of the pure substances sodium and chlorine.

There are many chemicals in the body but the one in the largest amount is water.

(1) Both "C" hands face out at shoulder level. Move both hands in alternate circular movements towards the center, then down and out to the sides. (MM)

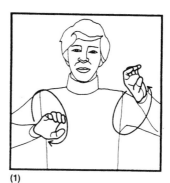

(1)

CHEMICAL BURN

An injury or burn on the skin caused by corrosive, caustic or irritating chemicals. Chemical burns include acid burns and alkali burns.

Chemical burns should be immediately flushed with lots of clean water to wash away the chemical.

(1) Sign CHEMICAL — both "C" hands face out at shoulder level. Move both hands in alternate circular movements towards the center, then down and out to the sides. (MM)

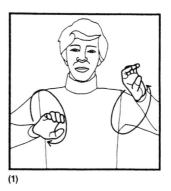

(1)

(Continued on next page)

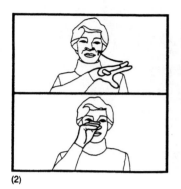

(2)

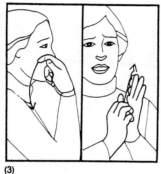

(3)

CHEMICAL BURN, *continued*

(2) The right "five" hand faces down at face level. Move the right hand in towards the nose, ending in a "flat-O" hand as if imitating inhaling something. (SM)

(3) The index finger of the right "one" hand moves from the nose down the right side of the throat. The right "claw" hand moves up the left "flat" hand. (SM)

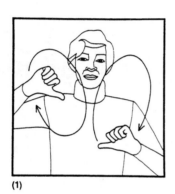

(1)

CHEMISTRY

The science that deals with the molecules and atoms that make up things.

A chemist is one who studies **chemistry.**

(1) Both "A" hands face out at shoulder level. Move both hands in alternate circular movements from center down and around to the sides. (MM)

CHEMOTHERAPY

The treatment of a disease using special chemicals which attempt not to affect the patient but to destroy the germs causing the disease.

Chemotherapy *is most often used when talking about treating cancer.*

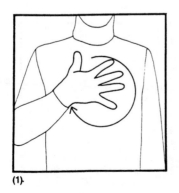

(1)

CHEST

Referring to the upper part of the trunk from the neck to the bottom of the ribs; the thorax. The major organs in the chest are the heart and lungs. *See Figure 1*

(1) The right "five" hand makes a circle on the chest area. (SM)

104

CHEW

The action of biting or grinding food with the teeth.
Masticate is another word for chew.
(1) The left "A" hand faces up at chest level. The right "A" hand faces down on the left hand. Move the right hand in small counterclockwise circles on the left palm a few times. (MM)

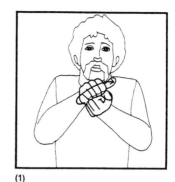

(1)

CHICKENPOX

A very contagious mild childhood disease caused by a virus; also called "varicella." The symptoms of chickenpox are a red rash, which should not be washed or scratched, itching and low fever.

Chickenpox does not leave scars if the small blisters are not scratched.

a. (1) Sign CHICKEN — the back of the right "G" hand touches the mouth. Open and close the index finger and thumb a few times as if imitating a beak. (MM)
(2) The fingertips of both "claw" hands move up the sides of the face. (MM)
b. (1) Sign CHICKEN — the back of the right "G" hand touches the mouth. Open and close the index finger and thumb a few times as if imitating a beak. (MM)
(2) Fingerspell "P-O-X".

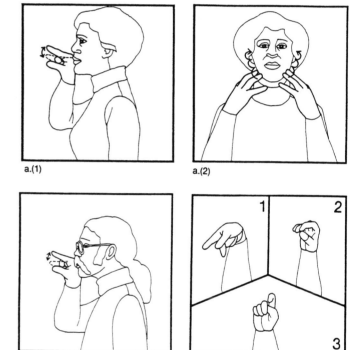

a.(1)   a.(2)

b.(1)   b.(2)

CHIGGER

A small insect which attaches to the skin of animals or man and eats the tissue in the area, causing a bump and itching.

People in chigger infested areas should wear clothes that are tight at the neck and arms, and tuck pant legs into shoes, to prevent getting these insects.

CHILBLAIN

A red, swollen area, which burns and itches, caused by cold damp weather. Chilblains result when the circulation to an area is slowed or stopped and are most common on the heels, back of the calves and ears.

Chilblains can be prevented by not wearing tight clothes, protecting yourself against cold and damp weather, and getting plenty of exercise.

CHILD

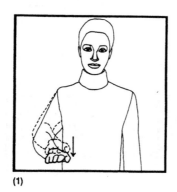
(1)

Any person between birth and puberty.

A child will usually be sick more often than an adult because it's immune system has not yet had a chance to be built up.

(1) The right "flat" hand faces down and pats the head of an imaginary child. (MM)

CHILDBIRTH

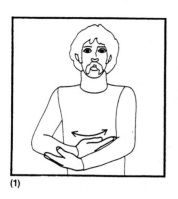
(1)

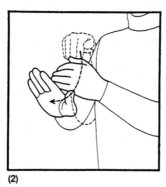
(2)

The process of giving birth, having a baby.

Childbirth is believed to be easier for women who attend classes which mentally and physically prepare them for it.

(1) Sign BABY — the right "flat" hand rests on the left forearm and the left "flat" hand rests under the right forearm. Rock both arms from left to right as if rocking a baby. (MM)

(2) Sign BORN — the left "flat" hand faces in at chest level. The right "cupped" hand faces down behind the left hand. Move the right hand down and under the left hand, then out forward. (SM)

CHILDHOOD DISEASES

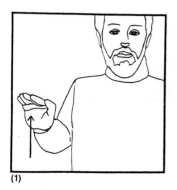
(1)

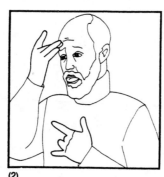
(2)

Diseases that are usually caught by young children.

Common childhood diseases are chickenpox and measles.

(1) Sign GROW UP — the right "cupped" hand faces down and moves up from waist level to chest level. (SM)

(2) Sign DISEASE — the middle finger of the right "eight" hand touches the forehead and the middle finger of the left "eight" hand touches the stomach. (SM)

* The facial expression should reflect sickness.

(Continued on next page)

(3) Sign MUMPS — both "claw" hands face in at the throat and open slightly. At the same time, the cheeks should puff out. (SM)

(4) Sign MEASLES — the fingertips of both "claw" hand move up the sides of the face, touching a few times. (MM)

(5) Sign WHAT — both "five" hands face up at chest level and shake slightly from left to right. (MM)

* *The facial expression should reflect questioning.*
* *To sign this idea sign GROW UP, DISEASE, MUMPS, MEASLES, WHAT. Any of the common childhood diseases could be used in this sequence, mumps and measles are only examples.*

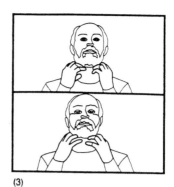
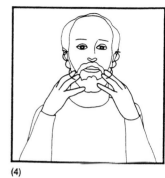

(3)

(4)

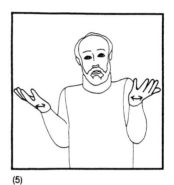

(5)

CHILL

A sudden shivering with a feeling of being cold.

Chills may be symptoms of a disease such as malaria or the first sign of an infection.

a. (1) Sign COLD — both "A" hands face each other at chest level. Shake both hands slightly as if imitating shivering. (MM)

b. (1) The left bent "V" hand faces up at chest level. The right bent "V" hand faces out on the left palm. Shake the right hand from side to side slightly as if imitating shivering. (MM)

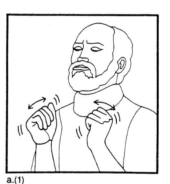
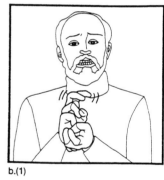

a.(1)

b.(1)

CHIN

The pointed, front part of the lower jaw.

See Figure 1

(1) The index finger of the right "one" hand circles the chin. (SM)

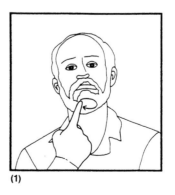

(1)

CHINESE RESTAURANT SYNDROME

An illness caused by eating food containing a lot of monosodium glutamate (MSG).

The symptoms of Chinese Restaurant Syndrome are burning sensations, headache, pressure in the face, sweating and chest pain.

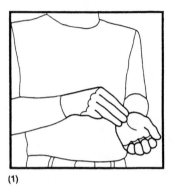
(1)

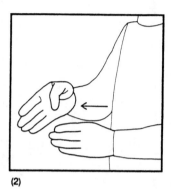
(2)

CHIROPODIST

A doctor who treats minor problems of the feet; also called a podiatrist.

Chiropodists usually treat corns, bunions and toenail problems.

(1) Sign DOCTOR — the right "M" hand touches the left inside wrist. (DM)

(2) Sign SPECIALIZE — the left "B" hand faces right at chest level. The right "B" hand faces left on top of the left hand. Move the right hand straight out on the left index finger. (SM)

(3) Fingerspell "F-O-O-T".

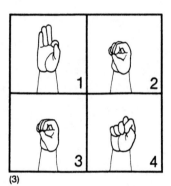
(3)

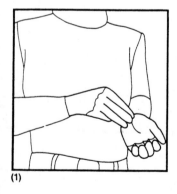
(1)

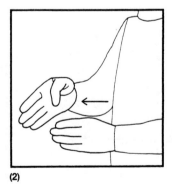
(2)

CHIROPRACTOR

A doctor who treats diseases and disorders by manipulating and adjusting the back and spinal column.

Chiropractors believe that some diseases are caused by spinal nerves being pinched or irritated.

(1) Sign DOCTOR — the right "M" hand touches the left inside wrist. (DM)

(2) Sign SPECIALIZE — the left "B" hand faces right at chest level. The right "B" hand faces left on top of the left hand. Move the right hand straight out on the left index finger. (SM)

(Continued on next page)

(3) Sign BACK — the right "flat" hand taps the back. (SM)
(4) The left "F" hand faces down at waist level. The right "F" hand faces down just above the left hand. Move the right hand straight up as if imitating the outline of the backbone. (SM)

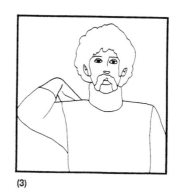

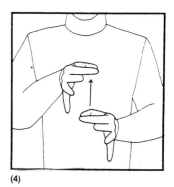

(3)   (4)

CHLORAL HYDRATE
A drug which acts as a sedative and causes a person to relax and sleep. Chloral hydrate is commonly called "knockout drops" when it is used in a drink.

Because chloral hydrate can cause addiction, it shouldn't be used for long periods of time and shouldn't be taken with alcohol because it can cause poisoning.

CHLORAMPHENICOL
An antibiotic originally made by a certain kind of bacteria and now made by man, which will stop an infection caused by some kinds of bacteria. Chloramphenicol is used to treat typhoid fever, meningitis, and some bacterial infections of the intestine.

Chloramphenicol should not be used for just any infection because it may cause upset stomach and problems with blood formation.

CHLORDIAZEPOXIDE
A mild tranquilizing drug which will make a person feel relaxed and less tense. Chlordiazepoxide is sold under the name of Librium® .

Chlordiazepoxide is used to treat anxiety and tension, nervousness before surgery and the symptoms of withdrawal from alcohol.

CHLORINATION
The treatment of water by adding chlorine (See CHLORINE).

Chlorination is used to disinfect water supplies and sewage of bacteria.

CHLORINE

A very irritating and poisonous gas used as a germ-icide and disinfectant. Chlorine, when added to sodium in the blood, helps metabolism, the osmotic pressure (water flow in the body), and regulation and stimulation of muscle action.

If chlorine is inhaled, it can cause damage to the mucus membranes in the respiratory passages.

CHLOROFORM

A clear liquid with a sweet taste and smell, widely used as a general anesthetic.

Chloroform is not used very much now because it can stop the heart, lower blood pressure and damage some organs.

CHLORPROMAZINE

A strong tranquilizing drug used to calm people with mental diseases, to control anxiety before surgery and in severe diseases, and to control nausea. It often takes seven to eight weeks for the drug to take affect. Chlorpromazine is often sold under the name of Thorazine® .

There are many possible side effects from taking chlorpromazine like severe depression, dizziness, tiredness, constipation, a change in urine color, dryness of the mouth and, if the drug is suddenly taken away, there can be withdrawal symptoms.

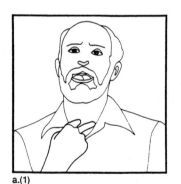

a.(1)

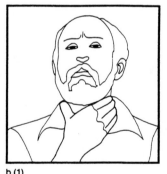

b.(1)

CHOKING

The slowing, stoppage or interference of breathing caused by blocking the trachea (windpipe).

When choking, a person will cough, the face will turn purple, the eyes will stick out and he may become unconscious.

a. (1) The fingertips of the right "V" hand touch the neck. (SM)

* *The facial expression should reflect choking.*

b. (1) The right hand grabs the throat. (SM)

* *The facial expression should reflect choking.*

CHOLERA

A severe disease caused by a bacteria which attacks the intestines. Symptoms of cholera are severe diarrhea, vomiting and cramps.

Cholera is more common in areas where sanitation is poor.

CHOLESTEROL

A substance which is found in animal tissue, egg yolks, some oils and fats and dairy products. Cholesterol is also made in the body by the liver, is found in the bile and helps to make some hormones.

Too much cholesterol in the blood can lead to arteriosclerosis.

CHOREA

A nervous disorder, especially of children, causing quick, jerky, uncontrollable movements.

Chorea, connected to a certain kind of bacterial infection, is becoming less common because of the increased use of antibiotics.

CHOROID

The brown-colored layer of the eye found inside the eyeball between the sclera and retina. The choroid carries the blood supply for the eye and prevents the passage of light. *See Figure 22*

CHROMOSOME

A very small structure found in the nucleus of a cell. Chromosomes are made up of genes which have the information needed to direct a person's development. Chromosomes determine the characteristics a person will have such as eye and hair color, the person's sex, whether a person will get a certain inherited disease such as sickle cell anemia or whether the person's hair will be straight or curly. (If the chromosomes of a baby are damaged by chemicals or radiation, birth defects will result.)

When an egg and sperm join to form a baby, each brings half the information or half the number of chromosomes needed to direct the baby's development, so a child is a blending of his ancestor's characteristics.

CHRONIC

A disease or injury that lasts a long time, that doesn't change much or that develops slowly.

Emphysema is a chronic disease.

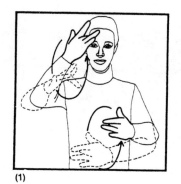
(1)

(1) The middle finger of the right "eight" hand touches the forehead. The middle finger of the left "eight" hand touches the stomach. Move both hands down and out forward in long, slow circles. (MM)

* The facial expression should show pain.

CICATRIX

Scar tissue that forms over a wound which has healed.

A cicatrix may be lighter than the skin around it because the cells that color the skin may be damaged.

CIGARETTE

Finely cut tobacco, rolled in paper for smoking and containing a poisonous alkaloid (nicotine). (See also SMOKE)

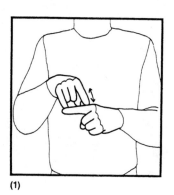
(1)

(1) The left "one" hand faces down at chest level. The index finger and little finger of the right hand tap the index finger a few times. (MM)

CILIA

Very small hair-like structures attached to some cells which can move in such a way that they can carry things in different directions.

Cilia on the cells lining the trachea and bronchi carry dust and mucus up toward the throat, away from the lungs, and cilia in the fallopian tubes carry the egg to the uterus.

CILIARY BODY

A structure inside the eyeball which connects the choroid to the edge of the iris. The ciliary body has a small muscle in it which can contract and cause a change in the shape of the lens of the eye, allowing us to focus on things at different distances. *See Figure 22*

112

CIRCULAR BANDAGE

A bandage which is wrapped around a body part.

A circular bandage may be used on a head injury.

(1) Sign BANDAGE — the left "B" hand faces in at chest level. The right "B" hand also faces in. Circle the right hand out and around the left hand a few times as if imitating wrapping a bandage. (MM)

* Fingerspell "C-I-R-C-U-L-A-R" before signing bandage. This can be signed at the area where the bandage is being applied.

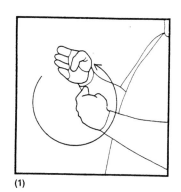

(1)

CIRCULATION

Referring to the movement of the blood through the heart, arteries, capillaries and veins of the body.

Circulation of the blood is caused by the beating of the heart.

(1) Sign BLOOD — The left "five" hand faces in at chest level. The right "five" hand faces in and touches the chin. Move the right hand up and down and at the same time, wiggle the fingers. (MM)

* This movement should be short, repeated and somewhat restrained.

(2) The left "five" hand faces in at chest level. The right "five" hand faces in and moves out and around the left hand, at the same time wiggle the fingers. (MM)

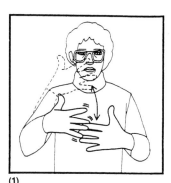

(1)

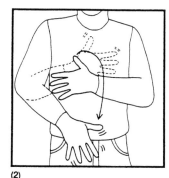

(2)

CIRCULATORY SYSTEM

The heart, blood vessels, veins, arteries, capillaries and the blood which moves through them. *See Figures 6 and 7*

CIRCUMCISION

The removal of the foreskin or fold of skin which covers the end of the penis, to prevent infection.

Men who had circumcision at birth have less chance of getting cancer of the penis than men who didn't.

(1) The middle finger of the right "P" hand taps the nose a few times.

(2) The left "A" hand with the thumb extended, faces in. The thumb of the right "A" hand circles around the left thumb. (SM)

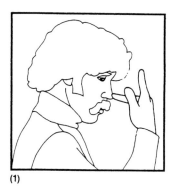

(1)

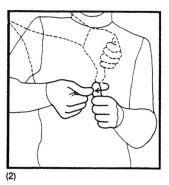

(2)

CIRRHOSIS

A chronic disease of the liver in which the cells are destroyed, scarring occurs and the organ becomes hard and doesn't work well.

Cirrhosis of the liver often occurs in people who drink too much alcohol or have a liver disease, such as hepatitis.

CITRIC ACID

A weak acid found in the juice of many fruits.

Citrus fruits such as oranges, grapefruits and lemons have a lot of citric acid, giving them a sour taste.

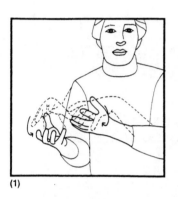
(1)

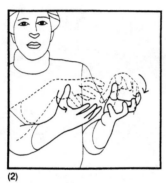
(2)

CLASSIFICATION

The orderly, systematic arrangement of information.

Classification of blood is done according to the kind of protein in the red blood cells.

(1) Both "claw" hands face down at the right chest level. Turn both hands so that they face up.
(2) Both "claw" hands then face down at the left chest level. Turn both hands so that they face up. (SM)

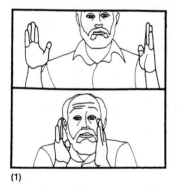
(1)

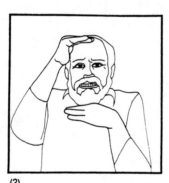
(2)

CLAUSTROPHOBIA

A great fear of being in small or tight places or places a person cannot get out of.

Sometimes people with claustrophobia can be treated by finding out why they are afraid and relaxing and practicing being in tight places.

(1) Both "flat" hands face each other at shoulder level and move towards each other. (SM)
(2) The right "flat" hand faces down at forehead level and the left "flat" hand faces down at chin level. Move both hands slightly towards each other. (SM)

* The facial expression should reflect that of being closed in.

(3) Sign FEAR — both "five" hands face in and move slightly towards the center. (SM)

* The facial expression should show fear.

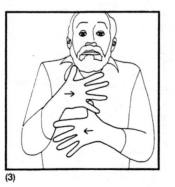
(3)

CLAVICLE

A rod-like bone that attaches the sternum (breastbone) to the scapula (shoulderblade). The clavicle is also called the collarbone. *See Figure 26*

(1) Fingerspell "B-O-N-E".

(2) The right index finger points to both sides of the clavicle.(DM)

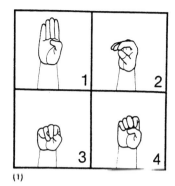

(1)

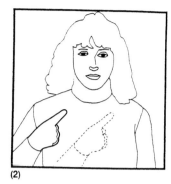

(2)

CLEAN

Not dirty or germ covered; to remove dirt from something.

Anything put on or near a wound should be clean to prevent an infection.

(1) The left "flat" hand faces up at chest level. The fingertips of the right "flat" hand move down the left palm. (SM)

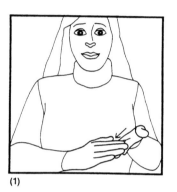

(1)

CLEANSE

To make something clean.

Liquids with germicides in them are used to cleanse some surgical instruments.

(1) Sign WASH — the left "flat" hand faces up at chest level. The fingertips of the right "flat" hand rub in a circular movement on the left palm. (MM)

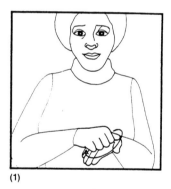

(1)

CLEAR

Easy to see; open or easy to look through.

Cataracts result when the normally clear lens of the eye becomes cloudy.

(1) Both "flat-O" hands face out at chest level. Move both hands out and up into "five" hands. (MM)

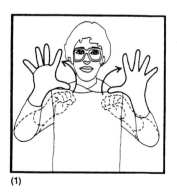

(1)

115

CLIMAX

See ORGASM

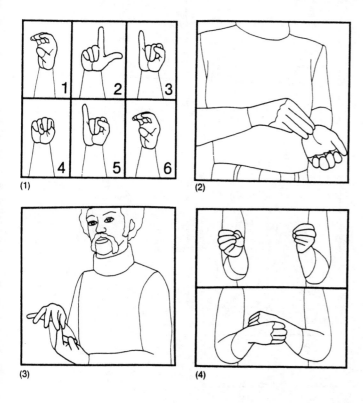

(1)
(2)
(3)
(4)

CLINIC

A place where patients are examined and treated but not hospitalized.

> A *clinic* may be run by several doctors specializing in one area, as an eye *clinic*.

(1) Fingerspell "C-L-I-N-I-C".
(2) Sign DOCTOR — the right "M" hand touches the left inside wrist. (DM)
(3) The left "one" hand points up at chest level. The thumb and index finger of the right "F" hand grab the left index finger. (SM)
(4) Sign OFFICE — both hands face each other at chest level. Move both hands towards the center with both hands facing in, the right hand slightly in front of the left hand. (SM)

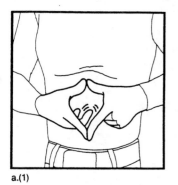

a.(1)

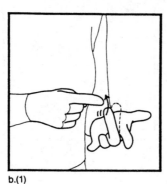

b.(1)

CLITORIS

A small structure which is part of a female's genitals. It is found at the upper end of the vulva and is very sensitive. (The clitoris of a woman is similar to the penis of a man in its origin and structure.) *See Figure 12*

a. (1) The fingertips of both "L" hands touch with the palms facing in at chest level. The middle finger of the right hand wiggles slightly a few times. (MM)
b. (1) The index finger of the right "one" hand flicks up the left middle finger a few times. (MM)

CLOSED FRACTURE

A broken bone with no wound going through to the skin.

> A *closed fracture* is also called a *simple fracture*.

CLOSED WOUND
See CONTUSION

CLOT

Blood which has become a somewhat solid mass, acting to stop the flow of liquid blood from or through a blood vessel.

A blood clot is also called a thrombus.

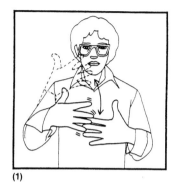

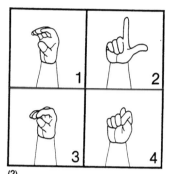

(1) Sign BLOOD — the left "five" hand is at chest level with the palm toward the body. The palm of the right "five" hand is toward the body with the middle fingertips touching the mouth. Move the right hand down the back of the left hand. Wiggle the fingers of the right hand as it moves. (MM)

* This movement should be short, repeated and somewhat restrained.

(2) Fingerspell "C-L-O-T".

CLOTTING

The process in which blood forms a somewhat solid mass; also called "coagulation."

Platelets found in the blood are important in starting the chain of chemical reactions involved in clotting.

COCAINE

A colorless or white narcotic drug taken from the leaves of the coca plant and used as a stimulant or an anesthetic to reduce surface pain.

Cocaine can cause addiction with symptoms of hallucinations, deep depression, nausea, dizziness, tingling in the hands and feet, rapid pulse, dilated pupils, and maybe convulsions and death.

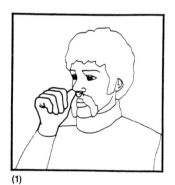

(1) The thumb of the right "A" hand touches both nostrils. (SM)

COAGULANT

Anything that causes blood to clot.

Vitamin K is a form of coagulant.

COAGULATION

Clotting of the blood.

Coagulation of blood is caused by formation of fibers in the blood which then act as a net and trap the red blood cells in them.

COBALAMINE

See VITAMIN B COMPLEX

COCCYX

The last, small bone at the bottom of the spinal column. The coccyx is usually made up of four vertebrae attached to each other. The coccyx is also called the tailbone. *See Figure 26*

COCHLEA

The spiral-shaped part of the inner ear which receives sound waves and turns them into nerve impulses which are sent to the brain. The cochlea is shaped like a snail's shell. *See Figure 20*

CODEINE

A drug made from opium that acts as an anesthetic or sedative.

Codeine is commonly used to help stop coughing.

COFFEE

A common drink which is made from the seeds of a certain kind of berry.

Coffee does not have calories in it but it does contain caffeine so it acts as a stimulant.

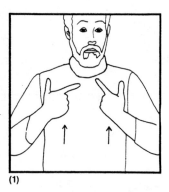
(1)

(1) The left "S" hand faces right at chest level. The right "S" hand faces left on top of the left fist. Move the right hand in counterclockwise circles on the left hand as if imitating a coffee grinder. (MM)

COHABITATION

Living together as husband and wife.

Cohabitation is usually used when referring to two people who are living together without being legally married.

(1) Sign LIVE — both "L" hands face in and move up the body from waist level to chest level. SM)

(Continued on next page)

118

(2) Both "A" hands are together at chest level. (SM)
(3) Both "S" hands are together facing down at chest level. Move both hands slightly forward into "H" hands pointing out. (DM)

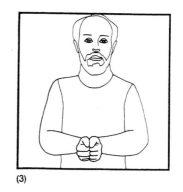

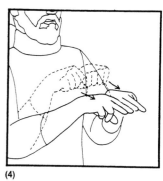

(3)

(4)

COHERENT

Understanding speech, writing or thoughts; being clear and making sense.

> *Accident victims should be watched closely because they may not be **coherent** and may do something dangerous.*

(1) Sign AWAKE — the fingers of both "G" hands are together at the sides of the eyes. Open the fingers of both hands and at the same time open both eyes wide. (MM)
(2) Fingerspell "O-K".

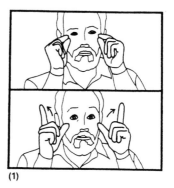

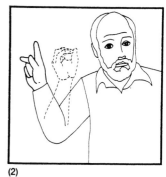

(1)

(2)

COITUS

Inserting the penis in the vagina with the release of sperm.

> *Coitus is also called sexual intercourse, mating or making love.*

(1) Sign INTERCOURSE — the left "V" hand faces up at chest level. The right "V" hand faces down at shoulder level. Move the right hand down to touch the left hand. (MM)

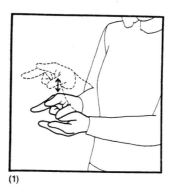

(1)

COITUS INTERRUPTUS

Removal of the penis from a woman's vagina before ejaculation in an effort to prevent pregnancy.

> *Pregnancy can still result if a couple uses **coitus inter-ruptus** as a means of birth control because some sperm may be present in the fluid that comes from the penis before ejaculation.*

(1) The index finger of the right "one" hand is inside the left "S" hand, both at chest level. Move the right hand out and to the right side with the finger pointing up. (SM)
(2) With the left hand still in place, the right "S" hand faces up and opens into a five hand. (SM)

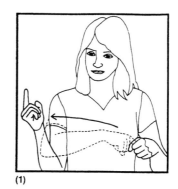

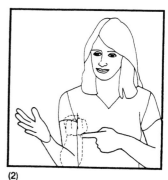

(1)

(2)

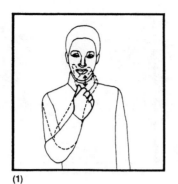
(1)

COLD

A contagious disease caused by many different kinds of viruses which attack the linings of the respiratory tract. Cold symptoms are a plugged up nose, runny eyes, coughing, a headache and perhaps a fever and body aches.

Antibiotics will not cure colds but decongestants, aspirin, rest and fluids will help the person feel better.

(1) The right "A" hand grabs down the nose a few times as if imitating wiping the nose. (MM)

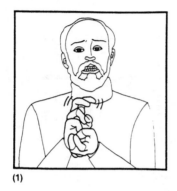
(1)

COLD EXPOSURE

Injury by being out in cold weather for too long. A person suffering from cold exposure will be shivering, numb, tired, will have a low temperature and may be confused.

The best way to avoid cold exposure is to dress in layers of wool and keep as dry as possible.

(1) The left "bent-V" hand faces up at chest level. The right "bent-V" hand faces out on the left palm. Pivot the right hand slightly from side to side a few times. (MM)
* The facial expression should reflect coldness.

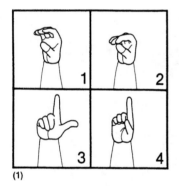
(1)

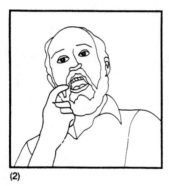
(2)

COLD SORE

An ulcer or sore which appears around the mouth when a person has a cold or fever or is under stress. Cold sores are caused by a virus (herpes) which lives in the nerves and attacks the skin when someone's resistance is low.

Cold sores are also called fever blisters.

(1) Fingerspell "C-O-L-D".
(2) The index finger of the right "one" hand points to the right corner of the mouth. (SM)
* This should be signed at the area of the cold sore.

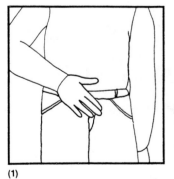
(1)

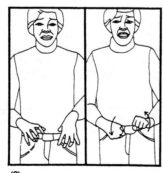
(2)

COLIC

Severe pain caused by a spasm or contraction of muscle in the digestive tract.

Colic is most often used for abdominal pain but it can refer to pain caused by a muscle contraction in any tube-like structure.

(1) The right "flat" hand touches the abdomen area. (SM)
(2) Sign CRAMP — both "claw" hands are at stomach level with the palms facing in. Move both hands into "S" hands, then twist in opposite directions as if wringing out a cloth. (SM)
* The facial expression should show pain or cramping.

120

COLITIS

Inflammation of the colon (large intestine), usually causing pain and diarrhea.

Colitis can be caused by parasites, nervousness or an infection.

COLLAPSE

The breakdown of a system; loss of consciousness or extreme weakness caused by exhaustion or some organ's failure.

Shock can cause someone to collapse because the tissue is not getting enough blood.

a. (1) Both "flat" hands face each other at chest level, with the fingertips touching and forming a peak. Drop both hands down as if the peak has collapsed. (SM)

b. (1) The index finger of the right "one" hand touches the forehead. (SM)

(2) Both "five" hands face each other at chest level, the fingers meshed together. Drop both hands down as if indicating something collapsing. (SM)

* These signs would be used when referring to mental collapse or breakdown.

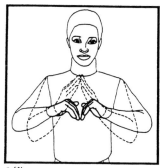

a.(1)

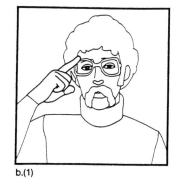

b.(1)

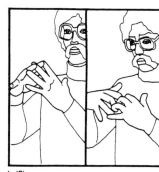

b.(2)

COLLARBONE

See CLAVICLE

COLLES' FRACTURE

A common fracture of the lower end of the radius bone just above the wrist.

A Colles' fracture is usually caused by a fall in which the wrist is bent back too far.

COLON

The part of the digestive tract which starts at the end of the small intestine and goes to the rectum. The major activity of the colon is removing fluid from digested food as it passes through. The colon is also called the large intestine. *See Figure 9*

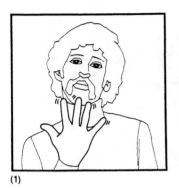
(1)

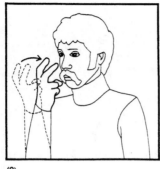
(2)

COLOR BLINDNESS

The inability to see red, blue or yellow correctly. Color blindness is caused by a problem in the cones in the retina of the eyes. It is more common in men than women.

The most common type of color blindness is the inability to recognize the difference between red and green.

(1) Sign COLOR — the right "five" hand faces in under the chin and the fingers wiggle. (SM)
(2) Sign BLIND — the right bent "V" hand faces in and moves towards the eyes slightly. (SM)

COMA

An abnormally deep state of unconsciousness caused by a disease, poisoning or injury.

A person in a coma cannot be awakened by anything and may stay in it for a long time.

COMBINE

To blend or mix.

One should never combine drugs without a doctor's approval because their effects may be made stronger when they are mixed.

(1) Sign MIX — both "claw" hands face each other at chest level, with the right hand on top. Move the right hand in clockwise circles above the left hand a few times. (MM)

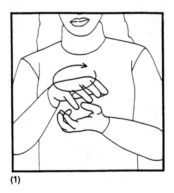
(1)

COMMINUTED FRACTURE

A fracture in which the bone has been broken or shattered into many small pieces.

A comminuted fracture usually occurs from a crushing blow and should be treated quickly so it doesn't become infected.

COMMUNICABLE

Referring to a disease which can be passed from one person to another; contagious.

Colds, chickenpox and influenza are examples of very communicable diseases.

(1) Sign SICK — the middle finger of the right "eight" hand touches the forehead. The middle finger of the left "eight" hand touches the stomach. Twist both hands slightly. (SM)
* *The facial expression should show pain.*

(2) Sign SPREAD — both "flat-O" hands face down at shoulder level. Move both hands out forward into "five" hands as if imitating something spreading. (SM)

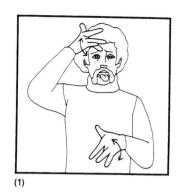

(1)

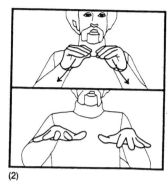

(2)

COMPLEX

Very complicated or difficult. The word "complex" is also used in psychiatry for a group of ideas or fears which a person may not be aware of but which cause him to behave in certain ways.

An example of a complex is an inferiority complex, wherein a person feels that he is not as good as other people, resulting in his being either very timid and shy or very aggressive and loud.

COMPLICATION

A disease or accident added to a person's already sick or injured condition making the first problem worse.

One reason for the vaccination of older people against the flu is that if they get it, they could easily get pneumonia as a complication.

(1) Sign PROBLEM — the right bent "V" hand faces in at shoulder level. The left bent "V" hand faces in at chest level. Alternately change the positions of both hands crossing in the center at the knuckles. (MM)

(2) Sign INCREASE — the left "H" hand faces down at chest level. The right "H" hand faces up at chest level. Turn the right hand over to face down with the fingers touching the top of the left fingers. (SM)

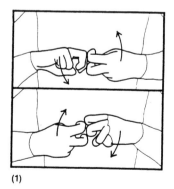

(1)

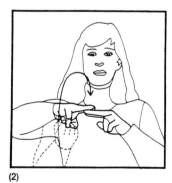

(2)

123

COMPOUND

A substance made up of more than one thing; a mixture.

Most medicines are not a single drug in pure form but are a compound of several substances.

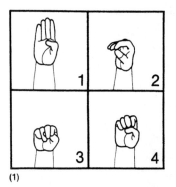
(1)

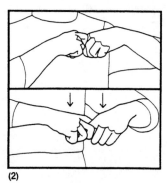
(2)

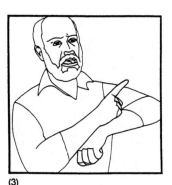
(3)

COMPOUND FRACTURE

The fracture of a bone where the broken end has penetrated the skin.

A compound fracture is more serious than one where the skin is not broken because infection may occur.

(1) Fingerspell "B-O-N-E".
(2) Both bent "V" hands face down at chest level with the fingers between each other. Drop both hands down slightly. (SM)
(3) The left arm is bent at the elbow, facing down. The right "one" hand points left on the left arm. Move the right hand to the left slightly as if imitating something puncturing or going through the skin. (SM)

* This should be signed at the area of the compound fracture.

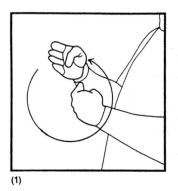
(1)

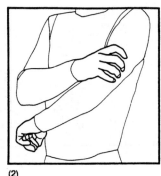
(2)

COMPRESS

A pad or cloth which is firmly pressed on an area to stop bleeding, cover a wound, or hold a medication in place.

A compress can be hot or cold, wet or dry, depending on what it is used for.

(1) Sign BANDAGE — the left "B" hand faces in at chest level. The right "B" hand also faces in. Circle the right hand out and around the left hand a few times as if imitating wrapping a bandage. (MM)

* This should be signed at the area where the bandage is being applied.

(2) The right "claw" hand grabs the left upper arm. (SM)

* This could be signed at the area.

COMPRESSION

Squeezing or pressing one or more structural parts together.

Compression of a lung may be caused by blood, fluid or air collecting around a lung.

(1) Both "claw" hands face in, the right on top of the left hand. Close both hands into "S" hands. (SM)
* Pat the area of the wound following the sign PRESSURE.

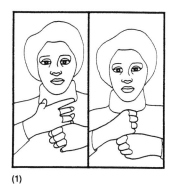
(1)

CONCEIVE

To become pregnant.

When a couple wants to have a baby but the woman is not able to conceive, the couple should see a doctor to find out what they can do.

(1) Sign PREGNANT — both "five" hands face each other at stomach level. Move both hands in so that the fingers mesh together. (SM)

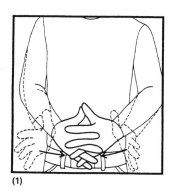
(1)

CONCENTRATION

To center one's thoughts or attention totally.

Concentration is also used to describe the amount of something in a liquid or the strength of a substance.

(1) Both "flat" hands face each other at the sides of the head. Move both hands straight forward. (SM)

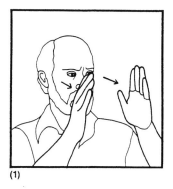
(1)

CONCEPTION

The union of sperm and ovum; fertilization.

Conception is the event that starts the formation of a baby.

(1) Sign PREGNANT — both "five" hands face each other at stomach level. Move both hands in so that the fingers mesh together. (SM)

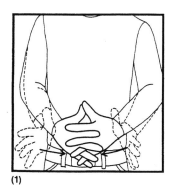
(1)

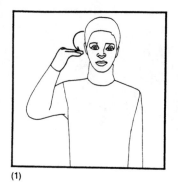
(1)

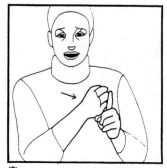
(2)

CONCUSSION

A common injury caused by a blow to the head or a fall in which the brain is rocked inside the skull. A person with a concussion may be dizzy, confused, or unconscious. The person may be unconscious for a few minutes or longer and often after waking may have headaches, a loss of memory or a change in personality.

In general, concussion *refers to an injury of any soft part but is most commonly used for injury to the brain.*

(1) Sign HEAD — the fingertips of the right "cupped" hand touch the top of the head and then move down slightly to touch the lower head. (SM)

(2) Sign HIT — the left "one" hand points up at chest level. The right "S" hand faces in and moves to sharply hit the left index finger. (SM)
* *The lips should mouth "POW".*

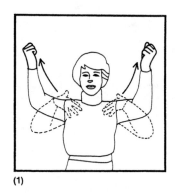
(1)

CONDITION

The state a person is in; how healthy one is.

The treatment given to an accident victim depends on his condition.

(1) Sign HEALTH — both "five" hands face in at chest level. Move both hands up and out into "S" hands. (SM)
* *It may be clearer to sign HOW before signing HEALTH.*

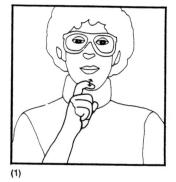
(1)

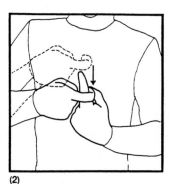
(2)

CONDOM

A thin rubber covering which is rolled over the penis before sexual intercourse as a method of birth control and as a way to prevent venereal disease; also called "rubbers" and prophylactics.

A condom *stops sperm from entering the vagina and fertilizing an egg.*

(1) Sign RUBBER — the knuckle of the right "X" hand brushes down the chin a few times. (MM)
(2) The left "one" hand points up at chest level with the palm facing in. The index finger of the right "X" hand hooks over the left index finger. (SM)

126

CONE

One of the special kinds of cells which make up the retina of the eye. Along with the rods, the cones detect light and color and send small electrical messages to the brain so we can see.
See Figure 22

CONFIDENTIAL

Not to be told to others or made public; secret.

> *Doctors keep the information a patient gives them confidential.*

(1) Sign SECRET — the right "A" hand faces left and the back of the thumb taps the lips. (MM)

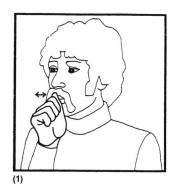

(1)

CONFINEMENT

Restriction to a certain place, usually away from others.

> *When someone has a very dangerous, communicable disease such as smallpox, they are usually placed in confinement.*

(1) The left "H" hand faces up at chest level. The right "H" hand also faces up on top of the left hand. Move both hands in a circular movement forward and around a few times. (MM)

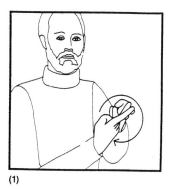

(1)

CONFUSION

A state of mental disorder where someone is mixed up, makes frequent mistakes or is unable to think clearly.

> *Confusion may result from an epileptic fit or a blow to the head.*

(1) Sign MIND — the index finger of the right "one" hand touches the forehead. (SM)
(2) Both "claw" hands are at head level and twist alternately from left to right a few times. (MM)
* The facial expression should reflect confusion.

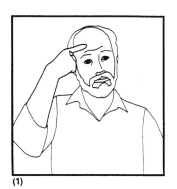 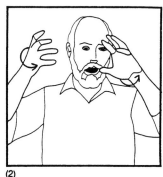

(1) (2)

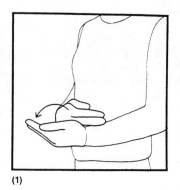

(1)

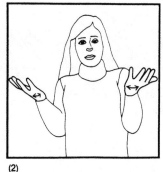

(2)

CONGENITAL

A mental or physical condition present at birth. Drug addiction and syphilis may be congenital.

Congenital defects occur during the development of a baby inside the mother.

(1) Sign BORN — the left "flat" hand faces up at stomach level. The right "flat" hand faces in. Move the right hand down to rest in the left palm. (SM)
(2) Sign WHAT — both "five" hands face up at chest level. Shake both hands from left to right a few times. (MM)

* The facial expression should reflect questioning. To sign this idea, sign BORN and WHAT, then DEAF, BLIND, HEMOPHILIA or any other possible congenital condition.

CONGESTION

Too much build-up of a fluid in an organ, tissue or cavity.

Congestion occurs in sinuses when there is too much mucus in these air spaces in the bones of the face.

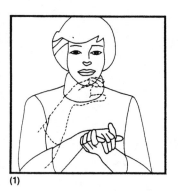

(1)

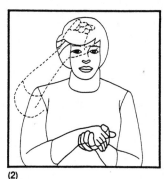

(2)

CONJUGAL

Referring to a husband and wife or a marriage.

Some prisons now allow conjugal visits for inmates who are married.

(1) Sign WIFE — the left "cupped" hand faces up at waist level. The back of the right "cupped" hand touches the chin and then moves down to touch the left hand. (SM)
(2) Sign HUSBAND — the left "cupped" hand faces up at waist level. The back of the right "cupped" hand touches the forehead, then moves down to touch the left hand. (SM)

CONJUNCTIVA

The thin membrane which lines the inside of the eyelids and covers the white part of the eyeball. *See Figure 22*

CONJUNCTIVITIS

Inflammation of the conjunctiva of the eye. Conjunctivitis can be caused by an infection, allergy or a foreign substance in the eye. The person's eye will be red, sore, itchy and sensitive to light.

When a person has conjunctivitis, the eye becomes red because of the tiny blood vessels in the conjunctiva dilating and letting more blood into the area.

(1) Sign RED — the index finger of the right "one" hand taps down the chin a few times. (MM)
(2) Sign EYE — the index finger of the right "one" hand points to the right eye. (SM)
(3) Sign INFECTION — the left "I"hand faces out at shoulder level and shakes slightly from left to right a few times. (MM)

* Mouth the word "infection" while signing.

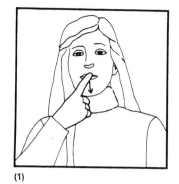 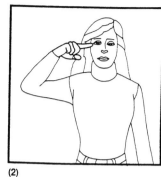
(1) (2)

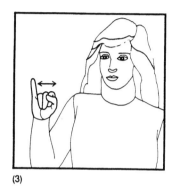
(3)

CONNECTIVE TISSUE

A type of tissue found throughout the body that supports and holds organs or structures together. Connective tissue is made up of cells and different types of fibers embedded in a material which varies from gel-like to solid.

Cartilage, tendons, ligaments and fat are all examples of connective tissue.

CONSCIOUS

Being awake and aware of what is happening.

Drugs which act as stimulants may make a person more active and more conscious of his surroundings.

(1) Sign AWAKE — the fingers of both "G" hands are together at the sides of the eyes. Open the fingers of both hands and at the same time open both eyes wide. (MM)
(2) Sign KNOWN — the fingertips of the right "flat" hand tap the right forehead a few times. (MM)

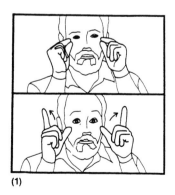 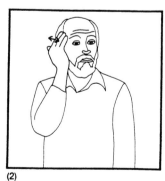
(1) (2)

129

CONSCIOUSNESS

Awareness, in which a person knows who and where he is. Consciousness is also used to describe the memories, emotions, personality and beliefs which make up a person's mind.

There are different levels of consciousness depending on how alert a person is.

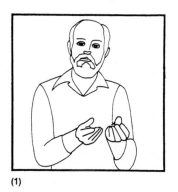

(1)

CONSISTENCY

The firmness or texture of a substance.

The consistency of feces depends on what is eaten, on the state of health and on the presence or absence of parasites.

(1) Both "flat-O" hands face up at chest level. Rub the thumb of both hands along the fingertips a few times. (MM)

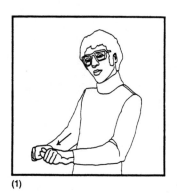

(1)

CONSTANT

A steady or unchanging state.

A constant pain may be the sign of disease or abnormality and the person should see a doctor.

(1) Sign CONTINUE — the thumb of the right "A" hand is on top of the thumb of the left "A" hand, both hands face down at chest level. Move both hands out forward. (SM)

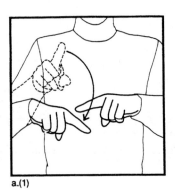

a.(1)

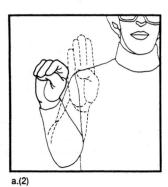

a.(2)

CONSTIPATION

Difficulty of bowel movements; unable to go to the bathroom. Constipation can be caused by improper diet, not enough physical activity, a blockage in the intestines or not drinking enough fluids. Fresh fruits and vegetables, liquids and whole grains can help relieve constipation.

In constipation, the feces are usually hard and dry.

a. (1) Sign CAN'T — the left "one" hand is palm down at waist level. The index finger of the right "one" hand strikes down on the left index finger. (SM)
(2) Fingerspell "B-M".

(Continued on next page)

b. (1) Sign CAN'T — the left "one" hand is palm down at waist level. The index finger of the right "one" hand strikes down on the left index finger. (SM)

(2) Sign FECES — the left "A" hand faces right at chest level. The thumb of the right "A" hand is inside the left fist. Move the right hand down. (SM)

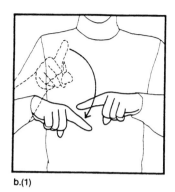 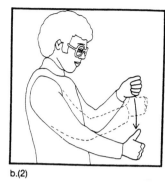

b.(1)   b.(2)

CONSTRICT

To shrink, get smaller or reduce in size.

*Arteries have the ability to **constrict** to control blood flow in the body.*

(1) The right "claw" hand faces in on top of the left "claw" hand, also facing in, both are at chest level. Close both hands into "S" hands. (SM)

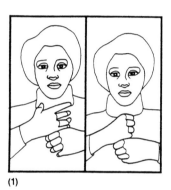

(1)

CONSTRICTION

The narrowing of an opening or vessel.

Constriction of the pupil of the eye will occur to reduce the amount of light reaching the retina.

CONSULT

To get advice or information.

*If in doubt about health care, a drug, condition, treatment or disease it is best to **consult** with a doctor.*

(1) Sign ADVISE — the left "flat" hand faces down at chest level. The fingertips of the right "flat-O" hand touch the back of the left hand and move forward. (SM)

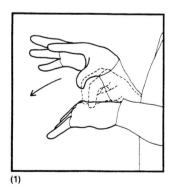

(1)

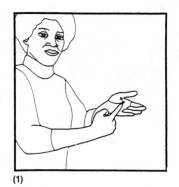

(1)

CONSULTATION

Two or more people getting together to discuss something or exchange ideas.

When a doctor has a patient whose disease or treatment he is unsure about, he may call another doctor for consultation.

(1) Sign DISCUSS — the left "flat" hand faces up at chest level. The index finger of the right "one" hand brushes up the left palm a few times. (MM)

CONSUMPTION

See TUBERCULOSIS

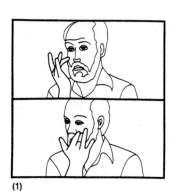

(1)

CONTACT LENS

A small, thin, round bowl-shaped piece of plastic which is worn on the cornea of the eye to correct vision defects.

A contact lens can be hard, made out of a stiff plastic, or soft, made out of plastic which is very flexible.

(1) The middle finger of the right hand taps under the right and then the left eyes. (SM)

CONTACT POISONING

Poisoning resulting from the skin touching different chemicals, plants or animals.

Harsh chemicals, poison oak or ivy, some pesticides and some jellyfish can cause contact poisoning.

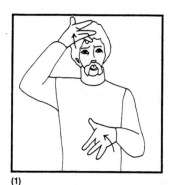

(1)

CONTAGIOUS

Referring to a disease which is easily passed from one person to another; communicable.

An epidemic can result when there is a very contagious virus going around.

(1) Sign SICK — the middle finger of the right "eight" hand touches the forehead. The middle finger of the left "eight" hand touches the stomach. Twist both hands slightly. (SM)

* The facial expression should show pain.

(Continued on next page)

(2) Sign EASY — the left "cupped" hand faces up at chest level. The fingertips of the right "cupped" hand brush up the back of the fingers of the left hand twice. (DM)

(3) Sign SPREAD — both "flat-O" hands face down at shoulder level. Move both hands out forward into "five" hands as if imitating something spreading. (SM)

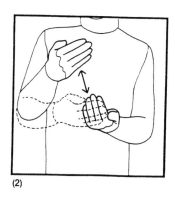
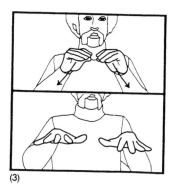

(2)

(3)

CONTAMINATE

To make something dirty, harmful or unusable through contact with something that is unclean or dangerous.

It is not safe to drink out of lakes or streams in crowded areas because the water may be contaminated with feces.

(1) Sign BECOME — the right "flat" hand is on top of the left "flat" hand. Twist both hands so that the left hand ends up on top of the right hand. (SM)

(2) Sign DIRTY — the right "five" hand faces down under the chin and the fingers wiggle. (SM)

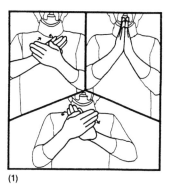
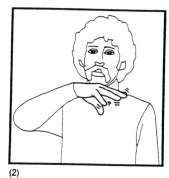

(1)

(2)

CONTAMINATION

The state of being dirty or unclean.

Contamination is usually used when disease-causing germs get on a sterile object.

CONTRACEPTION

The use of certain methods or procedures by a man and woman to prevent pregnancy. Contraception is another word for birth control.

Some forms of contraception are the use of condoms, the contraceptive pill, the diaphragm and sterilization.

(1) Sign PREGNANT — both "five" hands face in at stomach level with the fingers meshed together. Move both hands out slightly as if imitating the stomach growing. (SM)

(2) Sign PREVENT — both "flat" hands cross at chest level and move slightly forward. (SM)

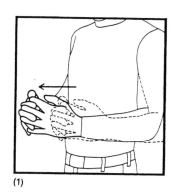
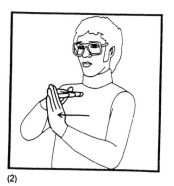

(1)

(2)

CONTRACEPTIVE

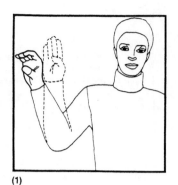

(1)

A device or drug used to prevent pregnancy.

A contraceptive will keep a man's sperm from uniting with and fertilizing a woman's ovum.

(1) Fingerspell "B-C".

CONTRACEPTIVE FOAM

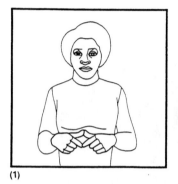

(1)

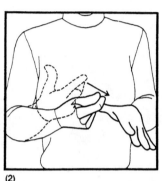

(2)

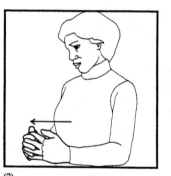

(3)

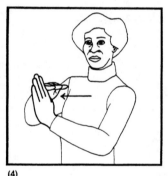

(4)

A substance injected into the vagina before intercourse, used as a form of birth control; spermicide. Contraceptive foam kills the sperm and is thought to be 85% effective in preventing pregnancy.

When buying a contraceptive foam, a woman should read the label to be sure it doesn't contain mercury or boric acid, which can be harmful.

(1) Sign VAGINA — the fingers of both "L" hands touch at waist level. (SM)

(2) Sign INJECT — the left "flat" hand faces down at chest level. The right "L" hand faces in at chest level. The thumb of the right hand closes as if injecting something in the thumb of the left hand. (SM)

(3) Sign PREGNANT — the fingers of both "five" hands are together at the stomach with the fingers meshed together. Move both hands out foward as if imitating the stomach growing. (SM)

(4) Sign PREVENT — both "flat" hands cross at chest level and move forward. (SM)

CONTRACEPTIVE PILL

See BIRTH CONTROL PILL

CONTRACTION

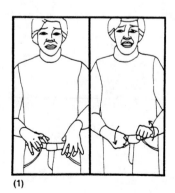

(1)

A shortening or tightening of something, as a muscle.

Contraction is often used for the muscle-tightening in a woman's uterus and abdomen during labor which moves the baby out of the uterus.

(1) Sign CRAMP — both "claw" hands are at stomach level with the palms facing in. Move both hands into "S" hands, then twist in opposite directions as if wringing out a cloth. (SM)

* The facial expression should show pain or cramping.

134

CONTRAINDICATION

A sign, condition or warning which states that the treatment or drug being used should be stopped during special times because it could be harmful. Some examples of contraindication are taking drugs during pregnancy and allergies to taking a specific drug. Other examples are for people with high blood pressure who must limit the amount of salt they eat and for people with heart or blood vessel diseases who must limit the amount of cholesterol they eat.

Most drugs, including those sold without a prescription, have an information sheet containing a list of contraindications which should be read carefully and understood.

CONTRAST MEDIA

A substance which is injected or eaten in order to outline a body space or organ, making them visible on an x-ray.

An example of a contrast media is barium sulfate, which is eaten or given as an enema to outline a region in the digestive tract.

CONTROL

To regulate, manage or direct someone or something.

The nervous system allows someone to control his body.

(1) Both "modified-A" hands face each other at chest level. Move both hands alternately forward and back a few times. (MM)

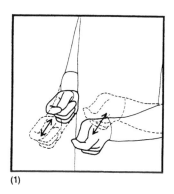

(1)

CONTUSION

An injury in which the skin is not broken; a bruise. A contusion may result in pain, swelling and a change in skin color to purple in the area.

Applying a cold pack to a contusion may reduce swelling and prevent pain.

(1) The left "S" hand faces down at waist level. The index finger of the right "one" hand makes a small bump on the left hand. (SM)

* This could be signed at the area of the contusion.

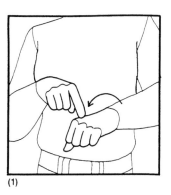

(1)

(Continued on next page)

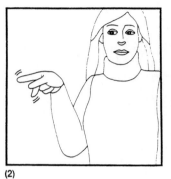

(2)

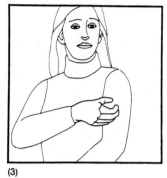

(3)

CONTUSION, *continued*

(2) Sign PURPLE — the right "P" hand faces out at shoulder level and pivots from left to right slightly a few times. (MM)

(3) The right "C" hand faces in on the left upper arm. (SM)

* *This should be signed at the area of the contusion.*

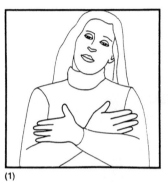

(1)

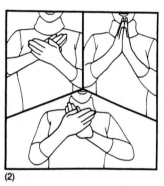

(2)

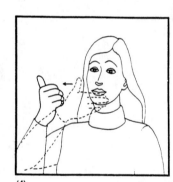

(3)

(4)

CONVALESCENCE

The time after an injury, operation or disease in which a person recovers, heals or becomes well.

The length of someone's convalescence will usually depend on the overall health before the injury and how bad the injury was.

(1) Sign RELAX — both "flat" hands cross on the chest.(SM)

* *The facial expression should reflect relaxation.*

(2) Sign BECOME — the right "flat" hand faces out on the left "flat" hand which faces in; the hands are crossed. Twist both hands so that the left hand ends facing out and the right hand ends facing in. (SM)

(3) Sign HEALTH — both "five" hands face in at chest level. Move both hands up into "S" hands. (SM)

(4) Sign BETTER — the fingertips of the right "flat" hand touch the chin, the thumb is extended. Move the hand to the right ending in an "A" hand with the thumb extended. Repeat this three times. (MM)

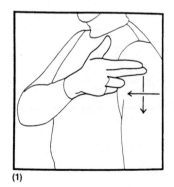

(1)

CONVALESCENT CENTER

A facility or hospital where older people or people recovering from an illness or injury can get special care.

A person who needs special care for long periods of time may stay in a convalescent center.

(1) Sign HOSPIAL — the fingers of the right "H" hand move from left to right on the left upper arm and then down, making a cross. (SM)

(Continued on next page)

(2) The right "flat" hand is on top of the left "flat" hand. Twist both hands so that the left hand ends up on top of the right hand. (SM)
(3) Sign HEALTH — both "five" hands face in at chest level. Move both hands up into "S" hands. (SM)

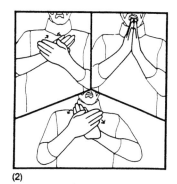
(2)

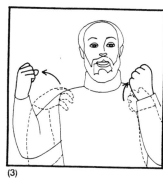
(3)

CONVULSION

A severe, uncontrollable contraction or tightening of the muscles in the body caused by abnormal brain activity. Some causes of convulsions are epilepsy, infections or damage in the brain, poisoning, and high fevers.

> When someone is having a *convulsion,* it is important to see that he doesn't injure himself by hitting his head against something.

(1) Both "claw" hands face in at chest level, the right above the left. Shake both hands slightly. (MM)
* The facial expression should reflect having a convulsion.

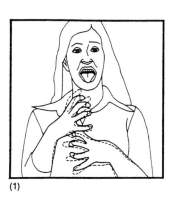
(1)

COOL

Slightly cold; not warm or hot.

> When a person feels faint, he will be *cool,* weak and nauseated.

(1) Both "flat" hands face in at shoulder level. Move both hands in and out a few times as if fanning yourself to keep cool. (MM)

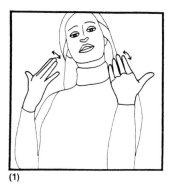
(1)

COORDINATION

The ability of muscles to work together and bring about certain smooth, controlled movements.

> When someone is under the influence of drugs, such as alcohol or barbiturates, is very cold or has problems with the inner ear, bodily *coordination* will be poor.

(1) The thumbs and index fingers of both "F" hands lock. Move both hands in a clockwise circular movement. (SM)
(2) Sign BODY — both "flat" hands face in. The fingertips of both hands touch the chest and then the stomach. (SM)

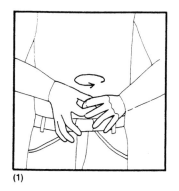
(1)

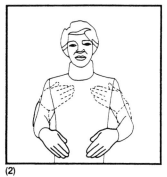
(2)

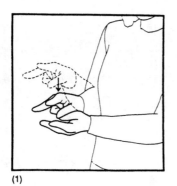
(1)

COPULATION

The act of placing the penis in the vagina and releasing sperm. Copulation may also be called coitus, mating, sexual intercourse and making love.

Copulation is usually used to mean sexual intercourse between animals more than between people.

(1) Sign INTERCOURSE — the left "V" hand faces up at chest level. The right "V" hand faces down and moves down to touch the left hand. (SM)

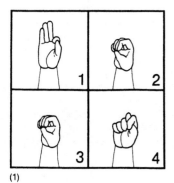
(1)

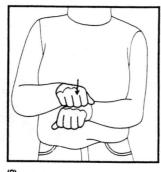
(2)

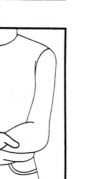
(3)

CORN

A painful hardening and thickening of the skin on a part of the foot.

Corns can be treated by wearing comfortable shoes, using medicine to soften them and wearing pads on them to protect them.

(1) Fingerspell "F-O-O-T".

(2) Sign HARD — the left "A" hand faces down at chest level. The right "A" hand faces down and moves down to tap the top of the left hand. (SM)

(3) The right "F" hand faces in at the area of the corn.

CORNEA

The clear, round front part of the eye which covers the pupil and iris. The cornea is more curved than the rest of the eye, so it sticks out a little. *See Figure 22*

CORNEAL LENS

See CONTACT LENS

CORONARY

Referring to something which goes around or encircles something; also used when referring to the heart.

Coronary is a shortened name for coronary thrombosis or a heart attack.

138

CORONARY THROMBOSIS

The blockage of one of the arteries, which take fresh blood to the heart, by a blood clot. A coronary thrombosis will cause damage to a part of the heart. The symptoms are a squeezing pain in the chest which may spread to the neck and left arm, nausea, sweating and a shortness of breath.

Heart attack is another name for **coronary thrombosis.**

(1) Sign HEART — the middle finger of the right "eight" hand taps the chest a few times.
(2) The left "flat" hand faces right. The right "A" hand moves down to sharply hit the palm of the left hand. (SM)

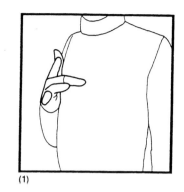
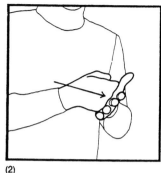

CORONER

An official who checks into the death of people who die violently or whose cause of death is unknown.

A **coroner** *may or may not be a doctor, depending on the laws of the state.*

CORPSE

A dead body.

Corpse is another word for cadaver.

(1) Sign DEAD — the left "flat" hand faces up at chest level. The right "flat" hand faces down at chest level. Turn both hands to the right so that the left hand ends facing down and the right hand ends facing up. (SM)
(2) Sign BODY — the fingertips of both "flat" hands touch first the chest and then the stomach. (SM)

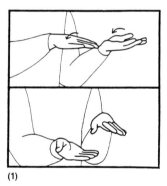
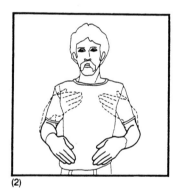

CORPULENT

The state of being overweight or fat; obese.

Corpulent people are more likely to get heart diseases, high blood pressure and diabetes.

(1) Sign FAT — both "five" hands face in and move out forward from the body. At the same time, the cheeks puff out. (SM)

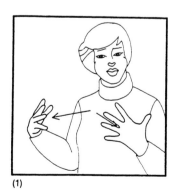

139

CORPUSCLE

A small rounded structure; a blood cell.
Erythrocytes are red blood corpuscles and leukocytes are white blood corpuscles.

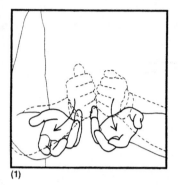
(1)
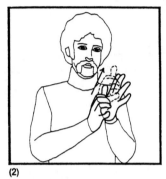
(2)

CORRODE

To slowly wear or eat away, especially by chemicals.
In some forms of arthritis the joint is corroded.
(1) Both "A" hands face each other at chest level. Drop both hands down forward into "five" hands, facing up. (SM)
(2) The left "five" hand faces right at chest level. The fingertips of the right "claw" hand move up the palm of the left hand a few times. (MM)

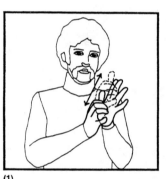
(1)
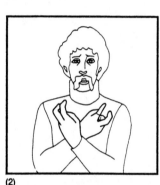
(2)

CORROSIVE POISONING

Poisoning caused by strong chemicals such as strong acids or alkalis, strong antiseptics, chemical drain openers, toilet bowl cleaners, bleaches and strong detergents. Corrosive poisoning causes shock and deep chemical burns of the mouth, throat and digestive tract which may cause swelling and choking or starvation.

When someone has swallowed a corrosive poison, the poison should be diluted with milk or water and the person should be taken to a physician or hospital immediately.

(1) The left "five" hand faces right at chest level. The fingertips of the right "claw" hand move up and down the palm of the left hand three times. (MM)
(2) Sign POISON — both bent "V" hands cross at the wrists and face in on the body. (SM)

CORTISOL

See CORTISONE

CORTISONE

A hormone made by the adrenal glands which controls the body's use of fats, carbohydrates, proteins and some minerals.
Cortisone is given to ease joint inflammation and to counteract some severe allergies.

COSMETIC SURGERY

See PLASTIC SURGERY

140

COUGH

A sudden, quick forcing of air through the throat from the lungs.

People cough to clear their throat or respiratory tract of mucus or other irritating substances.

(1) The fingertips of the right "claw" hand touch the chest. While keeping the fingertips in place, drop the hand slightly. (MM)
* *Imitate a cough while signing.*

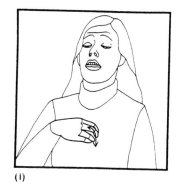
(1)

CRAB LOUSE

A small, wingless insect which attaches to hairs in the pubic region, on the lower abdomen or in the armpit; (See PEDICULOSIS).

A person gets crab louse by having sexual intercourse with an infested person or by using their clothes, towels or bed.

(1) The thumb of the right "three" hand touches the nose, the palm faces left. Bend and straighten the fingers of the right hand a few times and at the same time, the left "claw" hand scratches the pubic area. (MM)
* *The left hand should scratch at the area of the infestation, in this example, the pubic area.*

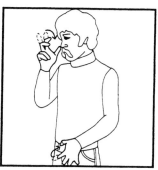
(1)

CRAMP

A sudden, steady tightening of a muscle, which is usually painful.

A cramp can be caused by over-exercising a muscle, stretching a muscle, poisoning, menstruation or working in hot weather.

(1) Both "claw" hands are at stomach level with the palms facing in. Move both hands into "S" hands, then twist in opposite directions as if wringing out a cloth. (SM)
* *This could be signed at the area of the cramp and the facial expression should reflect pain or cramping.*

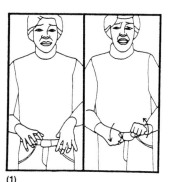
(1)

CRANIUM

The part of the skull around the brain. The cranium acts as a protective case for the brain.
See Figure 26

(1) The fingertips of the right "cupped" hand touch the top of the head and then move down to touch the bottom of the head. (SM)

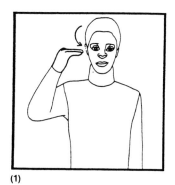
(1)

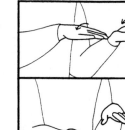
(1)

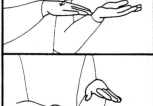
(2)

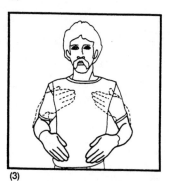
(3)

CRAVAT BANDAGE
A triangular bandage which can be folded into a band.

A cravat bandage can be used for an arm sling.

CREMATION
The burning of a dead person's body.

Some people prefer cremation to burial.

(1) Sign BURN — both "five" hands face in with the fingers pointing up at chest level. Wiggle the fingers of both hands. (MM)
(2) Sign DEAD — the left "flat" hand faces up at chest level. The right "flat" hand faces down at chest level. Turn both hands to the right so that the left hand ends facing down and the right hand ends facing up. (SM)
(3) Sign BODY — the fingertips of both "flat" hands touch the chest and then the stomach. (SM)

CREPITUS
Grating or crackling heard or felt when the ends of broken bones rub together.

Crepitus may also be the noise of gas being discharged from the intestines.

CRIB DEATH
See SUDDEN INFANT DEATH SYNDROME

CRIPPLED
The state of being injured or hurt as a result of a disease or accident so a part of the body doesn't work normally.

It is important to be immunized against polio because polio is a disease which attacks the nervous system, leaving a person crippled.

(1) Both "one" hands face in, pointing down at chest level. Alternately move both hands up and down a few times with the right hand moving slightly inward. (MM)

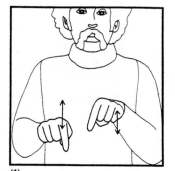
(1)

CRISIS

A sudden change in a disease or condition either for the better or worse; also the sharp drop in a high temperature or the pain involved with a disease or illness.

An abdominal crisis is a condition where there is severe pain in the abdomen.

CRITICAL

In medicine, a term used to describe a condition in which a person's life is in danger because of a disease or injury.

Patients in a hospital in critical condition are watched closely and are often placed in intensive care units.

(1) Sign DANGEROUS — the left "flat" hand faces in at chest level. The back of the thumb of the right "A" hand brushes up, out and around in a circular movement against the back of the left hand. (SM)

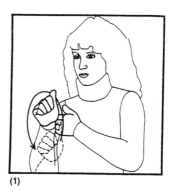
(1)

CROOKED

Curved, bent or not straight.

People wear different kinds of braces to straighten crooked parts of their bodies such as teeth or backs.

CROUP

A disease caused by an infection, allergy or inflammation in which the airways become narrower. A person with croup will have difficult, noisy breathing and a harsh cough.

Croup is treated by applying hot, wet packs to the throat and breathing steam.

CROWN

In dentistry, it is the part of the tooth which can be seen or an artificial cap made of porcelain, gold or silver fitted over a natural tooth; also called a cap.

A crown is placed on a tooth that has had root canal treatment or has a large filling in it to prevent it from cracking or breaking away.

(1) The index finger of the right "one" hand points to a tooth. (SM)
(2) The right "claw" hand moves down to cover the left fist. (SM)

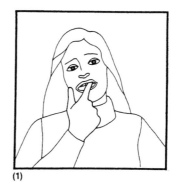
(1)

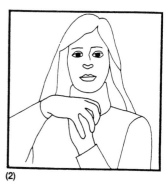
(2)

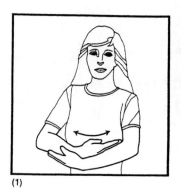
(1)

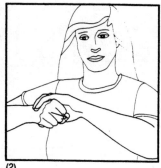
(2)

CROWNING

The stage in giving birth where the baby's head is first seen.

*Once **crowning** has occurred, delivery of the baby is usually anywhere from a few minutes to half an hour.*

(1) Sign BABY — the right hand and forearm face up, resting on the left hand and forearm which also face upwards. Both are then rocked back and forth as if holding a baby. (MM)

(2) The left "C" hand faces down at chest level. The right "S" hand moves through the left hand as if imitating the baby's head moving through the birth canal. (SM)

CRUSHING INJURY

An injury in which a part of the body is pressed so hard by something that it is damaged.

***Crushing** injuries are most common in car accidents, where a driver may be crushed by the steering wheel.*

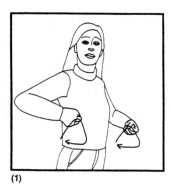
(1)

CRUTCH

A device to help a person in walking who is weak or who has leg injuries.

*The modern **crutch** can be adjusted to different sizes and has pads that fit under the armpit and on the hand grip.*

(1) Both "S" hands are at the sides of the body and move in a triangular movement as if imitating walking with crutches. (MM)

CRYSTAL

A solid having the parts arranged in a certain, regular way. Crystal is also a slang word for the drug methedrine or methamphetamine.

*Water can form ice **crystals** when it freezes and salt water leaves salt **crystals** when it evaporates.*

CRYSTALLINE LENS

See LENS

CULTURE

In medicine, bacteria grown in containers on special kinds of substances.

***Cultures** may be grown from specimens taken from a person and then examined to see if the person has a certain kind of bacterial infection.*

CUMULATIVE

Small amounts being added to increase the total amount.

Certain substances, such as lead and mercury, when taken into the body even in small amounts, can cause eventual poisoning by a cumulative effect because the body doesn't get rid of them quickly.

(1) The left "flat" hand faces up at waist level. The right "H" hand faces up at waist level. Turn the right hand over so that the hand faces down and the fingers touch the left palm a few times, at the same time, both hands move up to chest level. (MM)

* This can be signed with both "flat" hands and the same movement to mean a larger quantity.

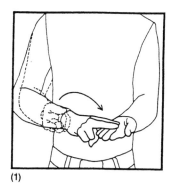

(1)

CURE

To heal an injury or disease; to make healthy.

There is no proven cure for cancer yet, so one should be cautious when someone is promising a treatment which will give quick and complete recovery from it.

(1) Sign BECOME — the right "flat" hand is on top of the left "flat" hand. Twist both hands so that the left hand ends up on top of the right hand. (SM)
(2) Sign HEALTH — both "five" hands face in at chest level. Move both hands down into "S" hands.

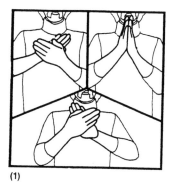 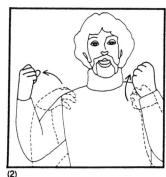

(1)   (2)

CUSP

In dentistry, the top, pointed part of the tooth. *See Figure 25*

CUSPID

A kind of tooth. There are four cuspids in the adult mouth, two on the top and two on the bottom. They are found near the front of the mouth and have a single sharp point which is why they are also called canine teeth. Cuspids are used for cutting and tearing. *See Figure 24*

(1) Fingerspell "C-U-S-P-I-D".
(2) The index finger of the right "one" hand points to a tooth. (SM)

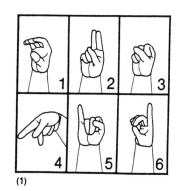 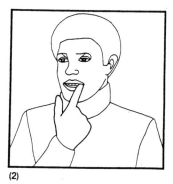

(1)   (2)

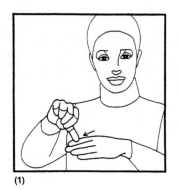
(1)

CUT

To pierce something with a sharp edge; an injury caused by breaking the skin with something sharp.

How much a cut bleeds depends on how big and how deep it is.

(1) The left "flat" hand faces in at chest level. The thumb of the right "A" hand move across the back of the left hand as if cutting. (SM)

CUTICLE

Referring to the thin strip of skin at the base of the fingernails or toenails.

Cuticle is also used for the epidermis of the skin.

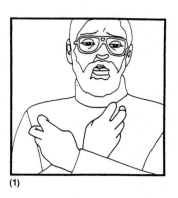
(1)

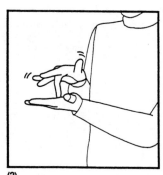
(2)

CYANIDE

A very poisonous chemical. Cyanide poisoning is one of the most common and dangerous types of poisoning. The seeds of certain stone fruits (jetberry bush and toyon) contain chemicals that turn to cyanide in the digestive tract. Symptoms of cyanide poisoning usually start within a few seconds and may include rapid pulse and breathing, convulsions, a choking feeling, anxiety, dizziness, confusion, headache and foaming of the mouth.

If not treated immediately, cyanide poisoning can cause death.

(1) Sign POISON — both bent "V" hands cross at the wrists and face in on the body. (SM)
(2) Sign MEDICINE — the left "flat" hand faces up at chest level. The middle finger of the right "eight" hand touches the left palm and pivots slightly from left to right a few times. (MM)

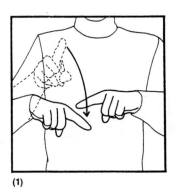
(1)

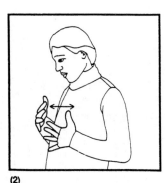
(2)

CYANOSIS

A bluish discoloration of the skin resulting from insufficient oxygen in the blood.

Cyanosis may result from an airway obstruction or an overdose of drugs.

(1) Sign CAN'T — the left "one" hand is palm down at waist level. The right "one" hand is chest level with the index finger pointing up. The right index finger strikes down on the left index finger. (SM)
(2) Sign BREATHE — both "flat" hands move in and out from the body a few times as if imitating breathing. (MM)

(Continued on next page)

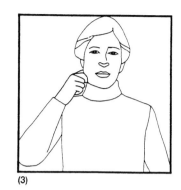

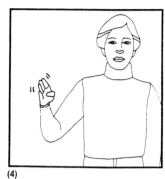

(3) Sign SKIN — the index finger and thumb of the right hand grab the right cheek. (SM)
(4) Sign BLUE — the right "B" hand faces out at shoulder level and pivots slightly from left to right a few times. (MM)

(3)

(4)

CYCLE

A regularly repeated sequence of events.

The menstrual **cycle** *takes 28 days on the average.*

CYST

An abnormal pouch or sac beneath the skin which contains a liquid or semisolid substance.

Cysts *often form when a gland becomes blocked.*

CYSTIC FIBROSIS

A hereditary disease caused by an abnormal gene which affects children and young adults. Cystic fibrosis affects the exocrine glands in the body, like the sweat glands and part of the pancreas. Cystic fibrosis causes chronic lung disease, problems breathing, a cough, diarrhea with greasy stools, cramps in the abdomen, an increased appetite and poor growth. The chances of living beyond adolescence are poor and there is no cure, but treatment with antibiotics may help infections that come back.

If a person has **cystic fibrosis,** *his skin will usually taste extra salty because the disease affects the sweat glands.*

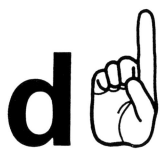

DAILY

Occurring every day.

Dental floss should be used daily to prevent tooth decay and gum disease.

(1) The right "A" hand faces left at the right side of the face. The thumb of the right hand brushes the right cheek a few times. (MM)

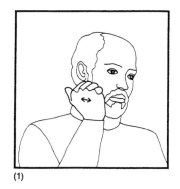
(1)

D&C

An abbreviation for dilation and curetage of the cervix.

D&C is a surgical procedure commonly done after an abortion or as a means of abortion.

(1) Fingerspell "D-C".

* This term may need to be explained more fully before fingerspelling "D-C".

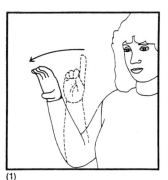
(1)

DALMANE

A sedative drug used to help someone relax or sleep; sold under the name of Flurazepam®

Dalmane, closely related to valium, should be used carefully because the drug stays in the body for a long time and its effects can bulid up.

DAM

In dentistry, a thin sheet of rubber used to prevent fluid or saliva from flowing into an area.

When filling a cavity, a dentist may use a dam to keep the tooth or teeth he is working on dry.

(1) Sign RUBBER — the index finger of the right "X" hand brushes down the chin a few times. (MM)

* This can also be signed by brushing down the right cheek a few times. (MM)

(Continued on next page)

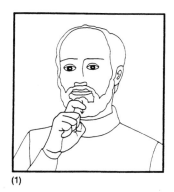
(1)

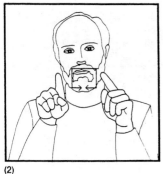

(2)

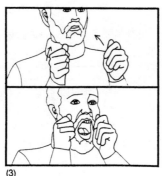
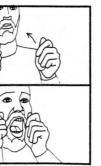

(3)

DAM, *continued*

(2) The index fingers of both "one" hands draw an imaginary square. (SM)

(3) Both "A" hands face each other at shoulder level. Move both hands towards the mouth as if putting something into the mouth. (SM)

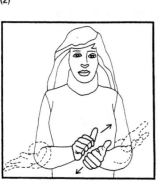

(1)

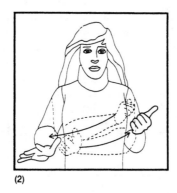

(2)

DAMAGE

Injury or harm.

> *Damage to the nervous system is dangerous because nerve cells cannot reproduce themselves.*

(1) The left "five" hand faces up at chest level. The right "five" hand faces down at chest level. Move both hands towards the center, ending in "A" hands with thumbs extended, facing each other.

(2) Continue moving the right hand through to the left and the left through to the right until they cross at the arms. At the same time, move the right hand back ot it's original position, ending in a "five" hand facing down and the left hand back to it's original position ending in an "A" hand facing down. (SM)

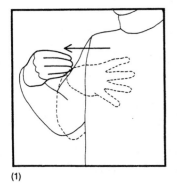

(1)

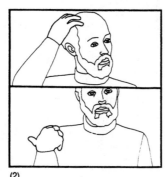

(2)

DANDRUFF

Small, white pieces of skin that flake off the scalp. Dandruff may be made worse by disease.

> *Some kinds of dandruff can be cured by using medicated shampoos.*

(1) Sign WHITE — the right "five" hand touches the chest and moves out ending in a "flat-O" hand. (SM)

(2) The fingers of the right "claw" hand scratch the head. Then, move the hand down to tap the shoulder a few times.

DANGEROUS

Able to cause harm or injury.

> *Smoking can be dangerous to your health.*

(1) The left "flat" hand faces in at chest level. The back of the thumb of the right "A" hand brushes the back of the left hand in an up, out and around circular movement. (SM)

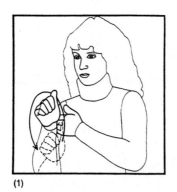

(1)

DARK ADAPTATION

The changes that occur in the pupil and retina of the eye that allow us to see in dim light.

In dark adaptation the pupil of the eye dilates to let more light into the eye.

(1) Sign BLACK — the index finger of the right "one" hand moves across the forehead from left to right. (SM)
(2) Sign EYES — the index finger of the right "one" hand points to both eyes. (SM)
(3) Both "S" hands face each other in front of the eyes. Open both hands slightly as if imitating the pupils dilating. (SM)

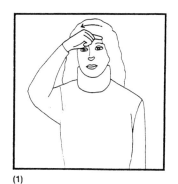

(1)

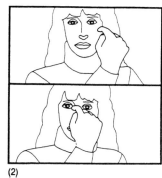

(2)

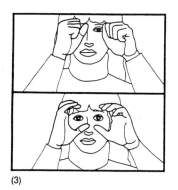

(3)

DEADLY NIGHTSHADE

See BELLADONNA POISONING

DEAF

In legal medicine, a hearing loss of 25 decibels or more. A severe hearing loss in which one cannot learn an oral language through the auditory channel with or without a hearing aid.

Some ear infections can cause a person to be deaf if not treated properly.

a. (1) The index finger of the right "one" hand touches the right ear then touches the mouth. (SM)
b. (1) The index finger of the right "one" hand touches the right ear then moves down to chest level, both "one" hands face down. (SM)

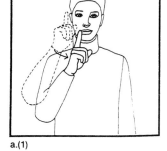

a.(1)

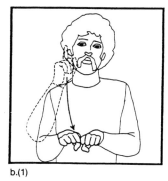

b.(1)

DEATH

The permanent and complete stopping of the body's activities; the end of life. There are many arguments about when death actually occurs and its exact definition.

Some people believe death occurs when the brain stops its activities and some believe it is when the heart and breathing stop and can't be started again.

(Continued on next page)

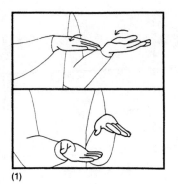
(1)

DEATH, *continued*

(1) The left "flat" hand faces up at chest level and the right "flat" hand faces down at chest level. Turn both hands over to the right, with the left hand ending palm down and the right hand ending palm up. (SM)

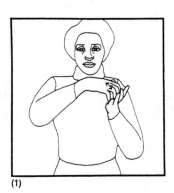
(1)

DEBILITY

Weakness or infirmity.

An injury or disease damaging the body will cause a certain amount of debility.

(1) Sign WEAK — the left "flat" hand faces up at chest level. The fingertips of the right "claw" hand rest in the left palm. Keeping the fingertips in place, bend and straighten the fingers of the right hand a few times. (MM)

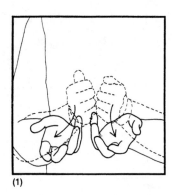
(1)

DECAY

Rotting, wasting away or falling apart.

Teeth will decay if a person has a poor diet, eats a lot of sweets, or doesn't brush the teeth or use dental floss regularly.

(1) Both "A" hands face each other at chest level. Drop both hands forward into "five" hands, palms up. (SM)

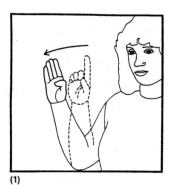
(1)

DECIBEL

A unit of measurement used in describing differences in loudness.

Normal sound is measured at 0-20 decibels.

(1) Fingerspell "D-B".

* *This may need to be explained before fingerspelling "D-B".*

DECIDUOUS TEETH

The "milk" teeth, "baby" teeth, or temporary teeth which a child has between 6 months and the time they begin to be replaced by permanent teeth, at about 6 years. There are 10 deciduous teeth in the upper jaw and 10 in the lower jaw. *See Figure 24*

(1) Sign BABY — the right hand and forearm face up, resting on the left hand and forearm which also face upwards. Both are then rocked back and forth as If holding a baby. (SM)
(2) Sign TEETH — the right index finger points to the teeth. (SM)

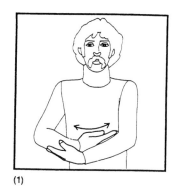
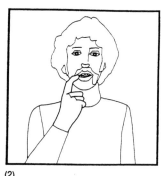

(1)   (2)

DECOMPRESSION

The lowering or removal of pressure on a body.

Deep sea divers must undergo decompression by coming up slowly or entering a special chamber which slowly decreases pressure so they can adjust gradually to the lower pressure of the atmosphere.

DECONTAMINATION

The cleaning or freeing of a person, object or area from harmful material.

Decontamination would be done to a person who has been exposed to radioactivity, to things which have come into contact with someone who has a very dangerous disease or to surgical instruments.

DECREASE

To lower, lessen or make smaller.

When there is a decrease in blood flow to an area, damage and death can occur in the area because of a lack of oxygen and a build-up of wastes.

a. (1) The left "cupped" hand faces up at waist level. The right "cupped" hand faces down at waist level. Move the hands slightly towards each other without touching. (SM)
b. (1) The left "one" hand faces up at waist level. The right "one" hand faces down at waist level. Move the hands slightly towards each other without touching. (SM)

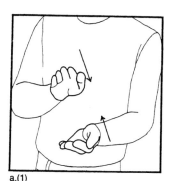
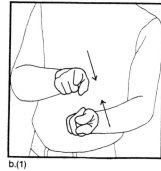

a.(1)   b.(1)

DEEP

Below the surface, far down or inside.

The amount of bleeding from a wound will depend on how deep it is.

(Continued on next page)

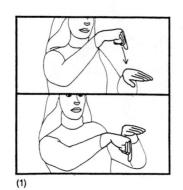
(1)

DEEP, *continued*

(1) The left "flat" hand faces down at chest level. The index finger of the right "one" hand points down and moves down past the left hand. (SM)

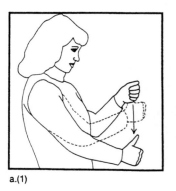
a.(1)

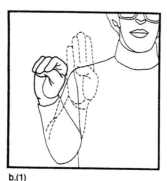
b.(1)

DEFECATION

The release of solid wastes from the rectum through the anus.

Defecation is another word for a bowel movement.

a. (1) The left "A" hand faces right at chest level. The thumb of the right "A" hand is inside the left fist, the hand faces left. Move the right hand down from the left hand, keeping the left hand still. (SM)
b. (1) Fingerspell "B-M".

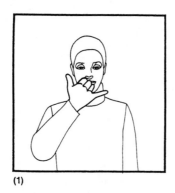
(1)

DEFECT

A mistake or abnormality.

A congenital defect is an abnormality that occurs at birth.

(1) Sign WRONG — the right "Y" hand faces in and brushes down the chin in a small circular movement a few times.

DEFIBRILLATION

Returning the heartbeat to normal when, for some reason, it is twitching or not contracting as a whole.

Defibrillation is usually done by using a device which sends an electrical shock through the heart causing the heart to start beating as a unit.

DEFICIENCY DISEASE

A disease caused by the failure to get enough of a substance needed for normal body activity.

A deficiency disease may be caused by not eating enough of what is needed, by a digestive problem where the substance isn't taken in by the intestines, or by the substance being used by a parasite before the body can use it.

DEFORMITY

A part of the body not shaped normally. A deformity may be present at birth or a person may get one through disease or injury.

If an injured person has a visible deformity in an area, there may be a fracture or dislocation.

(1) Sign NOT — the right "A" hand faces left. The thumb brushes under the chin out forward. (SM)
(2) Sign NORMAL — the left "S" hand faces down at chest level. The right "N" hand faces down. The right hand makes a clockwise circle above the left hand, then moves down to touch the top of the left hand. (SM)
(3) Sign WRONG — the right "Y" hand faces in and brushes down the chin a few times. (MM)

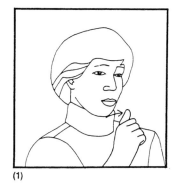

(1)

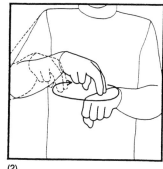

(2)

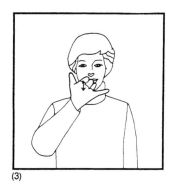

(3)

DEGENERATION

Failure of a structure to work well because it has fallen apart or deteriorated.

Degeneration of a part of the body may lead to death of the area.

a. (1) Sign DECLINE — both "A" hands with thumbs extended face each other at the sides, at chest level. Move both hands down in a wavy movement. (SM)
b. (1) Sign DECAY — both "A" hands face each other at chest level. Drop both hands forward and down into "five" hands. (SM)

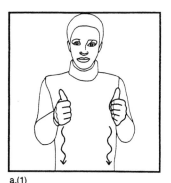

a.(1)

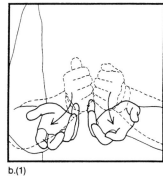

b.(1)

DEHYDRATION

A lack of water in the body. Dehydration is caused by more fluids leaving the body than are taken in.

Dehydration can be caused by not drinking enough fluids, diarrhea, vomiting, a lot of bleeding or extended sweating.

(1) Sign DRY — the right "one" hand faces down and points left under the chin. Move the hand to the right and, at the same time, the right index finger bends. (SM)
(2) The index finger of the right "one" hand moves down the throat. (SM)

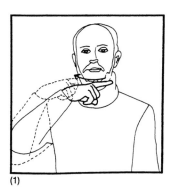

(1)

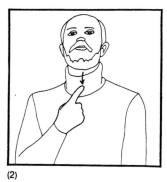

(2)

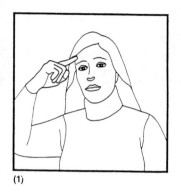
(1)

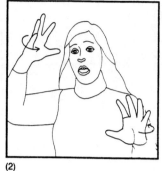
(2)

DELIRIUM

A state in which a person is confused, excited, restless and hallucinatory.

Delirium may be caused by many things, some of the most common being certain mental diseases, alcoholism, high fever, poisoning, and drug abuse.

(1) Sign MIND — the index finger of the right "one" hand touches the forehead. (SM)
(2) Sign CONFUSED — the right "claw" hand is at head level, the left "claw" hand is at chest level. Twist both hands from left to right a few times. (MM)
* The facial expression should reflect confusion.

DELIRIUM TREMENS

A severe mental condition caused by using alcohol in large amounts for a long time; also called potomania. A person with delirium tremens will be confused, shaking, afraid, excited and hallucinating. Delirium tremens are also called "D.T.'s".

People with delirium tremens may be given sedatives and may have to be restrained.

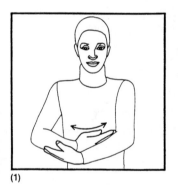
(1)

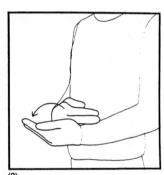
(2)

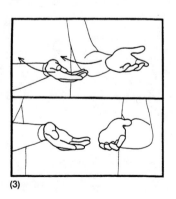
(3)

DELIVER

To give birth or to assist in giving birth.

Most women have a doctor help them deliver their babies.

(1) Sign BABY — the right hand and forearm face up, resting on the left hand and forearm which also face upwards. Both are then rocked back and forth as if holding a baby. (SM)
(2) Sign BORN — the left "cupped" hand faces in at stomach level. The right "cupped" hand also faces in behind the left hand. Move the right hand down to rest in the palm of the left hand. (SM)
(3) Both "flat" hands face up at the left side of the body. Move both hands in towards the body. (SM)

DELIVERY

The movement of a baby from a woman's uterus through the vagina to the outside; giving birth.

An obstetrician is a doctor who takes care of pregnant women and helps them during delivery.

(1) Sign BABY — the right hand and forearm face up, resting on the left hand and forearm which also face upwards. Both are then rocked back and forth as if holding a baby. (SM)

(2) Sign BORN — the left "cupped" hand faces in at stomach level. The right "cupped" hand also faces in behind the left hand. Move the right hand down to rest in the palm of the left hand. (SM)

(3) Both "flat" hands face up at the left side of the body. Move both hands in towards the body. (SM)

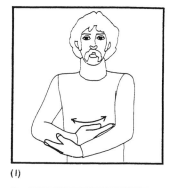
(1)

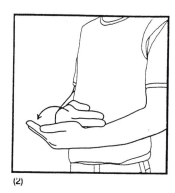
(2)

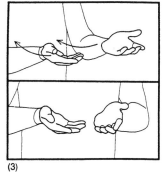
(3)

DELIVERY ROOM

A special room in a hospital where women give birth.

A delivery room has special equipment in it which a doctor may need to help a woman have a baby.

(1) Sign ROOM — both "flat" hands face each other at the sides. Move both hands to the center so that they both face in, the right hand in front of the left. (SM)

(2) Sign BABY — the right hand and forearm face up, resting on the left hand and forearm which also face upwards. Both are then rocked back and forth as if holding a baby. (SM)

(3) Sign BORN — the left "cupped" hand faces in at stomach level. The right "cupped" hand also faces in and moves down to rest in the left palm. (SM)

(4) Both "flat" hands face up at the left side of the body. Move both hands in towards the body. (SM)

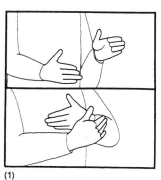
(1)

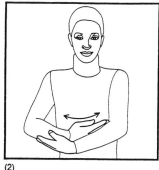
(2)

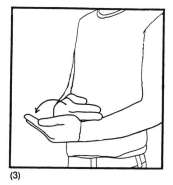
(3)

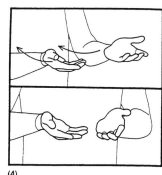
(4)

DELTOID

The thick muscle over the top of the shoulder used to lift the arm. *See Figure 4*

157

DELUSION

A persistent belief or idea held in spite of evidence to the contrary. Delusions are a symptom of some mental diseases.

*An example of a **delusion** is a **delusion** of grandeur in which a person thinks he has great wealth or power.*

DEMEROL

A drug used to calm a person and to prevent pain while delivering a baby; sold under the name of Meperidine.®

Demerol should be taken in the smallest possible amounts and for the shortest possible time because it can cause addiction.

DEMONSTRATE

To show or explain something.

*An oral hygienist or dentist can **demonstrate** how to correctly use dental floss and brush your teeth.*

(1) The left "flat" hand faces out at chest level. The index finger of the right "one" hand touches the left palm. Move both hands out forward. (SM)

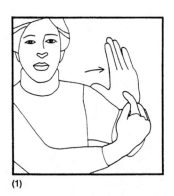

(1)

DENTAL

Referring to the teeth.

*A **dental** prosthesis is an artificial structure used to replace natural teeth.*

(1) Sign TEETH — the index finger of the right "one" hand taps the teeth a few times.

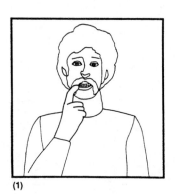

(1)

DENTAL FLOSS

Waxed or unwaxed thread which is worked into the spaces between the teeth and then rubbed up and down to clean between teeth and gums by removing food particles.

*The use of **dental floss** can help prevent cavities between the teeth and gum disease.*

(Continued on next page)

DENTAL FLOSS, *continued*

(1) Both "I" hands face in with the little fingers touching. Move both hands to the sides. (SM)
(2) Both "F" hands face out and imitate flossing. (MM)

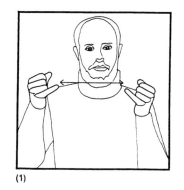

(1)

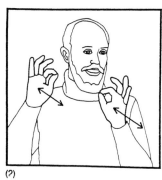

(?)

DENTIFRICE

A powder or paste used to clean the teeth.

Children should use a dentifrice containing fluoride to help prevent cavities.

(1) The right hand imitates spreading toothpaste on a brush.
(2) The index finger of the right "one" hand imitates brushing the teeth. (MM)

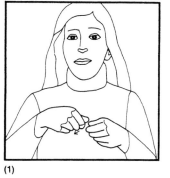

(1)

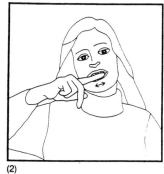

(2)

DENTIN

The hard bone-like substance making up the body of the tooth. The dentin surrounds the pulp of the tooth and is covered by enamel. *See Figure 25*

DENTIST

A doctor who prevents, diagnoses and treats disease and injuries of the teeth and mouth.

"Odontologist" is another name for dentist.

a. (1) The right "D" hand taps the mouth a few times. (MM)

* This is a newer sign and the meaning should be clarified before the sign is used.

b. (1) The right index finger moves across the teeth. (MM)
(2) Sign PERSON — both "flat" hands face each other at chest level. Move both hands down to waist level. (SM)

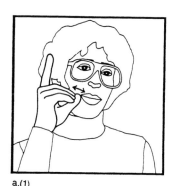

a.(1)

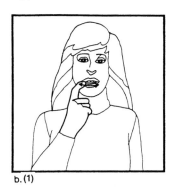

b. (1)

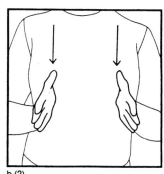

b.(2)

159

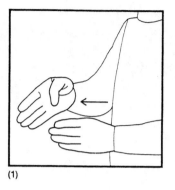
(1)

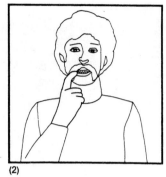
(2)

DENTISTRY

The area of medicine which prevents, diagnoses and treats diseases of the mouth and teeth, and injuries or deformities of the mouth.

Dentistry is also called odontology.

(1) Sign SPECIALIZE — the left "B" hand faces right at chest level. The right "B" hand faces left on top of the left hand. Move the right hand straight out on the left index finger. (SM)

(2) Sign TEETH — the index finger of the right "one" hand points to the teeth. (SM)

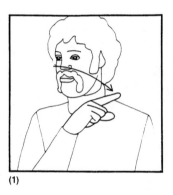
(1)

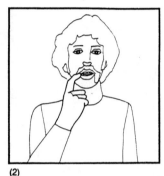
(2)

DENTURE

A set of natural or artificial teeth made to replace missing or damaged natural teeth.

Dentures are usually made out of plastic and metal, and should be brushed regularly just like real teeth.

(1) Sign FALSE — the right "L" hand faces left and brushes past the nose. (SM)

(2) Sign TEETH — the index finger of the right "one" hand points to the teeth. (SM)

(3) The index finger and thumb of the right hand imitate putting a denture in the mouth. (SM)

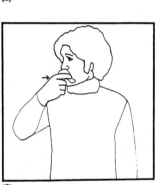
(3)

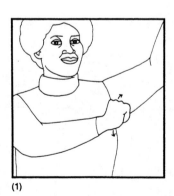
(1)

DEODORANT

Something used to destroy or cover up odors.

Many people use deodorants on their armpits to kill bacteria which cause odors.

(1) The right hand imitates spraying deodorant under the left armpit. (MM)

DEOXYRIBONUCLEIC ACID

The long name for DNA, a nucleic acid found in the cells which makes up chromosomes.

The deoxyribonucleic acid molecule is the structure which holds the information that directs our physical development and controls what we will be.

(1) Fingerspell "D-N-A".

* This is a very complex idea and should be explained before fingerspelling "D-N-A".

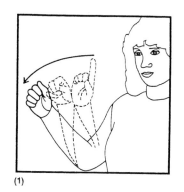
(1)

DEPENDENCE

In medicine, it is used for the mental or physical need a person has to use a certain drug in order to feel temporarily free from a craving for that drug.

Dependence on a drug will usually involve using larger and larger amounts of a drug in order to satisfy the desire for it.

(1) Sign MEDICINE — the left "flat" hand faces up at chest level. The middle finger of the right "eight" hand touches the left palm and pivots slightly from left to right a few times. (MM)

(2) Sign INJECT — the index finger of the right "L" hand taps the left upper arm a few times. (MM)

Sign PILL — the thumb and index finger of the right hand touch, the palm faces the mouth. Flick the index finger towards the mouth as if popping a pill into the mouth. (SM)

* Sign INJECT or PILL if the specific is known.

(3) Sign HABIT — both "five" hands cross at the wrists then move down slightly into "S" hands. (SM)

* This should be signed with intense vigor.

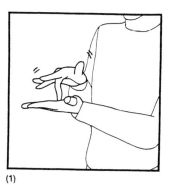
(1)

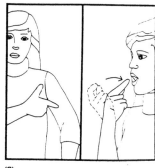
(2)

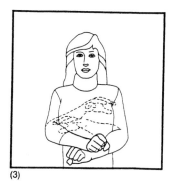
(3)

DEPOSIT

Any substance that settles out of a liquid and collects in an area.

Gallstones and kidney stones are hard deposits made from the fluids normally found in the gall bladder or kidney.

DEPRESSANT

Any substance that slows the body's activities and acts on the nervous system to cause relaxation and sleep. "Downers" is a slang word for depressants.

The most common depressants are barbiturates and alcohol.

(Continued on next page)

161

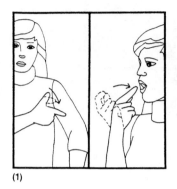
(1)

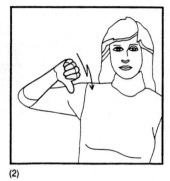
(2)

DEPRESSANT, *continued*

(1) Sign INJECT — the index finger of the right "L" hand taps the left upper arm a few times. (MM)

Sign PILL — the thumb and index finger of the right hand touch, the palm faces the mouth. Flick the index finger towards the mouth as if popping a pill into the mouth. (SM)
* *Sign INJECT or PILL if the specific is known.*

(2) Sign DOWNER — the right fist with the thumb pointing down moves down at shoulder level twice. (DM)

* *This is a general sign for depressants ("downers"). The specific type of drug should also be fingerspelled and all side effects explained.*

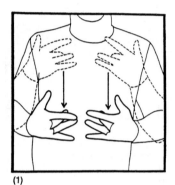
(1)

DEPRESSION

In psychology, a mental state with symptoms of sadness and a loss of hope and cheerfulness.

Sometimes depression is treated with drugs which make the person more active and feel better.

(1) The middle fingers of both hands touch at chest level and move down to waist level. (SM)

* *The facial expression should reflect depression. This sign only refers to the psychological state of depression.*

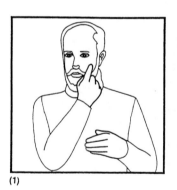
(1)

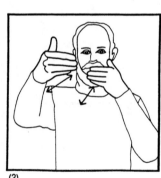
(2)

DEPTH PERCEPTION

The ability to see the distance between things, especially the ability to tell how far away things are.

We have depth perception because each of our eyes sees an object from a different angle and when the two pictures are put together in the brain, we can tell how far away from us things are.

(1) The index finger of the right "one" hand points to the left eye. (SM)

(2) Both "flat" hands face in at eye level, the right in front of the left. Move both hands alternately in and out from eye level a few times. (MM)

DERMATITIS

A general term for inflammation of the skin with itching, redness and perhaps bumps.

Dermatitis may be caused by an allergy, poisons or dangerous chemicals on the skin, too much sun or an infection.

(Continued on next page)

DERMATITIS, *continued*

(1) Sign SKIN — the index finger and thumb of the right hand grab the right cheek. (SM)
(2) Sign RED — the index finger of the right "one" hand brushes down the chin a few times. (MM)
(3) Sign ITCH — the right "claw" hand scratches the left upper arm a few times. (MM)

This can be signed at the area of the dermatitis.

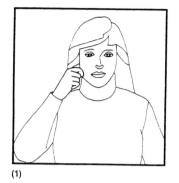
(1)

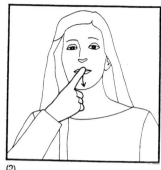
(2)

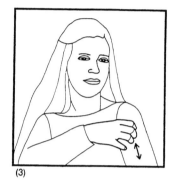
(3)

DERMATOLOGIST

A doctor who specializes in treating diseases of the skin.

> *Dermatologists are sometimes able to help people with bad acne.*

(1) Sign SKIN — the index finger and thumb of the right hand grab the right cheek. (SM)
(2) Sign DOCTOR — the right "M" hand touches the left inside wrist. (DM)

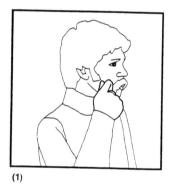
(1)

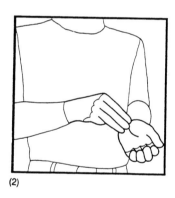
(2)

DERMATOLOGY

The study of the skin, how it works, its diseases and how to treat them.

> *Eczema and psoriasis are some disorders of the skin studied in dermatology.*

(1) Sign SPECIALIZE — the left "B" hand faces right at chest level. The right "B" hand faces left on top of the left hand. Move the right hand straight out on the left index finger. (SM)
(2) Sign SKIN — the index finger and thumb of the right hand grab the right cheek. (SM)

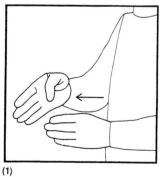
(1)

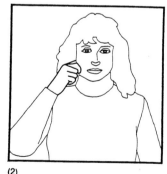
(2)

163

DERMIS

One of the two layers of skin, the inner layer of the skin.

The dermis contains fat deposits, hair roots, glands, nerves and blood vessels.

DESENSITIZE

To make less sensitive.

Some asthma patients or people allergic to drugs, such as penicillin, are desensitized by giving them small amounts of the protein they are sensitive to.

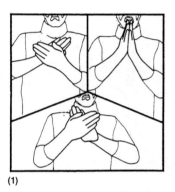

(1)

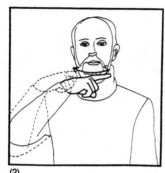

(2)

DESICCATE

To dry up.

Mucus is produced so that certain areas are not able to desiccate.

(1) Sign BECOME — the right "flat" hand is on top of the left "flat" hand. Twist both hands so that the left hand ends up on top of the right hand. (SM)
(2) Sign DRY — the right "one" hand faces down and points left under the chin. Move the hand to the right and, at the same time, the right index finger bends. (SM)

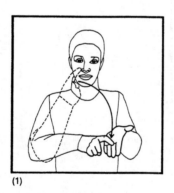

(1)

DETECT

To discover something or find something out.

When a culture is taken of a part of the body or a substance is taken from the body, such as urine, the doctor is trying to detect the presence of something that shouldn't be there.

(1) The left "flat" hand faces out at chest level. The index finger of the right "one" hand points to the right eye then moves down to touch the left palm. (SM)

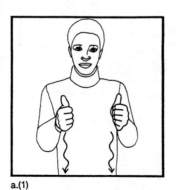

a.(1)

DETERIORATE

To fall apart, break up or wear away.

After about four months, a red blood cell will begin to deteriorate and be taken out of circulation by the spleen or liver.

a. (1) Both "A" hands face each other at shoulder level. Move both hands down in wavy motions to waist level. (SM)

(Continued on next page)

b. (1) Sign DECLINE — the right "flat" hand faces in and moves down the left arm, touching it several times. (MM)

c. (1) Sign DECAY — both "A" hands face each other at chest level. Drop both hands forward and down into "five" hands. (SM)

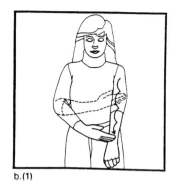
b.(1)

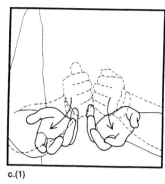
c.(1)

DEVELOPMENT

To grow or become more complex.

Development is the growth from an egg to an adult state.

(1) Sign GROW — the right "flat-O" hand is inside the left fist. Move the right hand up through the left fist, ending in a "five" hand. (SM)

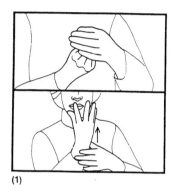
(1)

DEVIANT

A thing or person that differs from the normal, especially one who acts differently from others.

Deviate is another word for deviant.

(1) Both "one" hands face out at chest level with the index fingers crossing. Move both hands to the sides. (SM)

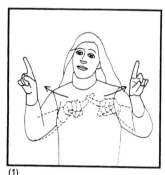
(1)

DEVITALIZE

To destroy or kill. In dentistry, to destroy the pulp and nerve of a tooth.

A tooth will be devitalized when it is chipped or injured so badly that the nerve is exposed or when a cavity goes to the nerve.

(1) Sign DESTORY — the left "five" hand faces up at chest level. The right "five" hand faces down at chest level. Move both hands towards the center, ending in "A" hands with thumbs extended, facing each other.

(2) Continue moving the right hand through to the left and the left through to the right until they cross at the arms. At the same time, move the right hand back to it's original position, ending in a "five" hand facing down and the left hand back to it's original position, ending in an "A" hand facing down.(SM)

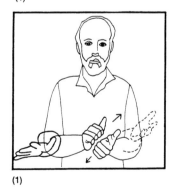
(1)

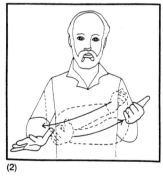
(2)

165

DEXEDRINE

The short name for dextroamphetamine.

Dexedrine is a common drug found in weight reducing pills.

DEXIES

See DEXTROAMPHETAMINE

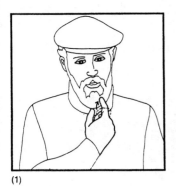
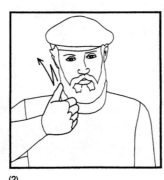

(1)   (2)

DEXTROAMPHETAMINE

A drug which acts as a stimulant. Dexedrine and "dexies" are the short names for dextroamphetamine.

Dextroamphetamine is used to treat depression and is sometimes used in weight reducing pills because it causes loss of hunger.

(1) Sign PILL — the thumb and index finger of the right hand touch, the palm faces the mouth. Flick the index finger towards the mouth as if popping a pill into the mouth. (SM)

(2) Sign UPPER — the right fist, with the thumb pointing up, moves up at shoulder level twice. (DM)

* *This is a general sign for stimulants ("uppers"). The specific type of drug should also be fingerspelled and all side effects explained.*

DEXTROSE

See GLUCOSE

DIABETES

A disease where insulin, which helps get a form of sugar called dextrose or glucose into the cells, isn't made in large enough amounts; also called diabetes mellitus. The sugar is used inside the cells to make energy and when it cannot be moved into the cells, the cells starve. A person with diabetes will have extra sugar in the blood and urine, need to urinate often, be thirsty, lose weight, and be nervous and weak.

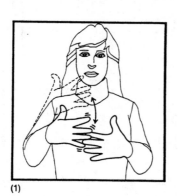

(1)

Diabetes is usually treated with diet control, exercise and insulin injections.

(1) Sign BLOOD — the left "five" hand is at chest level with the palm towards the body. The palm of the right "five" hand is towards the body with the middle fingertips touching the mouth. Move the right hand down the back of the left hand. Wiggle the fingers of the right hand as it moves. (MM)

* *This movement should be short, repeated and somewhat restrained.*

(Continued on next page)

DIABETES, *continued*

(2) Sign TOO MUCH — the left "cupped" hand faces down at chest level. The right "cupped" also faces down at chest level. Move the right hand up to shoulder level. (SM)

(3) Sign SUGAR — the fingertips of the right "flat" hand brush down the chin a few times. (MM)

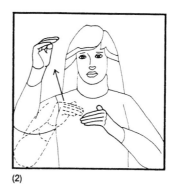
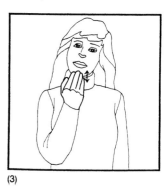

(2)   (3)

DIABETIC COMA

A comatose state people with diabetes may go into if they are not being treated or do not take enough insulin. Without insulin, which helps move sugar into the cells to be used to make energy, the cells starve. This starvation causes the body to use fats for energy, and the resulting by-products can build up, causing a form of poisoning called ketoacidosis. This poisoning causes the person to go into a coma, in which he becomes very quiet and appears to be asleep.

*A person in a **diabetic coma** needs insulin very badly and should be taken to a hospital immediately.*

DIAGNOSIS

A doctor's analysis of an illness, based on the patient's symptoms and medical history, a physical examination and appropriate tests.

A doctor may use blood tests and urinalyses to make a diagnosis.

(1) Sign DOCTOR — the right "M" hand touches the left inside wrist.(DM)

(2) Sign ANALYZE — both "V" hands face down at chest level. Drop both hands down into bent "V" hands a few times. (MM)

(3) Sign DECIDE — the index finger of the right "one" hand touches the forehead. Then, both "F" hands face down at chest level and move down to waist level. (SM)

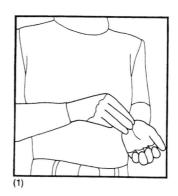
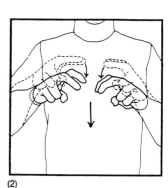

(1)   (2)

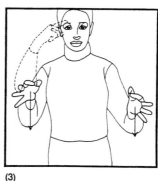

(3)

167

DIALYSIS

The separation of suspended particles from a liquid. It is done by placing the liquid in a sack made up of a membrane with holes in it small enough to hold back certain substances and let others pass through.

When a person's kidneys don't work well, dialysis may be done by a machine to clean the blood of wastes.

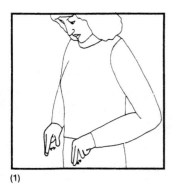
(1)

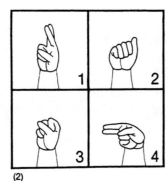
(2)

DIAPER RASH

Redness and inflammation of a baby's skin caused by wearing diapers soaked with urine for long periods of time.

Diaper rash can be prevented by changing diapers often, using an antiseptic on diapers and keeping the baby's bottom clean and dry.

(1) The index and middle fingers of both hands touch the thumbs of both hands at the area of diaper pins. Open and close the fingers of both hands a few times. (MM)
(2) Fingerspell "R-A-S-H".

DIAPHRAGM

A thin, flexible wall of muscle which separates the abdomen from the chest cavity. Hiccups are caused by spasms of the diaphragm.

See Figure 4

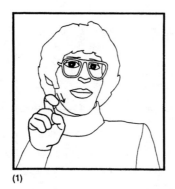
(1)

DIAPHRAGM, contraceptive

A cup-shaped piece of rubber placed over the cervix in a woman's vagina as a form of contraception. A diaphragm is used with a cream or jelly which kills sperm.

A woman must be fitted with a diaphragm by a doctor to be sure she gets the correct size.

(1) Sign RUBBER — the index finger of the right "X" hand brushes down the right cheek a few times. (MM)

(Continued on next page)

(2) The index fingers and thumbs of both hands form a circle. (SM)
(3) The right "flat-O" hand faces up and moves up into the left "S" hand. (SM)

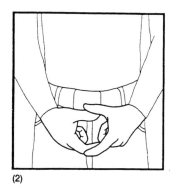

(2)

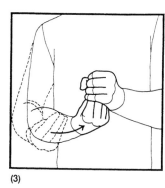

(3)

DIARRHEA

Frequent and watery bowel movements.

Diarrhea can be caused by a viral or bacterial infection, a parasite, strange food or certain drugs.

(1) The left "S" hand faces right at chest level. The thumb of the right "five" hand is inside the left fist. Move the right hand down from the left fist a few times, leaving the left hand in place. (MM)

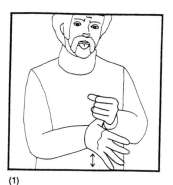

(1)

DIAZEPAM

A tranquilizing drug used to calm a person and reduce stress or excitement. Diazepam is sold under the name of Valium.®

Use of diazepam for a long time can cause addiction.

(1) Sign PILL — the thumb and index finger of the right hand touch, the palm faces the mouth. Flick the index finger towards the mouth as if popping a pill into the mouth. (SM)
(2) Sign DOWNER — the right fist with the thumb pointing down, moves down at shoulder level twice. (DM)

* This is a general sign for depressants ("downers"). The specific type of drug should also be fingerspelled and all side effects explained.

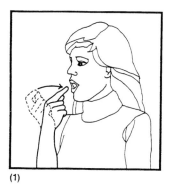

(1)

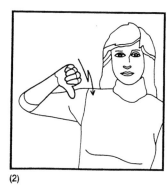

(2)

DIET

In general, the things a person eats and drinks regularly. A diet can also be certain foods a person eats to lose weight or to help control a disease.

Some diabetics can control the disease by following a certain diet.

a. (1) Sign EAT — the fingertips of the right "flat-O" hand tap the mouth a few times. (MM)

(Continued on next page)

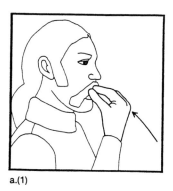

a.(1)

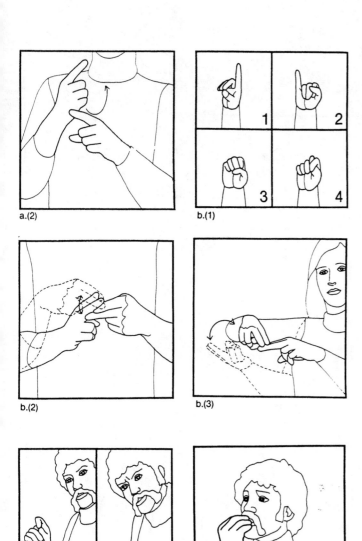

a.(2)   b.(1)

b.(2)   b.(3)

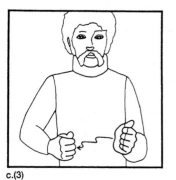 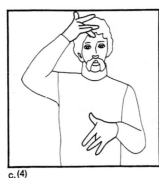

c.(1)   c.(2)

c.(3)   c.(4)

DIET, *continued*

a. (2) Sign REGULAR — the left "one" hand points out, the palm facing right and the right "one" hand points out, the palm facing left on top of the left hand. Tap the hands in a circular movement, at the same time, both hands move across the body from left to right. (MM)

* *These should be signed only if referring to a person's regular diet.*

b. (1) Fingerspell "D-I-E-T".

(2) The left "H" hand faces down at chest level. The right "H" hand also faces down on top of the left hand. Pivot the right hand slightly a few times. (MM)

(3) The left "H" hand faces down at chest level. The fingertips of the right "H" hand touch the fingers of the left hand. Turn the right hand over so that it faces up a few times. At the same time, both hands should move down to waist level. (MM)

* *These should only be signed when referring to a weight-control diet.*

c. (1) Both "modified-G" hands face each other at chest level and touch. (SM)

(2) Sign EAT — the fingertips of the right "flat-O" hand tap the mouth a few times. (MM)

(3) The left "A" hand faces right at chest level. The right "A" hand faces left and moves back from the left hand towards the body in a wavy movement. (SM)

(4) Sign DISEASE — the middle finger of the right "eight" hand touches the forehead and the middle finger of the left "eight" hand touches the stomach. (SM)

* *These should only be signed when referring to a specific disease controlling diet.*

170

DIETICIAN

A person specially trained in nutrition.

Most hospitals have a dietician who prepares meals for patients who must control what they eat.

(1) Sign PERSON — both "flat" hands face each other at chest level. Move both hands down to waist level. (SM)
(2) Sign SPECIALIZE — the left "B" hand faces right at chest level. The right "B" hand faces left on top of the left hand. Move the right hand straight out on the left index finger. (MM)
(3) Sign EAT — the fingertips of the right "flat-O" hand tap the mouth. (SM)
(4) Sign REGULAR — the left "one" hand points out, the palm facing right and the right "one" hand points out, the palm facing left on top of the left hand. Tap the hands in a circular movement, at the same time, both hands move across the body from left to right. (MM)

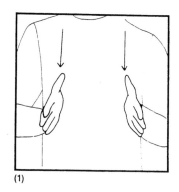

(1)

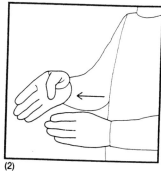

(2)

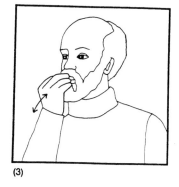

(3)

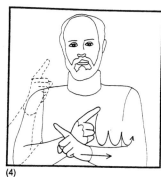

(4)

DIETHYLSTILBESTROL

A man-made drug (estrogen) used for treating menstrual disorders and other disorders due to estrogen problems; also called D.E.S. or "stilbestrol". Diethylstilbestrol was at one time given to pregnant women until it was discovered that the daughters of women given the drug during pregnancy developed vaginal disorders.

Diethylstilbestrol should never be taken during pregnancy!

DIET PILLS

Pills that usually contain stimulants which temporarily cause a person not to feel hungry.

Diet pills have proven to be bad for a person's health and a poor substitute for the right food and exercise.

a. (1) Fingerspell "D-I-E-T".
(2) Sign MEDICINE — the left "flat" hand faces up at chest level. The middle finger of the right "eight" hand touches the left palm and pivots slightly from left to right a few times. (MM)

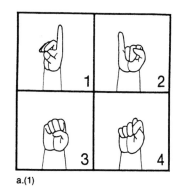

a.(1)

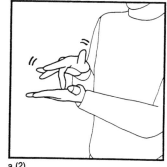

a.(2)

(Continued on next page)

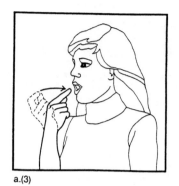
a.(3)

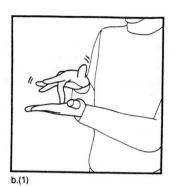
b.(1)

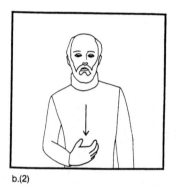
b.(2)

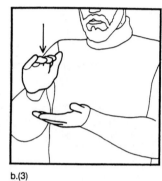
b.(3)

DIET PILLS, *continued*

a. (3) Sign PILL — the thumb and index finger of the right hand touch, the palm faces the mouth. Flick the index finger towards the mouth as if popping a pill into the mouth. (SM)

b. (1) Sign MEDICINE — the left "flat" hand faces up at chest level. The middle finger of the right "eight" hand touches the left palm and pivots slightly from left to right a few times. (MM)
(2) Sign HUNGER — the right "C" hand faces in and brushes down the chest a few times. (MM)
(3) Sign REDUCE — the left "flat" hand faces up at chest level. The right "flat" hand faces down at shoulder level. Move the right hand down to the left hand. (SM)

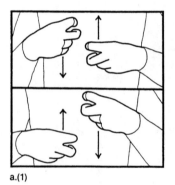
a.(1)

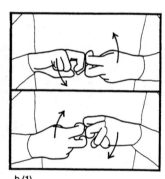
b.(1)

DIFFICULTY

A trouble or worry, or something which is not easy to do or understand; problem.

*An infection of the respiratory tract, such as a cold, can cause **difficulty** in breathing because of the mucus which is produced.*

a. (1) Sign PROBLEM — the fingers of both "V" hands are bent with the palms facing in. The right hand is at chest level and the left hand is at waist level. Hit the knuckles together while alternately changing the levels of the hands. (MM)

b. (1) Sign PROBLEM — the fingers of both "V" hands are bent and touching knuckles to knuckles. The left palm is up and the right palm is down. Twist the hands so that the palms face the opposite directions as from the beginning. (MM)

DIGEST

To change food by muscular and chemical action into a form the body can take in and use.

*Enzymes are very important in helping us **digest** our food.*

(Continued on next page)

(1) Sign EAT — the fingertips of the right "flat-O" hand tap the mouth a few times. (MM)
(2) Both "A" hands are together at chest level. Move both hands in alternating circles a few times. (MM)

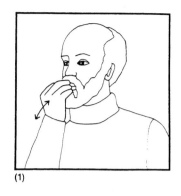
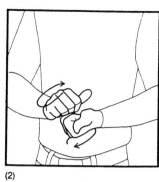

(1) (2)

DIGESTION

The breaking down of food into smaller and simpler parts by the mouth, stomach and intestines. When the food is broken down, it is taken into the bloodstream and used as energy or to make body structures.

> During the process of *digestion*, the mouth breaks the food into pieces that can be swallowed and adds saliva to moisten it, the stomach mixes it and adds acid and the intestine adds chemicals which break the food up into tiny pieces that can be absorbed into the blood.

(1) Sign EAT — the fingertips of the right "flat-O" hand tap the mouth a few times. (MM)
(2) Both "A" hands are together at chest level. Move both hands in alternating circles a few times. (MM)

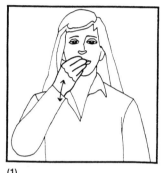
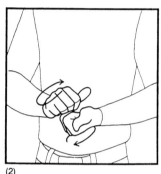

(1) (2)

DIGESTIVE TRACT OR SYSTEM

The glands, organs and structures that help move food in the body and break it down so it can be absorbed. The digestive tract begins at the mouth and includes the esophagus, the stomach, the small and large intestines, and the rectum; it ends at the anus.
See Figures 9 and 10

DIGIT

A toe or finger.
> There are five *digits* on each hand and five *digits* on each foot.

(1) The right index finger points to a finger or toe. (SM)

* Sign FOOT if referring to the foot.

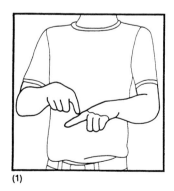

(1)

173

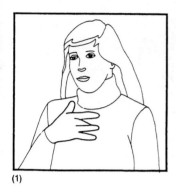
(1)

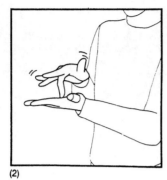
(2)

DIGITALIS

A drug made from the dried leaves of the foxglove plant and used for heart disorders to strengthen or slow down the heartbeat.

Digitalis poisoning or overdose can cause symptoms of nausea, vomiting, headache, weakness, fatigue, drowsiness, confusion, hallucinations, vision problems and possible death.

(1) Sign HEART — the middle finger of the right "eight" hand taps the chest a few times.

(2) Sign MEDICINE — the left "flat" hand faces up at chest level. The middle finger of the right "eight" hand touches the left palm and pivots slightly from left to right a few times. (MM)

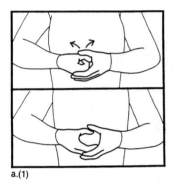
a.(1)

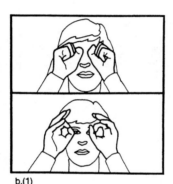
b.(1)

DILATE

To make wider or larger.

*During labor, a woman's cervix will **dilate** to allow the baby to pass through.*

a. (1) The right "S" hand is inside the left "C" hand. Open both hands slightly. (SM)

* *This should be signed only if referring to the cervix dilating.*

b. (1) Both "S" hands are in front of the eyes. Open both hands slightly. (SM)

* *This should be signed only if referring to the pupils dilating.*

DILAUDID

A narcotic drug made from morphine and used to calm a person, cause sleep and relieve pain.

*There is a very high "street demand" for **dilaudid** and if it is taken for a long time, it can cause addiction.*

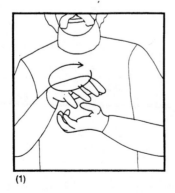
(1)

DILUTE

To make something weaker or thinner by adding a liquid.

When a solution is injected into a vein, the blood will dilute it.

(1) Sign MIX — both "claw" hands face each other at chest level. Move the right hand in a circular movement, keeping the left hand still. (MM)

DILUTE, *continued*

(2) Sign BECOME — the right "flat" hand is on top of the left "flat" hand. Twist both hands so that the left hand ends on top of the right hand. (SM)

(3) Sign WEAK — The left "flat" hand faces right at chest level. The fingertips of the right "claw" hand touch the left palm. Pivot the right hand slightly, keeping the fingers in place. (MM)

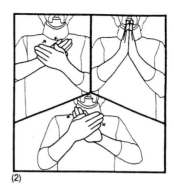
(2)

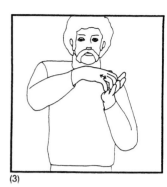
(3)

DIMETHYL SULFOXIDE

A colorless liquid with little odor used as a solvent on machines; better known as D.M.S.O.. Dimethyl sulfoxide is also used by veterinarians and in some cases, humans have used it for aches and pains.

Although **dimethyl sulfoxide** *has no real odor, after it is absorbed into the skin, the breath will have a strong smell of oysters.*

DIPHTHERIA

A severe, infectious disease caused by a bacteria which attacks the respiratory tract and makes a poison. A membrane may form in the throat, causing breathing trouble. Symptoms of diphtheria are a headache, fever, sore throat and weakness.

Diphtheria can be vaccinated against and a baby should start getting shots by three months of age.

(1) The right "D" hand faces in and brushes down the throat a few times. (MM)

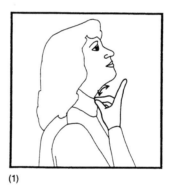
(1)

DIPLOPIA

A vision disorder causing objects to be seen as double; also called double vision.

Diplopia may be caused by astigmatism, a lens which is not in place or the muscles which control eye movement not working correctly.

(1) Sign SEE — the right "V" hand faces in at eye level and moves slightly forward. (SM)

(2) Sign TWICE — the left "flat" hand faces up at chest level. The middle finger of the right "V" hand brushes up the left palm. (SM)

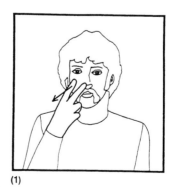
(1)

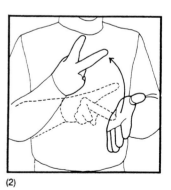
(2)

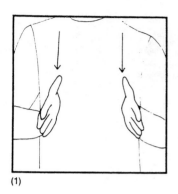
(1)

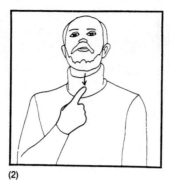
(2)

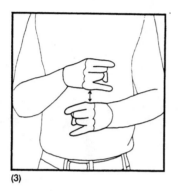
(3)

DIPSOMANIAC

A person who has an uncontrollable craving for alcohol.

Dipsomaniac is another word for an alcoholic.

(1) Sign PERSON — both "flat" hands face each other at chest level. Move both hands down to waist level. (SM)
(2) The index finger of the right "one" hand moves down the throat. (SM)
(3) The index fingers and little fingers of both hands are extended, both hands facing in at chest levels. Tap the hands a few times. (MM)

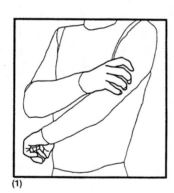
(1)

DIRECT PRESSURE

The action of pushing down on top of something.

Severe bleeding can usually be controlled with direct pressure over the wound.

(1) The right "claw" hand grabs the left upper arm. (SM)

* *This should be signed at the area where direct pressure is applied.*

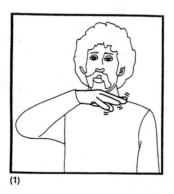
(1)

DIRTY

Soiled or not clean.

Dirty wounds, surgical instruments, needles or bandages can all lead to infections.

(1) The right "five" hand faces down under the chin. Wiggle the fingers. (SM)

DISABILITY

A physical or mental condition in which a person's ability to function has been changed and may interfere with normal living. In legal medicine, partial or total loss of mental or physical abilities due to injury or disease.

All living things, especially humans, have the ability to adapt to a disability or handicap and live useful, rewarding lives.

a. (1) Both "D" hands cross at chest level. (SM)
b. (1) Fingerspell "D-A".

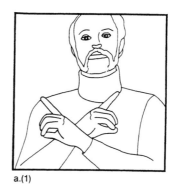
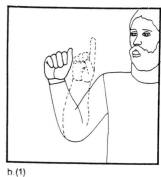

a.(1)   b.(1)

DISCHARGE

The flowing away of something from the body.

A discharge may be made up of mucus, blood, pus, urine or feces.

(1) The fingertips of the right "five" hand touch the right ear and move out away from it, the fingers wiggle at the same time. (MM)

* This refers only to discharge from the ear. This can be signed at the area of the discharge.

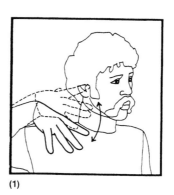

(1)

DISCHARGED (FROM HOSPITAL)

The act of being released from a hospital.

Usually a doctor will suggest a patient be discharged from the hospital when it is no longer necessary to closely watch his medical condition.

(1) The left "flat" hand faces up at chest level. The right "flat" hand brushes out on the left palm. (SM)

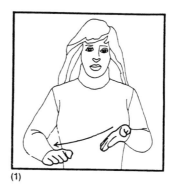

(1)

DISCOLORATION

An abnormal change of color.

Discoloration may occur when a part of the body is hit by a hard object because small blood vessels under the skin are broken and blood leaks out into the area.

(1) Sign CHANGE — the right "A" hand is on top of the left "A" hand. Twist both hands so that the left hand ends on top of the right hand. (SM)
(2) Sign COLOR — the right "five" hand faces in under the chin. Wiggle the fingers. (MM)

* The specific thing, such as eye or skin, should be signed before CHANGE and COLOR if known.

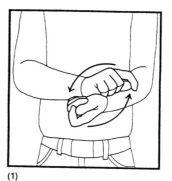
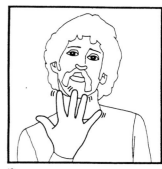

(1)   (2)

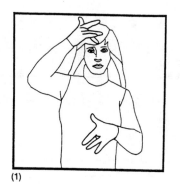

DISEASE

A sickness, illness or infection which makes a person not healthy and causes the body or a part of the body not to work normally.

A person can help avoid disease by improving his diet, exercising and changing his style of living.

(1) The middle finger of the right "eight" hand touches the forehead and the middle finger of the left "eight" hand touches the stomach. (SM)

* The facial expression should show pain or sickness.

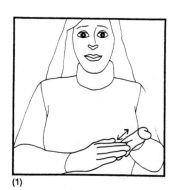

DISINFECT

To rid something of germs which could cause an infection or disease.

Hospitals disinfect everything to prevent diseases from being spread.

(1) Sign CLEAN — the left "flat" hand faces up at chest level. The right "flat" hand brushes down the palm of the left hand. (MM)

* The facial expression should reflect exaggerated "cleanliness".

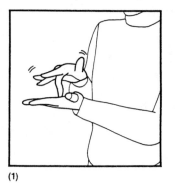

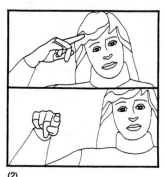

DISINFECTANT

A substance which kills germs that could cause an infection or disease. Disinfectant is another name for a germicide.

Common disinfectants are chlorine, formaldehyde, alcohol, hydrogen peroxide and boric acid.

(1) Sign MEDICINE — the left "flat" hand faces up at chest level. The middle finger of the right "eight" hand touches the left palm and pivots slightly from left to right a few times. (MM)

(2) Sign FOR — the index finger of the right "one" hand touches the forehead, then turns out so that the finger points out. (SM)

(3) Sign CLEAN — the left "flat" hand faces up at chest level. The right "flat" hand brushes down the palm of the left hand. (SM)

* The facial expression should reflect exaggerated "cleanliness".

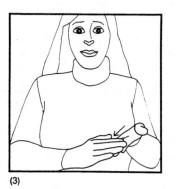

DISK

A flat, round structure.

Disks made of cartilage act as cushions between the vertebrae of the spinal column.

(1) Both bent index fingers and thumbs touch imitating the shape of a disk. Then the index finger and thumb of the right hand move slightly up and down between the index finger and thumb of the left hand. (MM)

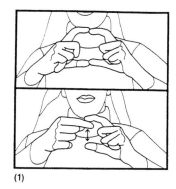

(1)

DISLOCATION

The movement of a part of the body out of its normal place, especially when a bone moves out of its place in a joint. The dislocation of a joint results in pain and swelling, and the joint will look deformed.

Dislocations are usually caused by a fall or a blow.

(1) Both bent "V" hands face in at chest level, the knuckles touching. Drop the right hand down slightly. (SM)

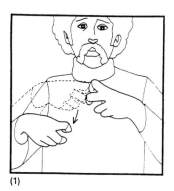

(1)

DISORDER

In medicine, an upset in physical or mental health resulting in a part of the body not working normally.

Nearsightedness and farsightedness are common vision disorders.

(1) The right bent "V" hand faces out and the left bent "V" hand faces in, both at chest level. Twist both hands in opposite directions a few times. (MM)

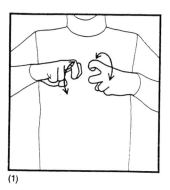

(1)

DISORGANIZATION

The state of being broken up or poorly arranged.

When a virus attacks a cell, it will cause disorganization of the cell by making new viruses.

(1) The right "claw" hand faces out at chest level and the left "claw" hand faces in at chest level. Twist both hands in opposite directions a few times. (MM)

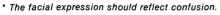
* The facial expression should reflect confusion.

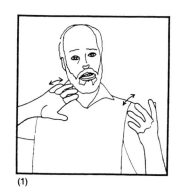

(1)

179

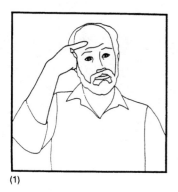
(1)

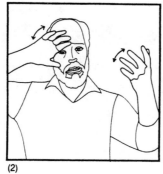
(2)

DISORIENTATION

The state of not knowing where one is or not recognizing familiar things.

A blow to the head, unconsciousness and high fevers can all cause disorientation.

(1) Sign MIND — the index finger of the right "one" hand touches the forehead. (SM)

(2) Sign CONFUSED — the right "five" hand faces out and the left "five" hand faces in, both at head level. Twist the hands from left to right a few times. (MM)

* The facial expression should reflect confusion.

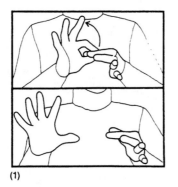
(1)

DISPLACEMENT

A movement of a structure from its normal or usual place or position.

A dislocation is the displacement of a bone.

(1) The left "F" hand faces down at chest level. The right "F" hand faces out with the fingers locking. Move the right hand away from the left ending in a "five" hand. (SM)

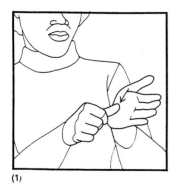
(1)

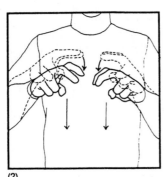
(2)

DISSECTION

The cutting up or cutting away of a structure so it can be studied.

Dissection is used to teach students how organs, structures and tissues are put together and what they look like.

(1) Sign CUT — the left "flat" hand faces right at chest level. The thumb of the right "A" hand moves down the left palm as if imitating cutting. (SM)

(2) Sign ANALYZE — both bent "V" hands face down at chest level. Drop both hands down slightly a few times and at the same time, moving them down to waist level. (MM)

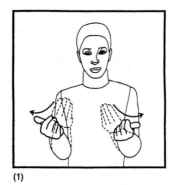
(1)

DISSOLVE

To cause a solid to break up and be absorbed by a liquid.

When doing surgery inside the body, a surgeon may use special stitches (sutures) that will dissolve inside the body after healing.

(1) Sign MELT — both "flat-O" hands face up at chest level. While moving the hands down sideways, brush the thumbs across the other fingers, ending in "A" hands. (SM)

DISTENTION

Being inflated or stretched out.

Distention of the uterus occurs during pregnancy as the baby grows.

(1) Both "C" hands face each other at chest level and move slightly out towards the sides. (SM)

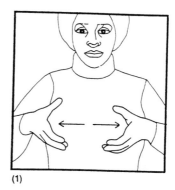

(1)

DISTORTION

The act or condition of being twisted or bent out of shape.

Astigmatism will cause distortion of images.

(1) The right "V" hand faces in at chest level. The left "V" hand faces out at chest level. Twist both hands so that the right hand faces out and the left hand faces in. (SM)

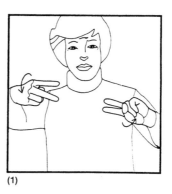

(1)

DIURETIC

A substance which causes the body to produce more urine.

Diuretics act by causing the cells in the kidneys to let more fluid out or by sending more blood to the kidneys to be filtered and cleaned, resulting in more urine being made.

(1) Sign MEDICINE — the left "flat" hand faces up at chest level. The middle finger of the right "eight" hand touches the left palm and the pivots slightly from left to right a few times. (MM)

(2) Sign CAUSE — both "A" hands face up at chest level. Open both hands to the left side, ending in "five" hands. (SM)

(3) The right "T" hand faces out at chest level and shakes from left to right a few times. (MM)

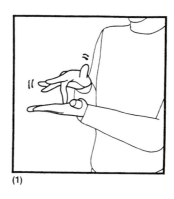

(1)

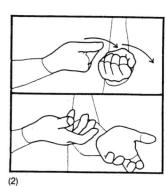

(2)

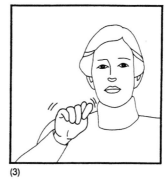

(3)

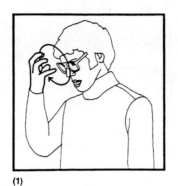
(1)

DIZZINESS

A feeling of spinning or falling.

Dizziness may be caused by an ear infection, alcohol, poisoning, some diseases and some drugs.

(1) The right "claw" hand faces in at head level and moves in counterclockwise circles a few times. (MM)

DMSO

See DIMETHYL SULFOXIDE

DNA

See DEOXYRIBONUCLEIC ACID

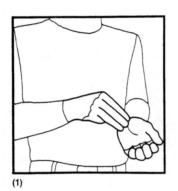
(1)

DOCTOR

A person who is trained in a certain field and has been licensed to dispense drugs, diagnose and treat injuries and diseases and educate people.

Physicians, surgeons, dentists, ophthamologists and veterinarians are all doctors.

(1) The right "M" hand touches the left inside wrist. (DM)

DOLOPHINE®

See METHADONE

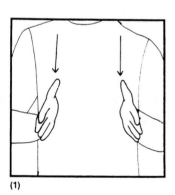
(1)

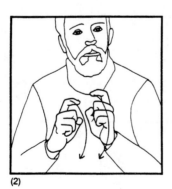
(2)

DONOR

A person who gives blood, tissue or an organ to be used in another person.

In most cases except blood donors, the donor of a body part is someone who has recently died.

(1) Sign PERSON — both "flat" hands face each other at chest level. Move both hands down to waist level. (SM)

(2) Both bent "V" hands face each other at chest level. Drop both hands down slightly. (SM)

* The specific thing, such as blood, an organ, or a body part, should be signed or fingerspelled first before these signs, if known.

DOPE

The slang term for a narcotic or drug used illegally.

Marijuana is also called **dope**.

a. (1) Sign MARIJUANA — the fingertips of the right "F" hand touch the mouth. (SM)

b. (1) The right "S" hand repeatedly hits the left inside elbow. (MM)

* *These are two slang signs for dope, marijuana and a heroin fix. The specific drug should be signed or fingerspelled.*

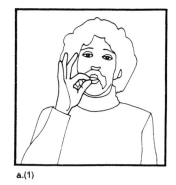

a.(1)

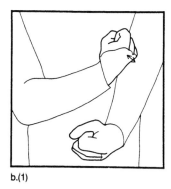

b.(1)

DORIDEN®

A drug used to help people sleep and to relax someone before surgery; the trade name under which glutethimide is sold.

Using large amounts of **Doriden®** *for a long time can cause addiction.*

DORSAL

Referring to the back or an area near the back. Dorsal is the opposite of ventral. The vertebral column runs down the dorsal side of the body.

DOSE

A certain amount of a medicine which is taken at one time.

It is important to take the prescribed **dose** *of a medicine because if too much is taken, an overdose could occur and if not enough is taken, the medicine may not do what it is supposed to.*

(1) Sign MEDICINE — the left "flat" hand faces up at chest level. The middle finger of the right "eight" hand touches the left palm and the hand pivots slightly from left to right a few times. (MM)

(2) Sign HOW MANY — both "S" hands face up at chest level and move up into "five" hands, facing in. (SM)

(3) The left "flat" hand faces right at chest level. The index finger of the right "one" hand touches the left palm. Move both hands back. (SM)

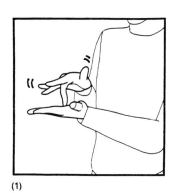

(1)

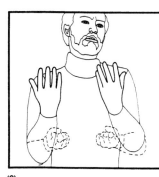

(2)

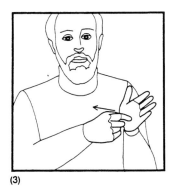

(3)

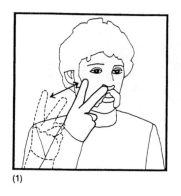
(1)
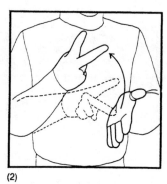
(2)

DOUBLE VISION

A vision disorder causing objects to be seen as double.

Diplopia is another word for double vision.

(1) Sign SEE — the right "V" hand faces in at eye level. Move the hand out. (SM)
(2) Sign TWICE — the left "flat" hand faces up at chest level. The middle finger of the right "V"' hand brushes up the left palm. (SM)

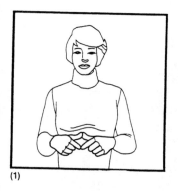
(1)
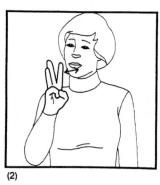
(2)

DOUCHE

The pouring of a stream of medicated or plain water into or on a part of the body to clean the area or to treat a problem.

Use of a douche in the vagina is not an effective form of birth control.

(1) Sign VAGINA — the index fingers and thumbs of both "L" hands touch, the palms face in. (SM)
(2) Sign WATER — the index finger of the right "W" hand taps the mouth, the palm faces left. (SM)
(3) The index finger of the right "one" hand moves into the left "S" hand. (SM)
(4) Sign CLEAN — the left "flat" hand faces up at chest level. The right "flat" hand brushes down the left palm. (SM)

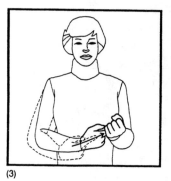
(3)
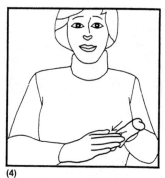
(4)

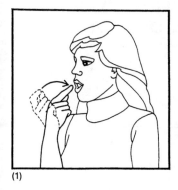
(1)
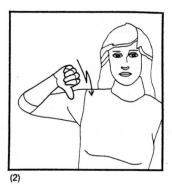
(2)

DOWNERS

The slang name for sedative or depressant drugs which force a person to relax and sleep.

Downers are especially dangerous to a person's health when taken along with alcoholic drinks.

(1) Sign PILL — the thumb and index finger of the right hand touch, the palm faces the mouth. Flick the index finger towards the mouth as if popping a pill into the mouth. (SM)
(2) Sign DOWNER — the right "A" hand with the thumb pointing down, moves down at shoulder level twice. (DM)

* This is a general sign for depressants ("downers"). The specific type of drug should also be fingerspelled and all side effects explained.

184

DOWN'S SYNDROME

A kind of mental retardation caused by an extra chromosome in the cells. Some symptoms of Down's Syndrome are a below normal intelligence, a broad nose, a smaller body size, slanted, almond-shaped eyes and short fingers. Down's Syndrome is also called mongolism but Down's Syndrome is the preferred term.

The chance of having a baby with Down's Syndrome goes up as the age of the mother increases.

DRAINAGE

In medicine, removing or letting fluid flow from a wound or space.

Drainage of an area can be helped by placing the patient in a position that will allow free flow of a fluid or by inserting a tube into the area.

(1) The left "four" hand faces in at chest level. The right "four" hand also faces in. The index finger of the right hand touches the little finger of the left hand, then moves down. (MM)

* This should be signed at the area of the drainage.

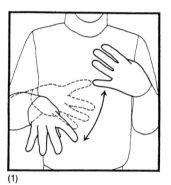
(1)

DREAM

A series of images, ideas, and emotions occurring in certain stages of sleep.

During some dreams, the eyes will move (rapid eye movements).

(1) The index finger of the right "one" hand touches the forehead and moves out, at the same time, bend and straighten the index finger a few times. (SM)

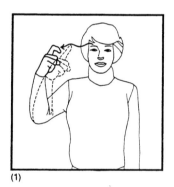
(1)

DRESSING

A covering placed over a wound or injured part to help stop bleeding, absorb blood or secretions, to keep the area clean or to lessen pain.

A dressing should be sterile or as clean as possible.

(1) Sign BANDAGE — the left "B" hand faces in at chest level. The right "B" hand also faces in and moves around the left hand as if imitating wrapping a bandage. (MM)

* This can be signed at the area where the bandage is being applied.

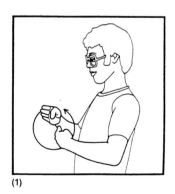
(1)

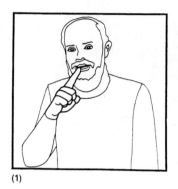
(1)

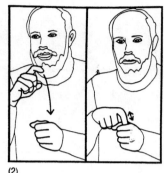
(2)

DRILL

A tool which spins an attachment very rapidly to make holes in something.

In dentistry, a drill is used to make holes in a tooth where it has decayed so a filling can be put in or to wear away part of the tooth so a crown can be put on.

(1) The index finger of the right "one" hand points to a tooth. (SM)
(2) The left "S" hand faces in at chest level. The index finger of the right "one" hand moves down into the left fist and taps a few times. (MM)

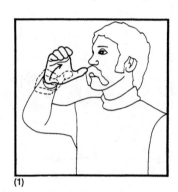
(1)

DRINK

To take in a liquid through the mouth, to swallow a liquid.

It is important to drink plenty of water and fluids because they are needed for normal body activities.

(1) The right "C" hand moves towards the mouth as if taking a drink. (SM)

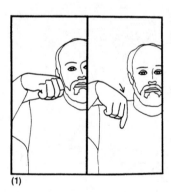
(1)

DRIP

The release of a liquid drop by drop.

A tube may be placed in a vein to drip a medicine into the body slowly.

(1) The right "S" hand faces down at shoulder level. Flick the index finger down several times. (MM)

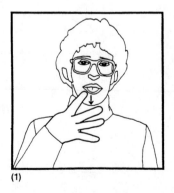
(1)

DROOL

To let saliva or another fluid run from the mouth.

After having dental work done, a person may drool because the mouth is numb.

(1) The index finger of the right "four" hand touches the mouth and moves slowly down and the tongue sticks out. (SM)

186

DROOPING EYELIDS

Eyelids that are not all the way open.

When a person has overdosed on a drug, he may have droopy eyelids.

(1) Both "G" hands face out at the eyes. The eyes should droop. (SM)

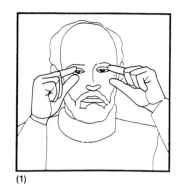
(1)

DROPSY

A collection of fluid in the spaces or tissues of the body. Dropsy is an old term for edema.

The person with dropsy may appear bloated or swollen all over.

(1) Sign BODY — the fingertips of both "flat" hands touch the upper chest and then move down to touch the stomach area. (SM)
(2) Sign WATER — the index finger of the right "W" hand taps the mouth, the palm faces left. (MM)
(3) Both "five" hands face in and move out from the body. The cheeks should also puff out. (SM)

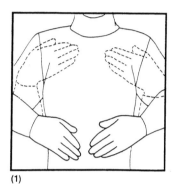
(1)

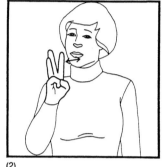
(2)

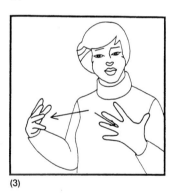
(3)

DROWNING

To die by suffocation in water. (The person cannot breathe because of water being in the airways and lungs, or a reflex closing off the larynx while the person is under water.) A person who is drowning will be unconscious, not breathing and his skin may be blue.

Drowning may be caused by an accident occuring in the water like a head injury, a heart attack, a stroke, exhaustion, fainting or muscle cramps.

a. (1) The left "flat" hand faces down at chest level. The right "A" hand with the thumb extended faces left and moves down from the left hand. (SM)

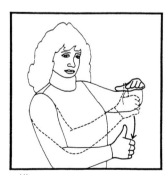
a.(1)

(Continued on next page)

187

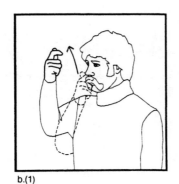

b.(1)

DROWNING, *continued*

b. (1) The index finger and thumb of the right fist grab the nose then move up and out. (SM)

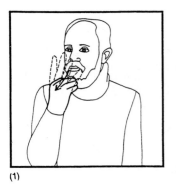

(1)

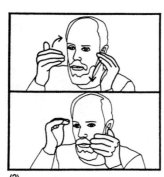

(2)

DROWSINESS

A feeling of sleepiness.

The night before an operation, people may be given a drug that causes drowsiness to relax them and help them sleep.

(1) The right "five" hand faces in at eye level. Move the hand out slightly, ending in a "flat-O" hand. (SM)

(2) Both "cupped" hands face down at eye level. Alternately twist both hands in and out a few times. (MM)

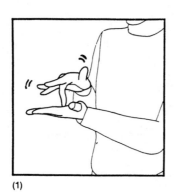

(1)

DRUG

A substance which changes the body's or mind's activities and is used to diagnose, prevent or treat a disease.

A drug may provide needed temporary help to a sick or injured person but used incorrectly, may only relieve symptoms and do nothing for the cause of a problem.

(1) Sign MEDICINE — the left "flat" hand faces up at chest level. The middle finger of the right "eight" hand touches the left palm and the pivots slightly from left to right. (MM)

DRUG TREATMENT CENTER

A place where a person can get help because he uses a drug a lot, is addicted to a drug or has had a drug overdose.

Drug Treatment Centers are located in most large cities.

DRUNK

A condition caused by drinking too much alcohol.

A person can be tested to see how drunk *he is by checking how much alcohol is in the blood or how much alcohol is in the air breathed out.*

a. (1) The right fist with the thumb and index finger extended, faces out and moves down in front of the body. (SM)

b. (1) The right "A" hand with the thumb extended faces out and moves down in front of the body. (SM)

c. (1) The right "five" hand faces down and moves across the forehead from left to right, and at the same time, wiggle the fingers. (SM)

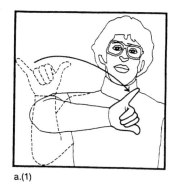

a.(1)

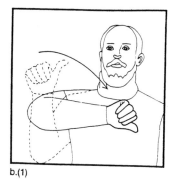

b.(1)

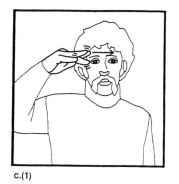

c.(1)

D.T.'S

See DELIRIUM TREMENS

DUCT

A narrow tube.

Duct is usually used for a passageway that takes the secretions made in a gland to another part of the body.

DULL

Not sharp; not mentally alert.

When referring to aches or pain, a doctor may ask if the pain is dull *or sharp.*

DUODENUM

The first part of the small intestine. The duodenum, about 10 inches long, is where various chemicals are mixed with the food to further the process of digestion. *See Figure 9*

189

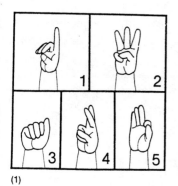
(1)

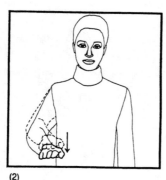
(2)

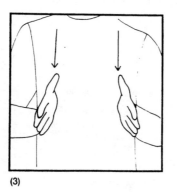
(3)

DWARF

An abnormally short person.

> A person could be a **dwarf** because of a bone growth problem, a hormone or gland abnormality or lack of a nutrient.

(1) Fingerspell "D-W-A-R-F".
(2) Sign SHORT — the right "flat" hand faces down at chest level. Move the hand down slightly. (SM)
(3) Sign PERSON — both "flat" hands face each other at chest level. Move both hands down to waist level. (SM)

DYSENTERY

A disorder of the intestines in which the lining is irritated. Symptoms are pain in the abdomen, diarrhea with mucus or blood in it, straining to have a bowel movement and perhaps dehydration.

> **Dysentery** can be caused by bacteria, viruses or parasites.

DYSMENORRHEA

Difficult or painful menstruation.

> **Dysmenorrhea** may be caused by an infection in the pelvis, bad mental attitudes towards menstruation, muscle cramps in the uterus or a build-up of blood and fluids in the area.

DYSMNESIA

Problems with or damage to the memory.

> Amnesia traumatica is a form of **dysmnesia**, caused by an injury.

(1) Sign THINK — the index finger of the right "one" hand touches the forehead. (SM)
(2) Sign MEMORIZE — the fingertips of the right "five" hand touch the forehead and then move the hand out slightly into a "S" hand. (SM)

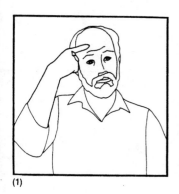
(1)

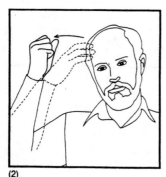
(2)

(Continued on next page)

(3) Sign DAMAGE — the left "five" hand faces up at chest level. The right "five" hand faces down at chest level. Move both hands towards the center, ending in "A" hands with thumbs extended, facing each other.

(4) Continue moving the right hand through to the left and the left through to the right until they cross at the arms. At the same time, move the right hand back to it's original position, ending in a "five" hand facing down and the left hand back to it's original position, ending in an "A" hand facing down. (SM)

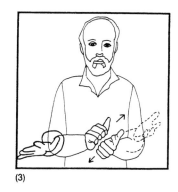
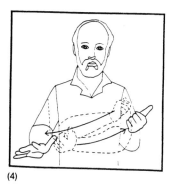

(3) (4)

DYSPLASIA

Abnormal development of tissue, organs or cells.

> *Dysplasia of the hip is a condition in which the socket of the joint is not deep enough to hold the ball of the femur correctly, resulting in pain and arthritis.*

(1) Sign GROW — the right "flat-O" hand moves up through the left fist into a "five" hand. (SM)

(2) Sign WRONG — the right "Y" hand faces in and brushes the chin in a small circular movement. (MM)

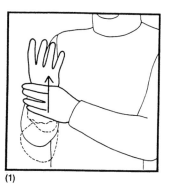
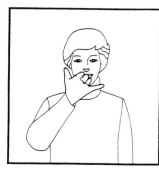

(1) (2)

DYSPNEA

Shortness of breath or difficulty in breathing.

> *Dyspnea is normal when caused by work or exercise, abnormal when caused by lung or heart disease.*

(1) Sign BREATH — both "five" hands move in and out from the chest a few times in short repeated movements. (MM)

* *The facial expression should reflect shortness of breath.*

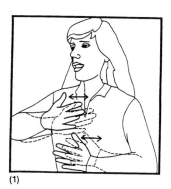

(1)

DYSTROPHY

A disorder caused by defects of nutrition.

> *Dystrophy may also be called dystrophia.*

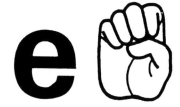

EAR

One of the two structures on either side of the head which enable us to hear. The ear is made up of the outer, middle and inner ear. Besides being the organ of hearing, the structures in the inner ear help us keep our balance. *See Figure 20*

a. (1) The right hand grabs the right ear and shakes it a little. (MM)

b. (1) The index finger of the right "one" hand points to the right ear. (SM)

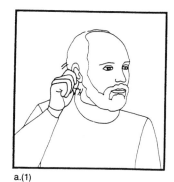

a.(1)

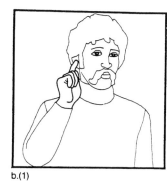

b.(1)

EARACHE

Pain in the ear; also called otalgia or otodynia.

Earaches are usually caused by infections, so a doctor should be seen before the infection causes a hearing impairment or spreads to the skull or brain.

(1) Both "one" hands point to each other and move in and out a few times at the right ear. (MM)

* The facial expression should reflect pain. This can also be signed by twisting both "one" hands in opposite directions a few times.

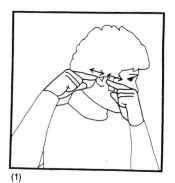

(1)

EARDRUM

The thin, oval membrane which separates the outer ear from the inner ear and which vibrates when sound waves hit it; also called the tympanic membrane. The movements of the eardrum are passed on by the three small bones in the middle ear to the inner parts of the ear, where the movements are sensed and impulses are sent to the brain and the sound is heard. Damage to the eardrum may cause scarring and lower a person's ability to hear. *See Figure 20*

EAR INFECTION

A condition where bacteria or a virus enters the ear and causes pain, irritation and perhaps damage. When someone has an ear infection, there may be pain, inflammation, swelling and perhaps a fever and difficulty in hearing. *(Continued on next page)*

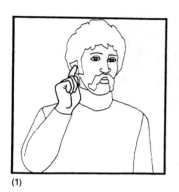

(1)

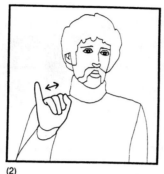

(2)

EAR INFECTION, *continued*

Ear infections can be caused by getting water in the ears, another disease spreading to the ear such as a cold, an ignored sore throat or not properly blowing the nose.

(1) The index finger of the right "one" hand points to the right ear. (SM)

(2) Sign INFECTION — the right "I" hand faces out at chest level and shakes from left to right a few times. (MM)

* Mouth the word "infection" while signing.

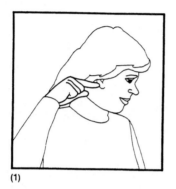

(1)

EAR LOBE

The soft, flexible lower part of the ear.

See Figure 20

People often pierce their ear lobes and then attach ear-rings through the holes.

(1) The index finger of the right "one" hand touches the right earlobe. (SM)

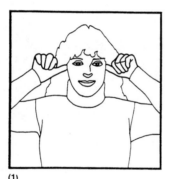

(1)

EAR PLUG

A small piece of plastic rubber or wax put into the opening of the ear to keep out loud noises.

Ear plugs should not be worn when swimming unless medically necessary because they prevent the pressure inside the ear from becoming the same with the pressure outside the ear.

(1) The thumbs of both hands stick in both ears. (SM)

EAR WAX

The waxy, orange colored substance made by special glands in the ear which protects the ear from things which may get in it like dust, bacteria or small insects.

Ear wax can collect in the ear, become hard, and ir-ritate the eardrum or plug the passage, causing tem-porary deafness.

EAT

To take food into the mouth, chew it and swallow it.

It is important to eat a well balanced diet so one gets all the vitamins, minerals, carbohydrates, fats and pro-teins needed for good health.

(Continued on next page)

194

(1) The fingertips of the right "flat-O" hand tap the mouth a few times. (MM)

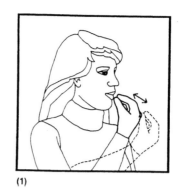

(1)

ECLAMPSIA

A disease a woman may get during pregnancy or just after having a baby. Symptoms of eclampsia are edema, high blood pressure, headaches, nausea, dizziness, having to urinate a lot, convulsions and perhaps coma.

*Good prenatal care will help to avoid getting **eclampsia**.*

ECTOPIC

An organ or structure being in an abnormal position or place.

*An **ectopic** pregnancy is one where the fertilized ovum has attached in the abdomen, ovaries or fallopian tubes (tubal pregnancy).*

ECZEMA

A skin disorder in which there may be inflammation, itching, swelling, blistering, scaling, a rash or a discharge. The cause of eczema is usually unknown but in some cases it is caused by an allergy, a fungal infection, not getting enough of a certain nutrient or uncleanliness.

***Eczema** is not contagious and people with thin, dry skin are more likely to get it.*

EDEMA

A condition where fluid collects in the body. A person with edema will appear puffy and when the skin is pressed in, a dent will be left. Edema may be caused by fluid leaking from the blood vessels into the tissues, heart failure, kidney failure, inflammation or malnutrition.

***Edema** is treated with rest, diuretics, cutting down on salt intake, not drinking many fluids and raising the part of the body with **edema**.*

(Continued on next page)

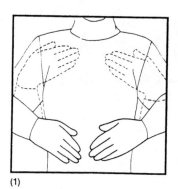

(1)

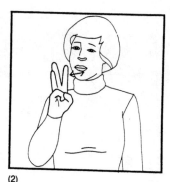

(2)

(1) Sign BODY — both "flat" hands touch the chest then the stomach areas. (SM)
(2) Sign WATER — the index finger of the right "W" hand taps the mouth a few times. (MM)
(3) Both "five" hands move out from the chest and at the same time, the cheeks should puff out. (SM)

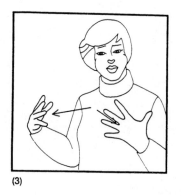

(3)

EEG

See ELECTROENCEPHALOGRAM

EFFECT

The result of an action.

> *Drugs are usually classified by their **effect**, such as stimulants, depressants, tranquilizers and hallucinogens.*

(1) The left "flat" hand faces down at chest level. The right "flat-O" hand is on top of the left hand and moves down into a "five" hand. (SM)

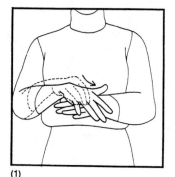

(1)

EFFUSION

The leakage of a body fluid into a space or area of the body.

> *Effusion can be the escape of pus, serum or blood into a cavity.*

EGO

In psychology, the part of the mind that deals with reality and controls behavior. Ego can also mean a person's image or beliefs about himself; self esteem.

(Continued on next page)

EGO, *continued*

In psychoanalysis, the **ego**, along with the id and superego, make up a person's personality.

(1) Fingerspell "E-G-O".

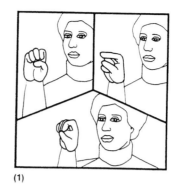

(1)

EGOCENTRIC

Someone not interested in the world around him and only concerned with himself.

Egocentric can also mean a very self-centered person.

a. (1) Both "I" hands face each other and alternately tap the chest a few times. (MM)

b. (1) The right "I" hand taps on the chest. (MM)
(2) The right "I" hand faces left on the chest. The left "C" hand faces in and moves from the right hand out and up. (SM)

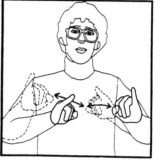

a.(1)

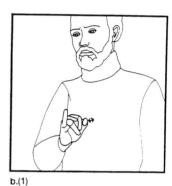

b.(1)

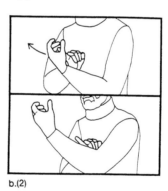

b.(2)

EJACULATION

The release of semen and sperm from a man's penis during orgasm.

Ejaculation occurs during sexual intercourse and masturbation.

(1) The left "one" hand points to the right at chest level. The right "S" hand faces left next to the left hand. Leaving the left hand in place, move the right hand out forward into a "five" hand. (SM)

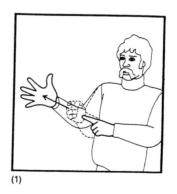

(1)

EKG

See ELECTROCARDIOGRAM

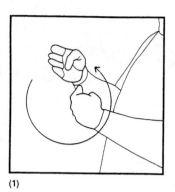
(1)

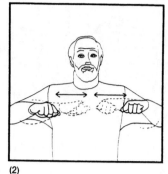
(2)

ELASTIC BANDAGE

A bandage made of a stretchy material and used to apply pressure.

Elastic bandages are easy to use because they are flexible, but care should be taken to not wrap them too tightly because they may interfere with circulation.

(1) Sign BANDAGE — the left "B" hand faces in at chest level. The right "B" hand also faces in and circles out and around the left hand as if imitating wrapping a bandage. (MM)

(2) Both "A" hands face down at chest level and move in and out towards the sides a few times indicating something stretchy. (MM)

ELAVIL®

A drug which acts as a sedative and is used to treat depression; the name under which amitriptyline is sold.

It takes about two or three weeks for Elavil® to work and there may be some common side effects like a dry mouth, tiredness, fainting, constipation, dizziness and eye problems.

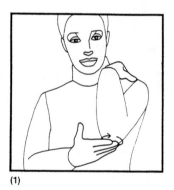
(1)

ELBOW

The joint between the arm and forearm which allows the arm to bend. *See Figure 3*

(1) The fingertips of the right "flat" hand make a small circle on the left elbow. (SM)

ELECTRA COMPLEX

In psychology, the sexual feelings a daughter has for her father.

The Electra complex is the reverse of the Oedipus complex.

ELECTRICAL BURN

An injury to tissues caused by electricity.

The damage caused by electrical burns is usually deeper than it appears.

(Continued on next page)

(1) Sign ELECTRICITY — both "X" hands face in at chest level. Move both hands in and out towards the sides a few times. (MM)
(2) Sign TOUCH — the middle finger of the right "eight" hand touches the back of the left "flat" hand. (SM)
(3) Fingerspell "B-U-R-N".

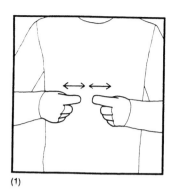
(1)

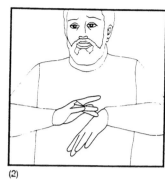
(2)

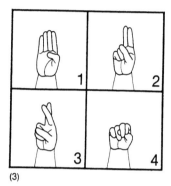
(3)

ELECTRICITY

A kind of energy caused by the movement of very small particles, which has a negative charge when moving through a substance (usually a liquid or metal).

Care should be taken using anything with electricity running through it because an electric shock can cause breathing and the heart to stop.

(1) Both "X" hands face in at chest level. Move both hands in and out towards the sides a few times. (MM)

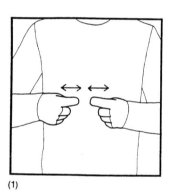
(1)

ELECTRIC SHOCK

The result of electricity passing through a part of the body. Injury caused by an electric shock may vary from a slight burn to unconsciousness caused by paralysis of the heart and respiratory muscles.

Care should be taken when touching or moving a victim of electric shock to see that electricity has been shut off.

(1) Sign ELECTRICITY — both "X" hands face in at chest level. Move both hands in and out towards the sides a few times. (MM)
(2) The index fingers of both "one" hands tap the sides of the head a few times.

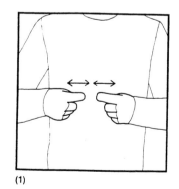
(1)

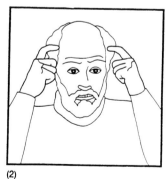
(2)

199

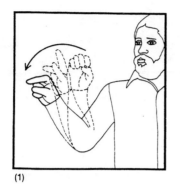
(1)

ELECTROCARDIOGRAM

The record or picture made by a machine which measures the electrical activity of the heart; also called E.K.G.

The electrocardiogram can help a doctor see if the heart is beating in a normal pattern or if there is any damage to the heart muscle.

(1) Fingerspell "E-K-G".

* *This may need to be explained fully before fingerspelling "E-K-G".*

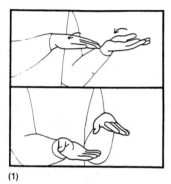
(1)

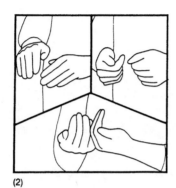
(2)

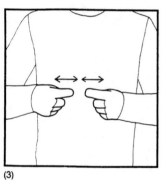
(3)

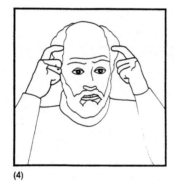
(4)

ELECTROCUTION

Killing a person or a tissue by using electricity.

Electrocution can occur in the home, even with low voltages, so when handling electric appliances, plugs or cords, a person should be careful.

(1) Sign DEAD — the left "flat" hand faces up at chest level and the right "flat" hand faces down. Turn both hands to the right so that the left hand ends facing down and the right hand ends facing up. (SM)

(2) Sign HOW — both "four" hands face down at chest level. Turn both hands down and around, pivoting on the fingertips then ending in "cupped" hands facing up. (SM)

* *The facial expression should reflect questioning.*

(3) Sign ELECTRICITY — both "X" hands face in at chest level. Move both hands in and out towards the sides a few times. (MM)

(4) The index fingers of both "one" hands tap the sides of the head a few times.

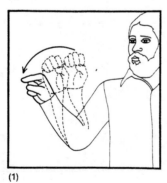
(1)

ELECTROENCEPHALOGRAM

The record or picture made by a machine which measures the electrical activity of the brain; also called E.E.G.

The electroencephalogram may allow a doctor to detect a brain disease or disorder such as epilepsy or a tumor.

(1) Fingerspell "E-E-G".

* *This may need to be explained fully before fingerspelling "E-E-G".*

ELECTROLYSIS

The killing of an area or tissue by passing electricity through it.

Electrolysis is often used to get rid of unwanted hair by destroying the root.

200

ELECTROSHOCK

Referring to producing shock by using electricity to the brain.

Electroshock is sometimes used when treating mental disorders.

(1) Sign ELECTRICITY — both "X" hands face in at chest level. Move both hands in and out towards the sides a few times. (MM)

(2) The index fingers of both "one" hands tap the sides of the head a few times.

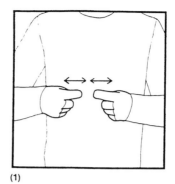 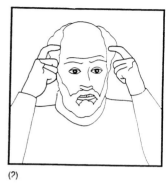

(1)   (?)

ELEVATE

To move something up or lift something higher.

If a person has bleeding or edema in an arm or leg, he should elevate that part.

(1) Sign RAISE — both "flat" hands face up at waist level and move up to chest level. (SM)

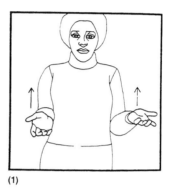

(1)

ELIMINATION

The removal of wastes from the body, done mostly by the kidneys and digestive tract.

Elimination of body wastes occurs through the lungs and skin but most wastes are gotten rid of through urination and bowel movements.

(1) The left "flat" hand faces up at chest level. The right "claw" hand grabs the left palm and then moves down into a "five" hand as if imitating grabbing something and throwing it away.(SM)

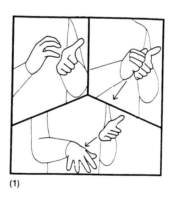

(1)

ELIXIR

A sweetened, good-smelling liquid, often containing alcohol, combined with a medicine.

Elixirs are a commonly used form of oral medication.

(1) Sign MEDICINE — the left "flat" hand faces up at chest level. The middle finger of the right "eight" hand touches the left palm and pivots slightly from left to right a few times. (MM)

(Continued on next page)

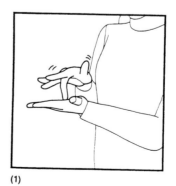

(1)

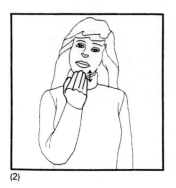

(2)

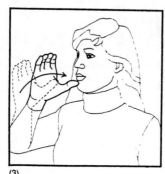

(3)

ELIXIR, *continued*

(2) Sign SWEET — the fingertips of the right "flat" hand brush down the chin a few times. (MM)
(3) Sign DRINK — the right "C" hand moves towards the mouth as if imitating taking a drink. (SM)

EMBOLISM

The blocking of a blood vessel by something being carried in the blood. An embolism could be caused by a clump of bacteria, air, fat, cells, parasites or more commonly a blood clot.

*When an **embolism** occurs, there is usually tissue death because the blood supply is cut off.*

EMBOLUS

A substance, moving in a clump through a blood vessel.

*An **embolus** may be made up of bacteria, air, fat, cells, parasites or a blood clot and when it plugs a vessel it is called an embolism.*

EMBRYO

A baby in the early stage of development in the mother's uterus. The embryo stage of development lasts from fertilization of the ovum until the third month. *See Figure 14*

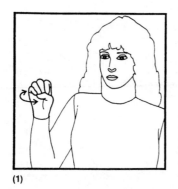

(1)

EMERGENCY

An event that happens unexpectedly and is very serious.

*In medicine, an **emergency** of any sort requires attention or action quickly.*

(1) The right "E" hand faces out at chest level and twists from left to right a few times. (MM)

EMERGENCY CHILDBIRTH

Giving birth to a baby before it is expected or when the mother cannot be taken to a hospital in time.

In emergency childbirth, one should try to find medical help or someone who is experienced in childbirth; once the baby has been born, the mother and baby should be taken to the hospital.

EMERGENCY ROOM

An area in a hospital or clinic where people who are injured or who suddenly become sick are taken to get immediate care.

A hospital's emergency room is usually open 24 hours a day and always has a doctor available.

(1) The right "E" hand faces out at chest level and twists from left to right a few times. (MM)
(2) Both "flat" hands face each other at the sides of the body. Move both hands towards the center so that they both face in, the right hand in front of the left hand. (SM)

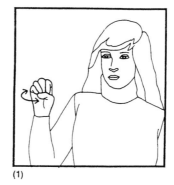
(1)

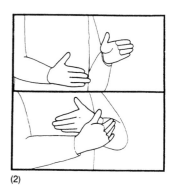
(2)

EMERGENCY SPLINT

A splint made with whatever materials are available at the time of an accident and which are used to hold a part of the body still until the injury can be seen by a doctor.

Emergency splints can be made from a pillow, blanket, cardboard, boards, newspapers or sticks.

(1) The right "E" hand faces out at chest level and twists from left to right a few times. (MM)
(2) The left "flat" hand faces down at chest level with the elbow bent. The right "flat" hand touches the top of the left arm and then turns over to touch the bottom of the left arm. (SM)

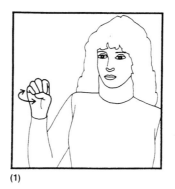
(1)

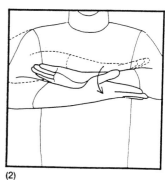
(2)

EMETIC

A substance that causes vomiting.

An emetic may cause vomiting by affecting the central nervous system or by irritating the stomach.

a. (1) Sign EAT — the fingertips of the right "flat-O" hand tap the mouth a few times. (MM)
b. (1) Sign DRINK — the right "C" hand moves towards the mouth as if imitating taking a drink. (SM)

* *Sign EAT or DRINK, whichever applies.*

(Continued on next page)

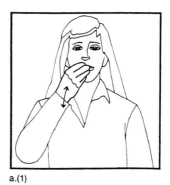
a.(1)

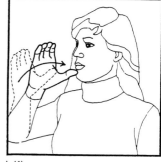
b.(1)

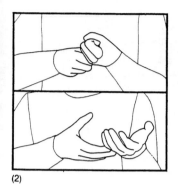
(2)

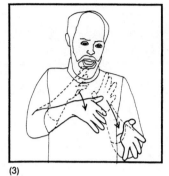
(3)

(2) Sign CAUSE — both "S" hands face up at chest level. Drop both hands down to the left side into "five" hands. (SM)

(3) Sign VOMIT — both "five" hands face each other and move out and down from the mouth as if imitating throwing up. (SM)

EMISSARY VEINS

Veins which go through the skull and carry blood from the sinuses inside the skull to the veins outside. These veins may enable an infection on the face to get inside the skull and to the brain.

An infection such as a boil on the cheek should get special attention because of the danger of it traveling along the emissary veins and affecting the brain.

EMOLLIENT

A substance that eases pain and softens an area of the body.

Hand lotions contain emollients to soften skin.

EMOTIONS

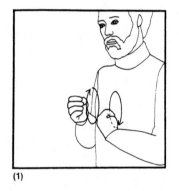
(1)

A group of mental states or feeling which, when they change, can also cause changes in the body's activities.

Some of the emotions are joy, hate, fear, love, and anger; when our feeling change from one to another our heart rate, breathing rate, blood flow or gland activity may change.

(1) Both "E" hands face out at chest level and move in alternating circles towards the center. (MM)

EMOTIONAL DISTURBANCE

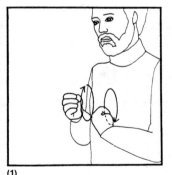
(1)

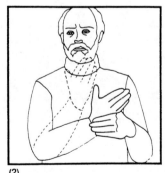
(2)

Another term for mental illness.

A person suffering from emotional disturbances may have a decrease in some emotions, may lose the ability to feel or express some emotions or the emotions he feels or expresses may not make sense.

(1) Sign EMOTIONS — both "E" hands face out at chest level and move in alternating circles towards the center. (MM)

(2) Sign DISTURB — the left "flat" hand faces in at chest level. The right "flat" hand faces in and moves down to touch the left hand. (SM)

204

EMPHYSEMA

A chronic lung disease in which the air spaces in the lungs become enlarged and the tissue between them becomes stiffer. A person with emphysema will have difficulty breathing and a cough, and the lungs will be larger than normal, causing a large, barrel-shaped chest.

Smokers have a greater chance of getting emphysema than non-smokers.

EMULSION

A combination of two liquids which won't mix together.

A mixture of oil and water is an emulsion because the oil will stay as small drops instead of blending with the water.

(1) Both "Y" hands face each other at chest level and turn in as if pouring something from the thumbs. (SM)

(2) Sign MIX — the left "claw" hand faces up at chest level. The right "claw" hand faces down and moves in a circular movement towards the left above the left hand. (MM)

(3) Sign SEPARATE — the left "cupped" hand faces up at chest level. The right "cupped" hand faces down, touching the left hand. Move the right hand up. (SM)

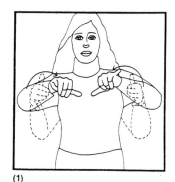
(1)

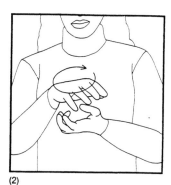
(2)

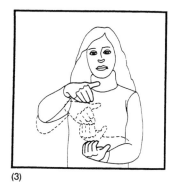
(3)

ENAMEL

The very hard, white substance covering the outside of the tooth. Enamel is the hardest substance in the body. *See Figure 25*

ENCEPHALITIS

Inflammation of the brain caused by a virus (togavirus) infecting the brain resulting from another disease such as measles, influenza or chickenpox. Symptoms of encephalitis are a fever, dizziness, nausea and sleepiness.

Encephalitis is dangerous because it can cause injury to the brain which may result in shaking, loss of control over movement, paralysis or loss of intelligence.

ENDOCRINE GLAND

A type of gland which puts its products directly into the blood, where they are carried to all parts of the body and have certain effects on other tissues or organs. Endocrine glands, also called ductless glands, secrete one or more hormones.

Some of the endocrine glands are the pituitary gland, the adrenal glands, the thyroid gland, the ovaries and the testes.

ENDOCRINOLOGY

The study of the ductless or endocrine glands; how they work and diseases associated with them.

Endocrinology has allowed us to discover the cause of some disorders, such as diabetes, dwarfism and goiter, and to find cures for them.

ENDODONTICS

An area of dentistry which deals with the causes, treatment and prevention of diseases affecting the pulp of a tooth.

A common endodontic procedure is a root canal treatment.

(1) Sign SPECIALIZE — the left "B" hand faces right at chest level. The right "B" hand faces left on top of the left hand. Move the right hand straight out on the left index finger. (SM)

(2) The index finger of the right "one" hand points to a tooth. (SM)

(3) Sign DISEASE — the middle finger of the right "eight" hand touches the forehead and the middle finger of the left "eight" hand touches the stomach. (SM)

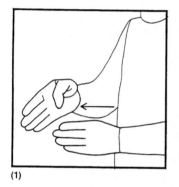
(1)

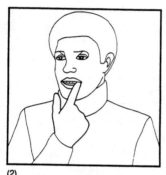
(2)

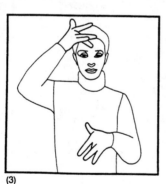
(3)

ENDOLABYRINTHITIS

Inflammation of the membranes in the ear.

ENDOLYMPH

Transparent fluid in the labrynth of the ear.

ENDOMETRIOSIS

A disease in which the tissue which usually lines the uterus is found in the abdominal cavity. Endometriosis may result in cysts or tumors forming on the fallopian tubes, ovaries or the lining of the abdominal cavity.

Endometriosis may cause painful menstrual periods.

ENDOMETRIUM

The mucus membrane lining in the uterus. After fertilization, the ovum attaches to the endometrium, later forming the placenta. *See Figure 12*

ENDOSCOPE

An instrument made up of a tube with a special design allowing a doctor to look inside an organ or space.

The use of an endoscope may prevent major surgery because it can be put into the body through a natural opening or a small incision to allow a doctor to see without making a large incision.

ENEMA

The insertion of a liquid into the rectum or lower colon through the anus.

Different kinds of enemas may be given to cause a bowel movement, to give a medication or anesthetic or to take an X-ray of the area.

(1) Sign WATER — the index finger of the right "W" hand taps the mouth a few times. (MM)
(2) The left "S" hand faces in at waist level. The thumb of the right "A" hand moves up into the fist of the left hand. (SM)

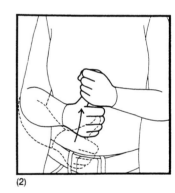

(1)

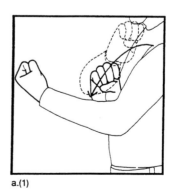

(2)

ENERGY

The ability or the power available to do work. Energy is produced in the body when oxygen combines with fats and sugars in the cells.

Energy comes in different forms such as motion, light, heat and sound.

a. (1) The left "S" hand faces in with the arm slightly bent at the elbow. The right "E" hand touches the left upper arm then arcs down to touch the elbow. (SM)

* This is a newer sign and may need to be explained before signing.

b. (1) The left arm is slightly bent at the elbow. The right "flat" hand touches the left upper arm then arcs down to touch the elbow. (SM)

* This is also a newer sign and may need to be explained before signing.

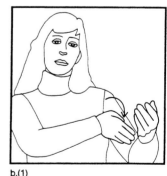

a.(1)

b.(1)

ENVIRONMENT

The surroundings or conditions around us that affect our bodies and lives.

A deaf person cannot hear sounds in his environment.

(1) The left "one" hand faces out with the index finger pointing up. The right "E" hand moves around the left index finger. (SM)

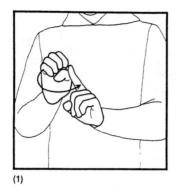

(1)

ENZYME

A type of protein made in the body which helps to change other molecules or substances. Enzymes help move materials into and out of cells, help carry out body activities and help make chemical reactions take place correctly and more quickly.

Digestive juices have many different kinds of enzymes in them which help break foods down into simple parts which can be taken into the body.

EPHEDRINE

A drug used to relieve asthma and lung problems, hay fever and some muscle disorders.

Ephedrine works much like adrenalin.

EPIDEMIC

The spread of an infectious disease which effects many people at the same time in the same area.

Epidemics can occur when people are in close contact with each other such as in schools or dormitories.

(1) Sign DISEASE — the middle finger of the right "eight" hand touches the forehead and the middle finger of the left "eight" hand touches the stomach.
(2) Sign SPREAD — both "flat-O" hands face down at chest level and move forward into "five" hands. (SM)

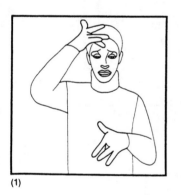

(1)

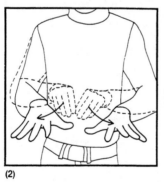

(2)

EPIDERMIS

One of the two layers of the skin, the thinner, outer layer.

The epidermis is made up of several layers of flattened, dead cells which are constantly being cast off and replaced from below.

(1) Sign SKIN — the index finger and thumb of the right hand grab the right cheek. (SM)

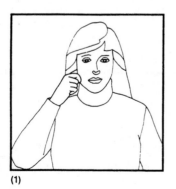

(1)

EPISIOTOMY

A cut made by the doctor into a woman's perineum, the area between the vagina and anus during labor, before the baby is born. Because a cut is easier to repair than a tear, an episiotomy is done to prevent tearing of the perineum and to make it easier for the baby to come out.

After the baby is delivered, the incision made by an episiotomy is stitched up.

(1) Sign VAGINA — the thumbs and index fingers of both "L" hands touch. (SM)
(2) The thumb of the right "A" hand moves down the index finger of the left "L" hand as if imitating cutting it. (SM)
(3) Sign SEW — the thumb and index finger of the right "F" hand imitate sewing on the index finger of the left "L" hand. (MM)

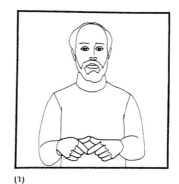
(1)

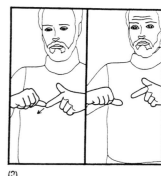
(2)

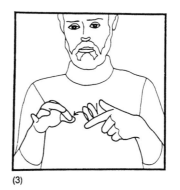
(3)

EPILEPSY

A disease in which the brain doesn't work correctly at times resulting in a partial or complete loss of consciousness and in some cases, convulsions. Epilepsy may be caused by many things, some of which are brain tumors, head injuries or having a history of the disease in the person's family.

Epilepsy can now be controlled with drugs, allowing the person to lead a normal and productive life.

EPILEPTIC ATTACK

The time when a person with epilepsy shows the disease's symptoms. An epileptic attack may be mild, lasting only a few seconds, with the person just stopping what they are doing and staring straight ahead or it may be worse. In more severe epileptic attacks, the person may feel strange (the "aura"), then lose consciousness, fall to the ground and go into convulsions.

When a person has an epileptic attack, one should not try to stop the attack, but one should protect them from falling and the person should be allowed to sleep if they want to.

209

EPIGLOTTIS

A thin flap of cartilage found in the throat at the base of the tongue. When we swallow, the epiglottis is tipped back over the opening of the trachea, covering it so food doesn't get into the windpipe, but instead is directed towards the esophagus. *See Figure 10*

EPINEPHRINE

A hormone made by the adrenal glands which acts as a stimulant and is produced when someone is excited, afraid or in danger. Epinephrine increases the heart beat, allows more blood to go to the muscles, puts nutrients into the blood and allows more air to go to the lungs. Epinephrine is also called adrenaline.

*Doctors may give **epinephrine** to a person who has an asthma attack.*

EPSOM SALTS

A chemical used to clean out the digestive tract, to relieve some ailments such as boils and to clean wounds.

The chemical name of Epsom salts is magnesium sulfate.

(1) Fingerspell "E-P-S-O-M".
(2) Sign SALT — the left "H" hand faces down at chest level. The fingers of the right "H" hand alternately tap the left index finger a few times. (MM)

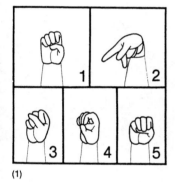
(1)

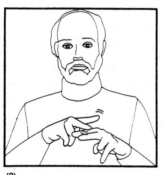
(2)

EQUANIL

See MEPROBAMATE

ERECTION

The time when a man's penis becomes larger and hard during sexual excitment. Erection must occur before the penis can be put into a woman's vagina.

*An **erection** occurs because the blood vessels leading to the penis open up and allow more blood into the penis while the blood vessels taking the blood out of the penis become smaller so that blood can't leave.*

a. (1) Sign PENIS — the middle finger of the right "P" hand taps the nose a few times.
(2) The right "S" hand faces up at chest level. The left "flat" hand is on the inside of the right elbow. Bend the right hand at the elbow. (SM)

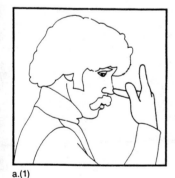
a.(1)

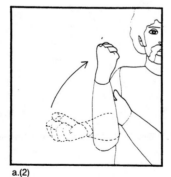
a.(2)

(Continued on next page)

b. (1) Sign PENIS — the middle finger of the right "P" hand taps the nose a few times. (MM)

(2) The right "one" hand points out at chest level. The index finger of the left "one" hand touches the right wrist. Bend the right hand up at the wrist. (SM)

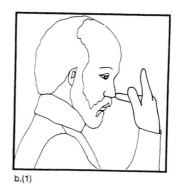
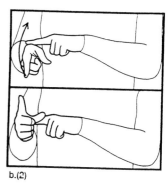

b.(1)

b.(2)

EROSION

The eating or wearing away of a structure by a chemical or something that is rough.

Erosion can occur on the teeth when the surface layer (enamel) is worn away.

(1) Both "S" hands face up at chest level. Drop both hands down into "five" hands. (SM)

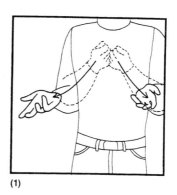

(1)

ERYTHROMYCIN

An antibiotic made by a certain kind of bacteria which stops an infection caused by many other types of bacteria.

Erythromycin is often used when someone is allergic to penicillin, another commonly used antibiotic.

ERYTHEMA

Redness of the skin. Erythema is caused by the small blood vessels just under the skin becoming larger.

Erythema may result from inflammation, heat, sun-burn, infections or poisons.

(1) Sign SKIN — the index finger and thumb of the right hand grab the right cheek. (SM)

(2) Sign RED — the index finger of the right "one" hand brushes down the chin a few times. (MM)

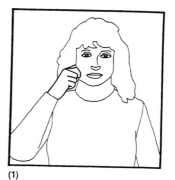
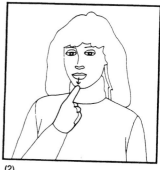

(1)

(2)

ERYTHROCYTE

See RED BLOOD CELL

211

ESOPHAGUS

The collapsible tube which goes from the back of the mouth down to the stomach. The esophagus is the part of the digestive system which carries food and liquid from the mouth to the stomach. *See Figure 10*

ESTABLISH

To set up, create, settle in a postion.

Some kinds of viruses reproduce very quickly and can establish an infection in two days.

(1) The left "S" hand faces down at chest level. The right "S" hand makes a circle above the left hand then moves down to touch the top of the left hand. (MM)

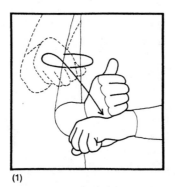

(1)

ESTROGENS

A group of hormones which are made by the ovaries or artificially. Estrogens are hormones which cause a girl to develop into a woman and also cause the monthly changes in the uterus preparing it for pregnancy and menstruation. Estrogens also help control pregnancy.

When a woman reaches menopause, estrogen is no longer produced, resulting in unpleasant symptoms which may be treated by giving her man-made estrogens.

ETHCHLORVYNOL

A drug which acts as a tranquilizer or sedative and is used to calm a person and lessen stress or excitement. Ethchlorvynol is sold under the name Placidyl .

If ethchlorvynol is used for a long time, it can cause addiction.

ETHER

An old-fashioned, sweet smelling, very flammable liquid anesthetic.

Ether may cause a person to salivate and feel nauseous.

(1) The right "claw" hand taps over the nose and mouth a few times. (MM)

(2) Sign SLEEP — the right "five" hand faces in at head level. Drop the hand slightly into a "flat-O" hand. At the same time, the eyes should close. (SM)

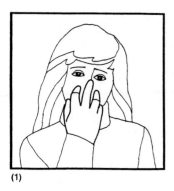 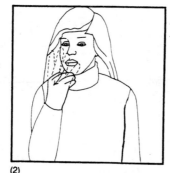

(1)   (2)

EUPHORIA

Feeling very good mentally and physically; well-being. In psychology, euphoria is a person's feeling good without reason for it.

Drugs such as marijuana can cause a feeling of euphoria.

(1) Both "flat-O" hands face in at chest level and move up the body into "five" hands. (SM)

* The facial expression should reflect happiness.

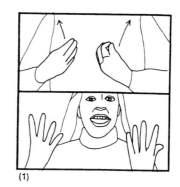
(1)

EUSTACHIAN TUBE

A small tube, about 1½ inches long which goes from the middle ear to the throat. The eustachian tube allows the pressure inside the ear to equal the pressure outside the ear so the eardrum isn't stretched and can move normally with sound waves. *See Figure 20*

EUTHANASIA

To die quietly without trauma. The practice of ending the life of an individual suffering from an incurable painful disease.

There is much controversy centered on whether euthanasia is legal or moral.

EVALUATE

To examine something and then decide what shape it is in; to judge something.

When a first-aider comes upon an accident scene with more than one injured person, he should evaluate them quickly to see who needs help the most.

a. (1) Both "V" hands face down at chest level and move in clockwise circles. (MM)
(2) Sign DECIDE — the index finger of the right "one" hand touches the forehead then moves down to chest level into a "F" hand facing down. The left "F" hand also faces down at chest level. (SM)
b. (1) Both "E" hands face out at chest level. Move both hands alternately in circular movements towards center then down and around a few times. (MM)

* This is an English version.

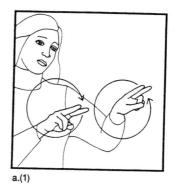
a.(1)

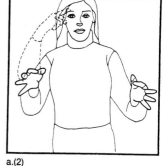
a.(2)

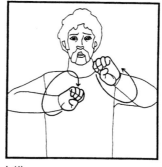
b.(1)

213

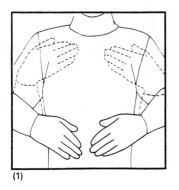
(1)

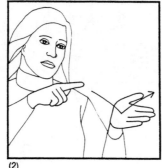
(2)

EXAMINATION

A doctor's inspection of a person's body, including checking the different parts of it and doing any tests needed to find out if a person has a disease.

*It is important to have regular **examinations** by your doctor and dentist because they can usually tell if there is something wrong with you and treat it before much damage is done.*

(1) Sign BODY — both "flat" hands touch the chest then the stomach areas. (SM)
(2) Sign CHECK — the index finger of the right "one" hand makes a check mark in the palm of the left "flat" hand. (SM)

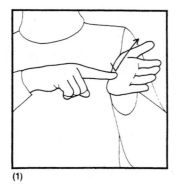
(1)

EXAMINE

To study or look at something.

*When we go to the dentist, he will **examine** our teeth and perhaps take X-rays to see if we have any cavities.*

(1) Sign CHECK — the index finger of the right "one" hand makes a check mark in the palm of the left "flat" hand. (SM)

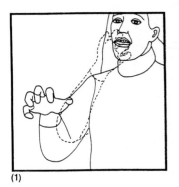
(1)

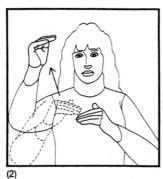
(2)

EXCESSIVE HEAT

Temperature that is above normal and possibly dangerous to one's health.

*A person can develop hyperthermia if exposed to **excessive heat**.*

(1) Sign HOT — the right "claw" hand faces in at mouth level then turns out and moves down slightly. (SM)
(2) Sign TOO MUCH — the left "cupped" hand faces down at chest level. The right "cupped" hand also faces down at chest level then moves up slightly. (SM)

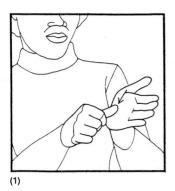
(1)

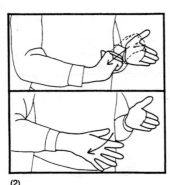
(2)

EXCISE

To cut out or remove something surgically.

*When a woman has a hysterectomy, only the uterus is **excised**, and not the ovaries.*

(1) Sign CUT — the left "flat" hand faces up at chest level. The thumb of the right "A" hand moves down across the left palm as if imitating cutting. (SM)
(2) Sign REMOVE — the left "flat" hand faces up at chest level. The right "A" hand touches the left palm then moves down into a "five" hand as if throwing something away. (SM)

214

EXCITE

To make something more active; to stimulate something.

A muscle will contract when a nerve excites it.

(1) The middle fingers of both "eight" hands touch the chest and then move alternately out in circular movements a few times. (MM)

* *The facial expression should reflect excitement.*

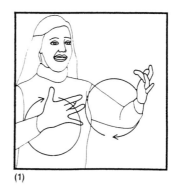
(1)

EXCREMENT

Wastes passed out of the body.

There are many different kinds of wastes made by the body but excrement usually means feces.

(1) Sign DEFECATE— the left "A" hand faces right at chest level. The thumb of the right "A" hand is inside the left fist. Drop the right hand down, leaving the left hand still. (SM)

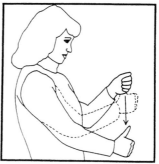
(1)

EXCRETE

To get rid of wastes from the body, blood or organs.

A person excretes wastes in the forms of feces, urine, and sweat.

(1) Sign DEFECATE — the left "A" hand faces right at chest level. The thumb of the right "A" hand is inside the left fist. Drop the right hand down, leaving the left hand still. (SM)

* *This sign refers only to bowel movements and urinating. Sweat should be signed if referring only to sweat.*

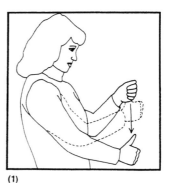
(1)

EXCRETORY SYSTEM

The system in the body which gets rid of wastes or things present in the body in too large amounts and cannot be used. The digestive tract, skin and lungs are important in getting rid of wastes but the most important part is the urinary system made up of the kidneys, ureters, bladder and urethra. *See Figure 9*

EXERCISE

The use of muscles; activity.

Exercise is important in keeping a person healthy, keeping his weight down, and is used to correct some ailments and improve coordination.

(Continued on next page)

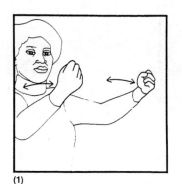
(1)

EXERCISE, *continued*

(1) Both "S" hands face in at shoulder level and move in and out a few times as if imitating doing exercises. (MM)

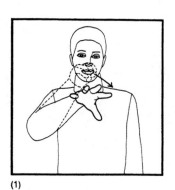
(1)

EXHALE

To breathe or to let air out of the lungs; expiration.

*When we **exhale**, the muscles in the rib cage relax, the ribs lower themselves and the diaphragm relaxes, causing the air to be pushed or forced out of the lungs.*

(1) The right "flat-O" hand faces down with the fingers pointing out at the mouth. Move the hand out forward into a "five" hand. (SM)

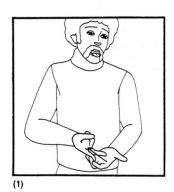
(1)

EXHAUSTION

Very tired or worn out.

Exhaustion is a sign that the body has been overworked.

(1) The right "V" hand faces up in the palm of the left "flat" hand. Move both hands back towards the body. (SM)

* The facial expression should reflect tiredness.

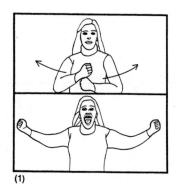
(1)

EXHIBITIONISM

In psychology, an abnormal need a person has to attract attention to himself by showing his genitals to a person of the opposite sex.

*A person can be arrested for **exhibitionism** and should get help from a psychologist.*

(1) Sign EXPOSE — both "A" hands face in at chest level. Move both hands to the sides as if opening a coat. (SM)

EXOCRINE GLAND

A type of gland which has ducts to carry material made by the gland to the outside of the body or to a body surface.

*Some kinds of **exocrine glands** are the salivary glands and sweat glands.*

EXPAND

To spread out, swell or become larger.

*When we breathe in, the rib cage will **expand**.*

(1) Both "S" hands face in at chest level, the right on top of the left. Open both hands slightly as if indicating something expanding. (SM)

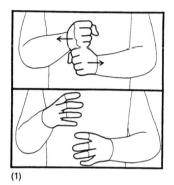

(1)

EXPERIMENT

A test done to find out how something works, to test an idea, to learn something or to show something.

*Before a new drug is tried on people, scientists often **experiment** with it on animals to make sure it is safe.*

(1) Both "E" hands face out at chest level. Alternately circle the hands down and to the sides a few times. (MM)

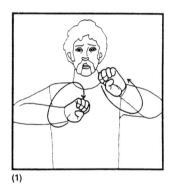

(1)

EXPIRE

To breathe out or let air out of the lungs; exhale. Expire can also mean "to die".

*When it takes someone longer to **expire** air than to breathe it in, a disease like asthma or emphysema may be present.*

a. (1) The right "flat-O" hand faces down with the fingers pointing out at the mouth. Move the hand forward into a "five" hand. (SM)

* *This should be signed only when referring to exhaling.*

b. (1) Sign DEAD — the left "flat" hand faces up at chest level and the right "flat" hand faces down at chest level. Turn both hands to the right so that the left hand ends facing down and the right hand ends facing up. (SM)

* *This should be signed only when referring to dying.*

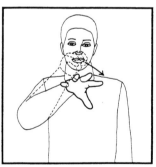

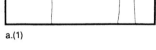

a.(1)

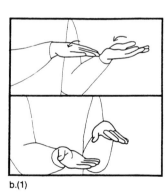

b.(1)

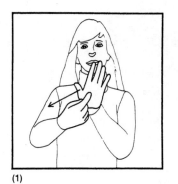
(1)

EXPOSE

To uncover or open something.

We should not look directly at the sun because if we expose the retina of the eye to such bright light, it could be dangerous.

(1) The index finger of the right "one" hand touches the palm of the left "flat" hand. Move both hands forward slightly. (SM)

EXPOSURE

The state of being in severe cold or heat without proper protection for a long time.

If a person is out in the cold weather for a long time, he could suffer from exposure or hypothermia.

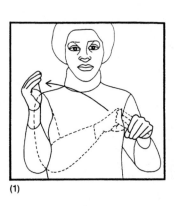
(1)

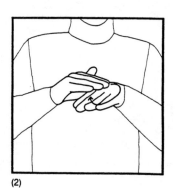
(2)

EXTERNAL

Referring to the outside or outer part of something.

The skin is the external covering of the body.

(1) Sign OUT — the fingers of the right "flat-O" hand are inside the left fist. Pull the right hand out. (SM)
(2) The fingertips of the right "flat" hand rub the back of the left "flat" hand. (SM)

EXTERNAL OBLIQUE

A large muscle in the abdomen region, attached to the front, lower part of the ribs. The external oblique presses the ribs down, flexes the vertebral column and presses the structures in the abdomen together. *See Figure 4*

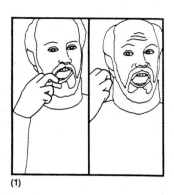
(1)

EXTRACTION

In dentistry, the removal of a tooth.

An extraction is usually done when a tooth is damaged so badly it can't be repaired, when it is very decayed or when there is severe gum disease.

(1) The right bent "V" hand moves from the mouth out as if imitating pulling a tooth. (SM)

EXTREMITY

An arm or leg.

> *The lower extremity is the leg and the upper extremity is the arm.*

a. (1) Sign ARM — the fingertips of the right "cupped" hand brush down the left arm. (SM)

b. (1) Sign LEG — both "flat" hands brush down the legs. (SM)

* *Sign ARM or LEG, whichever applies.*

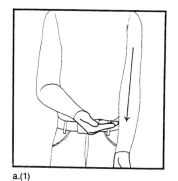

a.(1)

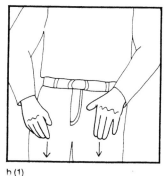

h (1)

EXTRICATE

To release or free something.

> *Sometimes special equipment is needed to extricate people from cars in bad accidents.*

(1) Sign FREE — both "S" hands face out and cross at the wrists. Move both hands to the sides. (SM)

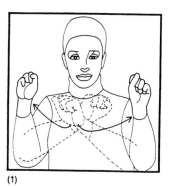

(1)

EYE

The organ which allows us to see. The eye includes many muscles, a nerve going to the brain and special structures to protect it from external damage. *See Figure 22*

(1) Sign EYE — the index finger of the right "one" hand points to the right eye. (SM)

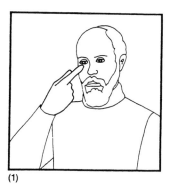

(1)

EYEBALL

The round part of the eye. *See Figure 22*

EYEBROW

The bony ridge extending over the eye and the arch of short hairs covering it. *See Figure 21*
(1) The index finger of the right "one" hand moves across the right eyebrow. (SM)

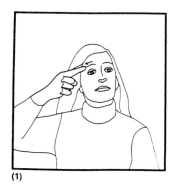

(1)

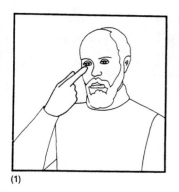
(1)

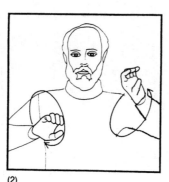
(2)

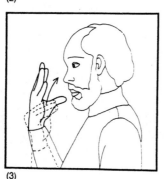
(3)

EYE BURN

Injury to the eye caused by irritating gases or strong chemicals like acids or alkalis.

Any eye burn should get immediate attention because the eyes are very delicate, valuable structures.

(1) Sign EYE — the index finger of the right "one" hand points to the right eye. (SM)

(2) Sign CHEMICAL — both "C" hands face out at chest level. Move both hands alternately towards the center then down and around in circular movements a few times. (MM)

(3) The right "flat-O" hand points to the face then opens into a "five" hand as if imitating splashing something on the face. (SM)

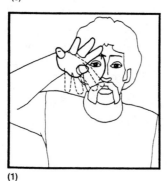
(1)

EYELASHES

The row of short, stiff hairs on the edges of the eyelid. The eyelashes help to keep things from getting into the eye. *See Figure 21*

(1) The right "four" hand faces down and moves up and down a few times in front of the right eye as if imitating eyelashes. (MM)

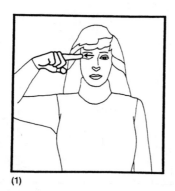
(1)

EYELIDS

The two movable folds of skin that can close and cover the eye. The eyelid protects the eye from dirt, from things which may hit the eye, from too bright light, and it also spreads tears over the eye to keep it from drying out. *See Figure 21*

(1) The index finger of the right "one" hand moves across the right eyelid. (SM)

EYEPATCH

A bandage or piece of cloth put over the eye.

An eyepatch is used to help an injury heal, to hold medication in place, or to protect an empty socket.

(Continued on next page)

(1) The right "flat" hand covers the right eye. (SM)

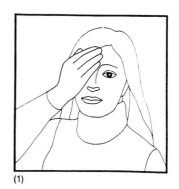

(1)

EYESTRAIN

Tiredness of the eyes caused by using them too much in poor lighting or by a vision defect.

Eyestrain will usually disappear after a good night's sleep.

(1) The index finger of the right "one" hand points to both eyes. (SM)

(2) Sign TIRED — the fingertips of both "cupped" hands touch the chest. Keeping the fingertips in place, drop both hands slightly. (SM)

* The facial expression should reflect tiredness.

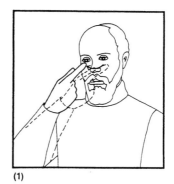

(1)

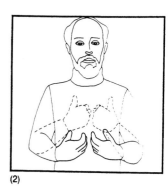

(2)

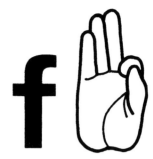

f

FACE

The front part of the head going from forehead to chin and from ear to ear. *See Figure 2*

(1) The right index finger circles left around the face. (SM)

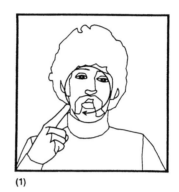

(1)

FACIAL

Referring to the face.

The eyes, nose and mouth are all facial structures.

(1) Sign FACE — the right index finger circles left around the face. (SM)

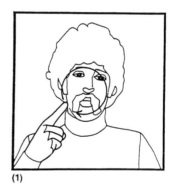

(1)

FACIAL ARTERY

The large blood vessel (carotid artery) which carries fresh blood to the skin and muscles of the face. *See Figure 6*

FACIAL BONES

The bones of the skull that make up the face. *See Figure 26*

(1) Sign FACE — the right index finger circles left around the face. (SM)

(2) Fingerspell "B-O-N-E".

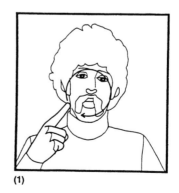

(1)

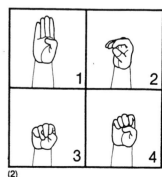

(2)

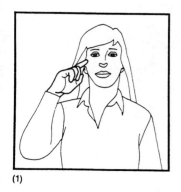
(1)

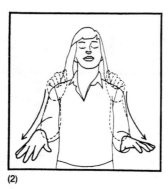
(2)

FAINT

Feeling dizzy, weak and nauseated and then losing consciousness. The person may be cool, sweating and have a weak and rapid heart beat.

A person may faint because not enough blood is getting to the brain.

(1) The right index finger points to the head. (SM)
(2) Both "A" hands face out at shoulder level. Move both hands down and out, ending in "five" hands palms down with the eyes closed. (SM)

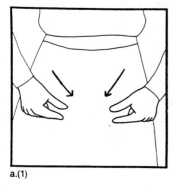
a.(1)

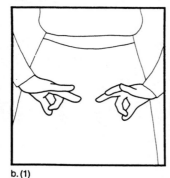
b.(1)

FALLOPIAN TUBES

The two tubes attached to the uterus and having their enlarged ends near an ovary. The fallopian tubes carry an ovum released from an ovary to the uterus. Most ova which are fertilized are fertilized in the fallopian tubes. *See Figure 12*

a. (1) Both "G" hands face in at the sides of the lower abdomen. Move both hands down slightly. (SM)
b. (1) Both "F" hands face out at the sides of the lower abdomen. (SM)

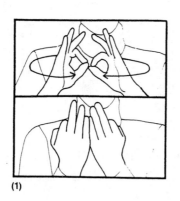
(1)

FAMILY

A group of people related by blood or marriage.

Family usually refers to parents and their children.

(1) Both "F" hands are together at chest level, palms facing out. Move both hands out and around, ending palms in. (SM)

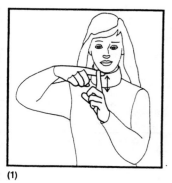
(1)

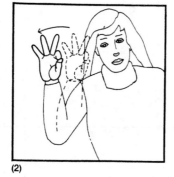
(2)

FARENHEIT

A system of measurement for temperature. 32°F is the temperature at which water freezes and 212°F is the temperature at which water boils.

The most common way of measuring temperature in North America is with the Farenheit scale, but the Centigrade scale is being used more and more.

(1) Sign TEMPERATURE — the left "one" hand faces right at chest level. The right "one" hand faces down, touching the inside of the left index finger. Move the right hand up and down along the left index finger. (MM)
(2) Fingerspell the number, in this example, "99".
* The specific temperature would be signed here.

(Continued on next page)

(3) The right "O" hand faces out and shakes slightly from left to right a few times indicating degrees.
(4) The right "F" hand faces out and shakes slightly from left to right a few times indicating farenheit.

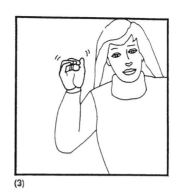

(3)

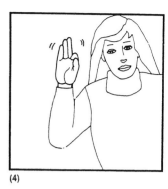

(4)

FARSIGHTEDNESS

A vision defect where the eye can focus on far away objects but not on objects that are close; also called hyperopia.

Farsightedness is caused by images being out of focus on the retina.

(1) Sign CAN'T — the left "one" hand faces down at chest level, pointing out. The right "one" hand faces down and moves down, the right index finger striking the left index finger. (SM)
(2) Sign SEE — the right "V" hand faces in at eye level and moves slightly forward. (SM)
(3) The right "flat" hand faces in and moves in towards the eyes. (SM)

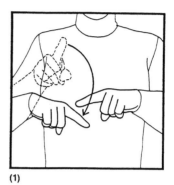

(1)

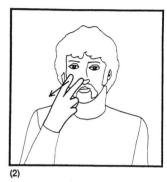

(2)

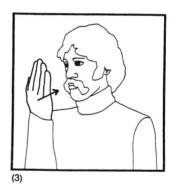

(3)

FART

See FLATULENCE

FAST

Not eating for a certain amount of time. When someone fasts, the fat stored in the body is used to supply energy.

People usually fast to lose weight, for religious reasons or to cleanse the body of wastes and toxins.

(1) The right "F" hand faces out and moves from the left to the right at the mouth. (SM)

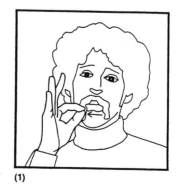

(1)

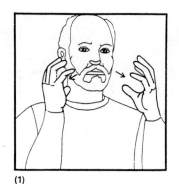

(1)

FAT

Overweight or obese. Fat is also used for a certain type of compound made up of carbon, hydrogen and oxygen arranged in a certain way. Fats are found in the body and are used to pad and protect some structures, to store up extra energy, and to help keep the body at normal temperature.

When we eat too much and don't exercise enough, some food is made into fat and stored.

(1) Both "claw" hands face in at the sides of the face and move slightly out, at the same time, the cheeks puff out. (SM)

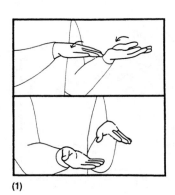

(1)

FATAL

Resulting in death; deadly.

Drug overdose, especially with barbiturates, can be fatal because the body's activities may be slowed down to the point where a person dies.

(1) Sign DEAD — both "flat" hands are at chest level, the right hand faces down and the left hand faces up. Flip both hands to the right, the right hand ending face up and the left hand ending face down. (SM)

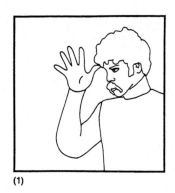

(1)

FATHER

A male parent or man whose sperm has fertilized an egg to help create a child, who has adopted a child or has developed a paternal relationship with someone.

Half of the chromosomes which direct a person's development come from the father's sperm and the other half comes from the mother.

(1) The thumb of the right "five" hand touches the forehead, the palm faces left. (SM)

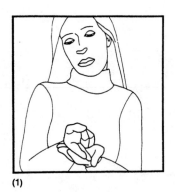

(1)

FATIGUE

Tiredness caused by activity or hard work.

Fatigue can result if wastes build up in the muscles, if a person is malnourished, if not enough oxygen is getting to the body's tissues, or if the person is sick.

(1) The left "flat" hand faces up at chest level. The right "V" hand faces up in the left palm. Move both hands back towards the body. (SM)

* The facial expression should show fatigue.

FEAR

The feeling of alarm or fright one gets when in danger, in pain or threatened.

When people feel fear, the hormone adrenaline is released, allowing them to be more active and to protect themselves.

(1) Both "S" hands face each other at chest levels. Move both hands in towards the center, ending in "five" hands facing in. (SM)

* *The facial expression should show fear.*

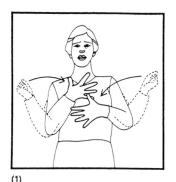
(1)

FEBRILE

Referring to a fever.

Measles, the mumps, influenza and chickenpox are all febrile diseases.

(1) Sign TEMPERATURE — the left "one" hand faces right at chest level. The right "one" hand faces down, touching the inside of the left index finger. Move the right hand up and down along left index finger, then stop slightly above the left hand, indicating "high." (MM)

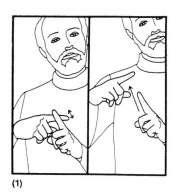
(1)

FECES

The solid waste matter left after digestion that is released from the rectum through the anus.

Besides unusable food, feces contain bacteria, cells from the lining of the intestines and mucus.

(1) The left "A" hand faces right at chest level. The thumb of the right "A" hand is inside the left fist. Move the right hand down leaving the left hand still. (SM)

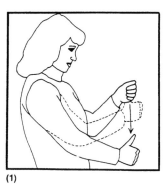
(1)

FEE

A charge, payment or the amount of money owed to someone for doing something.

Before one sees a doctor, arrangements should be made for payment of his fee.

(1) The left "flat" hand faces up at chest level. The index finger of the right "X" hand touches the left palm then moves down. (SM)

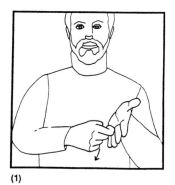
(1)

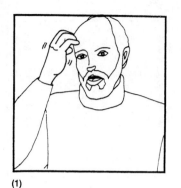
(1)

FEEBLEMINDED

Someone who is a slow learner or mentally retarded.

Good schools, teaching and a lot of patience can help most feebleminded people learn to take care of themselves.

(1) The fingertips of the right "claw" hand touch the forehead. Leaving the fingertips in place, bent and straighten the fingers at the knuckles a few times. (MM)

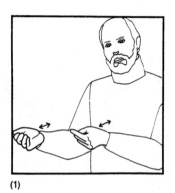
(1)

FEED

To give nourishment or food to someone.

Sometimes it is necessary to feed someone by putting a liquid food through a tube inserted through the nose or mouth into the stomach.

(1) Both "flat-O" hands face up at chest level and move in and out a few times. (MM)

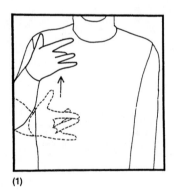
(1)

FEEL

To sense something by touch or to be aware of an emotion.

A person can feel pain from a shot and can also feel fear about having to get a shot.

(1) The middle finger of the right "eight" hand moves up the chest. (SM)

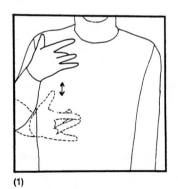
(1)

FEELING

An awareness, sensation or emotion.

A sick or injured person won't be feeling well.

(1) Sign FEEL — the middle finger of the right "eight" hand moves up and down the chest a few times. (MM)

FEET

See FOOT

FEMALE

The sex which produces ova or eggs and can have babies. In humans, females are women and girls.

A female (animal) has ovaries, a uterus, vagina and breasts or an udder.

(1) The thumb of the right "A" hand moves down the right side of the face from the ear to the chin. (SM)

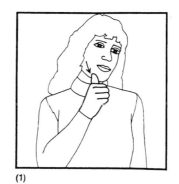

(1)

FEMORAL ARTERY

The major blood vessel supplying the lower extremity with fresh blood. The iliac artery becomes the femoral artery when it leaves the pelvic region and the femoral artery becomes the popliteal artery in the knee region. *See Figure 6*

FEMUR

The long bone which goes from the pelvis to the knee. The femur, also called the thighbone, is the longest and strongest bone in the body. *See Figure 26*

FENESTRATION

An opening in a structure. Fenestration is also the name of an operation done when someone has become deaf because of bone forming over the oval window.

Fenestration involves making a new opening into the cochlea so a person can hear.

FERTILE

Able to reproduce.

A fertile woman is one who can become pregnant.

a. (1) Sign WOMAN — the right "flat" hand faces down at the forehead. Move the hand down to a "five" hand facing left with the thumb touching the chest.(SM)
(2) Sign PREGNANT — both "five" hands mesh together at the stomach and move out forward as if imitating the stomach growing. (SM)

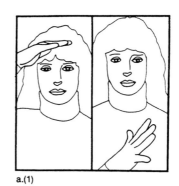

a.(1)

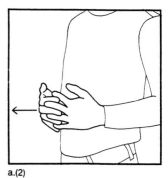

a.(2)

(Continued on next page)

229

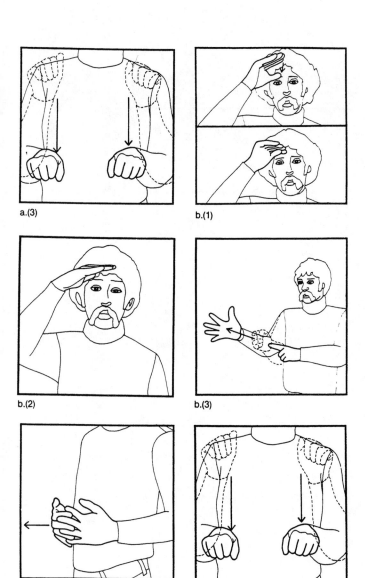

a.(3)

b.(1)

b.(2)

b.(3)

b.(4)

b. (5)

FERTILE, *continued*

a. (3) Sign CAN — both "A" hands face out at chest level. Drop both hands down to waist level, the palms facing down. (SM)

b. (1) Sign MAN — the right open "flat-O" hand faces down at the forehead. Move the hand slightly forward, closing the fingers into a "flat-O" hand. (SM)

(2) The right "flat" hand faces down at the forehead and moves slightly out forward. (SM)

(3) Sign EJACULATE — the right "S" hand faces left at chest level, the index finger of the left "one" hand touches the heel of the right palm. Keeping the left hand in place, move the right hand out into a "five" hand. (SM)

(4) Sign PREGNANT — both "five" hands mesh together at the stomach. Move both hands out forward as if imitating the stomach growing. (SM)

(5) Sign CAN — both "A" hands face out at chest level. Drop both hands down to waist level, the palms facing down. (SM)

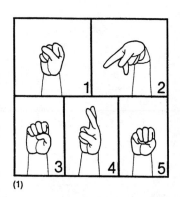

(1)

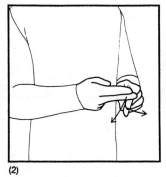

(2)

FERTILIZATION

The joining of a man's sperm and a woman's ovum.

*Once **fertilization** occurs, cell division begins and a baby starts to form.*

(1) Fingerspell "S-P-E-R-M".

(2) Both "H" hands face each other, the right on top of the left hand. Pivot both hands slightly so that the fingers face out then cross a few times in short repeated movements. (MM)

(Continued on next page)

230

(3) The thumbs and index fingers of both "F" hands join at chest level. (SM)

(4) The left "five" hand faces right at chest level. The index finger of the right "one" hand is between the left index and middle fingers. Twist the right hand slightly. (SM)

(5) Sign BABY — the right hand and forearm face up, resting on the left hand and forearm which also face upward. Both are then rocked back and forth as if holding a baby. (MM)

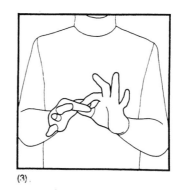

(3)

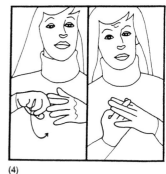

(4)

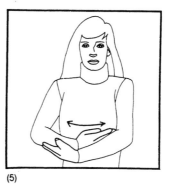

(5)

FESTER

An infection or inflammation where pus forms.

An abscess results when bacteria get under the skin and begin to fester.

(1) Sign CUT — the left "flat" hand faces in at chest level. The thumb of the right "A" hand moves down the back of the left hand as if imitating cutting. (SM)
* *This should be signed at the area of the cut.*

(2) Sign INFECTION — the right "I" hand faces out at shoulder level and moves slightly from left to right a few times. (MM)
* *Mouth the word "infection" while signing.*

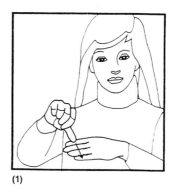

(1)

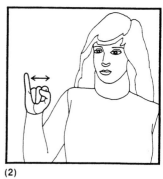

(2)

FETAL

Referring to a fetus or baby inside the uterus.

Fetal blood circulation changes when a baby is born so blood is sent to its lungs and the blood can get oxygen.

(1) Sign BABY — the right hand and forearm face up, resting on the left hand and forearm which also face upward. Both are then rocked back and forth as if holding a baby. (MM)

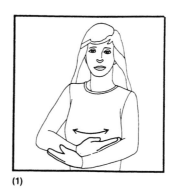

(1)

(Continued on next page)

231

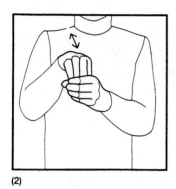
(2)

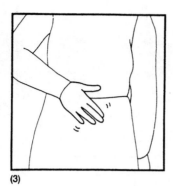
(3)

FETAL, *continued*

(2) Sign IN — the left "O" hand faces in at chest level. The fingertips of the right "flat-O" hand move into the left fist a few times. (MM)
(3) The fingertips of the right "flat" hand tap the stomach a few times. (MM)

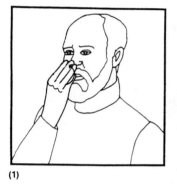
(1)

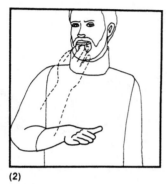
(2)

FETID

Bad smelling.

   An infected area will sometimes have a fetid odor.

(1) Sign SMELL — the fingertips of the right "flat" hand brush up the nose. (SM)
(2) Sign BAD — the fingertips of the right "flat" hand touch the mouth. Turn the right hand out and down. (SM)
* The facial expression should reflect bad smelling.

FETISHISM

Having abnormal sexual feelings of love for an object or part of a person.

   A person may have a fetishism for someone's hair, shoes, coat or other part of clothing.

FETUS

A baby in the mother's uterus from the 3rd month until birth. *See Figure 14*

(1) Sign BABY — the right hand and forearm face up, resting on the left hand and forearm which also face upward. Both are then rocked back and forth as if holding a baby. (MM)
(2) Sign IN — the left "O" hand faces in at chest level. The fingertips of the right "flat-O" hand move down into the left fist a few times. (MM)
(3) The fingertips of the right "flat" hand tap the stomach a few times. (MM)

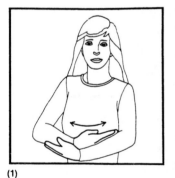
(1)

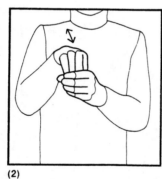
(2)

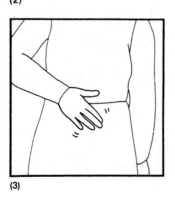
(3)

FEVER

Referring to a person's body temperature when it goes above normal (98.6°F).

Fevers can be caused by being in a hot environment, and by exercise, dehydration, infection or inflammation.

(1) Sign HOT — the right "claw" hand faces in at face level. Turn the hand out and slightly down. (SM)

(2) Sign TEMPERATURE — the index finger of the right "one" hand moves up and down on the index finger of the left "one" hand a few times, then stops above the left hand. (MM)

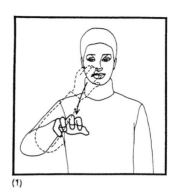 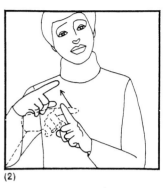

(1)   (2)

FEVER BLISTER

See COLD SORE

FIBRILLATION

An uncontrolled twitching or spasm of the cells in a muscle resulting in little or no movement in the whole muscle. When atrial fibrillation or ventricular fibrillation occurs in the heart, the heart jerks and twitches but doesn't pump blood well.

Fibrillation of the heart can be caused by plugged arteries in the heart itself, certain drugs or electrical shock.

FIBROSIS

The growth of fibers or tissue in an organ or structure, preventing it from working well.

Fibrosis usually results from injury, inflammation or disease.

FIBROUS

Something that is made up of fibers, has fibers in it or is like a fiber.

Scars are made up of fibrous tissue which replace injured structures.

FIBULA

The smaller of the two bones in the lower leg. *See Figure 26*

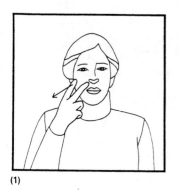
(1)

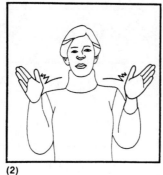
(2)

FIELD OF VISION

The area that can be seen with an eye without moving it or the head.

The field of vision is limited mostly by the structures around the eye.

(1) Sign SEE — the right "V" hand faces in at eye level and moves out slightly. (SM)
(2) Both "flat" hands face each other at the sides of the head and move out towards the sides; then, they bounce slightly. (MM)

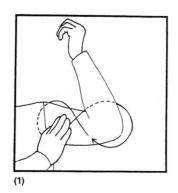
(1)

FIGURE OF EIGHT BANDAGE

A gauze bandage in which the turns cross each other like an eight.

Figure of eight bandages are used on joint areas and to hold splints in place.

(1) The left arm is bent at the elbow. The fingertips of the right "flat" hand imitate a figure eight movement on the left arm. (DM)
* This should be signed at the area where the bandage is applied.

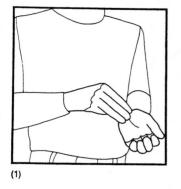
(1)

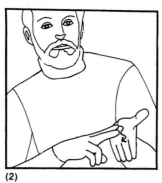
(2)

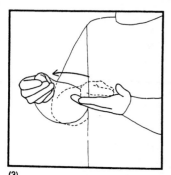
(3)

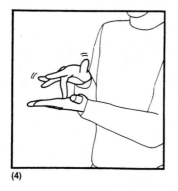
(4)

FILL (A PRESCRIPTION)

To buy drugs or medication from a druggist or pharmacist using a form with a doctor's signature and directions for taking the drug on it.

When having a pharmacist fill a prescription a person might see about getting generic drugs which are just as good as name brand drugs and usually less expensive.

(1) Sign DOCTOR — the right "M" hand touches the left inside wrist. (DM)
(2) The left "flat" hand faces up at chest level. The fingertips of the right "V" hand move down the left palm in a wavy movement. (SM)
(3) The left "flat" hand faces up at chest level. The right "flat-O" hand touches the left palm then moves out forward. (SM)
(4) Sign MEDICINE — the left "flat" hand faces up at chest level. The middle finger of the right "eight" hand pivots in the left palm from left to right a few times. (MM)

234

FILLING

In dentistry, the substance put in a cavity.

A filling is usually made of gold or amalgam.

(1) The right index finger touches the teeth. (SM)
(2) The left "S" hand faces in at chest level. The index finger of the right "one" hand touches inside the left fist, then the right "five" hand strikes the left hand. (SM)

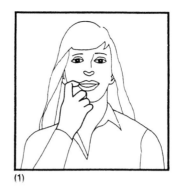
(1)

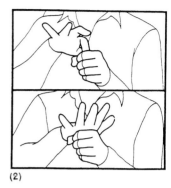
(2)

FILTER

To pass a substance through a screen or strainer to separate out a certain part. A filter is also the screen or strainer used to separate out a certain part from something.

*The kidneys are a **filter** which separates wastes from the blood.*

FIMBRIA

The long, finger-like endings on the fallopian tube which are near the ovary. The fimbria help to catch an ovum when it is released from an ovary and send it to the uterus. *See Figure 12*

FINGER

One of the five parts of the hand that allows us to hold things. *See Figure 1*

(1) The right index finger moves up the fingers of the left hand. (MM)

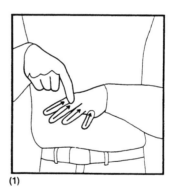
(1)

FINGERNAIL

The hard, flat structures found on top of the ends of the fingers.

*A **fingernail** grows about 1/36 of an inch per month.*

(1) The right index finger touches the left thumbnail. (SM)

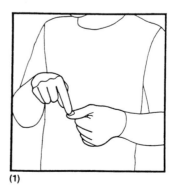
(1)

FINGERTIP BANDAGE

Bandages used on the ends of fingers.

(1) The left "H" hand faces in at chest level. The right "one" hand faces in and circles around the fingers of the left hand. (MM)

* This should be signed at the area the bandage is being applied.

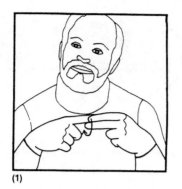
(1)

FIRE

Flames or the burning of something resulting in heat and light.

Fires are rapid chemical reactions in which the substance burned combines with oxygen.

(1) Both "five" hands face in at chest level. Move both hands up and at the same time, wiggle the fingers. (SM)

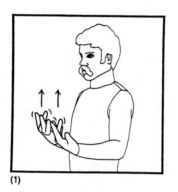
(1)

FIRST-AID

Emergency treatment given to injured or sick persons before professional medical care is available.

Some forms of first-aid are C.P.R. (cardiopulmonary resuscitation), the Heimlich Maneuver and applying splints.

(1) Sign FIRST — the right "one" hand points up at chest level and the palm faces out. Twist the hand to the left so that the palm faces in. (SM)
(2) Fingerspell "A-I-D".

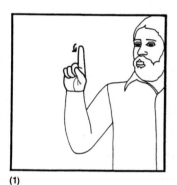
(1)
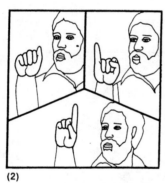
(2)

FIRST-AID KIT

Containers with bandages, tape, antiseptics, scissors, gauze, tweezers, and sometimes some medications which are used to treat someone who has suddenly gotten sick or had an accident.

It is a good idea to have a first-aid kit when going on a vacation, and also to have one in cars, in boats, in places where people work and places where people play sports.

(1) Sign FIRST — the right "one" hand points up at chest level and the palm faces out. Twist the hand to the left so that the palm faces in. (SM)
(2) Fingerspell "A-I-D".

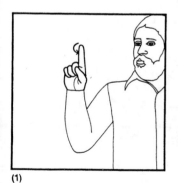
(1)
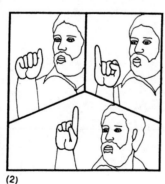
(2)

(Continued on next page)

(3) Both "flat" hands face each other at the sides. Move both hands in front of the body so that both face in, the right hand in front of the left hand as if imitating the shape of a box. (SM)

(4) The left "A" hand faces up at chest level. The right "A" hand faces down at chest level. Move the right hand up as if opening the box. (SM)

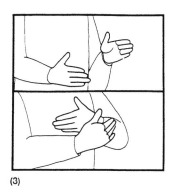

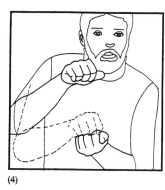

(3) (4)

FIRST DEGREE BURN

A burn which damages the outer skin layer or epidermis. They are not too severe and cause pain and redness but no blistering.

> A *first degree burn* can be caused by being in the sun too long, touching something hot or coming in contact with hot water or steam.

FIT

A sudden attack, convulsion or quick development of a symptom that lasts a short time.

> Grand mal epileptic attacks are sometimes called *fits* and a person having one should be kept from bumping into things.

(1) The left "flat" hand faces up at chest level. The right bent "one" hand faces up in the left palm and moves frantically as if indicating having a fit. (MM)

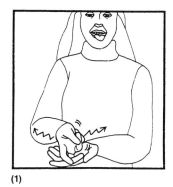

(1)

FISSURE

A deep groove or crack in a structure. In dentistry, a crack in the enamel of a tooth.

> A *fissure* is usually found on the top, flat part of the tooth.

(1) The right index finger points to a tooth. (SM)
(2) The left "flat" hand faces right at chest level. The fingertips of the right "cupped" hand make a sharp "S" in the left palm as if indicating a crack. (SM)

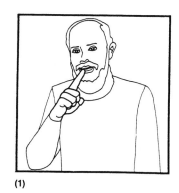

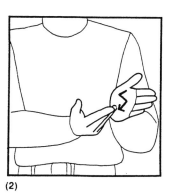

(1) (2)

237

FIX

Referring to the slang term for injection into the vein with heroin or some similar drug.

When injecting a fix, the person may get hepatitis because the needles used are often not sterile.

(1) The right "S" hand moves in and out from the inside of the left elbow. (MM)

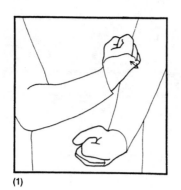
(1)

FIXATION

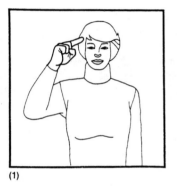
(1)

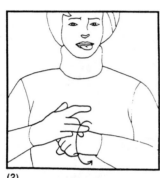
(2)

In psychiatry, referring to a person's personality when it stops developing before it should, causing the person to behave abnormally.

In fixation a person will often be too strongly attached to one or both of his parents.

(1) The right index finger points to the head. (SM)

(2) The left "S" hand faces down at chest level. The middle finger of the right "eight" hand touches the back of the left hand. Move both hands forward and around in a circular movement. (MM)

FIXATION SPLINT

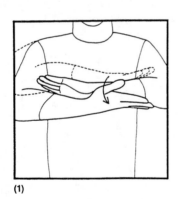
(1)

A kind of splint which is put on an injured limb to hold the broken bones and the joints still.

By using a fixation splint, pain can be decreased and damage to the structures around the break can be prevented.

(1) The left "flat" hand faces down with the elbow bent. The right "flat" hand touches the top of the left arm then the bottom of the arm. (SM)

FIXED PARTIAL DENTURE

A set of artificial teeth which replace one or more but not all of a person's natural teeth and can't be easily removed from the mouth.

A fixed partial denture is permanently attached to the natural teeth or roots of the teeth.

FLAGYL®

A man-made drug used to treat infections caused by some kinds of parasites. Flagyl is the name a drug called metronidazole is sold under. Flagyl is used to treat giardiasis, a certain kind of dysentery and most often trichomoniasis. Flagyl is a drug that works very well against these infections, but there have been tests done on it that show it may cause cancer. It would be wise to use Flagyl as seldom as possible, and then at the lowest dosage that will clear up the infection and for the shortest possible time.

A person taking Flagyl® should not have any drinks containing alcohol because the drug interferes with how the alcohol is used by the body and it may cause diarrhea, nausea, vomiting, headache, dizziness and perhaps shock.

FLANK

The part of the body between the pelvis and lower ribs; also used when referring to the outer side of the buttocks. *See Figure 3*

FLASHBACK

The return of mental images or hallucinations after a drug has worn off.

Flashbacks may occur a long time after the drug was taken and they are usually frightening.

(1) The right "K" hand faces in and moves past the right cheek back. (SM)
(2) Both "S" hands are at head level, the right hand behind the left hand. Open both hands into "C" hands. (SM)

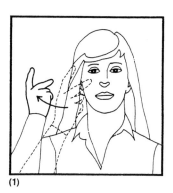
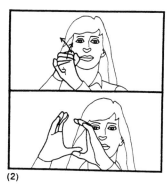

(1)   (2)

FLATULENCE

The passing of air or gas in the stomach or intestines out through the anus; also called "breaking wind", "passing gas", and the slang term "fart".

Flatulence may be caused by swallowing air when eating too rapidly or by gas formed by bacteria from the food in the intestines.

(1) The left "S" hand faces right at chest level. The right "flat" hand faces in, in front of the left hand. Pivot the right hand out slightly. (SM)

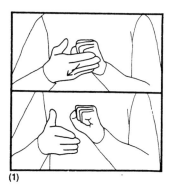

(1)

* *The lips should make a vibrating sound.*

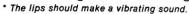

239

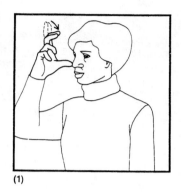

(1)

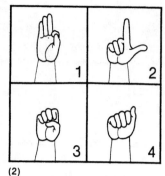

1 2 3 4

FLEA

A small insect which sucks blood from animals and man.

Fleas leave red, itchy bites and can transmit diseases and parasites from animals to man.

(1) Sign INSECT — the thumb of the right "three" hand touches the nose. Bend and straighten the fingers a few times. (MM)

(2) Fingerspell "F-L-E-A".

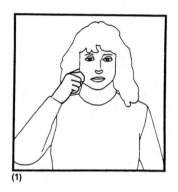

(1)

FLESH

The soft parts of the body, especially the muscles or skin.

We get much of the protein in our diet from animal flesh.

(1) Sign SKIN — the index finger and thumb of the right hand grab the right cheek. (SM)

FLOATERS

Small, dark things which float across our field of vision.

Floaters are caused by pieces of protein or cells floating in the vitreous humor.

FLU

See INFLUENZA

FLOATING KIDNEY

A kidney that has moved from its normal position.

A floating kidney is also called nephroptosis.

FLUID

A liquid or something which flows easily.

A person who is dehydrated, in shock or having surgery may have fluids injected into a vein.

* There is an English sign for this, however, the term is too general to translate into Ameslam. The specific fluid should be fingerspelled.

FLURAZEPAM

A sedative drug used to help a person relax or sleep. Flurazepam is sold under the name of Dalmane®

If flurazepam is used for a long time in large amounts, it can cause addiction.

FLUSH

Referring to the sudden redness of a person's skin. Flush can also mean the cleaning out or irrigating of a cavity with water.

A person can become flushed from fever, embarassment, strong emotions or hormone changes like those during menopause.

(1) Sign RED — the index finger of the right "one" hand brushes down the chin a few times. (MM)
(2) Both "L" hands face out at the sides of the face. (SM)

* *These signs refer to the face flushing.*

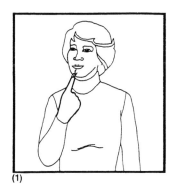
(1)

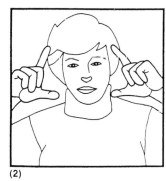
(2)

FLUTTER

Irregular, quick movements.

Flutter is usually used when talking about rapid regular beating of the heart.

(1) Sign HEART — the middle finger of the right "eight" hand taps the chest. (MM)
(2) The left "flat" hand faces in at chest level. The right "S" hand hits the left palm a few times, and at the same time, the cheeks should puff out. (MM)

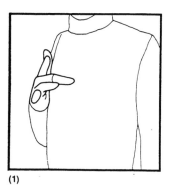
(1)

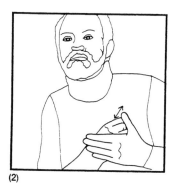
(2)

FOCUS

The place where light rays come together to make a complete, clear image after passing through a lens.

Fuzzy vision can be caused by the focus occuring in front of or someplace behind the retina and not directly on it.

FOLD

A ridge or something which has been bent over on itself.

A cravat is a very convenient bandage to have in a first-aid kit because one can fold it to fit many kinds of injuries.

(1) The left "flat" hand faces up at chest level. The right "flat" hand faces up at chest level and turns over to touch the left hand as if imitating folding something. (SM)

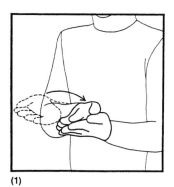
(1)

FOLIC ACID

A vitamin found in yeast, green vegetables and liver. Folic acid is needed to help make blood.

FOLLICLE

A small space, sac or gland.

A hair follicle is the small pit in the skin layers which produces and cares for a hair.

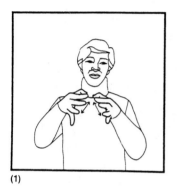
(1)

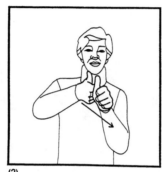
(2)

FOLLOW DIRECTIONS

To do something as told or directed.

It is a good idea to follow directions given to you by a doctor because they are well trained and experienced in their field.

(1) Both "F" hands face down at chest level and move alternately in and out a few times. (MM)
(2) Sign FOLLOW — the right "A" hand with the thumb extended is behind the left "A" hand with the thumb extended, both at chest level. Move both hands out forward. (SM)

FOMENTATION

A hot, wet dressing put on an area to relieve pain or inflammation.

Fomentation may be used to treat boils or abscesses by letting more blood go to the area to fight the infection.

FONTANELLE

See SOFT SPOTS

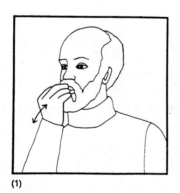
(1)

FOOD

The vegetables, meat, dairy products, grains and other things we eat which give us energy, minerals, vitamins and building materials to keep us healthy and active.

Because our bodies cannot make some substances we must eat enough of the different foods which will give us the needed nutrients.

(1) The fingertips of the right "flat-O" hand tap the mouth a few times. (MM)

FOOD POISONING

An illness which may develop very quickly and is caused by eating foods which contain toxins or poisons. The food may have a poison in a part of it, like some mushrooms and shellfish, or the poison may have been made by bacteria which got into the food and grew. Symptoms of food poisoning develop very rapidly and include pain in the abdomen, nausea, vomiting, diarrhea, a headache and perhaps vision trouble.

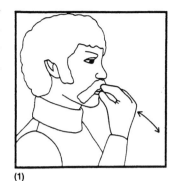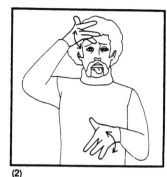
(1)　　　　　　(2)

Food poisoning may be confused with the flu but when several people suddenly get sick at the same time, after eating the same food, then it is probably food poisoning.

(1) Sign FOOD — the fingertips of the right "flat-O" hand tap the mouth a few times. (MM)

(2) Sign SICK — the middle finger of the right "eight" hand touches the forehead and the middle finger of the left "eight" hand touches the stomach. Twist both hands slightly. (SM)

* *The facial expression should show pain or sickness.*

FOOT

The lower part of the leg, which we stand on. A foot includes the toes, heel, arch and sole. *See Figure 1*

(1) The index finger of the right "one" hand points down to the feet. (SM)

(2) Fingerspell "F-O-O-T".

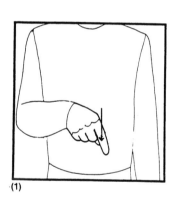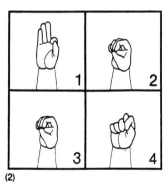
(1)　　　　　　(2)

FORAMEN

An opening or passage.

A foramen can be in the root of a tooth or between every two vertebrae, both allowing nerves and vessels to pass through.

FORBID

To prevent a person from doing something.

A doctor will forbid a person who has high blood pressure, heart disease or a blood vessel disease from smoking, drinking a lot of alcohol, eating salt, getting upset and eating food with a lot of fats.

(Continued on next page)

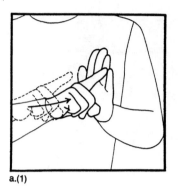

a.(1)

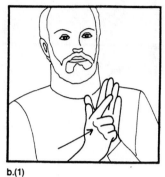

b.(1)

FORBID, *continued*

a. (1) The left "flat" hand faces out with the fingers pointing up. The right "one" hand moves to sharply hit the left palm then bounces off. (SM)
b. (1) The left "flat" hand faces out with the fingers pointing up. The right "L" hand moves to sharply hit the left palm then bounces off. (SM)

FORCEPS

A medical instrument, usually shaped like a pair of tweezers, used to hold, pull or remove things.

There are different sizes and shapes of forceps used for different operations.

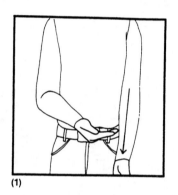

(1)

FOREARM

The part of the arm between the elbow and wrist. *See Figure 1*

(1) The right "cupped" hand brushes down the left arm. (SM)

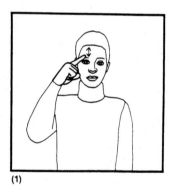

(1)

FOREHEAD

The upper part of the face above the eyes and below the hair. *See Figure 1*

(1) The index finger of the right "one" hand moves from the right eyebrow to the hairline a few times. (MM)

FOREIGN OBJECT OR BODY

Anything which gets into the skin, ears, eyes, nose or other parts of the body and causes irritation. A foreign object or body can be dirt, a piece of glass, wood splinters, pieces of food, small toys or slivers.

Foreign objects or bodies often cause the blocking of a passage or infections.

FORESKIN

The fold of skin which covers the end of the penis. Some men don't have a foreskin because it is removed during circumcision. *See Figure 13.*

(1) Sign PENIS — the middle finger of the right "P" hand taps the nose a few times. (MM)

(2) The left "one" hand faces down at chest level, the finger pointing right. The right "flat-O" hand moves out on the left index finger. (SM)

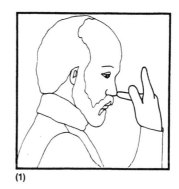
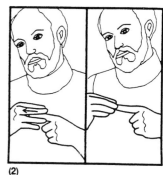

(1)　　　　　(2)

FORMULA

Liquid food given to an infant from birth until about 1 year of age, instead of breast feeding.

Most baby formulas contain the same nutrients as in a mother's breast milk except for antibodies and some trace minerals.

(1) Sign BABY — the right hand and forearm face up, resting on the left hand and forearm which also face upwards. Both are then rocked back and forth as if holding a baby. (MM)

(2) Sign MILK — the right "S" hand faces left at chest level. Open and close the hand slightly as if squeezing something. (MM)

(3) The left "flat" hand faces up at chest level. The right "C" hand faces in, resting in the left palm. Move the right hand up to the mouth into an "A" hand with the thumb extended as if imitating a bottle. (SM)

(4) The left arm is bent at the elbow. The right hand imitates feeding a baby from a bottle. (SM)

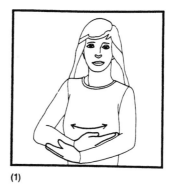
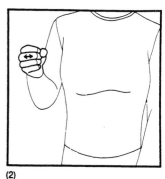

(1)　　　　　(2)

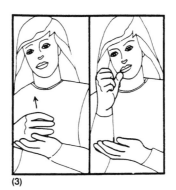
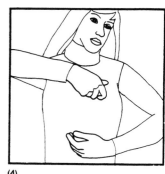

(3)　　　　　(4)

FOUR-TAILED BANDAGE

A strip of cloth with each end split into two halves, forming four tails.

The four-tailed bandage works well on parts of the body which stick out, such as the nose and chin.

FOVEA

See FOVEA CENTRALIS

FOVEA CENTRALIS

A small pit in the center of the retina which is the most sensitive part of the eye. The fovea centralis is contained in the macula lutea and it is made up of closely packed cones making vision very good in the area.

Our vision is best when looking directly at something because the light rays fall upon the fovea centralis.

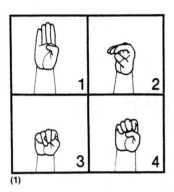 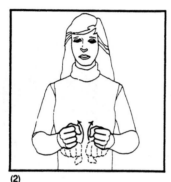

(1)　　　　　　　　　　(2)

FRACTURE

A broken bone. Fractures can be caused by sudden force being applied to a bone and in some diseases, bones may break by themselves. Symptoms of a fracture are pain, swelling, not being able to move the part and the part being shaped abnormally.

There are several different kinds of fractures depending on how the bone was broken and how much damage was done.

(1) Fingerspell "B-O-N-E".

(2) Sign BREAK — both "S" hands face down at chest level. Turn both hands up as if imitating breaking something. (SM)

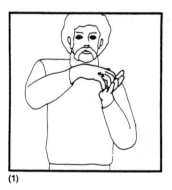 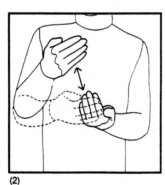

(1)　　　　　　　　　　(2)

FRAGILE

Easily broken or weak.

An older person's bones may break easily because the bones becomes more fragile and brittle.

(1) Sign WEAK — the left "flat" hand faces up at chest level. The fingertips of the right "claw" hand rest in the left palm. Keeping the fingertips in place, bend and straighten the fingers of the right hand a few times. (MM)

(2) Sign EASY — the left "cupped" hand faces up at chest level. The fingers of the right "cupped" hand brush up the back of the left fingers twice. (DM)

(3) Sign BREAK — both "S" hands face down at chest level. Turn both hands up as if imitating breaking something. (SM)

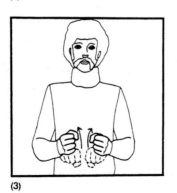

(3)

FRAGMENT

A part of something or a piece which has been broken off.

When a bone is broken, there are often bone fragments in the area.

FREEZE

To change from a liquid to a solid because of cold.

When we are in cold weather for a long time, we can freeze parts of our bodies, like our toes and fingers, causing death of the tissue.

(1) Both "five" hands face down at chest level. Move both hands up slightly into "claw" hands. (SM)

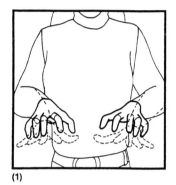
(1)

FRENZY

The state of being violently upset or excited; short time of craziness or madness.

During withdrawal from some drugs, a person may go into a frenzy.

(1) The right "five" hand faces out at shoulder level and twists from left to right a few times. (MM)
(2) The right "one" hand points up and rests on the back of the left hand. Move the finger frantically back and forth a few times. (MM)

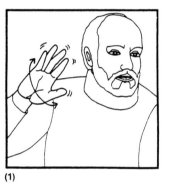
(1)
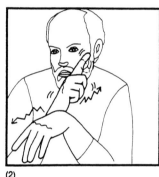
(2)

FREQUENT

Often.

If a person drinks a lot of water, he may have to make more frequent trips to the bathroom because more urine is made.

(1) Sign OFTEN — the left "flat" hand faces up at chest level. The fingertips of the right "cupped" hand touch and move up the left palm a few times. (MM)

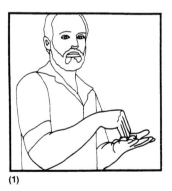
(1)

FRICTION

In medicine, a rubbing action.

Friction is used in massages and after hydrotherapy.

(Continued on next page)

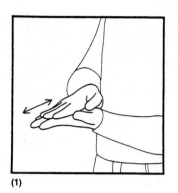
(1)

FRICTION, *continued*

(1) The left "flat" hand faces up at chest level. The right "flat" hand rubs back and forth on the left palm a few times. (MM)

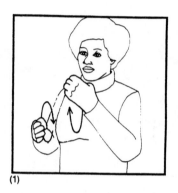
(1)

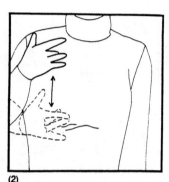
(2)

FRIGID

Not responding to emotions, cold feelings.

Frigid usually refers to a person not wanting to have sexual intercourse.

(1) Sign EMOTION — both "E" hands alternately move inward in circular movements at chest level.
(2) Sign FEEL — the middle finger of the right "eight" hand moves up and down the chest. (MM)
(3) Sign NONE — both "flat-O" hands face down at chest level and move out to the sides. (SM)

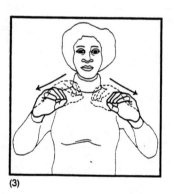
(3)

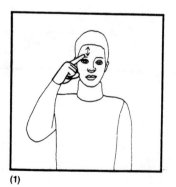
(1)

FRONTAL

Referring to the forehead; anterior.

The frontal bone is the forehead bone.

(1) The index finger of the right "one" hand moves from the right eyebrow to the hairline a few times. (MM)

FROSTBITE

Damage or destruction to a part of the body because it has been frozen. When frostbite occurs the part will first feel cold, tingle and turn red. Later the part will turn pale and the person won't be able to feel it.

Frostbite usually occurs on parts of the body which are a long way from the heart, like the fingers, toes and the nose.

(1) The right index finger points to the area affected by frostbite. (SM)

(2) Both "S" hands face down, the arms bent at the elbows. Drop both elbows down so that the hands face each other. (SM)

* The facial expression should reflect freezing.

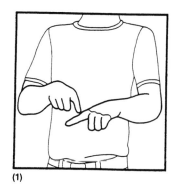

(1)

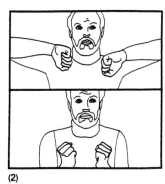

(2)

FROZEN

Having become stiff, turned to ice or unable to move freely.

Arthritis can cause a joint to be frozen in one position.

(1) Sign FREEZE — both "five" hands face down at chest level. Move both hands up slightly into "claw" hands. (SM)

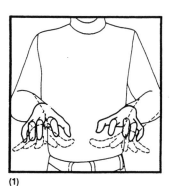

(1)

FRUCTOSE

A type of very sweet sugar; the common sugar found in honey and fruit.

Fructose is made in the body when carbohydrates are broken down to make energy.

(1) Sign SUGAR — the fingertips of the right "flat" hand move up and down on the chin a few times. (MM)

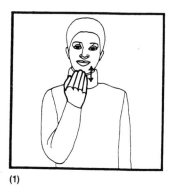

(1)

FRUSTRATION

The feeling of disappointment resulting from a person not being able to do or get what he wants.

Cancer patients sometimes have frustrations about their illness and may need help in dealing with those feelings.

(1) The back of the fingertips of the right "flat" hand tap the mouth a few times.

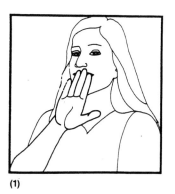

(1)

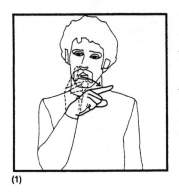
(1)

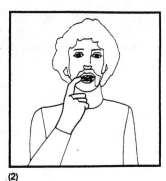
(2)

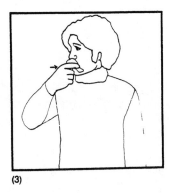
(3)

FULL DENTURE

A set of artificial teeth which replaces all of the natural teeth in both jaws.

Full dentures should be removed before sleeping, should be cleaned regularly and cared for like real teeth.

(1) Sign FALSE — the right "L" hand faces left and brushes past the nose. (SM)
(2) The index finger of the right "one" hand moves across the teeth from right to left. (SM)
(3) The right "modified-C" hand moves towards the mouth as if imitating putting a denture in. (SM)

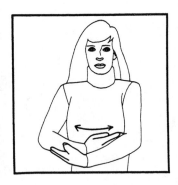

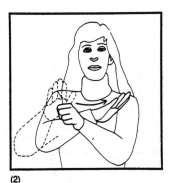
(2)

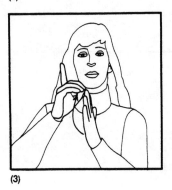
(3)

FULL TERM

The normal end of pregnancy where the fetus is well developed.

If a pregnancy is carried full term, the fetus is well developed having fingernails, toenails and testicles if it's a boy.

(1) Sign BABY — the right hand and forearm face up resting on the left hand and forearm, which also face upwards. Both are then rocked back and forth as if holding a baby. (MM)
(2) The left "S" hand faces right at chest level. The right "flat" hand brushes over the top of the left hand in towards the body. (SM)
(3) The left "flat" hand faces right at chest level. The right "D" hand faces left and moves from the bottom of the left hand to the fingertips. (SM)

FUNCTION

The activity of a structure.

If an organ does not function normally, it could be the result of a disease or disorder.

(1) Sign WORK — the left "S" hand faces down at chest level. The heel of the right "S" hand touches the left hand. (SM)

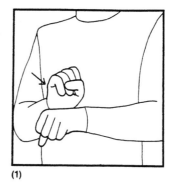
(1)

FUNGUS

A plant which lacks chlorophyll and can consist of a single cell or a group of cells. Fungi live off things which have died or are parasites on living things. Yeasts, molds and mushrooms are all types of fungus. Many types of fungus can cause diseases in plants and animals.

An infection caused by a fungus usually comes on slowly and affects the skin, hair or nails and is hard to treat or get rid of.

FUNNYBONE

The small area which sticks out on the inside of the humerus (elbow), where a nerve may be pressing, causing a tingling feeling.

When someone hits his elbow on something, he says he hit his funnybone.

(1) The left arm is bent at the elbow. The right "S" hand hits the left elbow. (SM)
(2) The right "claw" hand shakes slightly at the left elbow. (SM)

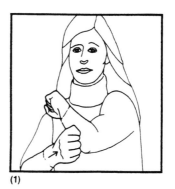
(1)

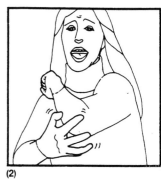
(2)

FUSION

The joining together of two substances. In medicine, fusion is the attaching of bones to each other to hold a part still or to straighten it.

Fusion is usually done to hold vertebrae still or to straighten the spine.

(1) The thumbs and index fingers of both "F" hand join and interconnect. (SM)

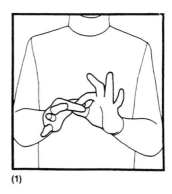
(1)

251

g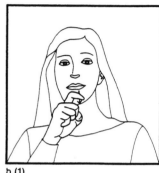

GAG

Trying to vomit; also in dentistry, a device put in the mouth to keep it open and to keep the jaws apart.

When something touches the back of the mouth or throat, a reflex makes us want to gag.

a. (1) The right "five" hand touches the chest and the facial expression should reflect gagging.

* *This should be signed only when referring to physical gagging.*

b. (1) Sign RUBBER the index finger of the right "X" hand brushes down the chin a few times. (MM)

(2) The thumb and index fingers of both hands outline the shape of the gag.(SM)

(3) The right hand imitates putting the gag in the corner of the mouth.

* *This should be signed only when referring to a dental gag.*

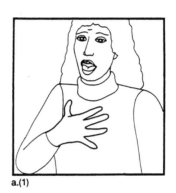
a.(1)

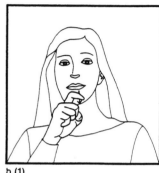
b.(1)

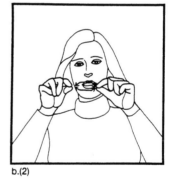
b.(2)

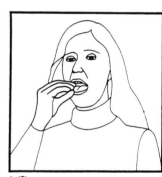
b.(3)

GAIN WEIGHT

Adding pounds to the body, weighing more or getting bigger.

People gain weight because they are growing, getting fatter or developing larger muscles.

(1) The left "H"hand faces down at chest level. The right "H" hand also faces down on top of the left hand. Pivot the right hand slightly a few times. (MM)

(2) The left "H" hand faces down at chest level. The right "H" hand faces up. Turn the right hand over so that the fingers of the right hand touch the fingers of the left hand a few times. (MM)

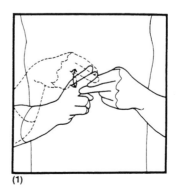
(1)

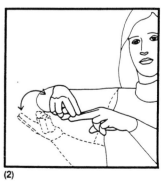
(2)

GALLBLADDER

A small, sack-like organ found under the liver that collects and concentrates the bile which is made in the liver. The gallbladder holds the bile until it is needed in the small intestine for digestion. *See Figure 9*

GALLSTONE

A small stone formed in the gallbladder from the concentrated bile stored there. Gallstones may stay in the gallbladder and cause no problems.

A gallstone could plug the duct going to the small intestine, causing pain and digestion problems and may need to be removed surgically.

GAMMA GLOBULIN

A protein in the blood made up mostly of antibodies.

The gamma globulin part of the blood attacks foreign substances in the body, such as bacteria or toxins.

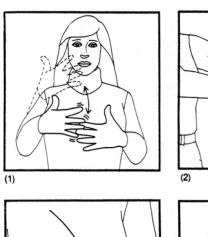

(1)

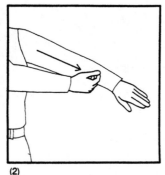

(2)

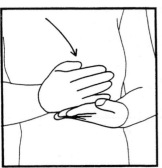

(3)

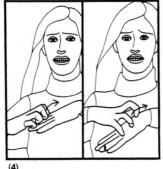

(4)

GANGRENE

Death of tissue because the blood supply is cut off. Gangrene can be caused by cutting a major artery to an area, infection and inflammation slowing the blood flow, frostbite or the blockage of the artery by something.

Before healing can occur, the part with gangrene must be removed or amputated.

(1) Sign BLOOD — the left "five" hand is at chest level with the palm toward the body. The palm of the right "five" hand is toward the body with the middle fingertips touching the mouth. Move the right hand down the back of the left hand. Wiggle the fingers of the right hand as it moves. (MM)

* *This movement should be short, repeated and somewhat restrained.*

(2) The back of the fingertips of the right "flat" hand brush down the left arm. (SM)

* *In this example, the arm is shown. However, the affected area should be shown when signing gangrene.*

(3) Sign STOP — the left "flat" hand faces up at chest level. The right "flat" hand faces left and moves down to sharply hit the left palm. (SM)

(4) The left "flat" hand faces down at chest level. The fingers of the right "claw" hand move up the left hand. (MM)

254

GARGLE

To wash the mouth and throat by holding a liquid in the mouth, tipping the head back, and blowing air out of the lungs through the liquid.

People gargle to help relieve a sore throat or to freshen breath.

(1) Sign DRINK — the right "C" hand imitates taking a drink. (SM)
(2) The fingers of the right "five" hand wiggle at the throat, imitating gargling. (MM)

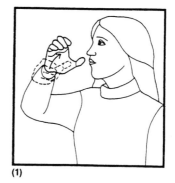
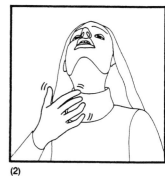

GAS

A substance that is neither solid or liquid and has no form or shape.

In dentistry, gas is used for an anesthetic which is inhaled and helps to relax and calm the patient.

(1) Fingerspell "G-A-S".
(2) The right "claw" hand faces in over the nose and mouth and taps a few times.
* These refer only to an anesthetic gas.

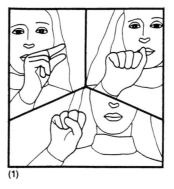
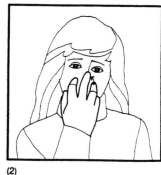

GASP

Difficult breathing, with short, quick inhalations and exhalations; also a quick inhaling of air.

Emotions, surprise or hard exercise can cause us to gasp.

(1) The right "five" hand touches the chest and the facial expression should reflect gasping. (SM)

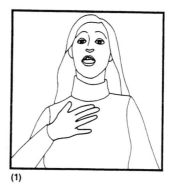

GASTRIC

Referring to the stomach.

Gastric juices are the fluids in the stomach which contain acids and enzymes and help us digest our food.

(1) The fingertips of the right "cupped" hand tap the stomach a few times.

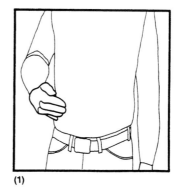

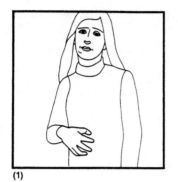
(1)

GASTRITIS

Inflammation of the stomach. Gastritis may be caused from an infection, drinking too much alcohol, or not eating the right foods.

*Symptoms of **gastritis** are pain or tenderness, nausea, vomiting and a coated tongue.*

(1) The fingertips of the right "claw" hand touch the stomach. Bend and straighten the fingers slightly. (MM)

* The facial expression should reflect pain.

GASTROCNEMIUS

The large muscle on the back of the lower leg which makes up the calf. The gastrocnemius is used to flex the foot. *See Figure 4 or 5* .

GASTROINTESTINAL ILLNESS

A disease affecting the stomach and intestine.

*The symptoms of a **gastrointestinal illness** are usually pain in the abdomen, nausea, vomiting and diarrhea.*

(1) The fingertips of the right "cupped" hand tap the stomach a few times.
(2) Sign DISEASE — the middle finger of the right "eight" hand touches the forehead and the middle finger of the left "eight" hand touches the stomach. Tap both middle fingers a few times.

* The facial expression should reflect illness or pain.

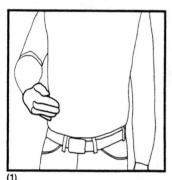
(1)
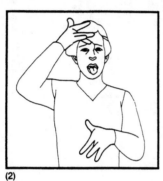
(2)

GAUZE

A thin, loosely woven material used in bandages and dressings.

*Many times **gauze** bandages are used because they absorb a lot.*

(1) The index finger and thumb of the right "F" hand touch the chin, then move down slightly. (SM)
(2) Both "flat-O" hands face up at chest level and open and close a few times. (MM)
(3) Sign BANDAGE — the left "B" hand faces in at chest level. The right "B" hand circles out and around the left hand, imitating wrapping a bandage. (MM)

* This could be signed at the area where the gauze or bandage is being applied.

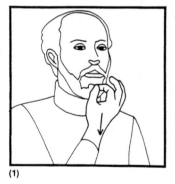
(1)
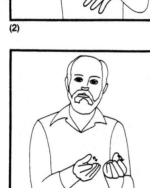
(2)

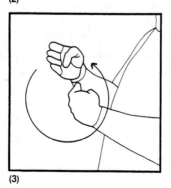
(3)

GENDER

The sex of someone.

A man's gender is male and a woman's is female.

(1) Sign MAN — the right open "flat-O" hand faces down at the forehead then closes. (SM)

(2) The right "flat" hand faces down at the forehead and moves out slightly. (SM)

(3) Sign WOMAN — the thumb of the right "A" hand moves down the right side of the face from the ear to the chin. Then move the right hand into a "flat" hand facing down at the forehead. (SM)

(4) Sign WHICH — both "A" hands with the thumbs extended face each other at chest level and move alternately up and down a few times. (MM)

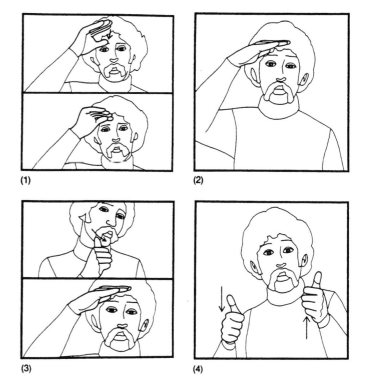

(1)   (2)   (3)   (4)

GENE

A tiny section of a chromosome in the cell. Each gene is responsible for directing the development of one thing. Genes are paired, with one set being inherited from a person's father and the other set from the mother.

Genes determine eye color, skin color, blood type and hair color, among many other traits.

GENERAL ANESTHETIC

A drug which causes a complete loss of feeling all over the body and also a loss of consciousness.

General anesthetics are commonly given before someone has surgery.

(1) Sign INJECTION — the index finger of the right "L" hand touches the left upper arm. Bend the thumb down as if injecting something into the left arm. (SM)

(2) Sign SLEEP — the right "five" hand is in front of the face. Move the hand down into an "A" hand on the left "A" hand. At the same time, the eyes should close. (SM)

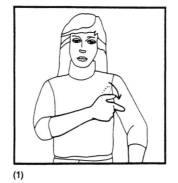

(1)

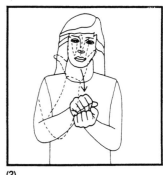

(2)

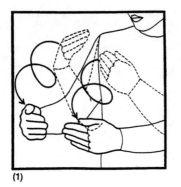

(1)

GENERATION

Any group of individuals born about the same time and having grown up together. Generation is also used for the time periods between the birth of parents and the birth of their children.

*For humans, a **generation** is about 30 years.*

(1) The fingertips of both "flat" hands touch the right shoulder. The hands alternately circle each other as they move forward and down. (SM)

GENERIC DRUG

Any drug prescribed and sold under its chemical name instead of under a special name from a certain company. Generic drugs are drugs that are not protected by a certain trademark. Generic drugs are the same as drugs with special names and are just as effective as the name-brand drugs.

Generic drugs are becoming more popular because their quality is good and they cost less.

GENITALS

The structures and organs involved in sex and reproduction. In a man, the genitals are the testes, penis, vas deferens, the seminal vesicles, prostate gland, and scrotum. In a woman, the genitals are the vulva, clitoris, vagina, uterus, fallopian tubes and ovaries. *See Figures 12 and 13*

GERIATRICS

The area of medicine which treats aging, older people and their diseases.

*Since the number of older people will be increasing greatly in the next 30 years, **geriatrics** is becoming a very important science.*

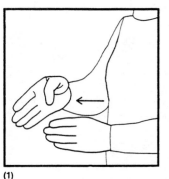

(1)

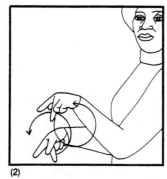

(2)

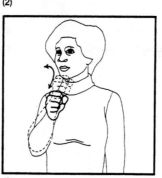

(3)

(1) Sign SPECIALIZE — the left "B" hand faces right at chest level. The right "B" hand faces left on top of the left hand. Move the right hand straight out on the left index finger. (SM)

(2) Sign PEOPLE — both "P" hands face down and move in alternate forward circles a few times. (MM)

(3) Sign OLD — the right "A" hand faces in and brushes down the chin a few times. (MM)

258

GERM

The general term for a very small living thing which can cause disease.

A germ can be a virus, fungus, bacteria or a very small parasite.

GERMAN MEASLES

An (acute) contagious disease caused by a virus. The disease lasts three to five days and has symptoms of a slight fever, a rash, sore throat and swollen glands in the neck and throat region. German measles is also called rubella.

German Measles is dangerous because if a pregnant woman gets this disease during the first three months of pregnancy, it can cause birth defects in her baby.

(1) Sign GERMAN — cross both "five" hands at the wrists and wiggle the fingers. (SM)
(2) The fingertips of both "five" hands move up the sides of the face, touching a few times. (MM)

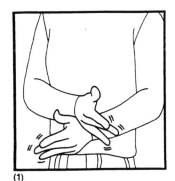
(1)

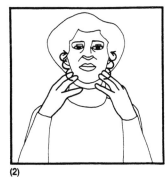
(2)

GERMICIDE

A substance which kills bacteria.

Germicide is another name for a disinfectant or bactericide.

GESTATION

The length of time from fertilization of an egg until birth.

The length of gestation for humans is about nine months.

(1) Sign PREGNANT — mesh the fingers of both "five" hands in front of the stomach and move both hands out forward slightly as if imitating the stomach growing. (SM)
(2) Sign NINE — the right "nine" hand faces out at chest level. (SM)
(3) Sign MONTHS — the left "one" hand points up and faces out at chest level. The index finger of the right "one" hand moves up and down on the left index finger a few times. (MM)

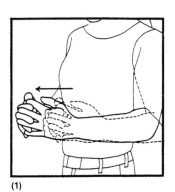
(1)

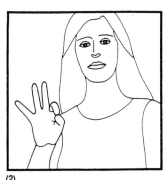
(2)

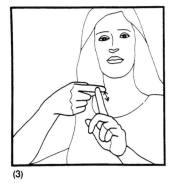
(3)

GIARDIASIS

A very common contagious disease caused by the parasite *Giardia lambia*, that lives in the small intestine. Symptoms of giardiasis are severe diarrhea, stomach pain, weight loss, gas and dehydration. Giardiasis spreads rapidly among people in close contact with each other but it can be treated with antibiotics.

*People usually get **giardiasis** by drinking water that has been contaminated with human feces or by drinking water from beaver ponds.*

GINGIVA

See GUMS

GINGIVECTOMY

The surgical cutting away of diseased gums that have pulled away (recessed) from the teeth due to inflammation.

*A **gingivectomy** may be done to get rid of pockets under the gums due to a disease such as pyorrhea.*

GLAND

An organ, structure or group of cells that make and put out a substance used in some other part of the body.

*Examples of **glands** are the lacrimal **glands**, which make tears, the salivary **glands**, which make saliva, the mammary **glands** or breasts, which make milk, the pancreas, which makes digestive juices and hormones, and the small **glands** lining the stomach and intestine, which make digestive juices.*

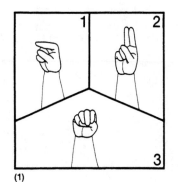
(1)

GINGIVITIS

Inflammation of the gums; Vincent's disease or trench mouth.

*Symptoms of **gingivitis** are redness, swelling and maybe some bleeding.*

(1) Fingerspell "G-U-M".

(Continued on next page)

GINGIVITIS, *continued*

(2) The index finger of the right "one" hand makes a small circle around the gums. (SM)
(3) Sign INFECTION — the right "I" hand faces out at chest level and shakes slightly from side to side a few times. (MM)

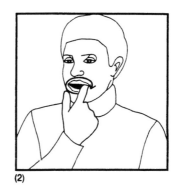

(2)

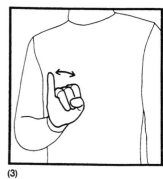

(3)

GLANDULAR FEVER
See MONONUCLEOSIS

GLASSES
A pair of glass or plastic lenses worn to correct a vision problem, protect the eyes from flying objects, or protect the eyes from bright light.

> *Glasses* or eyeglasses that are worn to help vision problems have to be prescribed by an optometrist and should only be worn by the person they are made for.

(1) Both "G" hands face each other at the eyes. Move both hands to the sides, with the thumbs and index fingers touching. (SM)

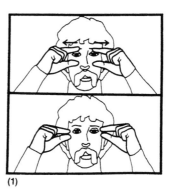

(1)

GLAUCOMA
A disease of the eye in which there is an increase in the pressure inside the eye, causing the eye to become hard and perhaps causing blindness. A person with glaucoma may have pain in the eyes, headaches and fuzzy vision.

> *Glaucoma, which can be discovered by an eye doctor during a checkup, can be treated with drugs or surgery.*

GLOBULIN
A group of proteins found in the blood.

> *One kind of* **globulin**, *the gamma* **globulin**, *helps us to fight infection.*

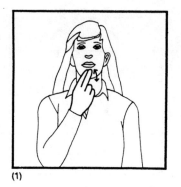

(1)

GLUCOSE

A kind of sugar found in starches, and most fruits; table sugar; dextrose. Glucose is made when some foods are broken down in the digestive tract and taken into the body, where it is used by the cells to make energy. When there is excess glucose in the body, it is stored in the liver or made into fat. When we don't have enough glucose in the body, fat stored in the body is made into glucose.

Glucose is often given to people by injection in cases of shock and as emergency energy to people who aren't eating.

(1) Sign SWEET — the fingertips of the right "H" hand brush down the chin a few times. (MM)

GLUTETHIMIDE

A non-barbiturate drug which acts as a sedative and makes a person relax and sleep.

Glutethimide is sold under the name of Doriden®.

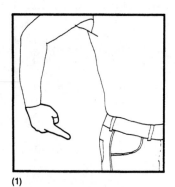

(1)

GLUTEUS MAXIMUS

The large muscle which helps make up the buttocks. The gluteus maximus is important in moving the thigh. *See Figure 5*

(1) The index finger of the right "one" hand points to the buttocks. (SM)

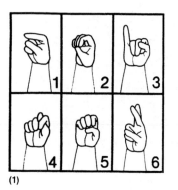

(1)

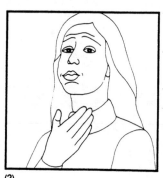

(2)

GOITER

An enlargement of the thyroid which causes a swelling at the front of the throat. A person with goiter may also be nervous, tremble, or sweating a lot, be skinny and have a high heart rate. A goiter is caused by a tumor in the thyroid gland or by not getting enough iodine in the diet which is needed by the thyroid gland to make a hormone.

To help prevent goiter, iodized salt should be used.

(1) Fingerspell "G-O-I-T-E-R".

(2) The right "C" hand moves out slightly from the throat, at the same time, the cheeks should puff out. (SM)

262

GONAD

A general term for the sex glands.

The gonads are the testes and the ovaries.

(1) Sign TESTICLES — both "flat-O" hands drop down slightly and bounce a few times. (MM)
(2) Sign OVARIES — both "F" hands face in on the lower abdomen area. (SM)

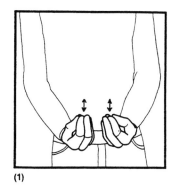

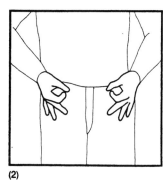

(1)　　　　　　　　　　　　　　(2)

GONORRHEA

A disease of the sex organs which is transmitted by sexual intercourse and caused by a bacteria. In men, there may be a yellowish discharge from the penis and difficult, painful urination. In women, there may not be any symptoms and if there are symptoms, they may not be bad enough to cause her to see a doctor. When a woman does have symptoms, they are a discharge from the vagina or urethra, painful urination and pain in the lower abdomen. Gonorrhea can be dangerous in a woman because it may damage her reproductive organs so badly that she can't have children.

Gonorrhea can be treated with antibiotics such as penicillin, tetracycline and ampicillin.

(1) Fingerspell "V-D".

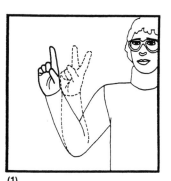

(1)

* *This is a general sign used for veneral disease. The specific type should be fingerspelled following "V-D".*

GOOFBALLS

See PHENOBARBITAL

GOUT

A disease caused by a build-up of a waste deposited in and around joints. Symptoms are pain, inflammation, redness and swelling around the joints, especially the big toe.

Gout can be treated with medication and by changing a person's diet.

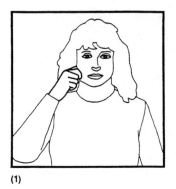
(1)

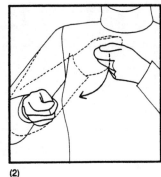
(2)

GRAFT

Transplanting a tissue or organ taken from another part of a person's body or from another person and used to replace a part that has been removed or damaged. Bone, skin, nerves and corneas are some structures that have been attached to people and used to replace a part of their bodies.

The major problem with a graft is that the person's body may recognize that it is not a natural part of the body and thus reject it.

(1) Sign SKIN — the index finger and thumb of the right hand grab the right cheek. (SM)
(2) Sign EXCHANGE — the left "A" hand faces in at chest level. The right "A" hand also faces in behind the left hand. Move the right hand down under the left hand then out forward. (SM)

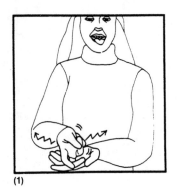
(1)

GRAND MAL SEIZURE

An epileptic attack, with loss of consciousness and convulsions. Before a grand mal, the patient may feel an aura, the strange feeling or warning a person gets before an attack. The person will become unconscious, fall to the ground, have convulsions and may go into a coma.

One should not try to stop a grand mal seizure but rather protect the person from hurting himself and afterwards let the person rest.

(1) The left "flat" hand faces up at chest level. The right bent "V" hand faces up in the left palm and moves frantically. (MM)

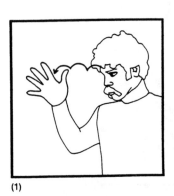
(1)

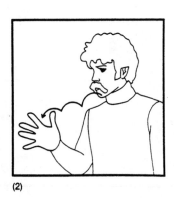
(2)

GRANDPARENTS

The parents of one's mother and father.

Grandmothers and grandfathers are grandparents.

(1) Sign GRANDFATHER — the thumb of the right "five" hand touches the forehead, then move the hand forward a few times. (MM)
(2) Sign GRANDMOTHER — the thumb of the right "five" hand touches the chin, then move the hand forward a few times. (MM)

GREENSTICK FRACTURE

A fracture where the bone has not broken completely through, caused by a fall or accident and more common with children.

A greenstick fracture should be treated immediately or a complete fracture may occur and possible deformity.

GRIEF

A feeling of great sadness and regret after someone has died or been lost.

People in a state of grief will first feel shock and disbelief; then they will feel depressed and not want to eat or sleep, and they may cry a lot.

(1) The middle finger of the right "eight" hand touches the chest.(SM)

* The facial expression should reflect sadness.

(2) Both "claw" hands are at chest level. Slightly twist them and then close them. (SM)

* The facial expression should also reflect sadness.

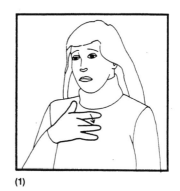

(1)

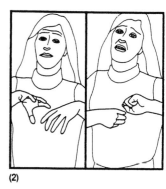

(2)

GROIN

The area where the thigh meets the body.
See Figure '1

GROWTH

An increase in size or the development of something.

Growth can be normal, as a person's becoming taller and larger until they are adults, or it can be abnormal, as the growth of a tumor.

(1) The right "claw" hand is on top of the left arm. Open the hand slightly, and at the same time, the cheeks should puff out. (SM)

* This could be signed at the area of the growth.

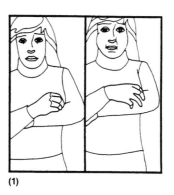

(1)

GUMS

The pink tissue that surrounds the bottoms of the teeth; also called the gingiva. *See Figure 25*

(1) Fingerspell "G-U-M".

(2) The index finger of the right "one" hand makes a small circle around the gums. (SM)

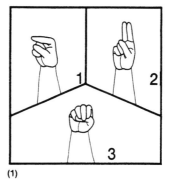

(1)

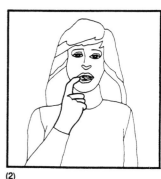

(2)

GUT

The bowel or intestine; the insides.

The gut may also be called the viscera.

(1) The fingertips of the right "cupped" hand tap the stomach a few times.

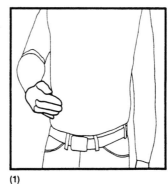

(1)

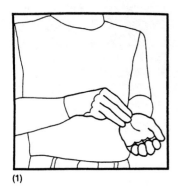
(1)

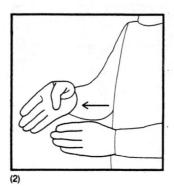
(2)

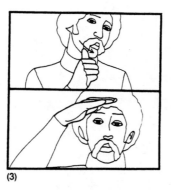
(3)

GYNECOLOGIST

A doctor who specializes in diseases of women, especially diseases of the reproductive organs.

Women should see a gynecologist regularly to have a Paps smear, a breast exam and a check to make sure they are healthy.

(1) Sign DOCTOR — the right "M" hand touches the left inside wrist. (DM)
(2) Sign SPECIALIZE — the left "B" hand faces right at chest level. The right "B" hand faces left on top of the left hand. Move the right hand straight out on the left index finger. (SM)
(3) Sign WOMAN — the thumb of the right "A" hand moves down the right side of the face from the ear to the chin. Then move the right "flat" hand to forehead level.(SM)

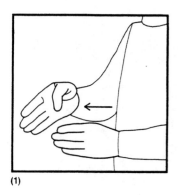
(1)

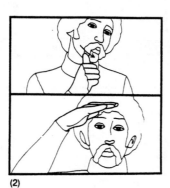
(2)

GYNECOLOGY

The area of medicine which deals with women's diseases.

Gynecology especially deals with diseases of the reproductive organs and the breasts.

(1) Sign SPECIALIZE — the left "B" hand faces right at chest level. The right "B" hand faces left on top of the the hand. Move the right hand straight out on the left index finger. (SM)
(2) Sign WOMAN — the thumb of the right "A" hand moves down the right side of the face from the ear to the chin. Then move the right "flat" hand to forehead level. (SM)

h

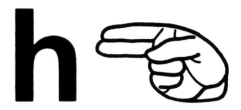

HABIT

An action we do frequently without really knowing we are doing it.

Habits are formed by doing something over and over again until the action becomes a reflex.

(1) The index finger of the right "one" hand touches the forehead, then moves down into an "S" hand crossing the left "S" hand at the wrist. (SM)

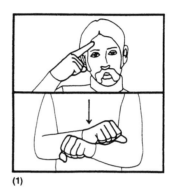

(1)

HAIR

A long, thin growth from the skin. Hair is a thread-like, bendable string of hardened, dead cells.

Different types of hair on the body have different growth rates; eventually they fall out and are replaced.

(1) The index finger and thumb of the right "F" hand grab some hair. (SM)

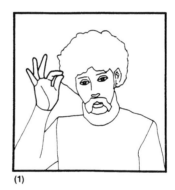

(1)

HALF RING TRACTION SPLINT

A kind of splint used to hold a broken bone still and prevent the broken ends from overlapping. A half ring traction splint is also called a Keller-Blake splint.

Half ring traction splints are very useful for a broken femur or thigh bone.

HALITOSIS

Bad smelling breath.

Halitosis can be caused by strong smelling foods, an unclean mouth or teeth, an upset stomach or an infection in the gums, teeth, mouth, throat or sinuses.

(Continued on next page)

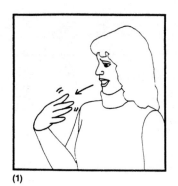
(1)

(1) The right "five" hand faces down and moves away from the mouth, at the same time the fingers wiggle. (SM)

* *The facial expression should reflect bad breath.*

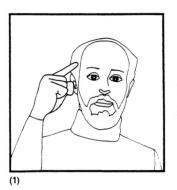
(1)

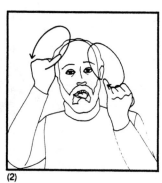
(2)

HALLUCINATION

The sensation that one sees, hears, feels, smells or tastes something that is not really there. The person usually cannot tell that what he is feeling is not real and so behaves as if it were real.

Hallucinations may be caused by mental illness, a head injury, disease of a part of the brain, or by certain drugs, such as LSD and alcohol.

(1) The index finger of the right "one" hand points to the head. (SM)

(2) Both "I" hands face in at head level. Move both hands alternately towards the center, then down and around in circular movements a few times. (MM)

HALLUCINOGEN

A drug that causes a person to see, hear, feel, smell or taste something that is not really there.

LSD, mescaline, and peyote are hallucinogens.

(1) Sign PILL — the thumb and index finger of the right hand touch, the palm faces the mouth. Flick the index finger towards the mouth as if popping a pill into the mouth. (SM)

(2) Both "I" hands face in at head level. Move both hands alternately towards the center, then down and around in circular movements a few times. (MM)

* *If the hallucinogen is taken a different way other than a pill, the specific should be fingerspelled or signed.*

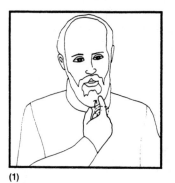
(1)

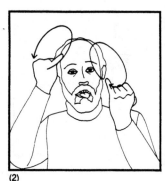
(2)

HAMMER

The common name for the malleus, one of the three tiny bones in the middle ear which helps carry sound waves from the eardrum to the inner ear. The movement is picked up by the auditory nerve as sound. *See Figure 20*

HAMSTRINGS

The muscles and tendons on the back of the thigh. The hamstrings bend the knee and help move it. *See Figure 5*

268

HAND

The lower part of the arm from the wrist to the tips of the fingers. The hand is made up of the wrist, palm and fingers. *See Figure 1*

(1) The left "flat" hand brushes down the back of the right "flat" hand and then the right "flat" hand brushes down the back of the left "flat" hand. (SM)

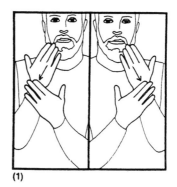

(1)

HANDICAP

In medicine, a term used to describe a condition in which normal mental or physical activity is limited without the help of aids. Also the way a person allows a disability to affect them or the interaction between a person's disability and their surrounding environment.

A person who adapts to a handicap with training and special equipment can live a useful, rewarding life.

(1) Fingerspell "H-C".

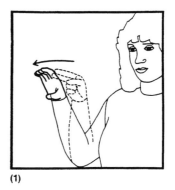

(1)

HANGNAIL

A piece of partly attached skin at the base of a fingernail.

Hangnails, sometimes caused by picking at the skin, should be left alone or they could become infected.

HANGOVER

A general word for the discomfort a person feels after drinking a certain amount of alcohol. A person will usually have a hangover after getting drunk but some people may get one after drinking a very small amount.

Symptoms of a hangover may be depression, a headache, nausea, thirst, tiredness or being easily upset.

(1) The right "A" hand with the thumb extended faces out at shoulder level and moves across and down in front of the body. (SM)

(2) Sign TOMORROW — the thumb of the right "A" hand brushes past the right cheek and slightly forward. (SM)

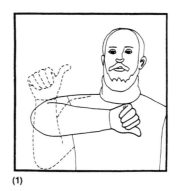

(1)

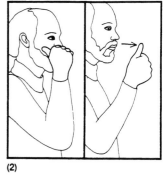

(2)

(Continued on next page)

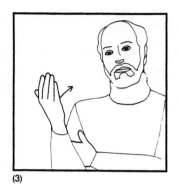

(3)

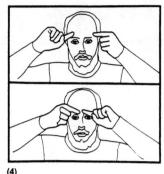

(4)

HANGOVER, *continued*

(3) Sign MORNING — the left "flat" hand touches the inside elbow of the right arm. The right "flat" hand faces up. Move the right hand up as if indicating the sun coming up in the morning. (SM)

(4) Sign HEADACHE — both "one" hands point to each other at the head and twist in opposite directions a few times. (MM)

* *The facial expression should reflect pain.*

HANSEN'S DISEASE

See LEPROSY

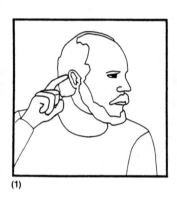

(1)

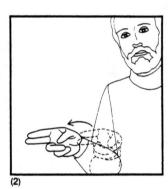

(2)

HARD OF HEARING

A partial loss of hearing in which a person is able to use hearing for learning and use an oral language with or without a hearing aid.

*It is common for a person who is **hard of hearing** to hear muffled sounds that would be clear to a person who has normal hearing.*

(1) The right index finger points to the right ear. (SM)

(2) The right hand signs "H" twice, moving to the side slightly. (DM)

HARDENING OF THE ARTERIES

A disease in which the walls of the arteries become thick and hard and lose their elasticity. Hardening of the arteries, or arteriosclerosis, usually takes place as people get older and is a major cause of death. Hardening of the arteries will make blood-flow difficult, causing high blood pressure.

*The exact cause of **hardening of the arteries** is unknown but eating fatty foods and not getting enough exercise are believed to help cause it.*

HARELIP

A tuck or cleft of the upper lip caused by a congenital (birth) defect.

Harelip may also be called cheiloschisis.

HASHISH

A concentrated and purified drug made from the marijuana plant (cannabis sativa). Hashish is usually smoked in a pipe or cigarette for its hallucinogenic effect.

The use and sale of hashish is illegal in most countries, including the United States.

(1) Fingerspell "H-A-S-H".
(2) The thumb and index finger of the right "F" hand touch the mouth. (SM)

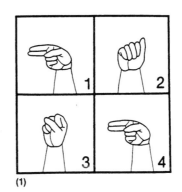

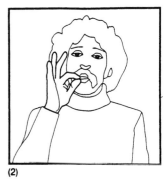

(1)   (2)

HAY FEVER

An allergy to pollen or dust, causing the nose, eyes and upper airways to become irritated.

A person with hay fever will sneeze, have a runny nose and sore, red, watery eyes during certain times of the year, especially during Spring and Fall.

(1) The index finger of the right "one" hand touches the nose. (SM)
(2) Sign OPPOSITE — both "one" hands point towards each other. Move the right hand back towards the body. (SM)

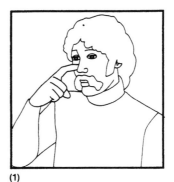

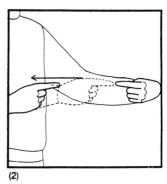

(1)   (2)

HEAD

The part of the body attached to the neck, containing the brain and the organs of sight, hearing, smell and taste.

The head is also made up of the skull and bones of the face.

(1) The fingertips of the right "cupped" hand touch the top of the head, then move down slightly to touch the lower part of the head. (SM)

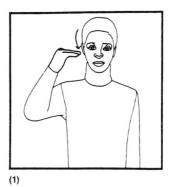

(1)

HEADACHE

A general pain inside the head. The pain can be in a certain area as behind the eyes, on one side of the head or in the back of the head or it can be spread out. The pain can be a dull ache or a sharp, stabbing one.

Headaches can be caused by any upset in the body, such as an infection, stress, poisoning, a blow to the head or a disease of the head.

(1) Sign HEADACHE — both "one" hands point to each other at the forehead. Twist both hands in opposite directions a few times. (MM)

* *The facial expression should reflect pain.*

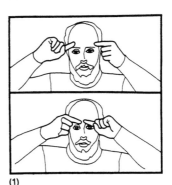

(1)

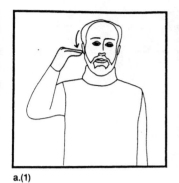

a.(1)

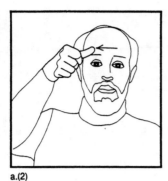

a.(2)

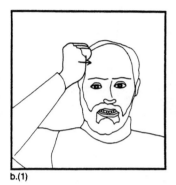

b.(1)

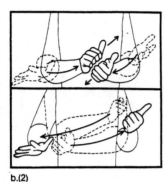

b.(2)

HEAD INJURY

A wound or damage to the head.

A head injury tends to bleed a lot and there is often the danger of brain damage.

a. (1) Sign HEAD — the fingertips of the right "cupped" hand touch the top part of the head then move down slightly to touch the lower part of the head. (SM)

(2) Sign CUT — the thumb of the right "A" hand moves from left to right across the forehead. (SM)

* *If the head is cut, these should be signed at the area of the cut.*

b. (1) Sign HIT — the right "A" hand hits the head. (SM)

(2) Sign DAMAGE — the left "five" hand faces up at chest level. The right "five" hand faces down at chest level. Move both hands towards the center, ending in "A" hands with the thumbs extended, facing each other. Continue moving the right hand through to the left and the left hand through to the right until they cross at the arms. At the same time, move the right hand back to its original position, ending in a "five" hand facing down and the left hand back to its original position, ending in an "A" hand facing down.

* *These should be signed if the head injury is a result of a blow.*

HEAL

Making something whole or healthy. Healing is curing the body or repairing damage caused by disease or injury.

The body will usually heal naturally but a doctor may have to help by speeding it up or correcting a defect.

(1) Sign HEALTH — both "claw" hands face down at shoulder level. Move both hands up slightly into "S" hands. (SM)

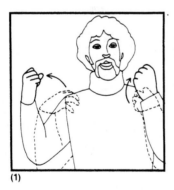

(1)

HEALTH

The state of well-being where the mind and all body functions are working normally.

For good health, a person should be comfortable physically, mentally and socially.

(1) Both "claw" hands face down at shoulder level. Move both hands up slightly into "S" hands. (SM)

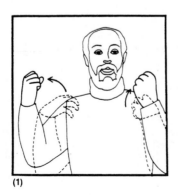

(1)

HEAR

Able to sense sounds.

Blind people can often hear sounds better than sighted people.

(1) The index finger of the right "one" hand points to the right ear. (SM)

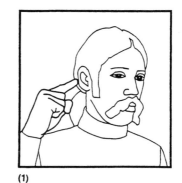

(1)

HEARING AID

A small electronic device placed in the ear which modifies sounds so that a person with a hearing loss can hear.

A hearing aid may help a person with a hearing loss.

a. (1) The right "F" hand touches the right ear and wiggles slightly. (MM)

b. (1) The index finger of the right "one" hand hooks over the right ear. (SM)

* The little finger could run down the chest to indicate a hearing aid with a wire, if referring to a specific type of hearing aid.

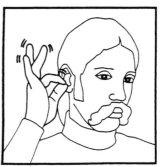

a.(1)

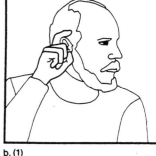

b. (1)

HEARING PERSON

A person who is able to hear sounds.

A hearing person is also usually able to speak.

(1) The index finger of the right "one" hand touches the mouth, then moves up and out in a small arc from the mouth. (MM)

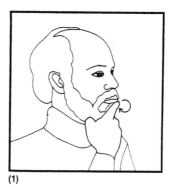

(1)

HEART

The hollow, muscular organ in the chest which contracts rhythmically to pump blood to all parts of the body. The heart has four chambers: two atria and two ventricles. There is an atrium sitting on top of each ventricle and there is a one-way opening between an atrium and ventricle. The two atria and the two ventricles do not have an opening between them so the heart is actually divided in half up and down. The atria are the part of the heart which collects blood from the body or lungs and holds it until they are full and then contracts to force the blood into the ventricles. The ventricles are very muscular;

(Continued on next page)

273

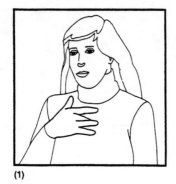
(1)

HEART, *continued*

when they get the blood from the atria, they contract and send the blood out to the general body or to the lungs. It is easier to understand how the heart works if it is thought of as two separate hearts. The atrium and ventricle on the right side gets used blood from the general body and sends it to the lungs to pick up oxygen and give off carbon dioxide. The atrium and ventricle on the left side get fresh blood with oxygen in it back from the lungs and sends it out to the general body. *See Figure 15 or 16*

(1) The middle finger of the right "eight" hand taps the chest a few times.

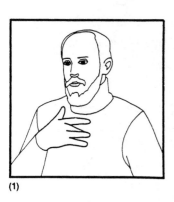
(1)

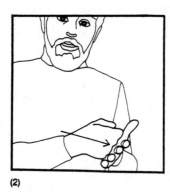
(2)

HEART ATTACK

A general term for the narrowing or plugging of an artery which takes fresh blood with oxygen in it to the muscle of the heart; cardiac arrest. A person having a heart attack will have a severe gripping pain in the chest, will be afraid, be sweating and nauseous, have shortness of breath and may be in shock. The pain in the chest may spread to the jaw, neck or left shoulder and arm. A heart attack is another name for a myocardial infarction.

*A person having a **heart attack** should be gotten to a hospital quickly because it may cause damage to the heart, resulting in death.*

(1) Sign HEART — the middle finger of the right "eight" hand taps the chest a few times.
(2) The left "flat" hand faces up at chest level. The right "S" hand faces in and sharply hits the palm of the left hand. (SM)

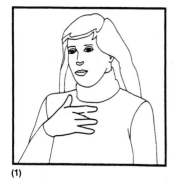
(1)

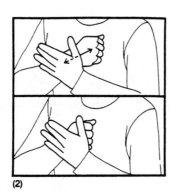
(2)

HEARTBEAT

The movement of the heart chambers. The heart chambers first contract (systole) and then relax (diastole). The two movements make one heartbeat or cardiac cycle.

*The result of a **heartbeat** is the movement of blood through the four chambers of the heart and the blood vessels of the body.*

(1) Sign HEART — the middle finger of the right "eight" hand taps the chest a few times.
(2) The left "flat" hand faces in at chest level. The right "S" hand sharply hits the left palm a few times as if imitating the heart beating. (MM)

HEARTBURN

A burning feeling behind the sternum (breastbone) caused by digestive juices from the stomach getting into the esophagus. The digestive juices contain acids that cause pain and irritation when they get out of the stomach.

Sometimes someone having a heart attack confuses the pain with a severe case of heartburn.

(1) Sign HEART — the middle finger of the right "eight" hand taps the chest a few times.
(2) Fingerspell "B-U-R-N".

* This should be explained because the term HEARTBURN is a slang expression.

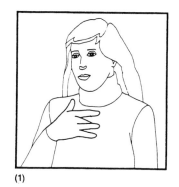
(1)

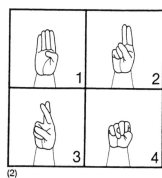
(2)

HEART DISEASE

Any of several diseases involving the heart.

Heart disease may be an infection of the heart, like rheumatic fever, or may be damage to the heart, like scarring after a heart attack.

(1) Sign HEART — the middle finger of the right "eight" hand taps the chest a few times.
(2) Sign DISEASE — the middle finger of the right "eight" hand touches the forehead and the middle finger of the left "eight" hand touches the stomach. (SM)

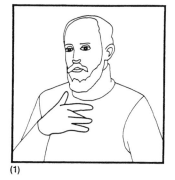
(1)

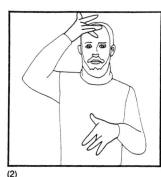
(2)

HEART FAILURE

See HEART ATTACK

HEART MURMUR

See MURMUR

HEAT CRAMPS

Painful tightening of muscles after working hard where it is hot. Heat cramps are caused by not getting enough salt and water to replace that lost by sweating.

Heat cramps can be prevented by adding a little salt to drinking water on hot days.

HEAT EXHAUSTION

A severe reaction to being in a hot place in which a person becomes very weak and may lose consciousness. The person will also be dizzy and have a headache; the skin will be cool, moist and pale and the body temperature will be normal.

Heat exhaustion is caused by the loss of body fluids and salt through sweating.

(Continued on next page)

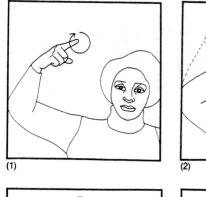
(1)

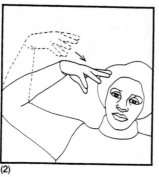
(2)

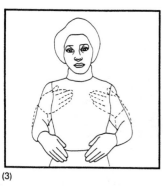
(3)

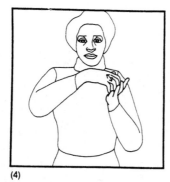
(4)

(1) Sign SUN — the index finger of the right "one" hand makes a small circle in the air as if indicating the sun. (SM)

(2) Sign SUN RAYS — the right "five" hand faces down and moves down slightly towards the body as if indicating the sun's rays coming down. (SM)

(3) Sign BODY — both "flat" hands touch the chest and then move down to touch the stomach area. (SM)

(4) Sign WEAK — The left "flat" hand faces up at chest level. The fingertips of the right "claw" hand touch the left palm. Keeping the fingertips in place, bend and straighten the fingers at the knuckles a few times. (MM)

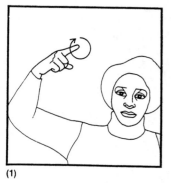
(1)

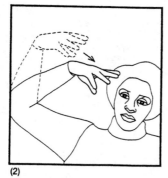
(2)

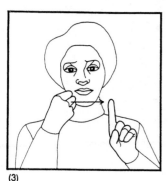
(3)

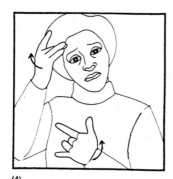
(4)

HEAT STROKE

A very severe, dangerous condition caused by being in high temperatures or the sun for a long time. The person will have a very high temperature, usually higher than 105°F, not be sweating, have a headache, and the skin will be hot, dry and red. In severe cases, coma and death may result unless the temperature is lowered. Heat stroke is also called sunstroke.

Heat stroke is caused by extreme heat causing the temperature controlling part of the brain to not work normally.

(1) Sign SUN — the index finger of the right "one" hand makes a small circle in the air as if indicating the sun. (SM)

(2) Sign SUN RAYS — the right "five" hand faces down and moves down towards the body slightly as if indicating the sun's rays coming down. (SM)

(3) The left "one" hand faces out with the finger pointing up. The right "S" hand sharply hits the left index finger. (SM)

(4) Sign SICK — the middle finger of the right "eight" hand touches the forehead and the middle finger of the left "eight" hand touches the stomach. Twist both hands slightly. (SM)

* The facial expression should reflect illness.

HEEL

The rounded part of the foot under the ankle. *See Figure 3*

HEIMLICH MANEUVER

A special way of removing an object from the trachea or pharynx when it is preventing flow of air from the lungs. When doing the Heimlich Maneuver, first wrap your arms around the victim's waist from behind. Make a fist with one hand and place it against the person's abdomen between the navel and rib cage. Grab the fist with the other hand and press in on the abdomen with a quick, upward movement. This should be repeated if necessary.

The Heimlich Maneuver is also known as the Heimlich Hug.

HELP

To assist or aid.

Nurses often help doctors when treating patients.

(1) The left "flat" hand faces up at waist level. The right "S" hand faces in on the left palm. Move both hands up to chest level. (SM)

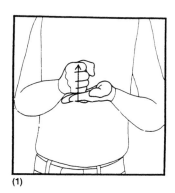
(1)

HEMATOMA

A swelling caused by the collection of blood from a broken blood vessel.

Hematomas, often caused by a blow which damages small blood vessels, are usually absorbed and go away by themselves.

(1) The right "S" hand hits the left arm. (SM)
(2) Sign BLOOD — the left "five" hand is at chest level with the palm toward the body. The palm of the right "five" hand is toward the body with the middle fingertips touching the mouth. Move the right hand down the back of the left hand. Wiggle the fingers of the right hand as it moves. (MM)

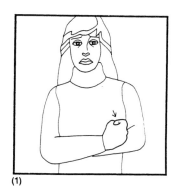
(1)

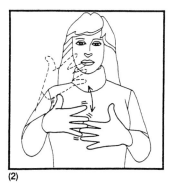
(2)

* This movement should be short, repeated and somewhat restrained.
* These should be signed at the area of the hematoma.

(Continued on next page)

277

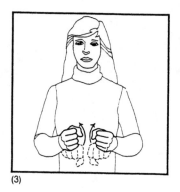
(1)

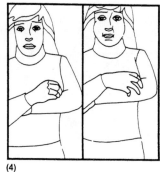
(2)

(3) Sign BREAK — both "S" hands are together at chest level with the palms facing down. Turn both hands up as if breaking something. (SM)

(4) The fingertips of the right "claw" hand touch the left forearm. Open the right hand slightly and at the same time, the cheeks should puff out, indicating swelling. (SM)

This could be signed at the location of the hematoma or point to the affected area following all four signs.

HEMOGLOBIN

A kind of protein containing iron found inside red blood cells and giving blood its red color. Hemoglobin can attach oxygen to itself and carry it through the bloodstream.

Hemoglobin picks up oxygen at the lungs and releases oxygen in the tissues.

HEMOPHILIA

An inherited blood disease wherein the blood takes a long time to clot, usually occuring in males; also called Bleeder's Disease or Bleeding Sickness. Symptoms of hemophilia are swelling in the joints or a cut that won't stop bleeding.

Hemophilia is caused by not having enough of a certain substance (antihemophilic globulin or antihemophilic factor) in the plasma which helps in clotting.

(1) Sign BLEED — the left "five" hand is at chest level with the palm toward the body. The palm of the right "five" hand is toward the body with the middle fingertips touching the mouth. Move the right hand down the back of the left hand. Wiggle the fingers of the right hand as it moves.(SM)

This movement should be long and slow.

(2) Sign DISEASE — the middle finger of the right "eight" hand touches the forehead and the middle finger of the left "eight" hand touches the stomach. (SM)

(3) Sign CUT — the left "flat" hand faces down at chest level. The thumb of the right "A" hand moves down the back of the left hand as if imitating cutting. (SM)

(4) Sign CAN'T — the left "one" hand faces down at chest level. The right "one" hand faces down and moves down to strike the left index finger. (SM)

(Continued on next page)

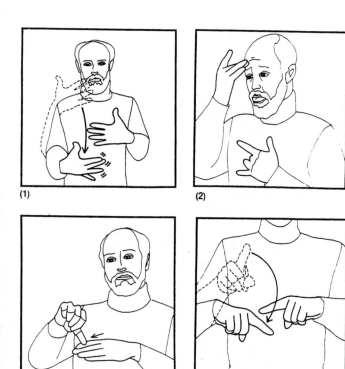
(3)

(4)

(5) Sign STOP — the left "flat" hand faces up at chest level. The right "flat" hand faces left and moves down to sharply hit the left palm. (SM)

(6) Sign BLOOD — the left "five" hand is at chest level with the palm toward the body. The palm of the right "five" hand is toward the body with the middle fingertips touching the mouth. Move the right hand down the back of the left hand. Wiggle the fingers of the right hand as it moves. (MM)

* This movement should be short, repeated and somewhat restrained.

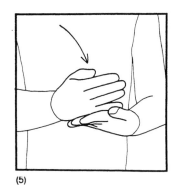
(5)

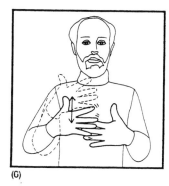
(6)

HEMORRHAGE

The abnormal escape of blood from an artery, vein or capillary, occuring inside or outside the body. When the hemorrhage is inside the body, the person will develop symptoms of shock, cold and moist skin, a pale face, and the pulse will be weak, rapid or irregular.

Although the body can lose one to two pints of blood without a great deal of harm, if a hemorrhage can be seen, pressure should be applied to stop it.

(1) Sign BLOOD — the left "five" hand is at chest level with the palm toward the body. The palm of the right "five" hand is toward the body with the middle fingertips touching the mouth. Move the right hand down the back of the left hand. (MM)

* This movement should be short, repeated and somewhat restrained.

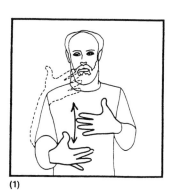
(1)

HEMORRHOID

A group of enlarged veins around the anus and rectum; piles. Hemorrhoids may bleed, be painful or itchy. They may be caused by not enough activity, being overweight, pregnancy or constipation.

Hemorrhoids can be treated with ointments or suppositories but in severe cases surgery may be needed.

(1) The right "one" hand points to the buttocks. (SM)
(2) Sign BLOOD — the left "five" hand is at chest level with the palm toward the body. The palm of the right "five" hand is toward the body with the middle fingertips touching the mouth. Move the right hand down the back of the left hand. (MM)

* This movement should be short, repeated and somewhat restrained.

(3) The right "O" hand is facing down on the left forearm. Open the hand slightly into a "claw" hand, at the same time, the cheeks should puff out. (SM)

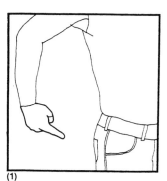
(1)

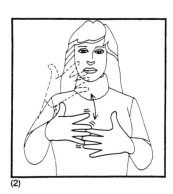
(2)

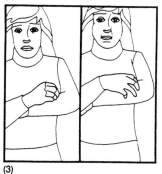
(3)

279

HEPARIN

An organic acid found in lung and liver tissue and used to prevent blood from clotting; anticoagulant.

Heparin may be used in treating thrombosis, embolism or frostbite.

HEPATITIS

Inflammation of the liver caused by a viral infection or poisoning. A person with hepatitis will usually have yellow colored skin, an enlarged sore liver, a fever, be very weak, nauseous and lose weight. There are two major kinds of viral hepatitis. The less severe is infectious hepatitis or Hepatitis A and the more serious kind is serum hepatitis or Hepatitis B, which can cause death.

Hepatitis is caught by having someone's blood who has the virus getting into your blood or by contact with someone's excretions who has the virus.

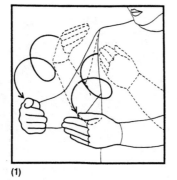

(1)

HEREDITARY

Characteristics inherited from a person's ancestors.

The way a person looks and acts is partly hereditary and partly environmental.

(1) The fingertips of both "cupped" hands touch the right shoulder. Alternately circle both hands forward and down. (SM)

HERNIA

The pushing of an organ or part of an organ through the wall of the area it belongs in; a rupture. Hernias are caused by weakness in the wall holding in the organ or by straining, as when lifting something heavy.

Hernias are dangerous because blood supply to the part forced out of its space may be cut off or movement of material through the forced-out part may be blocked.

HEROIN

A narcotic drug made from the poppy flower. Though heroin is a strong pain reliever and causes a person to feel very good, it isn't used much because it is very addictive.

Using heroin that has not been prescribed by a doctor, bringing heroin into the country, and selling heroin except in a registered pharmacy, are all illegal in the United States.

(Continued on next page)

(1) The right "S" hand hits the elbow of the left hand a few times. (MM)

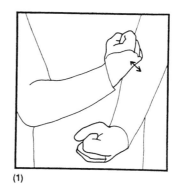

(1)

HERPES SIMPLEX

An infectious skin disease caused by one of the herpesviruses (herpesvirus hominis) causing eruptions of the skin or mucous membranes. Painful blisters usually occur on the head or face, on one side of the body. If herpes simplex returns, it usually occurs in the same spot as before.

Herpes simplex is also called "cold sores" or "fever blisters".

HERPES ZOSTER

An infectious skin disease caused by one of the herpesviruses (varicella-zoster); also called Shingles or Zoster. An area of the skin, usually on the head and only on one side of the body, becomes blistered and very painful. Herpes zoster is caused by the same virus which causes chickenpox staying in nerve cells and then, for some unknown reason, coming out and infecting the skin. Herpes zoster is thought to cause cancer of the cervix in women.

Herpes zoster can be dangerous if it affects the eye, in which case an ophthalmologist should be seen immediately.

HERPESVIRUS

Any of several viruses causing eruptions of the skin or mucous membranes; especially herpes simplex, herpes zoster and varicella (chickenpox). Other types of herpesviruses are herpes facialis (a form of herpes simplex occuring on the face), herpes genitalis (occuring on the male or female genitals), herpes labialis (a form of herpes simplex occuring on the lips), herpes menstrualis (occuring during the menstrual period), herpes praeputialis (occuring on the male genitals), herpes progenitalis (a form of herpes simplex occuring on the vulva), herpes simiae (spread from infected monkeys to man), and herpes opthalmicus (a form of herpes zoster occurring on the face, eye and nose.)

(Continued on next page)

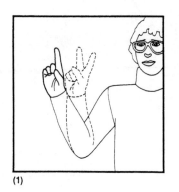
(1)

HERPESVIRUS, *continued*

(1) Fingerspell "V-D".

* *This is a general sign for VENEREAL DISEASE. The specific type should also be fingerspelled after signing "V-D".*

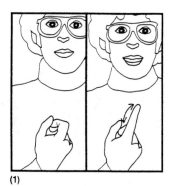
(1)

HICCUP

An uncontrollable, sudden inhalation of air which is stopped by closing the throat. Hiccups are caused by a quick contraction of the diaphragm. Irritation of the diaphragm, alcoholism, an upset stomach, nervousness, a brain problem or irritation of the nerve going to the diaphragm can cause hiccups.

If hiccups last for a long time, they may be the sign of a serious problem.

(1) The index finger of the right "S" hand flicks out a few times at chest level as if imitating hiccuping. (MM)

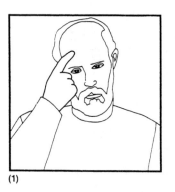
(1)

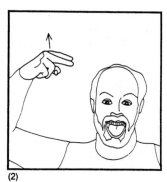
(2)

HIGH

The slang word for the good feeling, intoxication, happiness or hallucinations caused by using some drugs or drinking alcohol.

To get a high, people usually abuse a drug or use an illegal drug.

(1) Sign MIND — the index finger of the right "one" hand touches the forehead. (SM)
(2) Sign HIGH — the right "H" hand faces down and moves up. (SM)

HIGH BLOOD PRESSURE

Extreme force of the blood pushing against the walls of the arteries; hypertension. Some causes of high blood pressure are kidney problems, stress, arteriosclerosis (hardening of the arteries) and too much salt in the diet. Symptoms of high blood pressure don't happen often but they may be dizziness, headaches, bleeding from small blood vessels, vision problems and kidney inflammation.

Blood pressure is measured with a cuff wrapped around the arm and pumped up; when the reading is above 140 over 90, the person has high blood pressure.

(Continued on next page)

(1) The right "H" hand faces down at shoulder level and moves up slightly. (SM)

(2) Sign BLOOD — the left "five" hand is at chest level with the palm toward the body. The palm of the right "five" hand is toward the body with the middle fingertips touching the mouth. Move the right hand down the back of the left hand. Wiggle the fingers of the right hand as it moves. (MM)

* *This movement should be short, repeated and somewhat restrained.*

(3) The right hand grabs the left upper arm. (SM)

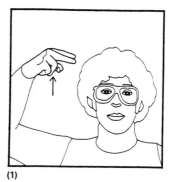

(1)

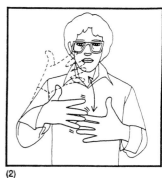

(2)

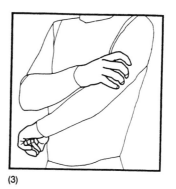

(3)

HIGH FEVER

Body temperature of 103 °F and above.

> *Some diseases that cause high fevers are yellow fever, typhoid fever and scarlet fever.*

(1) Sign TEMPERATURE — the index finger of the right "one" hand moves up and down on the back of the index finger of the left "one" hand. The right "one" hand then moves to just above the left hand indicating the temperature being high. (SM)

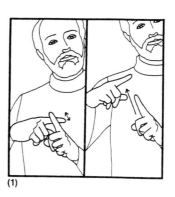

(1)

HIP

The upper part of the thigh and the area on each side of the pelvis. *See Figure 1*

(1) The right "flat" hand pats the right hip. (MM)

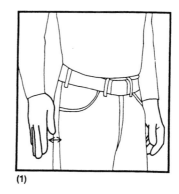

(1)

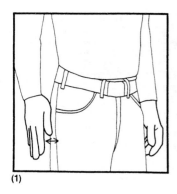
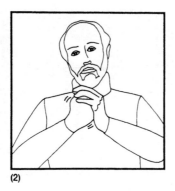

(1) (2)

HIP JOINT

The ball-and-socket joint between the femur (thighbone) and the pelvis. *See Figure 26*

(1) The right "flat" hand pats the right hip. (MM)
(2) The right "S" hand twists slightly in the left "C" hand. (MM)

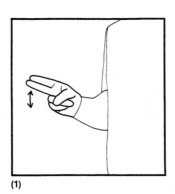

(1)

HISTORY

Medical information on a patient's physical conditions or past illnesses including any illnesses the ancestors may have had.

Doctors need to know their patient's history to sometimes help diagnose a current illness.

(1) The right "H" hand faces out at chest level. Drop the hand at the wrist twice. (DM)

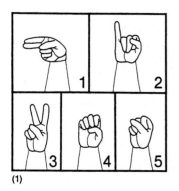
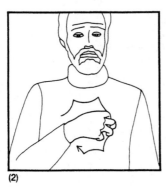

(1) (2)

HIVES

A skin condition in which very itchy bumps are caused by touching or eating something someone is allergic to.

Hives may be relieved with antihistamines, cortisone and soothing lotions.

(1) Fingerspell "H-I-V-E-S".
(2) The fingertips of the right "claw" hand touch the chest a few times indicating hives. (MM)
* This should be signed at the area of the hives.

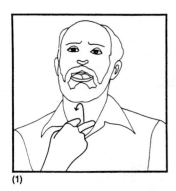
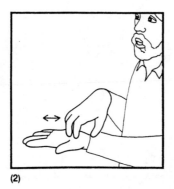

(1) (2)

HOARSENESS

Roughness of the voice.

Some things that may cause hoarseness are irritations such as tobacco, alcohol and chemicals and some diseases, like syphilis, tuberculosis and leprosy.

(1) Sign VOICE — the right "V" hand faces down and moves up the throat then out. (SM)
(2) The left "flat" hand faces up at chest level. The fingertips of the right "claw" hand move back and forth on the left palm as if scratching. (MM)

HOLISTIC MEDICINE

An approach to health in which all aspects of a person is involved including diet, mental and spiritual attitude, physical exercise, massage and movement, natural herbal and man-made medicine and counseling.

Many naturopathic physicians recommend holistic medicine as a life style in the prevention of disease and care of the body and mind.

HOME DELIVERY

Giving birth to a baby at home.

A woman planning to have a home delivery should have a doctor's care until she delivers to make sure she won't have any problems and she should have a trained midwife with her when she has the baby.

(1) Sign BABY — the right hand and forearm face up, resting on the left hand and forearm which also face upwards. Both are then rocked back and forth as if holding a baby. (MM)

(2) Sign DELIVERY — the left "flat" hand faces in at chest level. The right "flat" hand also faces in behind the left hand. Move the right hand down under the left hand then out forward. (SM)

(3) The right "one" hand faces out at chest level and shakes slightly from left to right. (MM)

(4) Sign HOME — the fingertips of the right "flat-O" hand touch the chin then the right cheek. (SM)

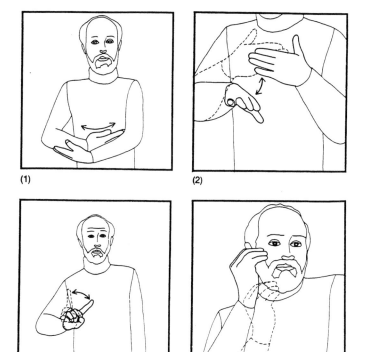

(1) (2)

(3) (4)

HOME REMEDY

Procedures or medicines made at home and passed on in a family which are used to cure diseases or stop pain.

A home remedy may be helpful in curing a condition but one should ask a doctor before using one to make sure no harm is done.

(1) Sign HOME — the fingertips of the right "flat-O" hand touch the chin then the right cheek. (SM)

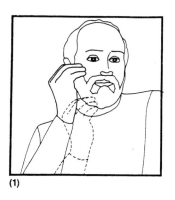

(1)

(Continued on next page)

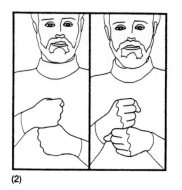
(2)

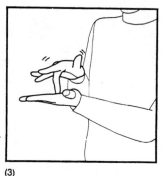
(3)

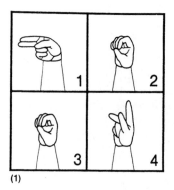
(1)

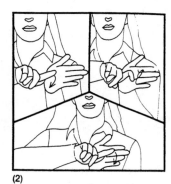
(2)

HOME REMEDY, *continued*

(2) Sign MAKE — both "S" hands face in, the right on top of the left. Twist both hands so that the left hand faces right and the right hand faces left. (SM)

(3) Sign MEDICINE — the left "flat" hand faces up at chest level. The middle finger of the right "eight" hand touches the left palm and pivots slightly from left to right a few times. (MM)

HOOKWORM

Small parasitic worms which get into the body through the skin and travel to the intestine where they attach to the lining and suck out blood. Young hookworms burrow through the skin of bare feet, hands or buttocks which touch soil containing them. Hookworms cause anemia, stomach pain, weakness and loss of appetite. They are found in warm moist areas like parts of the southern United States.

Hookworms are diagnosed by examining feces for their eggs and they can be gotten rid of by giving a person drugs to kill the worms.

(1) Fingerspell "H-O-O-K".

(2) Sign WORM — the left "flat" hand faces right at chest level. The index finger of the right "one" hand moves across the left palm, bending and straightening at the same time. (SM)

HORMONE

A substance made in an organ or gland which is carried by the blood through the body and causes another part of the body to become active, grow or to make and put out something else. Examples of hormones are insulin, adrenaline (epinephrine), estrogens and testosterone.

Hormones are effective in very small amounts.

HOSPICE

An institution or organization that deals with pa-teint's who are terminally ill (dying from cancer). Hospice have registered nurses and medical social workers who not only help relieve the patients physical pain, but also counsel the patient and his family to mentally prepare for death. The patients usually have 6 months or less to live.

A hospice can care for terminal patients either in their home or while in the hospital.

HOSPITAL

A special building used for the surgery, treatment, and care of people who are sick or injured. Hospitals have rooms for people to live in while they get better, special rooms for surgery or operations and other rooms for treating special diseases or disorders.

Most hospitals provide emergency medical care 24 hours a day.

a. (1) The right "H" hand faces left and moves from left to right across the forehead. (SM)

b. (1) The fingertips of the right "H" hand make a cross on the left upper arm. (SM)·

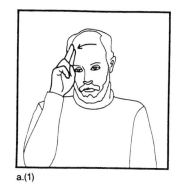

a.(1)

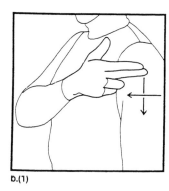

b.(1)

HOSPITALIZATION

Being put into a hospital for the treatment of an injury or disease.

A person should have insurance to help pay for any hospitalization, because it can be very expensive.

(1) Sign HOSPITAL — the fingertips of the right "H" hand make a cross on the left upper arm. (SM)
(2) Both "H" hands face up at right chest level. Move both hands to the left and slightly forward. (SM)

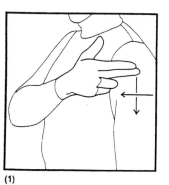

(1)

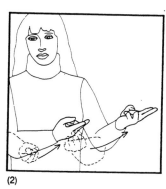

(2)

HOST

The animal on which a parasite lives, grows, reproduces and gets its food.

Most parasites do not damage their hosts much but when they do, they cause disease.

HOT

Being very warm; feverish.

Depending on how hot something is and how long someone touches it, a person can get first, second or third degree burns.

(1) The fingertips of the right "flat-O" hand touch the lips. Turn the hand out into a "five" hand facing down. (SM)

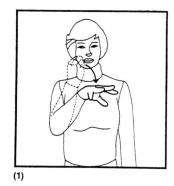

(1)

287

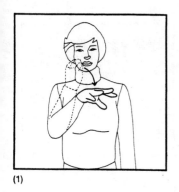 (1)
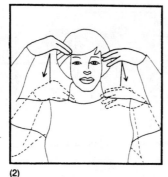 (2)

HOT FLASHES

A feeling of warmth caused by a sudden opening up of the blood vessels in the head and neck. Hot flashes usually occur in women after menopause and cause redness of the skin, sweating, and sometimes a feeling of suffocation.

Hot flashes and other menopause symptoms can be treated by hormones.

(1) Sign HOT — the fingertips of the right "flat-O" hand touch the lips. Turn the hand out into a "five" hand facing down. (SM)
(2) Both "cupped" hands face down at shoulder level. Move both hands up to head level, then back down to shoulder level. (SM)

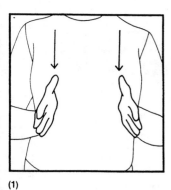 (1)
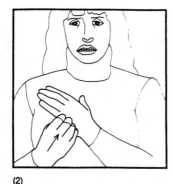 (2)

HUMAN BITES

Wounds caused by human teeth.

A person with a human bite should be seen by a doctor quickly because many dangerous bacteria live in people's mouths.

(1) Sign PERSON — both "flat" hands face each other at chest level. Move both hands down to waist level. (SM)
(2) The right "C" hand moves in on the left "flat" hand as if imitating biting it. (SM)
* This could be signed at the area of the bite.

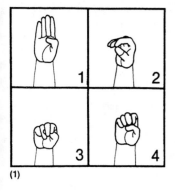 (1)
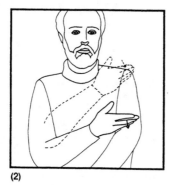 (2)

HUMERUS

The bone in the upper arm which goes from the shoulder to the elbow. *See Figure 26*
(1) Fingerspell "B-O-N-E"
(2) The right "flat" hand moves from the left shoulder to the elbow. (SM)

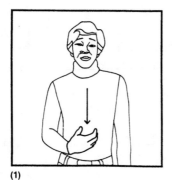 (1)

HUNGRY

Wanting or needing food. A hungry person may have weakness and a pain in the upper abdomen and the stomach may gurgle and make noises.

The pain in the abdomen of a hungry person is caused by strong contractions of the empty stomach.

(1) The right "C" hand faces in and moves from the throat down to waist level. (SM)

288

HUNTINGTON'S CHOREA

An inherited disease of the central nervous system which usually affects people between 30 and 50 years of age. A person with Huntington's Chorea has odd, quick, uncontrollable physical movements and mental deterioration which get worse.

There is no cure for Huntington's Chorea; death usually results.

HURT

To injure, wound, harm or cause pain.

People are often hurt on vacations so one should travel well prepared.

a. (1) Both "one" hands face in, the fingers pointing to each other. Move the hands in and out a few times. (MM)
b. (1) Both "one" hands face in, the fingers pointing to each other. Twist both hands in opposite directions a few times. (MM)

* *The facial expression should reflect pain.*
* *These should be signed at the area that hurts.*

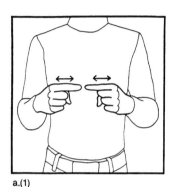 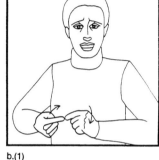

a.(1)   b.(1)

HUSBAND

The man a woman is married to.

Another word for a woman's husband is spouse.

(1) The right "flat-O" hand faces down and touches the forehead. Move the right hand down to clasp the left hand, palms together. (SM)

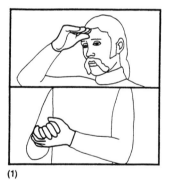

(1)

HYDROCORTISONE

See CORTISONE

HYDROGEN

A colorless, odorless gas that helps make up most organic compounds, including carbohydrates, fats and proteins. Hydrogen is also a part of all acids.

The most common source of hydrogen on earth is water, where it is combined with oxygen.

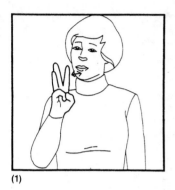
(1)

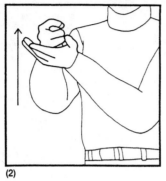
(2)

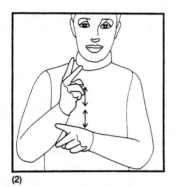
(1)

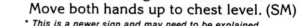
(2)

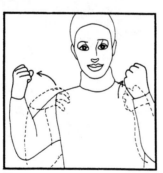
(3)

HYDROPHOBIA
See RABIES

HYDROTHERAPY
The use of water to treat disease. Some forms of hydrotherapy are hot baths, cold baths, showers or steam.

Hydrotherapy can cause relaxation, stimulation of a part, cool or warm the body, and relieve pain.

(1) Sign WATER — the index finger of the right "W" hand taps the mouth a few times. (MM)
(2) Sign THERAPY — the left "flat" hand faces up at waist level. The right "T" hand rests in the left palm. Move both hands up to chest level. (SM)

* This is a newer sign and may need to be explained.

HYGIENE
The science of staying healthy and preventing disease.

Good oral hygiene (keeping the mouth clean) can prevent cavities and gum disease.

(1) Sign SPECIALIZE — the left "B" hand faces right at chest level. The right "B" hand faces left on top of the left hand. Move the right hand straight out on the left index finger. (SM)
(2) The right "V" hand faces left and the left "V" hand faces right, both at chest level. Tap the hands together a few times. (MM)
(3) Sign HEALTH — the fingertips of both "claw" hands touch the chest and move up into "S" hands. (SM)

HYGIENIST
A person who specializes in hygiene (health).

A dental hygienist deals with the health of the mouth and is specially trained to clean the teeth and gums.

HYMEN
A fold of skin which partly covers the entrance of a woman's vagina. *See Figure 12*

HYPERACTIVE

Referring to increased or more than normal activity of an organ or of the whole person. When hyperactive is used for a person, it usually means a child who is always moving, always doing something, not able to concentrate on things and often aggressive.

Some researchers think that part of the reason some children are **hyperactive** *is that they eat too much sugar and other foods that aren't very good for them.*

(1) Sign PERSON — both "flat" hands face each other at chest level. Move both hands down to waist level. (SM)

(2) Sign CAN'T — the left "one" hand faces down at chest level. The right "one" hand faces down and moves down to strike the left index finger. (SM)

(3) Sign CONTROL — both "modified-A" hands face each other at chest level and move alternately in and out from the body a few times. (MM)

(4) The heel of the right "one" hand rests on the back of the left "flat" hand. Keeping the right hand on the left hand, move the right index finger around frantically. (MM)

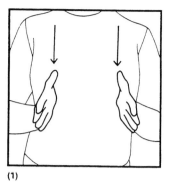
(1)

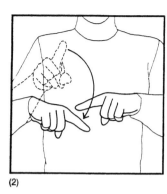
(2)

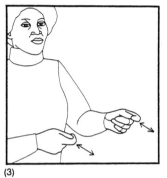
(3)

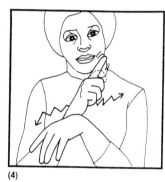
(4)

HYPERGLYCEMIA

A condition in which there is too much sugar (glucose) in the blood.

Hyperglycemia, affecting people with some kinds of diabetes, can cause a coma and make a person more likely to get an infection.

(1) Sign SUGAR — the fingertips of the right "H" hand brush down the chin a few times. (MM)

(2) Sign IN — the fingertips of the right "flat-O" hand move down into the left "O" hand a few times. (MM)

(3) Sign BLOOD — the left "five" hand is at chest level with the palm toward the body. The palm of the right "five" hand is toward the body with the middle fingertips touching the mouth. Move the right hand down the back of the left hand. Wiggle the fingers of the right hand as it moves. (MM)

* This movement should be short, repeated and somewhat restrained.

(4) Sign TOO MUCH — the left "cupped" hand faces down at chest level. The right "cupped" hand also faces down at chest level. Move the right hand up slightly. (SM)

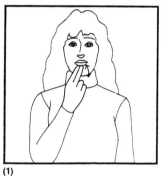
(1)

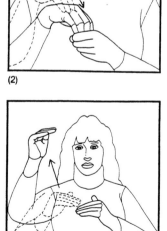
(2)

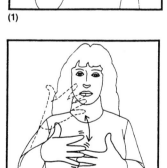
(3)

(4)

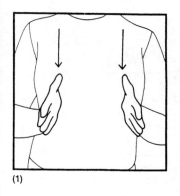
(1)

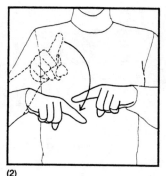
(2)

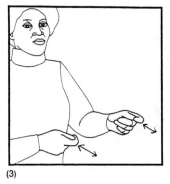
(3)

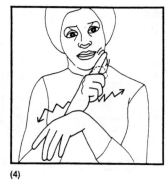
(4)

HYPERKINESIA

Excessive muscle activity and an increase in a person's movements; hyperactivity.

Hyperkinesia in children usually goes away when they reach adolescence.

(1) Sign PERSON — both "flat" hands face each other at chest level. Move both hands down to waist level. (SM)

(2) Sign CAN'T — the left "one" hand faces down at chest level. The right "one" hand faces down and moves down to strike the left index finger. (SM)

(3) Sign CONTROL — both "modified-A" hands face each other at chest level and move alternately in and out from the body a few times. (MM)

(4) The heel of the right "one" hand rests on the back of the left "flat" hand. Keeping the right hand on the left, move the right index finger around frantically. (MM)

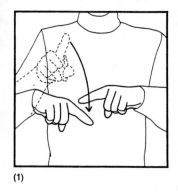
(1)

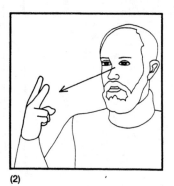
(2)

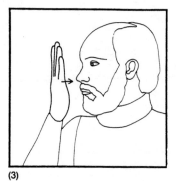
(3)

HYPEROPIA

Abnormal vision in which a person sees things far away better than things close to him; farsightedness.

Hyperopia is caused by the eye's being too flat or a mistake in the way light rays are focused on the retina, causing what is seen to be out of focus.

(1) Sign CAN'T — the left "one" hand faces down at chest level. The right "one" hand faces down and moves down to strike the left index finger. (SM)

(2) Sign SEE — the right "V" hand faces in at eye level and moves out forward. (SM)

(3) Sign CLOSE — the right "flat" hand faces in and moves in towards the eyes. (SM)

HYPERTENSION

Higher than normal force of the blood pushing against the walls of the arteries; high blood pressure. Symptoms of hypertension don't happen often but they may be dizziness, headaches, bleeding from small blood vessels, vision problems and kidney inflammation.

People with hypertension are more likely to have a heart disease or a stroke than people with lower blood pressures.

(1) Sign BLOOD — the left "five" hand is at chest level with the palm toward the body. The palm of the right "five" hand is toward the body with the middle fingertips touching the mouth. Move the right hand down the back of the left hand. Wiggle the fingers of the right hand as it moves. (MM)

* This movement should be short, repeated and somewhat restrained.

(2) The right "claw" hand grabs the left upper arm. (SM)

(3) The right "H" hand faces down at shoulder level and moves up slightly. (SM)

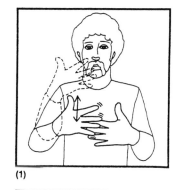 (1)
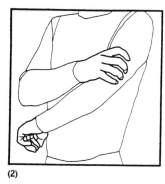 (2)
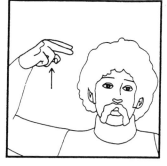 (3)

HYPERTHERMIA

A condition in which the body temperature is higher than normal. Hyperthermia is sometimes used as a treatment for disease by raising the body temperature.

Hyperthermia can be caused by injecting a malaria organism or foreign proteins into the body or, by being in excessive heat.

(1) Sign BODY — the fingertips of both "flat" hands touch the chest then move down to touch the stomach area. (SM)

(2) Sign TEMPERATURE — the index finger of the right "one" hand moves up and down on the index finger of the left "one" hand a few times, the right hand then stops above the left hand. (MM)

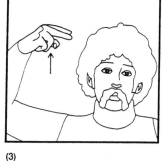 (1)
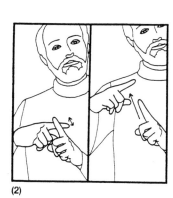 (2)

HYPERTROPHY

Enlargement of an organ or part. Hypertrophy occurs because the cells making up the part become larger.

Hypertrophy can also happen when a part is used more or becomes more active.

(1) Point to the area affected by hypertrophy.

(2) Sign BIG — both "claw" hands face each other at waist level. Move both hands to the sides, at the same time, the cheeks should puff out. (SM)

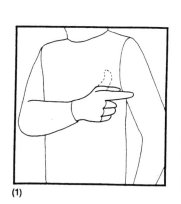 (1)
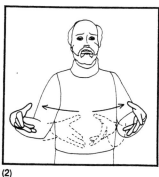 (2)

293

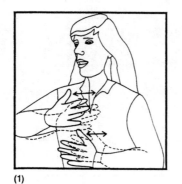

(1)

HYPERVENTILATE

Rapid or deep breathing without having exercised. When hyperventilating, a person may be very nervous and may pass out.

When a person hyperventilates, he should breathe into a paper bag and be calmed.

(1) Sign BREATHE — both "flat" hands move in quick, short movements in and out from the chest indicating rapid breathing. (MM)

HYPNOTICS

Drugs that cause a person to not feel pain, put people to sleep and have pleasant effects. Sedatives, analgesics and anesthetics are all hypnotics.

Hypnotics should not be taken unless a person is under a doctor's care.

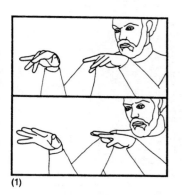

(1)

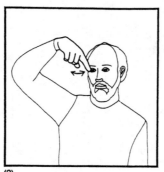

(2)

HYPNOTISM

An artificial, sleep-like condition in which consciousness is maintained. The patient may respond willingly to suggestions given him; hypnosis.

Hypnotism is sometimes used to help people stop smoking, lose weight and even as an anesthetic for minor surgery by giving post-hypnotic suggestions.

(1) Both "five" hands face down at chest level. Move both hands in and out a few times, at the same time, wiggle the fingers of both hands. (MM)

(2) The index finger of the right "one" hand points down in front of the eyes. Move the finger from left to right a few times indicating a clock or something moving in front of the eyes. (MM)

HYPOCHONDRIAC

A person who constantly believes he is ill or may become ill.

A hypochondriac can make himself believe that he is really sick so much that he can actually feel symptoms of an illness.

HYPODERMIC SYRINGE

A device used to place drugs or other things into or under the skin. It has a thin, hollow needle attached to a tube which holds the drugs. The needle is put into a vein, muscle or the area under the skin and the material in the tube is pushed out and into the body.

Hypodermic syringes are used to get a drug into the body quickly, when the drug would be destroyed in the stomach or when the drug should affect only a small area, as with a local anesthetic.

(1) Sign INJECTION — the index finger of the right "L" hand touches the left upper arm. Bend the right thumb down as if imitating injecting something into the left arm. (SM)
(2) The left "one" hand points to the right "L" hand and bounces alittle. (MM)

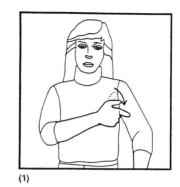
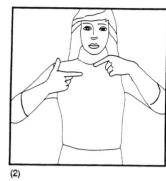

(1)   (2)

HYPOGLYCEMIA

An abnormally low level of sugar (glucose) in the blood. A person with hypoglycemia will get tired easily, be restless, weak, be easily upset, and in severe cases, may go into a coma and die.

A person with hypoglycemia may have a problem with the pancreas or may be a diabetic who has taken too much insulin.

(1) Sign SUGAR — the fingertips of the right "H" hand brush down the chin a few times. (MM)
(2) Sign IN — the fingertips of the right "flat-O" hand move down into the left "O" hand a few times. (MM)
(3) Sign BLOOD — the left "five" hand is at chest level with the palm toward the body. The palm of the right "five" hand is toward the body with the middle fingertips touching the mouth. Move the right hand down the back of the left hand. Wiggle the fingers of the right hand as it moves. (SM)
* This movement should be short, repeated and somewhat restrained.

(4) Sign NOT — the thumb of the right "A" hand touches under the chin and moves out forward. At the same time, the head should sh   "no." (SM)
(5) Sign ENOUGH — the left "S" hand faces right at chest level. The palm of the right "flat" hand brushes out across the left hand. (SM)

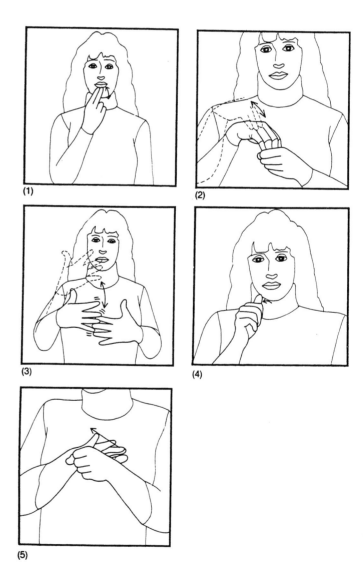

(1)   (2)

(3)   (4)

(5)

HYPOTHALAMUS

An important part of the brain which controls the body's temperature, some glands' activities, sleep and the body's use of water, sugar and fats. *See Figure 18*

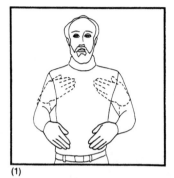
(1)
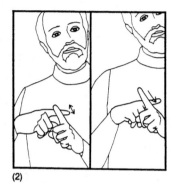
(2)

HYPOTHERMIA

A condition in which the body temperature is lower than normal. Hypothermia is sometimes caused on purpose to help with surgery but usually happens when someone is out in cold weather for a long time. People with hypothermia will not have just the outer parts of the body at a lower temperature but also the center of the body. They will be clumsy, confused, unable to think clearly, weak and will want to sleep.

Hypothermia can cause the center of the body to become so cold that the person may become unconscious and die of heart failure.

(1) Sign BODY — the fingertips of both "flat" hands touch the chest then move down to touch the stomach area.(SM)
(2) Sign TEMPERATURE — the index finger of the right "one" hand moves up and down a few times on the left index finger then stops down low on the left index finger. (MM)

HYSTERECTOMY

The surgical removal of a woman's uterus.

A woman may have a hysterectomy if she has very bad menstrual problems or if she has tumors in her uterus.

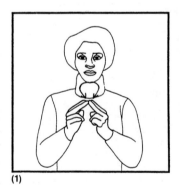
(1)
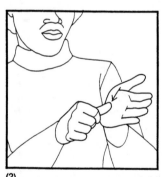
(2)

(1) Sign UTERUS — the fingertips of both "U" hands touch, then make the outline of the uterus. (SM)
(2) Sign CUT — the left "flat" hand faces up at chest level. The thumb of the right "A" hand moves down the left palm as if imitating cutting. (SM)
(3) The left "flat" hand faces right at chest level. The right "A" hand touches the left palm, then moves down into a "five" hand as if throwing something away. (SM)

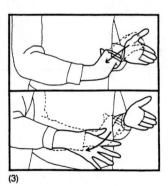
(3)

296

HYSTERIA

A mental condition in which a person shows symptoms of a disease without actually having the disease. What the person does is take the anxiety he has and turns it into periods of physical problems. The person with hysteria may cry or laugh without reason, may hallucinate, may have paralysis in a part of their body, have convulsions or become unconscious.

A person with hysteria should get attention from a psychiatrist.

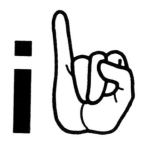

ICE

Water that has been frozen and changed from a liquid to a solid.

Ice is often used to treat an injury or burn because it will lessen blood flow to the damaged area, decreasing pain, swelling and irritation.

(1) Sign WATER — the right "W" hand faces left and the index finger taps the chin a few times. (MM)
(2) Sign FREEZE — both "five" hands face down at chest level and move up slightly into "claw" hands. (SM)

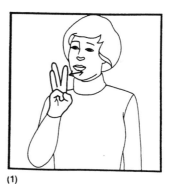

(1)

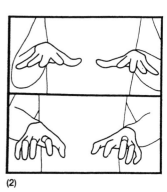

(2)

ID

In psychology, the part of our personality which contains our animal instincts and basic drives.

The id is the part of our personality which holds the desire to live, have children and have pleasure.

IDENTIFY

To establish or determine the origin or nature of something.

A doctor must identify a disorder before he can treat it properly.

(1) The left "flat" hand faces out at chest level. The right "I" hand touches the left palm then changes into an "O" hand. (SM)

* This is an English sign which usually means "identification" and may have to be explained. If "identify" is meant in any other context, this sign should not be used.

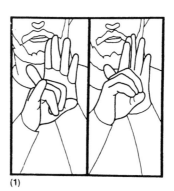

(1)

IDIOPATHIC

Disease or illness without cause or known origin.

Some diseases which are idiopathic are multiple sclerosis and leukemia.

299

IDIOSYNCRACY

The special ways a person looks, acts or thinks which makes him different from everybody else.

A person could have an idiosyncracy in which a certain drug affects him very differently from the way it affects most people.

ILEUM

The last part of the small intestine, about six feet long, just before the large intestine. *See Figure 10*

ILIAC ARTERY

The two large arteries that carry blood into the lower extremity or thigh. The iliac arteries are found where the aorta, which goes down the back of the body, branches. When the iliac arteries leave the abdomen and start down the thigh, they become the femoral arteries. *See Figure 6*

ILIUM

See HIP BONE

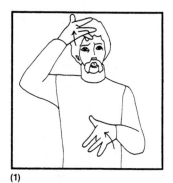
(1)

ILL

Sick; not healthy.

One way the body tells us that we are ill is by causing a fever.

(1) Sign SICK — the middle finger of the right "eight" hand touches the forehead and the middle finger of the left "eight" hand touches the stomach. Twist both hands slightly. (SM)

* The facial expression should reflect illness.

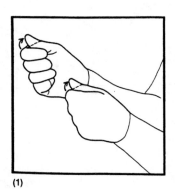
(1)

IMMEDIATELY

Without delay; as soon as possible.

If lumps are found during a breast self examination, a doctor should be seen immediately.

(1) Both "A" hands face each other at chest level with the thumbs inside the fists. Flick both thumbs out. (SM)

* The lips should also mouth "PE".

IMMERSE

To cover something with water or some other fluid.

When we immerse a burn in cold water quickly after it happens, pain is lessened and healing is helped.

(1) Sign WATER — the right "W" hand faces left and the index finger taps the chin a few times. (MM)
(2) Both "flat-O" hands point down at chest level and move down into "five" hands. (SM)

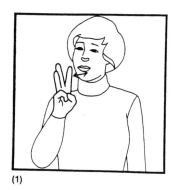
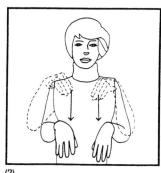

(1) (2)

IMMOBILIZE

To hold something so that it cannot move.

When a person may have a fracture, it is important to immobilize the part so there isn't any more damage to the part.

IMMUNITY

Resistance to or protection from a disease. A person gets immunity to a disease by having the disease, being vaccinated against the disease or inheriting protection in the genes. Having a disease or being vaccinated against it causes the body to make special proteins called antibodies which can attack and destroy the virus or bacteria that cause the disease. These antibodies stay in the body and when the person comes into contact with the virus or bacteria again, it is immediately attacked and destroyed so the disease doesn't even get started.

We may have to get shots against some diseases regularly because some kinds of immunity don't last very long.

IMMUNIZATION

Making someone resistant to a disease or protecting him from an infection by giving a weakened form of it. This will expose the body to substances which are like those in the "real" or severe form of the disease. The body makes special proteins called antibodies to destroy the mild form of the disease. These antibodies will also work on the severe form of the disease, so the person is protected against the disease without having had it.

There are several immunizations we should have to be protected against certain dangerous diseases.

(Continued on next page)

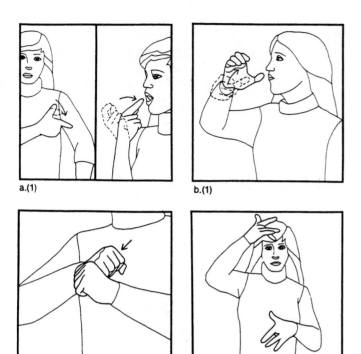

a.(1)

b.(1)

(2)

(3)

a. (1) Sign INJECTION — the index finger of the right "L" hand touches the left upper arm. Bend the thumb down as if imitating injecting something into the arm. (SM)

  Sign PILL — the right "modified-A" hand faces in at the mouth. Flick the index finger towards the mouth as if imitating popping a pill into the mouth. (SM)

b. (1) Sign DRINK — the right "C" hand faces left and moves towards the mouth as if imitating taking a drink. (SM)

(2) Sign PROTECT — both "S" hands cross at the wrists and move slightly forward and out. (SM)

(3) Sign DISEASE — the middle finger of the right "eight" hand touches the forehead and the middle finger of the left "eight" hand touches the stomach. (SM)

* Sign SHOT, PILL, or DRINK, depending on how the immunization is given, then sign PROTECT and DISEASE.

IMPACTED FRACTURE

A broken bone in which the two broken ends are wedged together, usually caused by a crushing force. There may be some discoloration or hemorrhaging in the area.

An impacted fracture should be put in a splint and then traction to hold it still or deformity may occur later.

IMPALED VICTIM

A person who has had an accident in which an object is forced into the body and is usually left sticking out.

An impaled victim should not have the object removed or more injury could be done.

IMPETIGO

A skin disease caused by bacteria (streptococci or staphylococci) in which the skin becomes inflamed, crusty, and bumps with pus form. Impetigo usually occurs first around the mouth and nose and spreads quickly.

Impetigo, which usually affects children, can be treated with antibiotics.

IMPORTANT

Something of great value.

It is important for all women to check their breasts for any lumps or changes after each menstrual period because most breast cancer can be treated if found early.

(1) Both "F" hands face each other at chest level. Move both hands around and up so that they touch, both hands facing down. (SM)

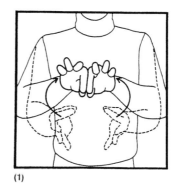

(1)

IMPOTENCE

Referring to a male not being able to have sexual intercourse. The problem is usually that the penis will not become erect.

Impotence can be caused by a mental disturbance, a disease, drugs or poor health.

(1) Sign ERECTION — the right "one" hand points down at waist level. The index finger of the left "one" hand touches the right wrist. Keeping the left hand in place, lift the right hand so that it points up. (SM)
(2) Sign CAN'T — the left "one" hand faces down with the index finger pointing out. The index finger of the right "one" hand strikes down the left index finger. (SM)

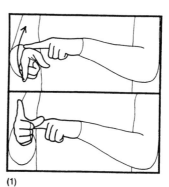

(1)

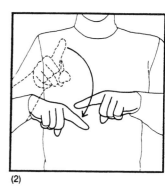

(2)

IMPREGNATE

To fertilize an egg; to make pregnant.

A man can impregnate a woman without having actual sexual intercourse because if semen get in the vulva near the vagina, they can swim up into the uterus and fertilize an egg.

(1) Fingerspell "S-P-E-R-M".
(2) Sign EGG — the right "H" hand faces left on top of the left "H" hand which faces right. Pivot both hands out. (SM)
(3) The index fingers and thumbs of both "F" hands join at chest level. (SM)
(4) Sign PREGNANT — both "five" hands mesh together at stomach level and move slightly forward. (SM)

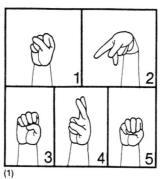

(1)

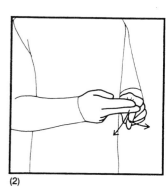

(2)

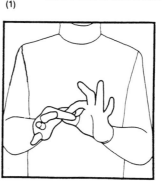

(3)

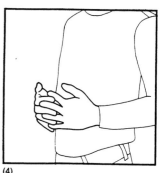

(4)

IMPRESSION

In dentistry, an imprint of a person's gums and teeth made by using gel or wax which becomes hard very fast.

Impressions are used to make dentures and other artificial teeth.

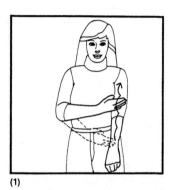

(1)

IMPROVE

To make or become better.

Proper diet and daily exercise will improve a person's health.

(1) The right "flat" hand faces in and moves up the left arm, touching a few times. (MM)

IMPROVISED SPLINT

An emergency splint made from whatever material is around to hold a broken bone still.

An improvised splint can be made from sticks or newspaper and is used until better medical help is available.

IMPULSE

In medicine, the tiny electrical charge which carries information along a nerve or muscle and results in activity.

The brain sends out impulses along nerves to muscles in a way that allows us to move smoothly and do things.

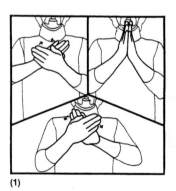

(1)

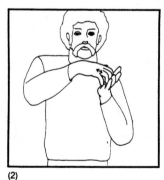

(2)

INCAPACITATE

To take away someone's strength or make him unable to do something.

Most diseases or infections will incapacitate a person to some degree.

(1) Sign BECOME — the right "flat" hand faces out on the left "flat" hand which faces in; the hands are crossed. Twist both hands so that the left hand ends facing out and the right hand ends facing in. (SM)
(2) Sign WEAK — the left "flat" hand faces up at chest level. The fingertips of the right "claw" hand touch the left palm. Keeping the fingertips in place, bend and straighten the fingers at the knuckles a few times. (MM)

INCEST

Sexual intercourse between closely related people. Incest is against the law and can be harmful to the people involved and the rest of the family.

Incest happens most often between a father and daughter and help should be gotten from a family child abuse specialist.

INCISAL EDGE

The lower or cutting edge of the front teeth.

*The **incisal edge** of the incisors or canine teeth can be chipped if they are struck hard enough.*

INCISION

A cut made into the body with a knife as a part of surgery.

Before an operation, the place where an incision is going to be made is shaved and cleaned with antiseptics.

(1) Sign KNIFE — the left "H" hand faces down at waist level. The fingertips of the right "H" hand brush down out across the fingers of the left hand. (SM)

(2) Sign CUT — the left "flat" hand faces up at chest level. The thumb of the right "A" hand is slightly extended and moves down the left palm as if cutting it. (SM)

* This could be signed at the area of the incision.

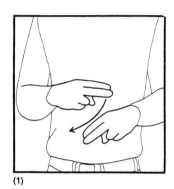

(1)

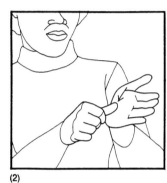

(2)

INCISOR

A kind of tooth. There are eight incisors in the front of an adult's mouth, four on the top and four on the bottom. Incisors are used to grab, hold and cut into food. *See Figure 24*

INCOHERENT

Unable to think or express thoughts clearly.

*A person will usually be **incoherent** because of something affecting the brain, such as drugs, or damage, like a blow to the head.*

(1) Both "five" hands face each other at eye level, the right hand on the inside. Shake both hands slightly in opposite directions a few times. (MM)

(2) Sign THINK — the index finger of the right "one" hand touches the forehead. (SM)

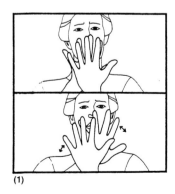

(1)

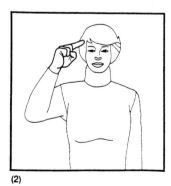

(2)

(Continued on next page)

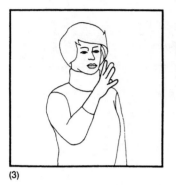
(3)

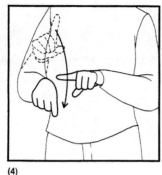
(4)

INCOHERENT, *continued*

(3) The right "four" hand faces left and moves out and in a few times. (MM)

(4) Sign CAN'T — the left "one" hand faces down at chest level, pointing out. The right "one" hand faces out and moves down to strike the left index finger. (SM)

INCOMPETENT

A person not able to do something or a part of the body not able to work normally.

> *If there is a problem in the heart preventing normal activity, the heart is said to be incompetent.*

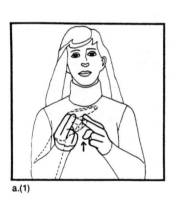
a.(1)

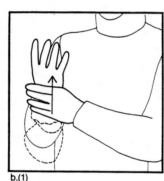
b.(1)

INCREASE

To become or make larger; to grow.

> *If a person regularly increases the amount of a drug he is taking, he could become addicted to it.*

a. (1) The left "H" hand faces in at waist level. The right "H" hand faces up and turns over to touch the left fingers a few times; at the same time, both hands move up to chest level. (MM)

* Use this sign if referring to something increasing in size.

b. (1) The right "flat-O" hand moves up through the left fist as if imitating something growing. (SM)

* Use this sign if referring to something increasing in quantity.

INCUS

One of the three small bones in the middle ear which helps carry sound waves from the eardrum to the inner ear, where the movement is picked up as sound. The incus is also called the anvil. *See Figure 20*

INDEX FINGER

The finger next to the thumb, also called the forefinger or the pointer finger. *See Figure 1*

INDIGESTION

A condition in which food is not digested or is not digested correctly. Indigestion can cause a feeling of fullness after eating, pain, nausea, vomiting, heart burn, gas formation and belching.

Indigestion can be caused by eating certain foods, by a problem in the digestive tract itself, like an ulcer, or by nervousness.

(1) Sign EAT — the fingertips of the right "flat-O" hand tap the mouth a few times. (MM)
(2) Sign WRONG — the right "Y" hand faces in under the chin. (SM)
(3) Sign DIGEST — both "A" hands face each other, the right hand on top, at chest level. Move both hands in alternate circles a few times. (MM)
(4) The right "claw" hand faces in at the stomach and moves in a circular movement a few times. (MM)

* *The facial expression should reflect illness.*

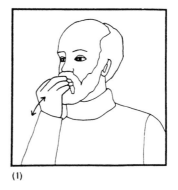
(1)

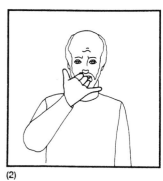
(2)

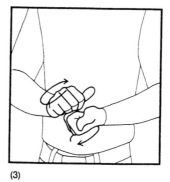
(3)

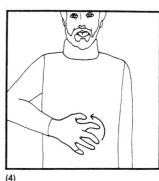
(4)

INDUCE

To produce something, start something or cause something to happen.

If a woman is overdue in having a baby, the doctor may induce labor.

(1) Sign CAUSE — both "A" hands face up at chest level. Move both hands out forward and slightly to the left side, ending in "five" hands facing up. (SM)
(2) Sign HAPPEN — both "one" hands face up, pointing out at chest level. Turn both hands in so that they face down. (SM)

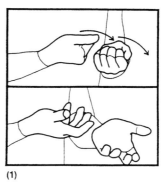
(1)

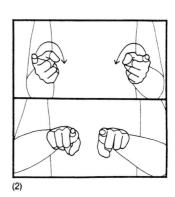
(2)

INFARCTION

The death of a part of the body or part of an organ because the blood supply has been cut off.

When an infarction occurs in the heart, part of the heart muscle dies and the heart may not work well; this condition is called a heart attack.

INFANT

A baby or a child less than two years old.

For the first couple of days after birth, an infant will lose weight but will then start to put weight on.

(Continued on next page)

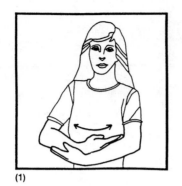
(1)

INFANT, *continued*

(1) Sign BABY — the right hand and forearm face up, resting on the left hand and forearm which also face upwards. Both are then rocked back and forth a few times as if holding a baby. (MM)

INFANTILE PARALYSIS
See POLIOMYELITIS

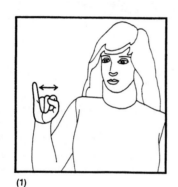
(1)

INFECTION
The growth of a virus, fungus, parasite or bacteria in the body or a part of the body, causing inflammation or disease. Symptoms of infection may be pain, swelling, redness, a fever, tiredness.

> *Infection can get into the body through a break in the skin, through the respiratory tract, or through the genitals.*

(1) The right "I" hand faces out at chest level and shakes slightly from left to right a few times. (MM)
* Mouth the word "infection" while signing.

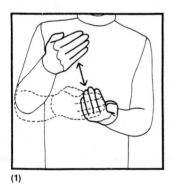
(1)

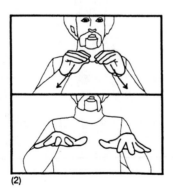
(2)

INFECTIOUS
Contagious, communicable diseases which can be passed easily from one person to another.

> *When someone has an infectious disease, he should stay away from other people so they don't get sick also.*

(1) Sign EASY — the left "cupped" hand faces up at chest level. The fingertips of the right "cupped" hand brush up the back of the left fingers twice. (DM)
(2) Sign SPREAD — both "flat-O" hands face down at chest level. Move both hands out forward into "five" hands facing down as if imitating something spreading. (SM)

INFECTIOUS MONONUCLEOSIS

An infectious disease caused by a virus which affects lymph glands, the liver, spleen and blood. A person with infectious mononucleosis may have a very high number of white blood cells in the blood, large and tender lymphnodes, a larger than normal spleen, a fever, sore throat and will be always tired. Infectious mononucleosis is also called "mono", glandular fever or just mononucleosis.

People, usually children or young adults, generally get infectious mononucleosis only once.

INFERIOR

Something lower or beneath something else. The feet and legs are the inferior part of the body.

INFESTATION

Having a large number of insect parasites, like ticks, fleas, lice or mites on or inside the body.

Infestation with ticks or fleas is dangerous because both can pass on dangerous diseases, such as spotted fever.

INFERTILITY

The condition of not being able to reproduce or become pregnant, occuring in the husband, the wife, or both. Some causes of infertility may be poor nutrition, abnormal reproductive organs, alcohol abuse or other drug abuse, or emotional problems.

If a couple wants to have a baby but the woman can't become pregnant, they should both see a doctor, who can give them tests to find out the reason for their infertility.

a. (1) Sign MAN — the right "open flat-O" hand faces left at the forehead. Move the hand out slightly, closing into a "flat-O" hand.
(2) The right "flat" hand faces down at the forehead and moves out slightly. (SM)
(3) Sign EJACULATE — the right "S" hand faces left at chest level. The index finger of the left "one" hand touches the right wrist. Keeping the left hand in place, move the right hand out forward into a "five" hand. (SM)
(4) Sign PREGNANT — both "five" hands mesh together at the stomach and move out slightly. (SM)

(Continued on next page)

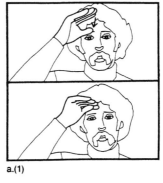

a.(1)

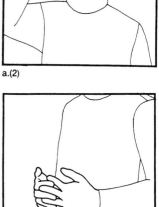

a.(2)

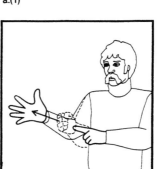

a.(3)

a.(4)

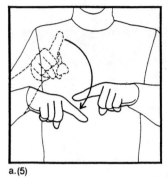
a.(5)

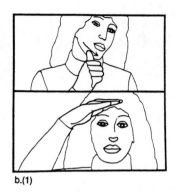
b.(1)

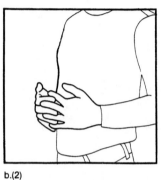
b.(2)

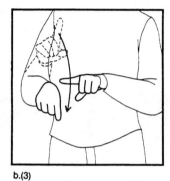
b.(3)

a. (5) Sign CAN'T — the left "one" hand faces down with the index finger pointing out. The index finger of the right "one" hand strikes down the left index finger. (SM)

b. (1) Sign WOMAN — the thumb of the right "A" hand moves down the right chin. The right "flat" hand then faces down at the forehead and moves out slightly. (SM)

(2) Sign PREGNANT — both "five" hands mesh together at the stomach and move out slightly. (SM)

(3) Sign CAN'T — the left "one" hand faces down with the index finger pointing out. The index finger of the right "one" hand strikes down the left index finger. (SM)

* Sign a.(1), (2), (3), (4), and (5) if referring to Male infertility and b.(1), (2), and (3) if referring to Female infertility.

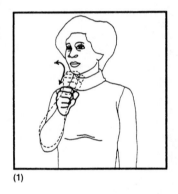
(1)

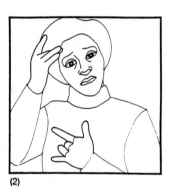
(2)

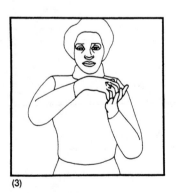
(3)

INFIRM

Being weak because of old age or disease.

An infirm person may need help walking or getting in and out of bed.

(1) Sign OLD — the right "S" hand faces left hand brushes down the chin a few times. (MM)

(2) Sign DISEASE — the middle finger of the right "eight" hand touches the forehead and the middle finger of the left "eight" hand touches the stomach. (SM)

(3) Sign WEAK — the left "flat" hand faces up at chest level. The fingertips of the right "claw" hand touch the left palm. Keeping the fingertips in place, bend and straighten the fingers at the knuckles a few times. (MM)

INFIRMARY

A small hospital or other place where sick or injured people are taken care of.

An infirmary is usually a part of another institution, such as a school or business, and usually has a nurse running it.

(1) The little finger of the right "I" hand makes a cross on the left upper arm. (SM)
* The sign for HOSPITAL may also be signed here.

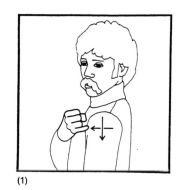
(1)

INFLAMMATION

The changes tissue goes through when it is injured, infected or irritated. When there is inflammation, there will be pain, redness, swelling and heat in the area.

Most of the symptoms of inflammation are caused by an increase in the amount of blood going to the area.

(1) The left "flat" hand faces out at chest level. The fingertips of the right "O" hand touch the left palm. Open the right hand into a "claw" hand and at the same time, the cheeks should puff out indicating swelling. (SM)
* This could be signed at the area of the swelling.

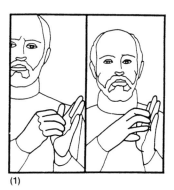
(1)

INFLUENZA

A contagious infection of the respiratory tract caused by several kinds of viruses; commonly called "the flu." There are cold-like symptoms which come on quickly, like a fever, headache, sore muscles, a cough, sore throat, runny nose and tiredness. The person may also be dizzy, be nauseous, or vomit.

If a type of influenza comes from another country, it will be named for the place it came from, such as the Hong Kong Flu.

(1) Fingerspell "F-L-U".
(2) Sign SICK — the middle finger of the right "eight" hand touches the forehead and the middle finger of the left "eight" hand touches the stomach. (SM)

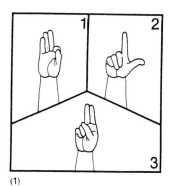
(1)

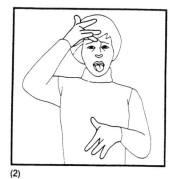
(2)

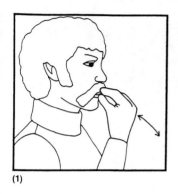
(1)

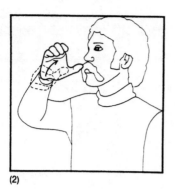
(2)

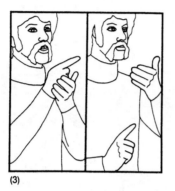
(3)

INGESTION

The process of taking something, usually food, into the mouth; eating or drinking.

After ingestion, food goes into the gastrointestinal tract.

(1) Sign FOOD — the fingertips of the right "flat-O" hand tap the mouth a few times. (MM)
(2) Sign DRINK — the right "C" hand faces left and moves towards the mouth as if imitating taking a drink. (SM)
(3) The left "flat" hand faces in at chest level. The right "one" hand points up with the hand touching the left palm. Drop the right hand down to waist level, keeping the right index finger pointing up as if indicating something being swallowed. (SM)

INGUINAL REGION

Referring to the groin area.

Hernias may occur in the inguinal region.

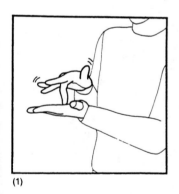
(1)

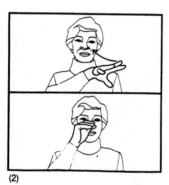
(2)

INHALANT

A medicine or some other substance that is gotten into the body by breathing it into the lungs.

Steam inhalants may be given to people with breathing problems to give heat and moisture to the membranes of the lungs.

(1) Sign MEDICINE — the left "flat" hand faces up at chest level. The middle finger of the right "eight" hand touches the left palm and pivots slightly from left to right a few times. (MM)
(2) Sign INHALE — the right "five" hand faces down at mouth level. Move the right hand in towards the nose and mouth, ending in a "flat-O" hand as if imitating inhaling something. (SM)

INHALE

To breathe in or take air into the body.

The muscles between the ribs lift the ribs, which help us inhale.

(Continued on next page)

INHALE, *continued*

(1) The right "five" hand faces down at mouth level. Move the right hand in towards the nose and mouth, ending in a "flat-O" hand as if imitating inhaling something. (SM)

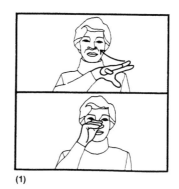

(1)

INHERITED

Referring to the physical and mental traits or characteristics that a person gets from his parents by gene transmission.

The development of our inherited characteristics is controlled by our genes.

(1) Sign GENERATION — the fingertips of both "flat" hands touch the right shoulder. Move both hands out and down in alternating circular movements. (SM)

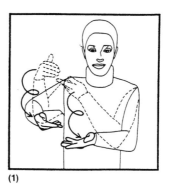

(1)

INJECT

To put something, usually a fluid, into the body using a needle and syringe.

Many diabetics must learn to inject themselves daily with insulin.

(1) The index finger of the right "L" hand touches the left upper arm. Bend the thumb down as if imitating injecting something into the arm. (SM)

* This could be signed at the area of the injection.

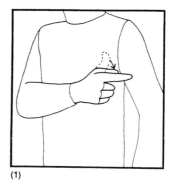

(1)

INJECTION

The fluid forced into a blood vessel, organ, or area under the skin, usually with a needle or syringe.

Everything used in giving an injection should be sterilized and the skin area the needle goes in should be cleaned with alcohol.

(1) The right "K" hand faces in at the left upper arm. Bend the thumb in as if imitating injecting something into the arm. (SM)

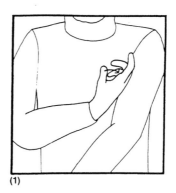

(1)

313

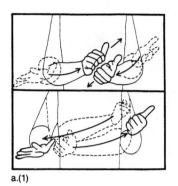

a.(1)

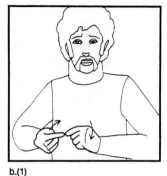

b.(1)

INJURE/INJURY

Damage, harm or a wound to the body.

A person with an injury should be watched closely to make sure he doesn't go into shock.

a. (1) Sign DAMAGE — the right "five" hand faces down at chest level and the left "five" hand faces up at chest level. Move both hands in towards the center of the body, the right "A" hand on top of the left "A" hand. Continue moving the hands through until they cross. Then move both hands back to their original positions, the left "A" hand facing up and the right "five" hand facing down. (SM)

b. (1) Sign HURT — both "one" hands point to each other and twist in opposite directions a few times. (MM)

* *This could be signed at the area of the injury. The facial expression should reflect pain.*

INLAY

In dentistry, a solid filling premade to fit into a cavity in a tooth and which is attached to the tooth.

An inlay may be made of porcelain, plastic or metal like gold.

INNER EAR

The part of the ear that is farthest inside the head, containing the cochlea and semicircular canals. The cochlea turns sound waves into nerve impulses that are sent to the brain and which we pick up as sound. The semicircular canals help us keep our balance. The inner ear is filled with fluid, while the middle and outer ear have air in them. *See Figure 20*

INOCULATION

Inserting a serum into the body to make a person immune to a disease.

Inoculation is usually done with a needle and syringe and usually has a weakened form of the disease virus which will protect us against the severe form of the disease.

314

INOPERABLE

A condition where a disease or illness cannot be cured by an operation or surgery. A disease may be inoperable due to its location, its advanced stage or the poor health of the patient.

If a cancer is not found early and if it spreads to other parts of the body, it usually becomes inoperable.

(1) Sign CAN'T — the left "one" hand faces down at chest level, pointing out. The right "one" hand faces out and moves down to strike the left index finger. (SM)
(2) Sign OPERATE — the left "flat" hand faces in at chest level. The thumb of the right "A" hand moves down the left palm as if imitating cutting. (SM)

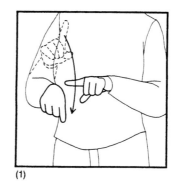
(1)

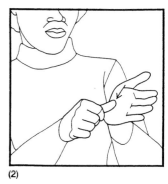
(2)

INORGANIC

Referring to any substance that doesn't come from plant or animal life; also a substance that doesn't have carbon in it.

A mineral is an inorganic substance.

INQUEST

An examination held by a coroner to decide the cause of a sudden or violent death.

An inquest is held so a death certificate can be made out for the person, naming the cause of death.

(1) Sign DEAD — the left "flat" hand faces up at chest level and the right "flat" hand faces down at chest level. Turn both hands over so that the left hand faces down and the right hand faces up. (SM)
(2) Sign BODY — the fingertips of both "flat" hands touch the chest then the stomach. (SM)
(3) Sign CHECK — the left "flat" hand faces in at chest level. The index finger of the right "one" hand makes a check on the left palm a few times. (MM)

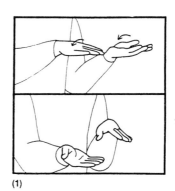
(1)

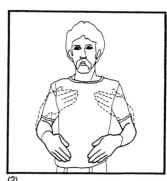
(2)

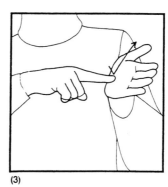
(3)

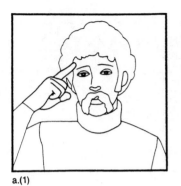

a.(1)

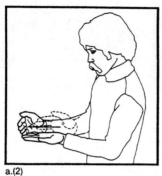

a.(2)

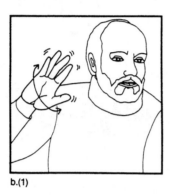

b.(1)

INSANITY

A term for severe mental disorders.

People suffering from insanity may have delusions or hallucinations, may be dangerous to themselves and others, may be unable to care for themselves, and may be unable to tell right from wrong.

a. (1) Sign MIND — the index finger of the right "one" hand touches the forehead. (SM)
(2) The left "flat" hand faces up at chest level. The right "flat" hand moves out over the left palm then turns to the left on the fingertips. (SM)

b. (1) The right "five" hand shakes from left to right a few times at the head. (MM)

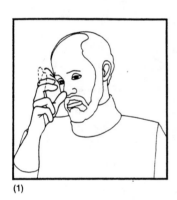

(1)

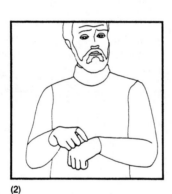

(2)

INSECT BITES OR STINGS

A bite or sting from an insect, especially flies, mosquitoes, lice, fleas, ticks, spiders, scorpions, bees, hornets and wasps (Anthropoda).

Sometimes, the poison injected by the insect can be more harmful than the venom from snakes, so if a person shows a reaction from an insect bite or sting, he should see a doctor.

(1) Sign INSECT — the thumb of the right "three" hand touches the nose. Bend and straighten the fingers a few times. (MM)
(2) Sign BITE — the left "S" hand faces down at chest level. The index finger of the right "one" hand taps the top of the left hand. (SM)

* *The facial expression should reflect pain.*

INSEMINATION

Inserting semen into a woman's vagina. (Artificial insemination is a doctor's placing semen from a woman's husband or a donor into her uterus.)

When the word insemination is used alone, it usually means semen being let out of a man's penis into a woman's vagina during sexual intercourse.

(Continued on next page)

316

(1) The index finger of the right "one" hand moves into the left "S" hand. (SM)
(2) Sign EJACULATE — the right "S" hand faces left at chest level. The index finger of the left "one" hand touches the right wrist. Keeping the left hand in place, move the right hand out forward into a "five" hand. (SM)

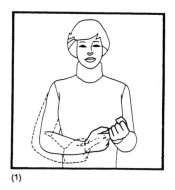
(1)

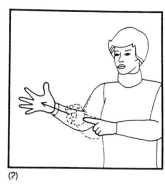
(2)

INSENSIBLE

Unconscious; unable to feel; to slight; to be noticed or sensed.

*Some people don't care or are **insensible** to other people's feelings.*

INSOMNIA

Not able to sleep.

Insomnia may be a symptom of many disorders or diseases but the most common causes are anxiety and pain.

(1) Sign CAN'T — the left "one" hand faces down with the index finger pointing out. The index finger of the right "one" hand strikes down the left index finger. (SM)
(2) Sign SLEEP — the right "five" hand faces in at face level. Move the hand down slightly into a "flat-O" hand. At the same time, the eyes should close. (SM)

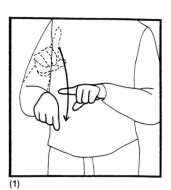
(1)

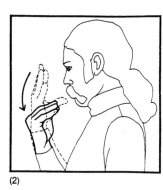
(2)

INSPECTION

An examination of the outside of the body.

*During an **inspection**, a doctor will check the person's posture and how the body moves.*

(1) The index finger of the right "one" hand points to the eye. (SM)
(2) The left "flat" hand faces up at chest level. The index finger of the right "one" hand moves back and forth a few times on the left palm. (MM)

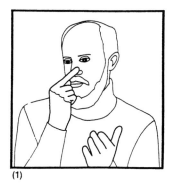
(1)

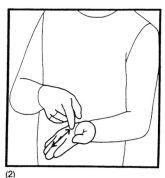
(2)

317

INSTEP

The inner, curved part of the foot; the arch. *See Figure 1*

INSTINCT

Inherited behavior. The person or animal does these things naturally, without thinking about it, and knows how to do them, without having any experience.

Instincts are reactions which have allowed generations of a type of animal to survive.

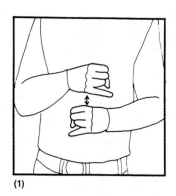
(1)

INSTITUTION

An established organization serving the public such as a university or hospital.

An institution may also mean a mental hospital.

(1) Both "I" hands face in at chest level, the right on top of the left. Tap the hands together a few times. (MM)

INSULIN

A hormone made in the pancreas which is put into the blood and used to help the right amount of glucose (dextrose) get into the cells.

When not enough insulin is made by the pancreas, glucose isn't used correctly and diabetes results.

INSULIN REACTION/SHOCK

A disorder caused by a diabetic's taking too much insulin. When there is too much insulin in the blood, the amount of glucose (dextrose) in the blood is lowered below the normal level. A person in insulin shock will have a rapid pulse, pale and moist forehead and be in a coma.

A person having an insulin reaction or shock should eat something sweet if conscious.

INSURANCE

The system of financially protecting or insuring people and property.

Due to rising medical costs, people should have medical insurance in case of long illnesses to help pay for those costs.

(1) The right "I" hand faces out at chest level and shakes slightly from side to side a few times. (MM)
* Mouth the word "insurance" while signing.

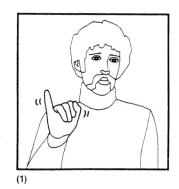
(1)

INTELLIGENCE

The ability to think, find an answer to problems, understand things, and to adjust to new situations.

No single test can measure intelligence because it is such a complex idea.

(1) The right "one" hand faces out and points up at the side of the head. Move the hand up and out. (SM)

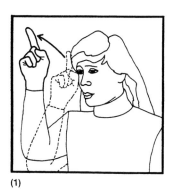
(1)

INTENSE

Large in amounts or strength.

Women in labor usually have intense pain and can take drugs or can use special breathing exercises to help lessen the pain.

(1) Both "S" hands face in at chest level. Move both hands out slightly. (SM)
* The facial expression should reflect intensity.

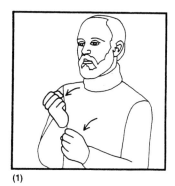
(1)

INTENSIVE CARE UNIT

A specially equipped area in a hospital for the care and treatment of very sick or badly injured patients.

The equipment and highly trained doctors and nurses in an intensive care unit can give special attention and frequent care to the patients until they are out of danger.

(1) Fingerspell "I-C-U".
* This may need further explanation before fingerspelling.

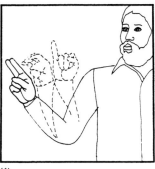
(1)

INTERFERON

A special protein made when someone is exposed to a virus. When some cells are infected with a virus, they will cause interferon to be made. The interferon will go through the body and protect cells that haven't been infected yet.

Much study is being done on interferon to see if it can be made for us by bacteria and then used to cure diseases such as some kinds of cancer.

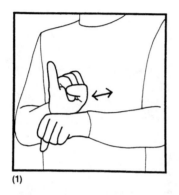
(1)

INTERN

A recently graduated doctor who is getting a year of training before getting his license.

An intern lives and works at a hospital, and helps treat patients.

(1) The left "S" hand faces down at chest level. The right "I" hand faces out and moves slightly from left to right a few times on the back of the left hand. (MM)

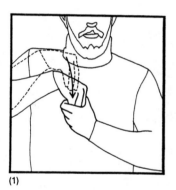
(1)

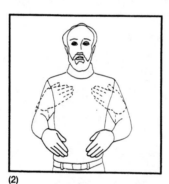
(2)

INTERNAL

Inside the body.

The liver, heart, intestines and kidneys are internal body structures.

(1) Sign IN — the right "flat-O" hand moves down into the left "O" hand. (SM)
(2) Sign BODY — the fingertips of both "flat" hands touch the chest then the stomach. (SM)

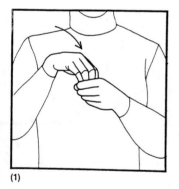
(1)

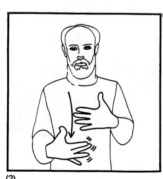
(2)

INTERNAL BLEEDING

Bleeding from an organ or place on the inside of the body.

Internal bleeding is dangerous because after an injury, people may not know they are bleeding inside and they could go into shock.

(1) Sign IN — the right "flat-O" hand moves down into the left "O" hand. (SM)
(2) Sign BLEED — the left "five" hand is at chest level with the palm toward the body. The palm of the right "five" hand is toward the body with the middle fingertips touching the mouth. Move the right hand down the back of the left hand. Wiggle the fingers of the right hand as it moves. (SM)
* This movement should be long and slow.

320

INTERVERTEBRAL

The area between two of the bones (vertebrae) that make up the spine. *See Figure 26*

INTERVERTEBRAL DISK

A flat piece of tough cartilage between two vertebrae. Intervertebral disks prevent friction between the bones and absorb shock.
See Figure 26

INTESTINE

The part of the digestive tract between the stomach and the anus. The intestine is like a long tube packed into the abdomen. Food moves through the intestine and is absorbed. The unused waste (feces) is held in the rectum until it is released in a bowel movement. The intestine is made up of two parts: the small intestine and the large intestine, or colon.
See Figure 9

(1) The right "F" hand faces out at stomach level and moves down in a wiggly movement as if imitating the outline of the intestines. (SM)

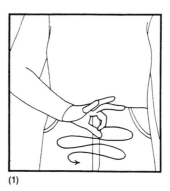
(1)

INTOXICATION

The condition caused by drinking too much alcohol.

> *Intoxication also refers to poisoning by a drug or some other substances.*

(1) The right "Y" hand faces out and moves down in front of the body. (SM)

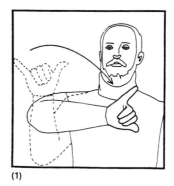
(1)

INTRAMUSCULAR INJECTION

A shot in which the needle of a hypodermic syringe is placed into a muscle, where the drug or medicine is released.

> *An intramuscular injection is usually given in the hip or shoulder and often hurts and makes the muscle sore.*

(1) Sign INJECTION — the index finger of the right "L" hand touches the left upper arm. Bend the thumb down as if imitating injecting something into the arm. (SM)

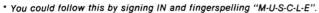
* You could follow this by signing IN and fingerspelling "M-U-S-C-L-E".

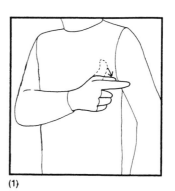
(1)

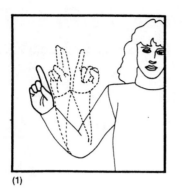

(1)

INTRAUTERINE DEVICE (IUD)

A contraceptive device used by women. An intrauterine device is a coil or loop of plastic placed in the uterus and left there. It has a thread hanging down into the vagina so the woman can be sure it is still in place.

A woman must have an examination to be sure she can use an intrauterine device and it must be put in place by a doctor.

(1) Fingerspell "I-U-D".

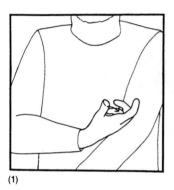

(1)

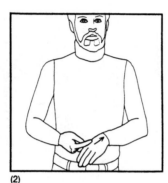

(2)

INTRAVENOUS INJECTION

A shot in which the needle of a hypodermic syringe is inserted into a vein and a drug or medication is released directly into the blood.

When someone gets an intravenous injection in the arm, a tight band is usually placed between the elbow and shoulder to make the vein stand out, making it easier to put the needle in.

(1) Sign INJECTION — the right "K" hand is at the left upper arm. Bend the thumb in as if imitating injecting something into the left arm. (SM)
(2) The index finger of the right "one" hand moves up the back of the left "flat" hand. (SM)

* You could sign IN and then fingerspell "V-E-I-N" after these two signs.

INTRODUCER

In medicine, a device used to put something into the body.

An example of an introducer may be a tube (intubator) placed in the trachea to let air into the larynx.

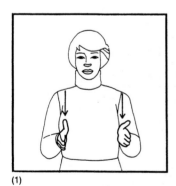

(1)

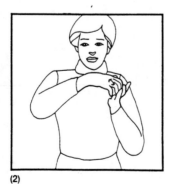

(2)

INVALID

A sick or weak person.

Invalid is usually used when referring to someone who is confined to a bed or wheelchair.

(1) Sign PERSON — both "flat" hand face in at chest level and move down to waist level. (SM)
(2) Sign WEAK — the fingertips of the right "claw" hand rest on the palm of the left "flat" hand, at chest level. Keeping the fingers in place, bend and straighten the fingers at the knuckles a few times. (MM)

(Continued on next page)

(3) Sign CAN'T — the left "one" hand faces down with the index finger pointing out. The index finger of the right "one" hand strikes down the left index finger. (SM)

(4) Sign WALK — both "flat" hands face down at chest level. Move both hands alternately forward and back a few times as if imitating walking. (MM)

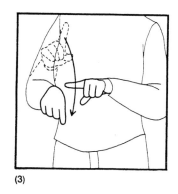
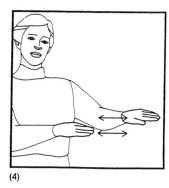

(3)   (4)

IODINE

A chemical needed in small amounts by the thyroid gland to make a hormone. Iodine is also mixed with alcohol to make tincture of iodine, used as a disinfectant.

*It is important to use iodized salt or buy vegetables and seafood with **iodine** in them to prevent goiter.*

IPECAC

The dried root of the ipecacuanha plant grown in Brazil and used an an emetic (causing vomiting).

Ipecac is sometimes used to cause vomiting as an emergency treatment for some poisonings.

(1) Sign MEDICINE — the left "flat" hand faces up at chest level. The middle finger of the right "eight" hand touches the left palm and pivots slightly from left to right a few times. (MM)

(2) Sign DRINK — the right "C" hand faces left and moves towards the mouth as if imitating taking a drink. (SM)

(3) Sign CAUSE — both "A" hands face up at chest level. Move both hands out forward and slightly to the left side, ending in "five" hands facing up. (SM)

(4) Sign VOMIT — the right "five" hand faces in and touches the mouth then moves down as if imitating vomiting. (SM)

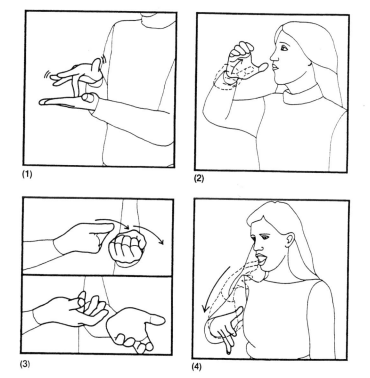

(1)   (2)

(3)   (4)

IRIS

The colored part of the eye behind the cornea and in front of the lens. By opening up and closing down, the iris can control the amount of light entering the eye through the pupil, the dark hole in its center
See Figure 21

IRON

A very common chemical needed by the body to make hemoglobin and some enzymes. Not getting enough iron can cause anemia.

Because women who menstruate or are pregnant need much more iron than men, they should take vitamins that have extra iron in them.

IRRATIONAL

Unable to think clearly, speak clearly, reason or control actions.

When people are afraid or injured badly, they should be watched carefully because they may be irrational.

IRRIGATE

To wash a wound or area out with a fluid.

An area is usually irrigated to get out things that shouldn't be there, such as pieces of dirt or dangerous chemicals.

IRRITATE

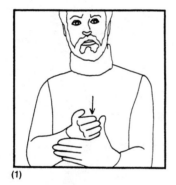

To rub, cause pain, upset or make uncomfortable.

When a substance irritates a person but doesn't bother most other people, that person may have an allergy.

(1) Sign BOTHER — the left "flat" hand faces in at chest level. The right "flat" hand faces left and moves down to touch the left hand between the thumb and index finger. (SM)

* The facial expression should reflect irritation.

IRRITATING GASES

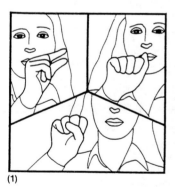
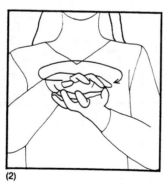

Gases that cause pain and damage to the body.

Irritating gases are most dangerous to the eyes and airways because their linings and coverings, being thin, are not able to protect against the substances in the gases.

(1) Fingerspell "G-A-S".
(2) Both "claw" hands face each other at chest level. Move both hands in opposite circles a few times. (MM)

(Continued on next page)

IRRITATING GASES, *continued*

(3) The thumbs of both "five" hands touch the chest. Move both hands in towards the body into "flat-O" hands. (SM)

(4) The left "S" hand faces in at chest level. The right "A" hand faces left and moves up to hit the back of the left hand. (SM)

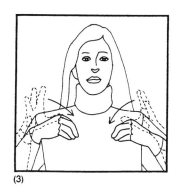
(3)

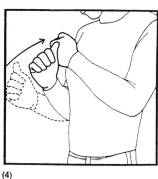
(4)

IRRITATION

Pain, soreness, roughness or sensitivity caused by something damaging the body.

Irritation may be the sign that inflammation is starting.

(1) Sign PAIN — both "one" hands point to each other at chest level and twist in opposite directions a few times. (MM)

* The facial expression should reflect pain.

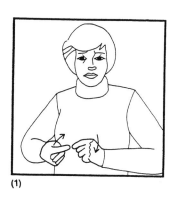
(1)

ITCH

An irritation making a person want to scratch.

An itch that won't go away may be a sign of an infection or allergy.

(1) The right "claw" hand moves up and down the left arm a few times as if imitating scratching or itching. (MM)

* This could be signed at the area of itch.

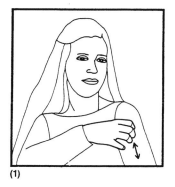
(1)

IUD

See INTRAUTERINE DEVICE

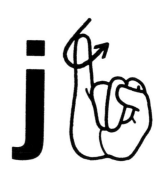

j

JAEGER TEST

A test for checking a person's near vision.

In the Jaeger test, a person reads lines of different size type off a card.

(1) Sign EYES — the index finger of the right "one" hand points to both eyes. (SM)
(2) Sign TEST — both "one" hands face out at shoulder level with the fingers pointing up. Move both hands down slightly and at the same time, bend and straighten the index fingers. Repeat this movement three times, ending at waist level. (MM)

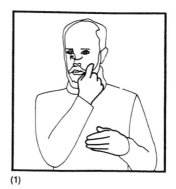
(1)
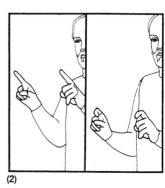
(2)

JAUNDICE

Yellowness of the skin, eyes and body fluids caused by too much bilirubin in the blood and tissues. Bilirubin is a yellow substance made from worn-out red blood cells. Jaundice can be a symptom of many problems, such as blockage in the liver or the passages to the gall bladder, the destruction of red blood cells or a disease of the liver.

Jaundice is a sign that something is wrong with the liver and if too much damage is done, a person could die.

(1) Sign YELLOW — the right "Y" hand faces out at chest level and shakes slightly from left to right a few times. (MM)
(2) Sign SKIN — the index finger and thumb of the right fist grab the right cheek. (SM)

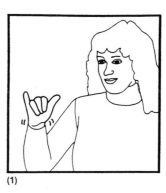
(1)
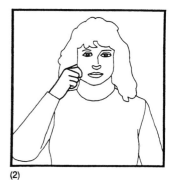
(2)

JAW

The bony parts of the mouth which hold the teeth and containing the maxilla and the mandibular bones. *See Figure 26*

(Continued on next page)

327

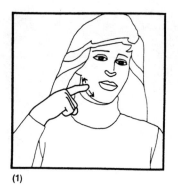
(1)

JAW, *continued*

(1) The index finger of the right "one" hand moves up and down on the right jaw. (MM)

JEJUNUM

The middle part of the small intestine, coming after the duodenum and before the ileum. The jejunum is a part of the digestive tract which absorbs a lot of food. *See Figure 9*

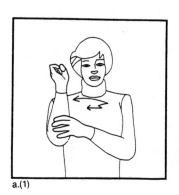
a.(1)

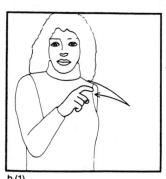
b.(1)

JERK

A sudden movement of part of the body caused by a muscle contracting suddenly.

A doctor will test our nervous system and reflexes by tapping certain tendons to see if a part of the body will jerk.

a. (1) The right "S" hand faces left with the arm bent, the left hand grabs the right arm. Move the right hand in a jerking movement towards the left then back to the right. (SM)

b. (1) The right "one" hand faces out and makes a jerking movement from left to the right. (SM)

JOINT

A place where two bones come together. Joints are usually made up of cartilage and tough connections called ligaments.

Because joints are used and stressed a lot, they are often injured and inflammed.

(1) The right "one" hand points to the left elbow. (SM)

* *This is just an example. The right hand should point to the area referred to.*

(2) Both "S" hands face in at chest level, touching at the knuckles. Move both hands down slightly. (SM)

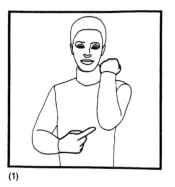
(1)

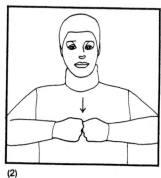
(2)

JUGULAR VEINS

The large veins in the neck which take blood from the face, brain and neck back to the heart. *See Figure 7*

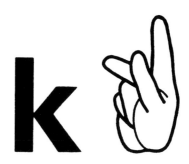

k

KELLER-BLAKE SPLINT

A splint used to keep a broken bone's ends from overlapping, also called a half-ring traction splint.

Keller-Blake splints are very useful in holding a broken femur still.

KELOID

See SCAR TISSUE

KIDNEYS

Two organs found on either side of the spinal column in the lower back which are very important parts of the excretory system. They act as filters and take wastes out of the blood and help control the amount of water in the blood. Urine, formed by the kidneys' activities, is sent to the bladder through the ureters, where it is held until we urinate. *See Figure 11*

(1) Fingerspell "K-I-D-N-E-Y".
(2) The right "F" hand faces out at the area of a kidney. (SM)

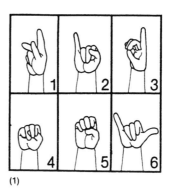

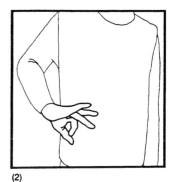

KIDNEY STONE

A hard, stone-like object made of urine that forms in the kidneys and may stop the flow of urine if it gets into a ureter and plugs it.

If the kidney stone is small enough, it may be passed down the ureters, through the bladder and down the urethra, causing severe pain.

(1) Fingerspell "K-I-D-N-E-Y".
(2) Sign STONE — the left "A" hand faces down at chest level. The right "A" hand faces down and taps the back of the left hand a few times. (MM)

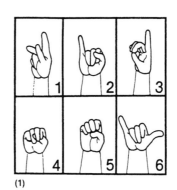

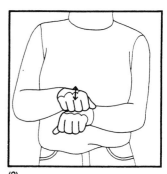

329

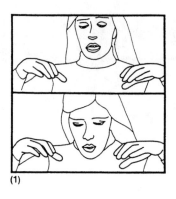

(1)

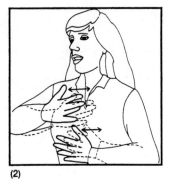

(2)

KISS OF LIFE

Another name for mouth-to-mouth resuscitation in which a person breathes air into another person's lungs through the mouth.

The Kiss of Life is a way to do artificial respiration.

(1) Both "C" hands face down at shoulder level. Imitate blowing into something. (MM)

(2) Sign BREATH — both "five" hands move in and out from the chest a few times as if imitating breathing. (MM)

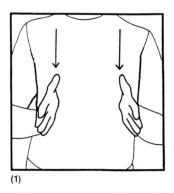

(1)

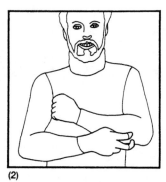

(2)

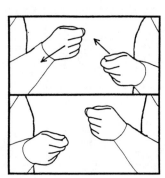

(3)

(4)

KLEPTOMANIAC

A person who has an uncontrollable need to steal things because of a mental problem.

After kleptomaniacs steal something, they are usually very sorry they did it.

(1) Sign PERSON — both "flat" hands face each other at chest level. Move both hands down to waist level. (SM)

(2) Sign STEAL — the left arm is bent. The right "bent-V" hand faces in at the left elbow. (SM)

(3) Sign CAN'T — the left "one" hand faces down at chest level, pointing out. The right "one" hand faces out and moves down to strike the left index finger. (SM)

(4) Sign CONTROL — both "modified-A" hands face each other and move alternately forward and back a few times at chest level. (MM)

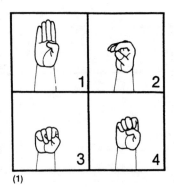

(1)

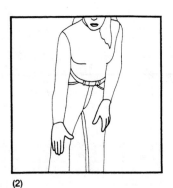

(2)

KNEE

The joint between the thigh and leg. *See Figure 1*

(1) Fingerspell "B-O-N-E".

(2) The right "flat" hand taps the knee a few times. (MM)

KNEECAP

The small, round bone that sits in front of the knee joint; also called the patella. *See Figure 26*

(1) The right "F" hand faces in on the kneecap. (SM)
(2) Fingerspell "B-O-N-E".
(3) The right "claw" hand is on top of the left fist. (SM)

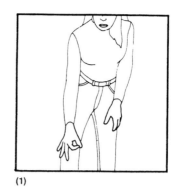

(1)

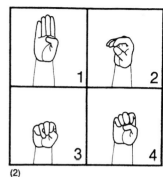

(2)

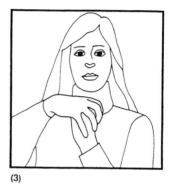

(3)

KNOCKOUT DROPS

A slang name for chloral hydrate, a drug that acts as a sedative and makes someone unconscious.

Knockout drops can be put in alcoholic drinks or water to put someone to sleep.

(1) Sign MEDICINE — the left "flat" hand faces up at chest level. The middle finger of the right "eight" hand touches the left palm and pivots slightly from left to right a few times. (MM)
(2) The left "C" hand faces right at chest level. The right "S" hand faces down above the left hand. Flick the index finger down a few times as if imitating dropping something into the left hand. (MM)
(3) Sign DRINK — the right "C" hand faces left and moves towards the mouth as if imitating taking a drink. (SM)
(4) The right "K" hand faces out at chest level then drops slightly down into an "O" hand. (SM)

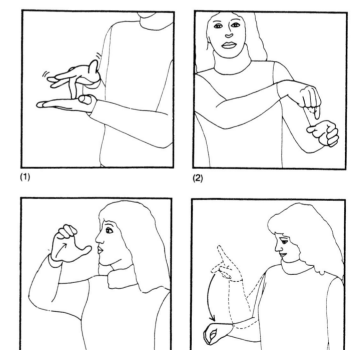

(1)

(2)

(3)

(4)

331

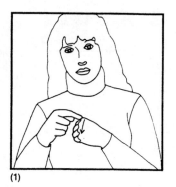
(1)

KNUCKLES

The joints of the fingers, especially those that stick out when the fist is closed. *See Figure 3*

(1) The index finger of the right "one" hand moves across the knuckles of the left hand. (SM)

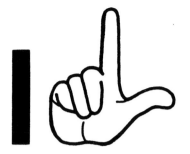

LABOR

In medicine, the physical process of giving birth. Labor starts with abdominal contractions and dilation of the cervix; then there is the birth of the baby; it ends with the placenta coming out of the uterus.

The muscular activities and changes that go on in a woman's body during labor are controlled by hormones.

(1) Fingerspell "L-A-B-O-R".

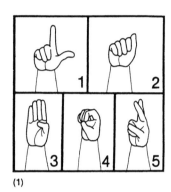

(1)

LABYRINTH

The loops and coil that make up the inner part of the ear. The labyrinth, surrounded by bone, includes the semicircular canals and cochlea and is filled with fluid.

LACERATION

A wound or ragged tear in a part of the body.

A laceration may be made by tearing or stretching the skin with a dull object.

(1) Sign CUT — the left "flat" hand faces in at chest level. The thumb of the right "A" hand moves down the back of the left hand a few times as if imitating cutting. (MM)

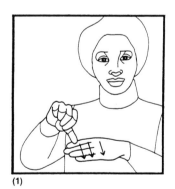

(1)

LACRIMAL GLAND

The gland above and to the side of the eye which makes tears. *See Figure 21 or 22*

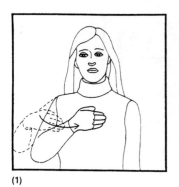

(1)

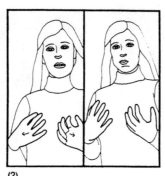

(2)

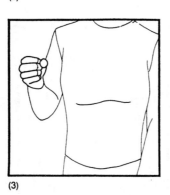

(3)

LACTATION

The forming of milk in a mother's breasts to feed a baby, starting when a baby is born and going on as long as a baby is fed from the breast.

During lactation, a woman needs extra calcium to replace that lost in the milk she makes for the baby.

(1) Sign BREAST — the fingertips of the right "cupped" hand touch the right then the left chest area. (SM)

(2) Both "claw" hands face in at chest level. Open and twist both hands slightly and at the same time the cheeks should puff out. (SM)

(3) Sign MILK — the right "S" hand faces left at chest level. Open and close the hand slightly as if squeezing something. (MM)

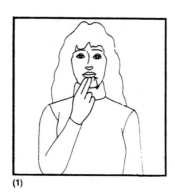

(1)

LACTOSE

A kind of sugar which has glucose (dextrose) in it.

Lactose is also called milk sugar because it is found in milk.

(1) Sign SUGAR — the fingertips of the right "H" hand brush down the chin a few times. (MM)

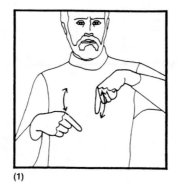

(1)

LAME

Disabled or crippled in one or more limbs.

Lame usually refers to a leg or foot that is damaged or weak that causes movement to be difficult.

(1) Both "one" hands face down at chest level. Rock both hands slightly up and down a few times. (MM)

LANCE

To pierce or cut the skin.

> *A doctor will usually **lance** a boil or abscess to let pus out and allow the area to drain and heal.*

(1) Sign CUT — the left "flat" hand faces in at chest level. The thumb of the right "A" hand moves down the back of the left hand a few times as if imitating cutting. (MM)

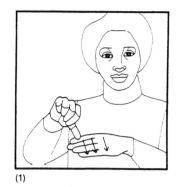

(1)

LARGE

Something big or bigger than normal.

> *When a part of the body suddenly starts to become **large**, it may be because of normal growth, the part is being used more, or there is disease in the area.*

(1) Both "L" hands with the index fingers and thumbs slightly bent face each other at chest level and move out towards the sides. (SM)

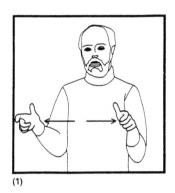

(1)

LARGE INTESTINE

The colon; that part of the digestive tract which goes from the end of the small intestine to the rectum. The major activity of the large intestine is removing fluid from the digested food that is in it.
See Figure 9

LARYNGECTOMY

Surgical removal of the larynx. The most common reason for removing the larynx is cancer of the larynx which is usually caused by drinking large amounts of alcohol, smoking or breathing dangerous gases.

> *A **laryngectomy** will affect breathing and speaking to different degrees depending on how much of the larynx is removed.*

(1) The thumb of the right "A" hand moves across the throat from left to right as if imitating cutting the throat. (SM)

(2) The right "S" hand touches the throat then turns out and down into a "five" hand as if throwing something down. (SM)

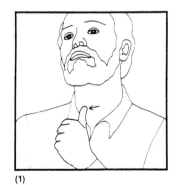

(1)

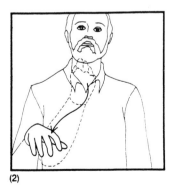

(2)

LARYNGITIS

Inflammation of the larynx. Symptoms of laryngitis may include a dry and sore throat, painful swallowing, hoarseness and sometimes a cough.

Laryngitis can have many causes, including talking too much, a cold or infection in the throat, breathing in harmful gases, and smoking.

LARYNX

The large. upper part of the trachea in back of and below the mouth. The larynx, made up of muscle, cartilage and membranes, holds the vocal cords, which allow us to speak. *See Figure 10*

LATENT

Hidden, quiet; not active.

*The virus which causes cold sores will be **latent** in the nerve cells until it travels down the nerve and attacks the skin.*

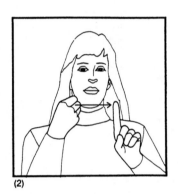

(1)   (2)

(1) Sign NOT YET — the right "cupped" hand faces back at the right side and moves forward and back a few times in a short repeated movement. (MM)
(2) The left "one" hand faces out at chest level, the index finger pointing up. The right "S" hand faces in and moves to sharply hit the left index finger. (SM)

LATERAL

To or on the side of a structure.

*The ears are on the **lateral** part of the head.*

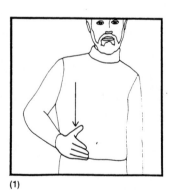

(1)

(1) The right "flat" hand moves down the right side of the body. (SM)

LATISSIMUS DORSI

A large, triangle-shaped, flat muscle which wraps around the back and side of the body. It covers all of the middle and lower back, and becomes narrow as it goes up where it attaches to the upper part of the humerus. The latissimus dorsi is used to move the arm and also the shoulder. *See Figure 5*

LAXATIVE

A substance which prevents or relieves constipation by making it easier for the feces to move out of the body. Laxatives work by making the intestines more active, by making the linings of the intestines slippery or by softening the feces by making them wetter.

Finding the cause of constipation and getting plenty of exercise and eating a diet with plenty of bulk or fiber in it may make using laxatives unnecessary.

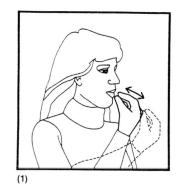 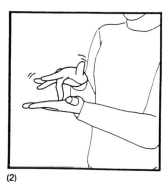

(1) Sign EAT — the fingertips of the right "flat-O" hand tap the mouth a few times. (MM)

(2) Sign MEDICINE — the left "flat" hand faces up at chest level. The middle finger of the right "eight" hand touches the left palm and pivots slightly from left to right a few times. (MM)

(3) Sign FOR — the index finger of the right "one" hand touches the forehead and turns out forward, the finger pointing out. (SM)

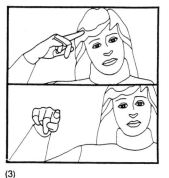 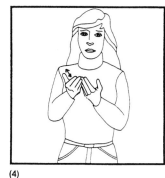

(4) Sign EASY — the left "cupped" hand faces up at chest level. The fingers of the right "cupped" hand brush up the back of the left hand twice. (DM)

(5) Sign FECES — the left "A" hand faces right at chest level. The thumb of the right "A" hand is inside the left fist. Keeping the left hand in place, move the right hand down from the left. (SM)

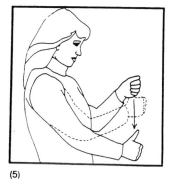

(5)

LEAD POISONING

Poisoning caused by eating or being exposed to lead or something that contains lead. Lead poisoning usually happens over a long time because lead builds up in the body. Most cases of lead poisoning occur in children who eat or suck on paint on walls, window sills or toys that have lead in them. A person could also get lead poisoning from working around it a lot, breathing it in or by using food containers which have lead in them. Symptoms of lead poisoning are loss of appetite, nausea, anemia, cramps in the abdomen and muscles, nervous system problems such as joint pain, brain damage and mental problems.

Most people recover from lead poisoning if they stop taking the lead into their bodies and if they get treatment for it soon enough.

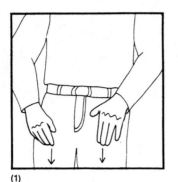
(1)

LEG

One of the two lower limbs which we stand on and which move us around. The leg includes the calf, ankle and foot. *See Figure 2*

(1) The fingertips of both "flat" hands brush down both legs. (SM)

LENS

The round structure in the eye behind the pupil and iris which is held in place by the ciliary body. The shape of the lens can be changed by small muscles in the ciliary body so things which are different distances from us can be focused on the retina. The lens is also called the crystalline lens. *See Figure 22*

LEPROSY

A communicable disease caused by a bacterium (Mycobacterium leprae) and found mostly in warm climates; also called Hansen's Disease. The disease progresses slowly and is very difficult to treat. Leprosy affects the nerves and skin, causing parts of the body to lose feeling and then die. Parts of the body become deformed and the person may become weak or paralyzed.

*If **leprosy** is found early, modern drugs can help the person live longer and possibly even be cured.*

LESION

Skin or tissue changed by an injury or a disease.

*When someone has any type of **lesion** on their genitals, they should have a check-up to see if they have a venereal disease.*

LESS

A smaller amount of something.

*A person who is not doing hard work or who isn't very active will need **less** food than someone who is.*

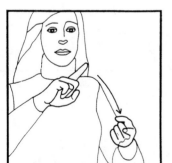
a.(1)   b.(1)

a. (1) The left "one" hand faces up at chest level. The right "one" hand faces down and moves down towards the left hand. (SM)
b. (1) The left "cupped" hand faces up at chest level. The right "cupped" hand fces down and moves down towards the left hand. (SM)

338

LETHAL

Having to do with or causing death.

Too much of a drug or chemical can be lethal.

(1) Sign CAUSE — both "A" hands face up at chest level. Drop both hands down to the left side into "five" hands. (SM)

(2) Sign DEATH — the left "flat" hand faces up at chest level and the right "flat" hand faces down at chest level. Turn both hands to the right so that the left hand ends facing down and the right hand ends facing up. (SM)

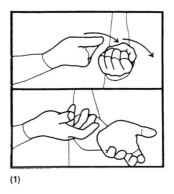

(1)

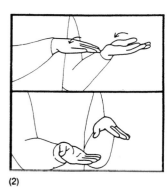

(2)

LEUKEMIA

Any of several usually fatal diseases which affect blood-making organs, causing too many white blood cells to be made. The symptoms may include poor appetite, weakness, enlarged spleen and liver, swollen lymph nodes, anemia, pain in the bones, bleeding and the inability to fight off infections.

The disease may be slowed by using drugs and chemicals but the cause of leukemia is not known.

(1) Sign BLOOD — the left "five" hand is at chest level with the palm toward the body. The palm of the right "five" hand is toward the body with the middle fingertips touching the mouth. Move the right hand down the back of the left hand. Wiggle the fingers of the right hand as it moves. (MM)
* This movement should be short, repeated and somewhat restrained.

(2) Sign WHITE — the fingertips of the right "five" hand touch the chest then move out forward into a "flat-O" hand. (SM)

(3) Fingerspell "C-E-L-L".

(4) Sign DISEASE — the middle finger of the right "eight" hand taps the forehead and the middle finger of the left "eight" hand taps the stomach. (MM)

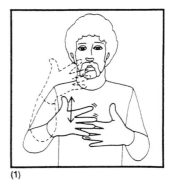

(1)

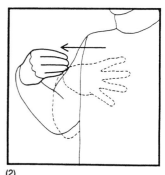

(2)

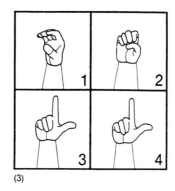

(3)

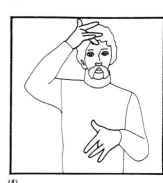

(4)

LEUKOCYTE

See WHITE BLOOD CELLS

LIBIDO

In psychology, the sexual drive, the desire to live and the desire for pleasure that are a part of a person's personality.

The libido is one part of our personalities that is responsible for our instinctual behavior.

(Continued on next page)

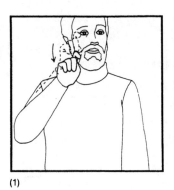
(1)

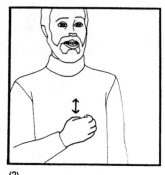
(2)

LIBIDO, *continued*

(1) Sign SEX — the right "X" hand faces out and the index finger touches the head at eye level then moves down to touch at the chin.(SM)
(2) Sign DESIRE — the fingertips of the right "C" hand brushes up and down the chest a few times in a short repeated movement. (MM)
* The facial expression should reflect desire.

LIBRIUM®

The name under which the drug chlordiazepoxide is sold. This drug is one of the most commonly used tranquilizers.

People taking large doses of Librium for a long time can become addicted to it and may have symptoms like restlessness, cramps, shaking, sweating, vomiting and perhaps convulsions when it is taken away.

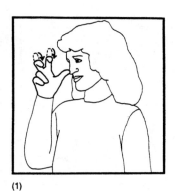
(1)

LICE

Small, wingless insects that live on animals, including man. Lice may live in the body hair or on clothing. (See PEDICULOSIS)

Lice bite and suck blood and may transmit diseases to people.

(1) Sign INSECT — the thumb of the right "three" hand touches the nose. Bend and straighten the fingers a few times. (MM)

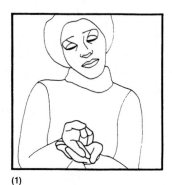
(1)

LIE DOWN

A prone position; to recline.

If a person is injured, he should lie down to avoid any additional injury.

(1) The right "H" hand faces up in the palm of the left "flat" hand. The eyes should also close. (SM)

LIFE

The time between birth and death of an organism. Biologically, the condition in which the organs of an animal or plant can perform all or any of their functions.

You can help protect your life from injury by learning first-aid and preventive medicine.

(1) Both "L" hands face in and move up the body from waist level to chest level. (SM)

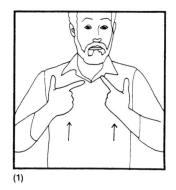

(1)

LIGAMENT

The strong fibers that hold the ends of bones together or hold organs or other structures in place.

Ligaments limit the amount of movement a part may have.

LIGHT ADAPTATION

The changes in the eye which allow us to see things comfortably in bright light after being in dim light.

When light adaptation occurs in the eye, the pupil becomes smaller to let in less light.

(1) Sign BLACK — the index finger of the right "one" hand moves across the forehead from left to right. (SM)
(2) Sign EYES — the index finger of the right "one" hand points to both eyes. (SM)
(3) Both "O" hands are in front of the eyes. Close both fists as if indicating the pupils closing. (SM)

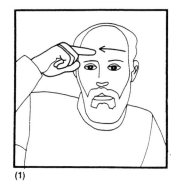

(1)

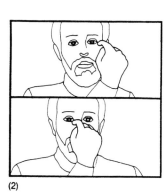

(2)

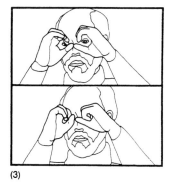

(3)

LIGHT PERCEPTION

The eye's ability to tell light from dark.

People may have a form of blindness because of problems with light perception.

341

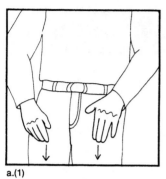
a.(1)

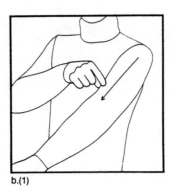
b.(1)

LIMB

An arm or leg.

The arms are the upper limbs and the legs are the lower limbs.

a. (1) The fingertips of both "flat" hands brush down both legs. (SM)

b. (1) The index finger of the right "one" hand moves down the left arm. (SM)

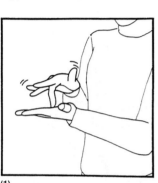
(1)

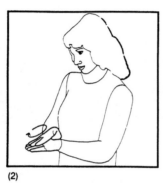
(2)

LINIMENT

A fluid containing medicine and applied on the outside of the body.

The medicine in liniments can also contain oil, water or alcohol.

(1) Sign MEDICINE — the left "flat" hand faces up at chest level. The middle finger of the right "eight" hand touches the left palm and pivots slightly from left to right a few times. (MM)

(2) Sign RUB — the left "flat" hand faces down at chest level. The right "flat" hand faces down and rubs the back of the left hand in a circular movement. (MM)

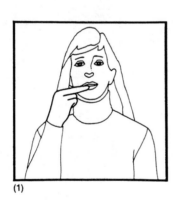
(1)

LIPS

The soft, fleshy, red structures around the opening of the mouth. *See Figure 23*

(1) The index finger of the right "one" hand touches the lips. (SM)

LIPID

Any one of different fats or fat-like substances.

Lipids form an important part of the membrane which holds a cell together.

LIP READING

Understanding what people say by watching their lips move as they talk.

Using signs and fingerspelling to communicate with the deaf is clearer than lip reading because there are many sounds which are not made with the lips.

(Continued on next page)

(1) The right "V" hand faces down in front of the mouth and moves from left to right a few times. (MM)

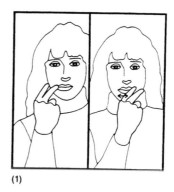

(1)

LIQUID

A substance that flows easily; a fluid.

> *All things, depending on their form, can be grouped as solids, gases or liquids.*

(1) Fingerspell "L-I-Q-U-I-D".

* *If referring to a specific liquid such as water, it should be signed or fingerspelled.*

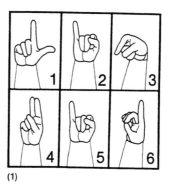

(1)

LIQUID DIET

Meals or foods that are fluids or liquid. A person may be put on a liquid diet after an operation or when easily digested food is needed.

> *Common foods in a liquid diet are soft drinks, coffee, tea, milk, fruit juices, soups and meat broths.*

(1) Fingerspell "D-I-E-T".
(2) Sign DRINK — the right "C" hand faces left and moves towards the mouth as if imitating taking a drink. (SM)
(3) Sign ONLY — the right "one" hand points up and faces out at chest level. Turn the hand to the left down and around in a circle, ending with the hand facing in. (SM)

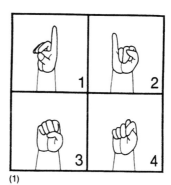

(1)

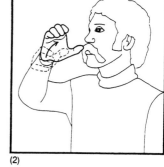

(2)

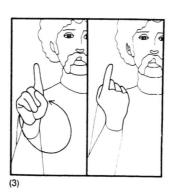

(3)

343

LIQUOR

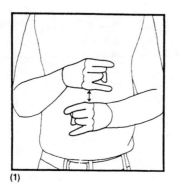
(1)

A drink with alcohol in it; also any fluid mixture or solution.

Drinking small amounts of liquor periodically is said to be good for the internal organs, however, too much may lead to physical damage.

(1) Sign ALCOHOL — the index and pinky fingers of both hands are extended, the hands face in at chest level with the right hand on top. Tap the hands together a few times. (MM)

LITTER

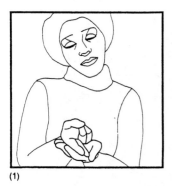
(1)

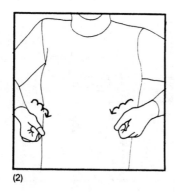
(2)

A device with handles big enough for a person to lie on and used to carry people who are sick or injured.

A litter is also called a stretcher.

(1) The right "H" hand faces up in the palm of the left "flat" hand, both at chest level. The eyes should be closed. (SM)

(2) Both "S" hands are at the sides of the body facing each other. Bounce the hands up and down slightly a few times as if imitating carrying a stretcher. (MM)

LITTLE

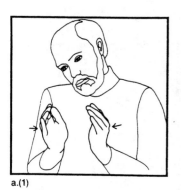
a.(1)

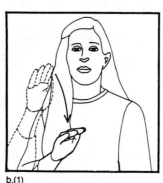
b.(1)

Small or short.

When a person is abnormally little and not growing properly, the cause may be a hormone problem, a poor diet, or an enzyme problem in the body.

a. (1) Sign SMALL — both "cupped" hands face each other at chest level and move in towards each other a little. (SM)

b. (1) Sign SHORT — the right "cupped" hand faces down at head level and moves down to shoulder level. (SM)

LIVER

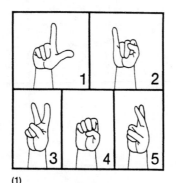
(1)

The largest organ in the body, found on the right side of the abdomen, beneath the lungs and above the stomach. The liver gets blood carrying nutrients from the intestines which have just been taken into the body from the food. These nutrients may not be in a form the body can use and the liver changes them into usable forms. The liver also makes bile which is sent to the gall bladder, where it is held until it is used to help digest food. *See Figure 9*

(1) Fingerspell "L-I-V-E-R".

LOBOTOMY

An incision made in the brain (frontal or prefrontal); cutting through the nerve fibers that pass from the frontal lobe of the cerebrum to the thalamus.

A lobotomy may be done to control certain mental disorders or to relieve pain that can not be treated otherwise.

(1) The index finger points to the head. (SM)

(2) Sign CUT — the left "flat" hand faces in at chest level. The thumb of the right "A" hand moves down the back of the left hand as if imitating cutting. (SM)

(3) Sign REMOVE — the left "flat" hand faces up at chest level. The right "A" hand touches the left palm then moves down into a "five" hand as if throwing something away. (SM)

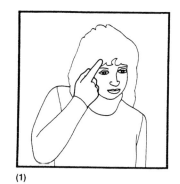
(1)

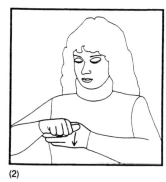
(2)

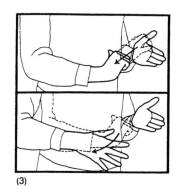
(3)

LOCAL ANESTHETIC

An anesthetic injected into a certain part of the body to prevent feeling or stop pain in that area only.

Local anesthetics work by stopping nerve activity in the area without making a person lose consciousness.

(1) Sign INJECTION — the index finger of the right "L" hand touches the left upper arm. Bend the thumb as if injecting something into the left arm. (SM)

(2) Sign FREEZE — both "five" hands face down at waist level. Move both hands up slightly into "claw" hands. (SM)

* This should be signed at the area where the anesthetic is being given.

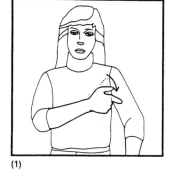
(1)

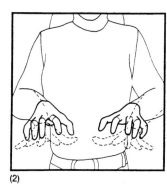
(2)

LOCKJAW

See TETANUS

LOIN

The lower part of the back and the sides between the ribs and pelvis. *See Figure 3*

LOOSE

Free; not tied down; not fastened securely.

A person's adult teeth can become loose if they aren't eating the right foods, if they are hit in the mouth or if they have a gum disease.

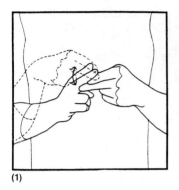

(1)

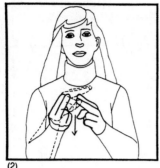

(2)

LOSE WEIGHT

To take pounds off the body, to weigh less or become smaller.

*People will **lose weight** if they use up more calories than they get in their food.*

(1) The left "H" hand faces down at chest level. The right "H" hand also faces down on top of the left hand. Pivot the right hand slightly a few times. (MM)

(2) The left "H" hand faces down at chest level. The fingertips of the right "H" hand touch the fingers of the left hand. Turn the right hand over so that it faces up a few times. At the same time, both hands should move down to waist level. (MM)

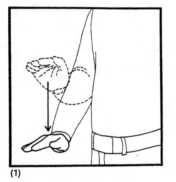

(1)

LOW

Short or below normal.

*A **low** body temperature will slow down the body's activities and affect the person's brain, causing one to be confused and want to sleep.*

(1) The right "cupped" hand faces down at chest level and moves down to waist level. (SM)

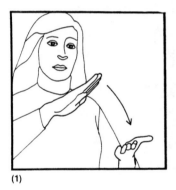

(1)

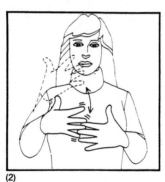

(2)

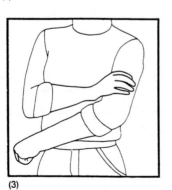

(3)

LOW BLOOD PRESSURE

Not enough force of the blood pushing against the walls of the blood vessels; hypotension. When someone has low blood pressure, the blood may not be pushed to the parts of the body that need it. Low blood pressure may occur in shock or when someone has lost a lot of blood.

*When someone has very **low blood pressure**, not enough blood may be getting to the brain, resulting in unconsciousness.*

(1) The left "flat" hand faces up at chest level. The right "flat" hand faces down at shoulder level and moves down to the left hand. (SM)

(2) Sign BLOOD — the left "five" hand is at chest level with the palm toward the body. The palm of the right "five" hand is toward the body with the middle fingertips touching the mouth. Move the right hand down the back of the left hand. Wiggle the fingers of the right hand as it moves. (MM)

* This movement should be short, repeated and somewhat restrained.

(3) The right "claw" hand grabs the left upper arm. (SM)

LOWER LEG

The part of the leg below the knee. *See Figure 1*

LSD

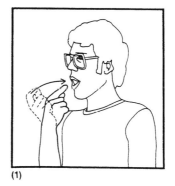 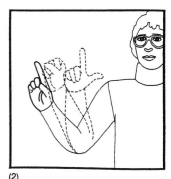

The initials and slang name for lysergic acid diethylamide, an hallucinogenic drug; also called acid. LSD is made from the fungus growing on grains and wet grass. It is used legally only for experiments.

The illegal use of LSD has increased so much that it is now a social and legal problem.

(1) Sign PILL — the thumb and index finger of the right hand touch, the palm faces the mouth. Flick the index finger towards the mouth as if popping a pill into the mouth. (SM)

(2) Fingerspell "L-S-D".

LUMBAGO

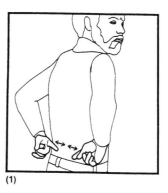

A dull ache in the lower back.

Lumbago may be caused by overworking muscles in the area or by problems with one of the disks between the vertebrae.

(1) Both "one" hands point to each other behind the back and move in and out from each other a few times. (MM)

* The facial expression should reflect pain. This can also be signed by twisting the hands in opposite directions.

LUMBAR

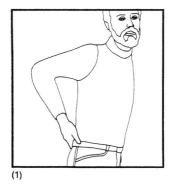

Referring to the lower back.

The kidneys are located in the lumbar region.

(1) The right "flat" hand touches the right lower back. (SM)

LUMBAR VERTEBRAE

The five bones of the spinal column just above the pelvis and below the chest region. *See Figure 26*

LUMP

A bump or an area which sticks out above the tissue around it.

A lump can be caused by abnormal cell growth in an area or by blood or fluid collecting in an area.

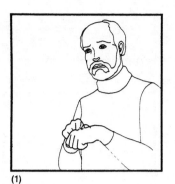
(1)

(1) The left "S" hand faces down at chest level. The index finger of the right "one" hand makes a small bump on the back of the left hand. At the same time, the cheeks should puff out. (SM)

* *This could be signed at the area of the lump.*

LUNACY

An old word for insanity.

The word lunacy comes from "luna," the Latin word for moon, as it was thought at one time that insanity was caused by the moon.

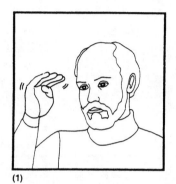
(1)

(1) The right cupped "four" hand faces the head and pivots slightly from left to right a few times. (MM)

LUNGS

Two spongy organs in the chest which hold air that has been inhaled. The lungs are made up of small tubes and sacs with blood vessels in the walls. Oxygen in the inhaled air passes into the blood in the blood vessels. Carbon dioxide which has been picked up from body cells by the blood and taken to the lungs will pass out of the blood into the air in the lungs and be exhaled. The lungs are connected with the mouth opening by the bronchi and the trachea. *See Figure 10*

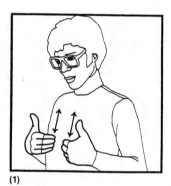
(1)

(1) The fingertips of both "cupped" hands brush up and down the chest a few times in short repeated movements. (MM)

LYMPH

A clear, slightly yellow fluid which is a part of the blood and which can leave the blood vessels and go out into the tissues and bathe the cells. The lymph is collected in special ducts after leaving the blood vessels and is carried back to the heart and put into the bloodstream. The lymph is like blood but it doesn't have any red blood cells in it.

The lymph carries white blood cells, takes nutrients to cells and carries away wastes and harmful bacteria.

LYMPH GLAND

See LYMPH NODE

LYMPH NODE

A small, round gland found along the ducts that carry lymph; also called lymph gland. Lymph nodes can be alone or in groups. Groups of lymph nodes are found in the armpit, groin and neck. Lymph nodes make white blood cells and filter out things that aren't supposed to be in the body like bacteria.

> *Lymph nodes* often swell when a person has an infection because they are working hard to stop the infection from spreading to other parts of the body.

LYSERGIC ACID DIETHYLAMIDE

See LSD

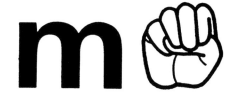

MACE

A mixture of chemical (methylchloraform, chloroacetophenone) in spray form and used as a weapon.

Mace causes intense, burning eye pain, bronchitis and irritation to the respiratory system.

(1) Sign CHEMICAL — both "C" hands face out at chest level. Move both hands in alternating circular movements a few times. (MM)
(2) The right "one" hand points up and faces out at chest level. Bend the index finger and at the same time the mouth should say "psst", indicating spraying.

* *It may be necessary to fingerspell "M-A-C-E" to clarify.*

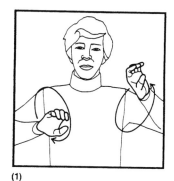
(1)

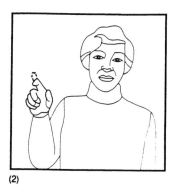
(2)

MACULA LUTEA

A yellow spot next to the place where the optic nerve leaves the eye.

The macula lutea contains the fovea centralis where there is a concentration of cones, and vision is best in this area.

MAINLINE

The slang word for injecting a drug into a large vein.

People who mainline with an illegal drug and use unclean needles or syringes may get a disease such as hepatitis.

(1) The right "S" hand moves in and out from the left inside elbow a few times. (MM)

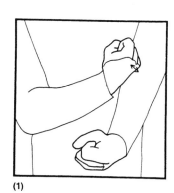
(1)

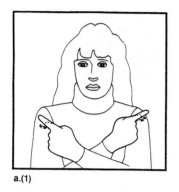

a.(1)

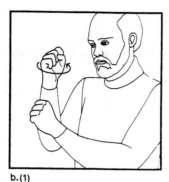

b.(1)

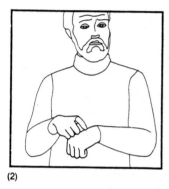

(2)

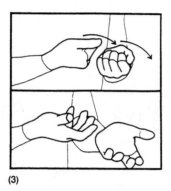

(3)

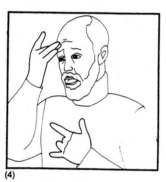

(4)

MALARIA

An infectious disease caused by a small parasite which gets into and destroys red blood cells. The disease is more common in warm climates and is passed between people by mosquitoes. People with malaria have a cycle of chills, fever and sweating which is repeated over and over again. They will also be tired and weak, anemic because of the destruction of red blood cells, and have enlarged spleens.

Before travelling to countries where malaria if found, a person should see a doctor and start taking drugs which can prevent the disease.

a. (1) Sign MOSQUITO — both "one" hands cross at the chest. Bend and straighten both index fingers a few times. (MM)

b. (1) Sign MOSQUITO — the left "S" hand faces right at chest level. The right "S" hand faces left above the left hand. Move the right hand in a counterclockwise circle. (SM)

(2) Sign BITE — the index finger of the right "one" hand taps the back of the left hand. (SM)

(3) Sign CAUSE — both "A" hands face up at chest level. Drop both hands down to the left, ending in "five" hands facing up. (SM)

(4) Sign SICK — the middle finger of the right "eight" hand touches the forehead and the middle finger of the left "eight" hand touches the stomach. Twist both hands slightly. (SM)

* The facial expression should reflect sickness.
* Sign a.(1) or b.(1) MOSQUITO, then sign BITE, CAUSE and SICK.

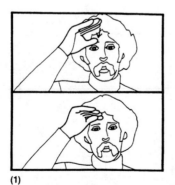

(1)

MALE

The sex which can make sperm to fertilize an egg. In humans, males are called men and boys.

A male animal has testes to make sperm and a penis to carry it into a female.

(1) The right open "flat-O" hand faces down at the forehead. Move the hand out slightly, also closing the hand to a "flat-O" hand. (SM)

352

MALIGNANT

The condition, in a disease or growth, of getting worse, spreading or resisting treatment.

Cancer is a malignant growth.

(1) Sign SICK — the middle finger of the right "eight" hand touches the forehead and the middle finger of the left "eight" hand touches the stomach. Twist both hands slightly. (SM)

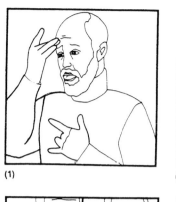
(1)

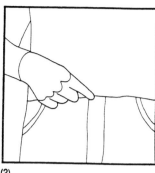
(2)

(2) The index finger of the right "one" hand points to the area of the growth. (SM)

(3) The fingertips of both "flat-O" hands touch the chest. Spread both hands on the chest into "five" hands. (SM)

* *This could be signed at the area of the growth.*

(4) Sign WORSE — both "K" hands cross at the wrists at waist level. Tap the hands with an arcing movement several times and at the same time, move both hands up to chest level. (MM)

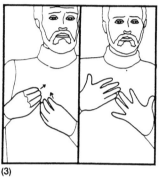
(3)

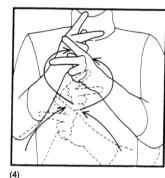
(4)

MALLEUS

One of the three small bones in the middle ear which moves and helps carry sound waves from the eardrum to the inner ear, where the movement is picked up as sound. The malleus (also called the hammer) is the largest bone, is attached to the eardrum, and is shaped like a hammer. *See Figure 20*

MALNUTRITION

The condition resulting from the body's not getting enough of certain types of food or not getting the right nutrients. Malnutrition may be caused by not eating enough food, not eating good foods, by the body not taking the food in from the intestine or by the body not using the food correctly.

Dieters should be sure to eat well balanced meals and take vitamins to prevent malnutrition.

MALOCCLUSION

In dentistry, a condition in which teeth are not in a normal position when they are brought together.

Abnormal growth of the jaws or the loss of teeth may cause malocclusion.

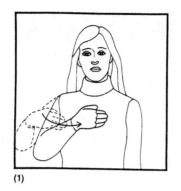
(1)

MAMMARY

Referring to a breast or milk-making structure.

Mammitis is a condition where there is inflammation of a mammary.

(1) Sign BREAST — the fingertips of the right "cupped" hand touch the right then the left chest. (SM)

MAMMARY GLANDS

Referring to the glands in breasts.

The mammary glands make up a woman's breast and can make milk.

MAMMECTOMY

See MASTECTOMY

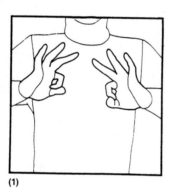
(1)

MAMMILLARY

Referring to the nipple of a breast or something like a nipple.

Mammillitis is the inflammation of the mammillary.

(1) Sign NIPPLES — both "F" hands face out at the nipples. (SM)

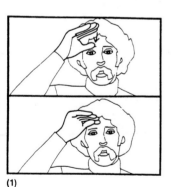
(1)

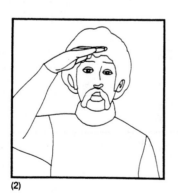
(2)

MAN

An adult male human being; also the general term for the species Homo-Sapien.

Man is the opposite of woman.

(1) The right open "flat-O" hand faces down at the forehead. Move the hand out slightly, closing to a "flat-O" hand. The right "flat" hand then faces down at the forehead and moves out slightly. (SM)

(2) The right "flat" hand faces down at the forehead and moves out slightly. (SM)

354

MANGE

An infectious skin disease of animals, including man, caused by a small insect which burrows into the skin. Mange causes itching, loss of hair, and dry, scaly skin.

An animal with patches of hair missing may have mange, and should be touched as little as possible and taken to a veterinarian.

MANIA

A mental disorder causing people to have a strong desire for something, rapidly changing ideas, extreme happiness and to be very active.

Mania can also cause people to show violent abnormal behavior.

MANDIBLE

The bone which makes up the lower jaw. *See Figure 26*

MANDIBULAR NERVE

A nerve which serves the lower part of the face, that is, the lower teeth, gums, jaw, skin of the cheek and two thirds of the tongue.

The mandibular nerve is often deadened with an anesthetic when a dentist does work on the lower teeth.

MANIPULATION

The skillful control or movement of something with the hands.

Manipulation is used to put a broken bone in the correct position or to put a dislocated bone back where it belongs.

(1) Sign SKILLED — the left "flat" hand faces right at chest level. The right hand grabs the pinky finger side of the left hand. Move the right hand down to an "A" hand. (SM)

(2) Sign MAKE — the right "S" hand faces left on top of the left "S" hand which faces right. Twist both hands so that they end facing in. (SM)

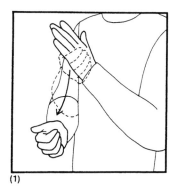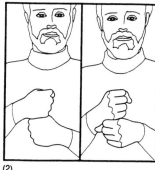

(1)   (2)

* *Mime the movement of manipulation.*

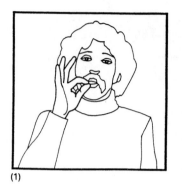
(1)

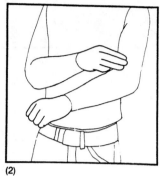
(2)

MARIJUANA

An intoxicating, illegal drug made from the leaves and flowers of the Indian hemp plant (Cannabis sativa); slang names include "pot", "grass", and "weed". When eaten or smoked in cigarette form, a chemical (Tetrahydrocannebinol, THC) caused a person to feel "light-headed". Marijuana may cause a psychological habit but in itself is not physically addictive.

Marijuana has been shown to lessen the symptoms of cancer chemotherapy.

a. (1) The thumb and index finger of the right "F" hand touch the mouth. (SM)
b. (1) The fingertips of the right "M" hand touch the inside of the left elbow. (SM)

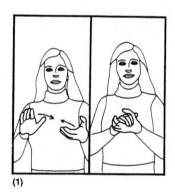
(1)

MARRIAGE

The state of being husband and wife by legal union.

If a husband and wife are having emotional problems, they should talk with a marriage counselor, who might be able to help them.

(1) Clasp the hands together with the right hand on top.(SM)

MARROW

The soft material found inside bones that helps make red blood cells.

In an adult, most blood formation occurs in the marrow of the sternum (breastbone), vertebrae and pelvis.

MASOCHISM

An abnormal sexual need in which a person gets sexual pleasure from being abused or suffering physical pain.

A masochist is a person who practices masochism.

MASSAGE

Rubbing, kneeding, stroking or manipulation of the body with the hands.

Massage is used to help a person relax, to help a part heal, to relieve pain, or to stimulate circulation in a part of the body.

(Continued on next page)

MASSAGE, *continued*

(1) Both hands face down and imitate massaging. (MM)

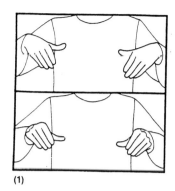

(1)

MASTECTOMY

The surgical removal of a breast; also called mammectomy.

> *Mastectomy combined with radiation is the most common treatment for breast cancer.*

(1) Sign BREAST — the fingertips of the right "cupped" hand touch the right and then the left chest. (SM)
(2) Sign CUT — the thumb of the right "A" hand moves down across the left breast. (SM)
(3) Sign REMOVE — the left "flat" hand faces right at chest level. The right "A" hand touches the left palm then moves down into a "five" hand as if throwing something away. (SM)

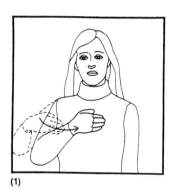

(1)

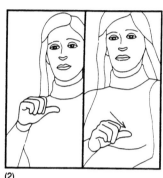

(2)

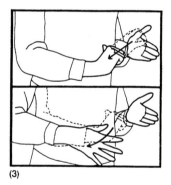

(3)

MASTITIS

Inflammation of a breast; also called mammitis. The first signs of mastitis are redness of a part of the breast and a fever.

> *Mastitis often occurs during lactation, when bacteria may enter the breast through the nipple or a scrape on the nipple.*

(1) Sign INFECTION — the right "I" hand faces out at chest level and shakes from left to right a few times. (MM)

* *Mouth the word "infection" while signing.*

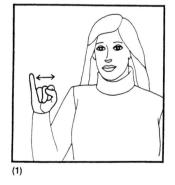

(1)

(Continued on next page)

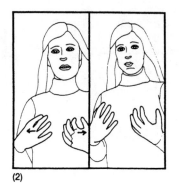
(2)

MASTITIS, *continued*

(2) Both "claw" hands face in at the chest and move slightly to the sides, at the same time, the cheeks should puff out. (SM)

MASTOID PROCESS

The part of the skull which sticks out, pointing down behind the ear. The mastoid process feels like a hard bump behind the ear. The mastoid process is a place where several muscles attach that move the head. A space inside the mastoid process is filled with air and is connected with the eardrum. Because of this connection, an infection in the ear may be passed to this part of the mastoid process and then go from there to the brain. *See Figure 26*

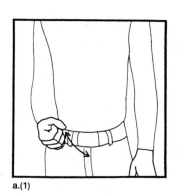
a.(1)

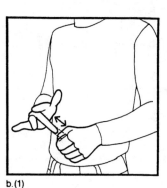
b.(1)

MASTURBATION

Manipulation of the sexual organs in some way other than sexual intercourse to cause sexual excitement or orgasm.

The possible harm done by masturbation comes from the guilt or shame it may cause and not the actual act.

a. (1) Male - the right "S" hand is slightly open with the palm facing left. Move the hand away and toward the body in front of the penis.(MM)
b. (1) Female - the left "S" hand is slightly open at hip level. The palm faces the right. The middle finger of the right "eight" hand moves in and out of the left hand.(MM)

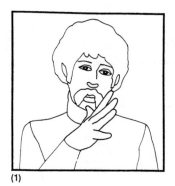
(1)

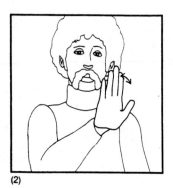
(2)

MATERNAL

Having to do with a mother.

The maternal half of the chromosomes that affect a child's development are found in the egg.

(1) Sign MOTHER — the thumb of the right "five" hand touches the chin. (SM)
(2) Sign HERSELF — the right "flat" hand faces out and moves out slightly a few times. (MM)

358

MATERNITY

The state of being a mother; motherhood.

A maternity ward is an area in a hospital where a woman stays after she has had a baby.

(1) Sign WOMAN — the thumb of the right "A" hand moves down the right cheek then to a "flat" hand facing down at the forehead. (SM)

(2) Sign PREGNANT — both "five" hands face in and mesh together at stomach level. Move both hands out slightly. (SM)

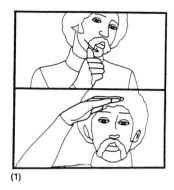

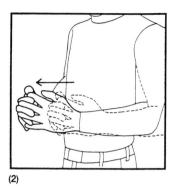

(1)   (2)

MATURE

Being fully grown or developed.

When an ovum in an ovary is mature, it will be released and travel down the fallopian tube to the uterus.

MAXILLA

The bone which makes up the upper jaw.
See Figure 26

MAXILLARY NERVE

A nerve which serves the upper part of the face, that is the upper teeth, gums, jaw, skin of the cheek and nasal pharynx.

The maxillary nerve is often deadened with an anesthetic when a dentist does work on the upper teeth.

MAXILLARY SINUS

A space or cavity in the maxillary bone (upper jaw) which makes up the opening into the nose.

If a person has a sinus infection or hay fever which plugs the maxillary sinus, it may cause the teeth to hurt.

MAXILLOFACIAL

Referring to the face and the upper jaw.

A person with an injury to the maxillofacial area may have their airways blocked, problems speaking and opening and closing the mouth, and problems swallowing.

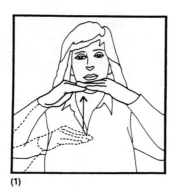
(1)

MAXIMUM

The highest or largest amount.

The maximum amount of blood a person can lose without harm is two pints; loss of more than this could cause shock.

(1) The left "flat" hand faces down at shoulder level. The right "flat" hand faces down at chest level. Move the right hand up even to the left hand. (SM)

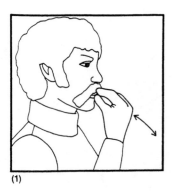
(1)

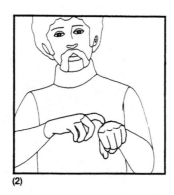
(2)

MEAL

A portion of food eaten during one particular period of time.

For good health, one should have three balanced meals each day.

(1) Sign EAT — the fingertips of the right "flat-O" hand tap the mouth a few times. (MM)
(2) Sign TIME — the index finger of the right "one" hand taps the left wrist a few times. (MM)

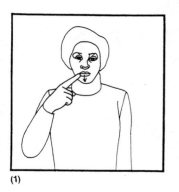
(1)

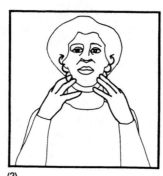
(2)

MEASLES

A very contagious disease caused by a virus; also called Rubeola or morbilli. A person with measles will have symptoms of a bad cold with a runny nose, tiredness, a temperature as high as 105° F, a cough and then a rash. Although a person will get over measles in about five days, there is a danger of the virus causing pneumonia or an inflammation of the brain which may cause death or permanent damage.

Children should be vaccinated against measles be-tween ten and twelve months of age.

(1) Sign RED — the index finger of the right "one" hand brushes down the chin a few times. (MM)
(2) The fingertips of the right "claw" hand move up the sides of the face, touching several times. (MM)

MEASURE

To determine the length, area, quantity or dimensions of something; the act of measurement.

A pelvimeter is an instrument used to measure the pelvis of a pregnant woman to see if she can deliver her baby normally.

(Continued on next page)

MEASURE, *continued*

(1) Both "Y" hands face down at waist level. Tap the thumbs together a few times. (MM)

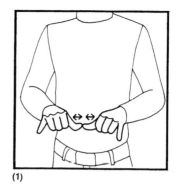
(1)

MECHANICAL OBSTRUCTION

An object stuck in a tube or passage in the body, blocking the movement of things through the tube or passage. Mechanical obstructions can be pieces of food, small toys, coins or collections of mucus, blood or saliva.

Mechanical obstructions often occur in the airways when food is inhaled and blocks the flow of air to the lungs.

MEDIC

A doctor, a medical student or a medical person in the military.

A medic is also called a medical corpsman.

MEDICAL

Referring to the study and practice of medicine; caring for the ill.

Medical assistants who help doctors are called physian's assistants.

(1) Sign MEDICINE — the left "flat" hand faces up at chest level. The middle finger of the right "eight" hand touches the left palm and pivots slightly from left to right a few times. (MM)

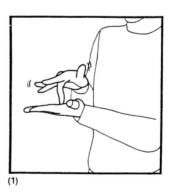
(1)

MEDICAL PRACTICE

A business having to do with medicine or caring for the sick or injured.

Medical practice is when a doctor uses his knowledge and skills to diagnose, treat or prevent illness.

(1) Sign MEDICINE — the left "flat" hand faces up at chest level. The middle finger of the right "eight" hand touches the left palm and pivots slightly from left to right a few times. (MM)

(Continued on next page)

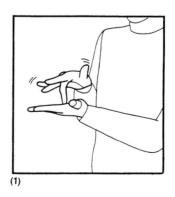
(1)

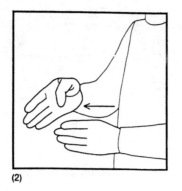
(2)

(2) Sign SPECIALIZE — the left "B" hand faces right at chest level. The right "B" hand faces left on top of the left hand. Move the right hand straight out on the left index finger. (SM)

MEDIC ALERT

An organization that makes an informational bracelet to be worn by a person with different medical conditions such as disease, allergy to penicillin, diabetes, contact lenses or a person who wishes to donate an organ after death.

A Medic Alert bracelet can be gotten by writing to Medic Alert, Turlock, California.

MEDICATION

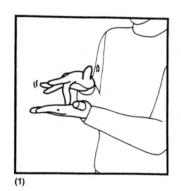
(1)

The use of a medicine to treat a problem.

A person can be given a medication by injecting, inhaling, or eating it, or by putting it on the skin.

(1) Sign MEDICINE — the left "flat" hand faces up at chest level. The middle finger of the right "eight" hand touches the left palm and pivots slightly from left to right a few times. (MM)

MEDICINE

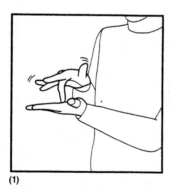
(1)

A drug or chemical used to treat or help cure disease or injury; also the science of preventing, diagnosing and treating diseases or injuries.

Before a medicine can be used to treat an injury or illness, it must be tested to be sure it's safe and must be approved by the Food and Drug Administration.

(1) The left "flat" hand faces up at chest level. The middle finger of the right "eight" hand touches the left palm and pivots slightly from left to right a few times. (MM)

MEDULLA OBLONGATA

The upper, enlarged part of the spinal cord inside the skull at the base of the brain. The medulla oblongata controls heart rate, blood pressure, respiration, coughing and vomiting.

See Figure 17 or 18

MELANIN

A dark brown or black substance made by skin and hair cells that gives us our skin and hair color. The amount of melanin made will determine whether we have light or dark colored skin or hair.

When we get a sun tan, the cells in the skin make more melanin to protect us from the sun's harmful rays, causing our skin to become darker.

MEMBRANE

A thin, soft, flexible layer of tissue in the body that lines a tube or space, covers an organ or separates areas or structures. Some of the functions of membranes are making and putting out substances like mucus, keeping a part from drying out, preventing friction between two things and acting to keep harmful things out of the body like bacteria.

Membranes that are exposed to the outside, like those in the nose, throat, lungs and eyes, all produce mucus to keep them from drying out and to trap bacteria or dust.

MEMORY

The ability to retain and recall past experiences.

An injury to the head (concussion), senility or alcoholism can cause a loss of memory.

(1) Sign REMEMBER — the left "A" hand faces right at chest level. The thumb of the right "A" hand touches the forehead then moves down to touch the thumb of the left hand. (SM)

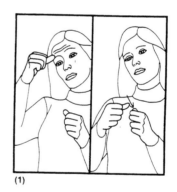
(1)

MENARCHE

The time when menstruation first occurs in a young woman.

Menarche almost always occurs between 10 and 17 years of age.

(1) Sign FIRST — the index finger of the right "one" hand flicks off the thumb of the left "A" hand. (SM)
(2) Sign MENSTRUATION — the right "A" hand taps the right cheek a few times. (MM)

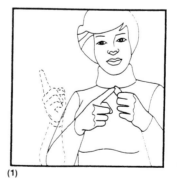
(1)

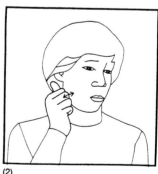
(2)

MENINGES

The three membranes that cover the brain and spinal cord, providing protection and nutrients. The three meninges are called the pia mater, arachnoid and dura mater. *See Figure 18*

MENINGITIS

Inflammation of the meninges which cover the spinal cord and brain, usually caused by bacteria or viruses from other parts of the body being carried to the meninges by the blood stream. Symptoms of meningitis are a fever, severe headache, inability to stand loud sounds and light, pain and stiffness in the back or neck, delirium, convulsions and coma. Meningitis is also called "brain fever".

Meningitis can be caused by an infection like a boil on the face or an ear infection travelling to the linings of the brain.

MENOPAUSE

The permanent stopping of menstruation, usually between 45 and 50 years of age. After menopause, a woman may have sudden feelings of being hot or cold (hot and cold flashes), weakness and depression. Menopause is also called the change of life or climacteric.

During menopause, the menstrual flow may stop suddenly, there may be a lowering of the amount of menstrual flow each month, or the length of time between periods may get longer and longer until it finally stops.

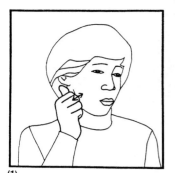
(1)
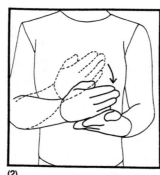
(2)

(1) Sign MENSTRUATION — the right "A" hand taps the right cheek a few times. (MM)
(2) Sign STOP — the left "flat" hand faces up at chest level. The right "flat" hand faces left and moves down to sharply hit the left palm. (SM)

MENSTRUAL CYCLE

The changes that regularly occur in a woman's uterus, ovaries and vagina that prepare her body for pregnancy. The average length of the menstrual cycle is 28 days with day number one being the first day of menstrual flow and the last day being the day before the next menstrual flow. The menstrual cycle involves a build-up of the inner lining of the uterus, the release of an ovum from an ovary and, if the egg isn't fertilized, the shedding of the lining (the blood, mucus and cell-containing flow that comes out).

The activities of the menstrual cycle are controlled by hormones from the pituitary gland of the brain and the ovaries.

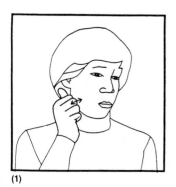
(1)
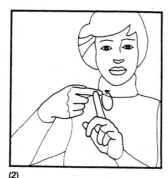
(2)

(1) Sign MENSTRUATION — the right "A" hand taps the right cheek a few times. (MM)
(2) Sign MONTHLY — the left "one" hand points up at chest level, the palm facing out. The index finger of the right "one" hand brushes the back of the left index finger in a circular movement several times. (MM)

MENSTRUATION

The regular discharge of blood, mucus and cells from the uterus through the vagina. Menstruation occurs about every four weeks and lasts about five days. Menstruation gets rid of the unused lining of the uterus when an egg hasn't been fertilized. Afterwards, the lining is built back up and prepared to receive and nourish a fertilized egg.

Menstruation usually starts between 10 and 17 years of age and stops between 45 and 50 years of age.

(1) The right "A" hand taps the right cheek a few times. (MM)

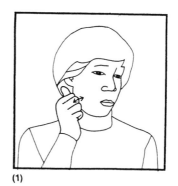

(1)

MENTAL

Referring to the mind.

A mental disorder is a disease of the mind.

(1) Sign MIND — the index finger of the right "one" hand touches the forehead. (SM)

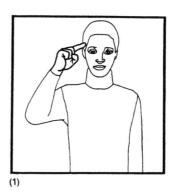

(1)

MENTAL DISEASE

A disorder or problem with the mind.

New drugs and therapy may help some people with mental disease.

(1) Sign MIND — the index finger of the right "one" hand touches the forehead. (SM)
(2) Sign DISEASE — the middle finger of the right "eight" hand taps the forehead and the middle finger of the left "one" hand taps the stomach. (MM)

* The facial expression should reflect sickness.

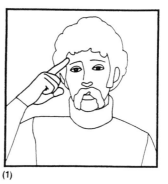 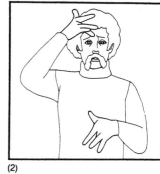

(1)   (2)

MENTAL RETARDATION

Less than normal or slower than normal development of intelligence; also called mental deficiency. People who are mentally retarded may not learn things as quickly.

With special training, patience and understanding, people with mental retardation can be taught skills and how to take care of themselves.

(1) The right "M" hand touches the forehead then changes to a "R" hand. (SM)

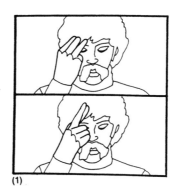

(1)

MEPERIDINE

A man-made narcotic drug used to relieve pain and calm someone. Meperidine is sold under the name of Demerol® .

If meperidine is used for a long time, it can cause addiction.

MEPROBAMATE

A certain drug which acts as a tranquilizer to calm a person and lessen stress or excitement. Meprobamate is also called Miltown or Equanil.

Meprobamate can cause addiction and even poisoning with symptoms of drowsiness, severe hypotension (abnormally low blood pressure), defect of the muscles, or coma.

MESCALINE

A certain drug that causes hallucinations, mood changes and abnormal behavior; also called "peyote".

Mescaline is the poisonous substance which comes from the mescal cactus.

METABOLISM

All of the physical and chemical activities that go on in a living thing. Metabolism involves the use of foods, the production of energy, the building of new body parts and the breaking down of old body parts.

The liver is an organ that is very active in body metabolism so if the liver is diseased, a person may be very sick.

METACARPUS

The part of the hand between the fingers and wrist; the palm. The metacarpus contains five bones called metacarpals. *See Figure 26*

METASTASIZE

The moving of a disease from one part of the body to another. Metastasize is usually used for the spread of cancer cells from one area to another through the lymph system or blood stream.

The reason it is very important to discover and treat cancer early is to get it out of the body before it can metastasize and affect other parts of the body.

(Continued on next page)

(1) Sign BODY — the fingers of both "flat" hand touch the chest then the stomach. (SM)

(2) Sign DISEASE — the middle finger of the right "eight" hand touches the forehead and the middle finger of the left "eight" hand touches the stomach. (SM)

* *The facial expression should reflect sickness.*

(3) The fingertips of both "flat-O" hands touch the body several times. (MM)

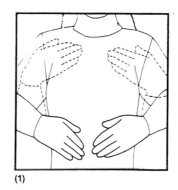

(1)

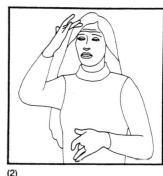

(2)

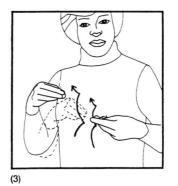

(3)

METATARSUS

The part of the foot between the ankle and the toes. *See Figure 26*

METHADONE

A man-made drug which prevents pain and is like morphine. Methadone is not as strong a narcotic as morphine but it can still cause addiction. Methadone is sold under the name of Dolophine® .

> *Methadone is sometimes given to people who are addicted to heroin or morphine to get them off of the more dangerous drugs and to make withdrawal easier.*

METHAMPHETAMINE

A certain drug which acts as a stimulant and keeps a person alert; also called methedrine. Other names for methamphetamine are meth, speed and crystal.

> *Because methamphetamine lessens a person's appetite, makes a person more active and reduces depression, it may be used to treat overweight people, narcolepsy and depression.*

(1) Sign PILL — the thumb and index finger of the right hand touch, the palm faces in. Flick the index finger towards the mouth as if popping a pill into the mouth. (SM)

(Continued on next page)

367

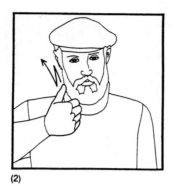

(2)

METHAMPHETAMINE, *continued*

(2) Sign UPPER — the right "A" hand with the thumb extended faces in at shoulder level and moves up twice. (DM)

* *This is a general sign for stimulants ("uppers"). The specific type of drug should also be fingerspelled and all side effects explained.*

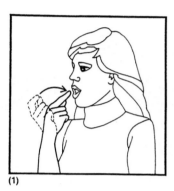

(1)

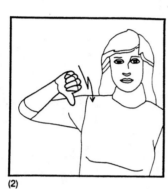

(2)

METHAQUALONE

A certain drug which acts as a sedative and is used to help a person sleep or relax; sold under the name of Quaaludde .

Someone who has been taking **methaqualone** *for a long time can become addicted to it and if they suddenly stop taking it, they may have withdrawal symptoms like nervousness, nausea, shaking, confusion, weakness and perhaps convulsions.*

(1) Sign PILL — the thumb and index finger of the right hand touch, the palm faces in. Flick the index finger towards the mouth as if popping a pill into the mouth. (SM)

(2) Sign DOWNER — the right "A" hand with the thumb extended faces out at shoulder level and moves down twice. (DM)

* *This is a general sign for depressants ("downers"). The specific type of drug should also be fingerspelled and all side effects explained.*

METHEDRINE

See METHAMPHETAMINE

METHYLPHENIDATE

A drug which acts as a stimulant and keeps a person alert; sold under the name of Ritalin® . It is often used to treat depression and narcolepsy.

If used for long periods of time, **methylphenidate** *can cause addiction and mental problems.*

METRONIDAZOLE

See FLAGYL

MICROBIOLOGY

The study of living things that are so small that special instruments like microscopes have to be used to see them.

Bacteria, viruses, fungi and very small parasites are studied in microbiology.

(1) Sign BIOLOGY — both "B" hands face out and move in alternating circular movements a few times. (MM)
(2) The right "O" hand faces in on top of the left "O" hand which also faces in. Twist the right hand a few times as if imitating looking through a microscope. (MM)
(3) Sign ANALYZE — both "bent-V" hands face down at chest level. Drop both hands slightly at the wrists a few times and at the same time, move the hands down to waist level. (MM)

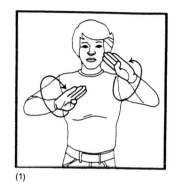

(1)

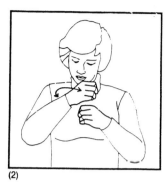

(2)

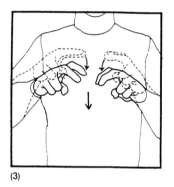

(3)

MICROORGANISM

A very tiny living thing which can't be seen with the eye alone. A microscope or other instrument which magnifies things must be used to see a microorganism. Microorganisms can be made up of just one cell.

Bacteria, fungi and some very small parasites are all microorganisms.

MICROSCOPE

An instrument which makes very small things appear large enough to be seen. A microscope is used to clearly see objects or structures that can't be seen with the eyes alone. Different kinds of microscopes work in different ways.

The most common kind of microscope has several lenses in it which bend light rays coming from the object being looked at in such a way that it looks larger.

(1) The right "O" hand faces in on top of the left "O" hand which also faces in. Twist the right hand a few times as if imitating looking through a microscope. (MM)

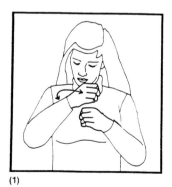

(1)

369

MILD

Slight, not severe or not harmful.

When a person is bitten by a mosquito and a bump forms which itches, the person is having a mild reaction to the substance the mosquito injected into him.

(1) Sign LITTLE BIT — the right "A" hand faces left at chest level. Flick the thumb up a few times. (MM)

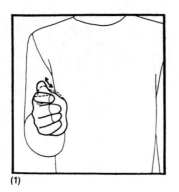
(1)

MIDDLE EAR

The part of the ear which goes from the eardrum to the inner ear. The middle ear has the eustachian tube opening into it and it also holds the malleus, incus and stapes. These three tiny bones, which are connected together, turn sound waves hitting the eardrum into movement which is passed on to the inner ear. *See Figure 20*

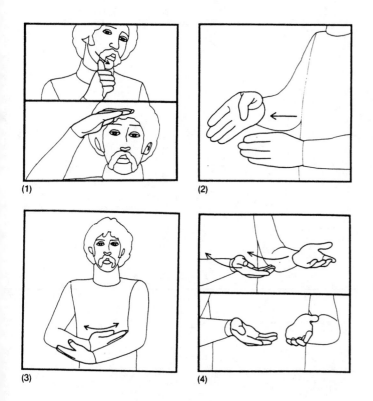
(1)   (2)

(3)   (4)

MIDWIFE

A woman who helps other women during labor.

Although a midwife is not a doctor, she has special training and is experienced in the art of helping a woman have a baby.

(1) Sign WOMAN — the thumb of the right "A" hand moves down the right cheek then to a "flat" hand facing down at the forehead. (SM)
(2) Sign SPECIALIZE — the left "B" hand faces right at chest level. The right "B" hand faces left on top of the left hand. Move the right hand straight out on the left index finger. (SM)
(3) Sign BABY — the right hand and forearm face up, resting on the left hand and forearm which also face upwards. Both are then rocked back and forth as if holding a baby. (MM)
(4) Both "flat" hands face up at the left chest level. Move both hands in towards the body. (SM)

MIGRAINE

A very severe throbbing headache which affects a person from time to time. The headache will usually be on one side of the head and the person may also have vision problems, unable to stand light, have an upset stomach and be sweating.

The exact cause of **migraines** *is unknown but they may be caused by blood vessels in the head suddenly expanding.*

(1) Sign PAIN — both "one" hands point to each other at the forehead and twist in opposite directions a few times. (MM)
* *The facial expression should reflect pain.*

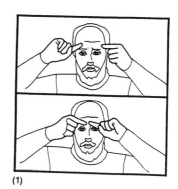
(1)

MINERAL

An inorganic substance found in nature. Minerals help to make up the hard parts of the body like the bones and teeth and they are also needed for many important body activities. Minerals are important in transporting things through the body, they are important parts of some enzymes, they allow muscles to contract, they allow nerves to pass on electrical impulses and they help keep the right amounts of water in different parts of the body. The important minerals found in the body are calcium, phosphorus, sodium, potassium, chlorine, magnesium, sulfur, iron, iodine and copper.

Minerals themselves don't supply energy but they are needed in certain amounts for a person to be healthy and for the body to work normally.

MINIMUM

The least or lowest amount.

Minimum lethal dose is the smallest amount of a substance that can cause death.

(1) Both "flat" hands face down at chest level. Move the right hand up to shoulder level. (SM)

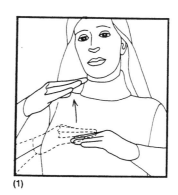
(1)

MISCARRIAGE

An occurrence during pregnancy in which the fetus is released from the uterus before it is able to live outside the mother, resulting in its death. A miscarriage is also called an accidental abortion.

(Continued on next page)

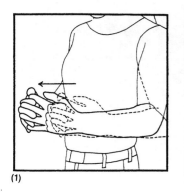
(1)

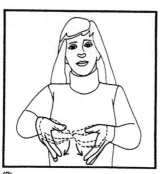
(2)

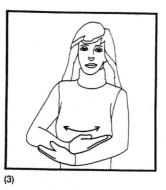
(3)

MISCARRIAGE, *continued*

In the early months of pregnancy, a miscarriage can happen without a woman's knowledge.

(1) Sign PREGNANT — both "five" hands face in and mesh together at stomach level. Move both hands out slightly. (SM)

(2) Sign LOST — the fingertips of both "flat-O" hands touch at chest level. Drop both hands open. (SM)

(3) Sign BABY — the right hand and forearm face up, resting on the left hand and forearm which also face upwards. Both are then rocked back and forth as if holding a baby. (MM)

MOLAR

The twelve largest teeth in an adult human mouth. Located in the back of the mouth, the molars are used for grinding and crushing food. The very last molars to appear are called wisdom teeth; not everyone gets them. *See Figure 24*

MOLE

A small tan, red, brown or black growth on the skin.
Most moles are caused by a collection of blood vessels or the collection of melanin.

(1) Sign DARK — both "flat" hands face in at the eyes. Drop both hands down slightly. (SM)

(2) The right "F" hand faces out on the right cheek. (SM)

* This could be signed at the area of the mole.

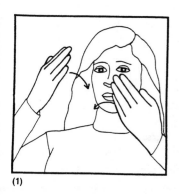
(1)

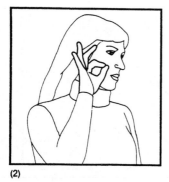
(2)

MONGOLISM

See DOWN'S SYNDROME

MONILIASIS

See CANDIDIASIS

MONONUCLEOSIS
See INFECTIOUS MONONUCLEOSIS

MOOD
An attitude or state of mind which is seen in one's thoughts and the things one does.

Depression can now be treated by doctors with mood changing drugs.

(1) Sign FEEL — the middle finger of the right "eight" hand moves up and down on the chest a few times. (MM)

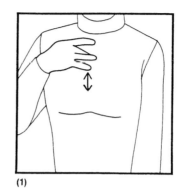

(1)

MORGUE
A place where dead bodies are kept until they are identified or buried.

Most large hospitals have a morgue in one of the lower floors.

(1) Both "flat" hands face each other at chest level. Move both hands to the center, both hands facing in, the right hand in front of the left hand. (SM)
(2) Sign DEAD — the left "flat" hand faces up at chest level and the right "flat" hand faces down at chest level. Turn both hands over so that the left hand ends facing down and the right hand ends facing up. (SM)
(3) Sign BODY — the fingers of both "flat" hands touch the chest and then the stomach. (SM)
(4) The left "C" hand faces out at chest level. The right "flat-O" hand moves into the left fist a few times. (MM)

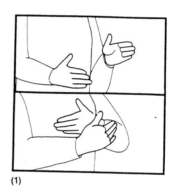

(1)

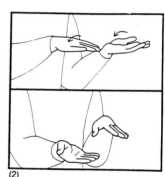

(2)

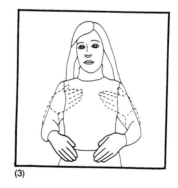

(3)

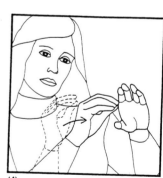

(4)

MORNING GLORY SEEDS
The seeds of the morning glory plant (Ipomoea).

When eaten, morning glory seeds can cause hallucinations and abnormal behavior.

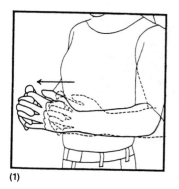
(1)

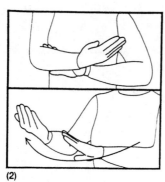
(2)

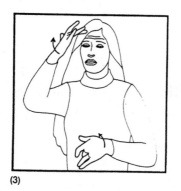
(3)

MORNING SICKNESS

The upset stomach and vomiting some women have during the first few months of pregnancy just after getting up in the morning. Continued vomiting during the day can be dangerous and a doctor should be seen.

Morning sickness, which affects about half of all pregnant women, usually stops around the third month of pregnancy.

(1) Sign PREGNANT — both "five" hands face in and mesh together at stomach level. Move both hands out slightly. (SM)
(2) Sign MORNING — the left "flat" hand faces down and touches the right inside elbow. The right "flat" hand faces up pointing to the left side. Move the right hand from the left to the right side, keeping the left hand in place. (SM)

(3) Sign SICK — the middle finger of the right "eight" hand touches the forehead and the middle finger of the left "eight" hand touches the stomach. Twist both hands slightly. (MM)

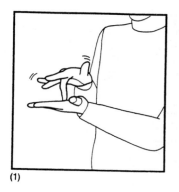
(1)

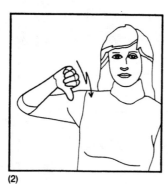
(2)

MORPHINE

A bitter-tasting, colorless narcotic drug made from opium which is used as a pain-killer and sedative. Morphine is like heroin and if used regularly, can cause addiction.

Symptoms of morphine poisoning include periods of excitement before drowsiness, nausea, vomiting, tiny pupils, relaxing of muscles, slow breathing, slow pulse, cyanosis (blue or purple discoloration of skin), coma, a fall in blood pressure, and respiratory failure causing death.

(1) Sign MEDICINE — the left "flat" hand faces up at chest level. The middle finger of the right "eight" hand touches the left palm and pivots slightly from left to right a few times. (MM)
(2) Sign DOWNER — the right "A" hand with the thumb extended faces out at shoulder level and moves down twice. (DM)
* Fingerspell "M-O-R-P-H-I-N-E" to clarify.

MORTALITY

The number of deaths; death rate.

The mortality rate in newborns is decreasing because of better medical techniques and educating the mother how to take care of herself.

(Continued on next page)

(1) Sign DEAD — the left "flat" hand faces up at chest level and the right "flat" hand faces down at chest level. Turn both hands over so that the left hand ends facing down and the right hand ends facing up. (SM)

(2) Sign HOW MANY — both "S" hands face up at chest level. Move both hands up to "five" hands. (SM)

* The facial expression should reflect questioning.

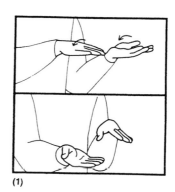
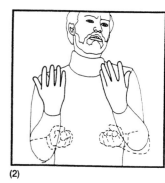

(1) (2)

MORTICIAN

A person who takes care of dead bodies and arranges funerals, burials and cremations; also called "undertaker" or "funeral director".

Morticians are specially trained to prepare bodies for burial.

(1) Sign FUNERAL — both "V" hands face out at chest level and move forward in a wavy movement. (MM)

(2) Sign CONTROL — both "modified-A" hands face each other at chest level. Move both hands alternately in and out from the body a few times. (MM)

(3) Sign PERSON — both "flat" hands face each other at chest level and move down to waist level. (SM)

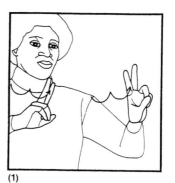
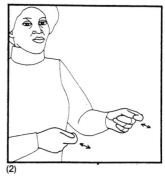

(1) (2)

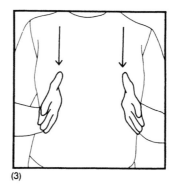

(3)

MOTHER

A female parent or a woman who has had a child, adopted or otherwise established a maternal relationship with another person.

Half of the chromosomes which direct a person's development come from the mother.

(1) The thumb of the right "five" hand taps the chin a few times. (MM)

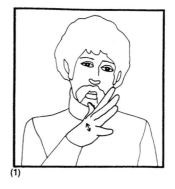

(1)

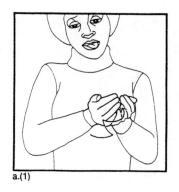
a.(1)

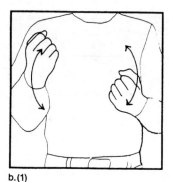
b.(1)

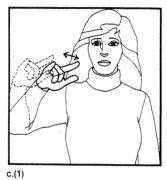
c.(1)

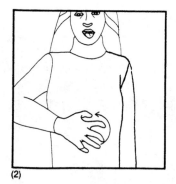
(2)

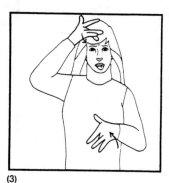
(3)

MOTION SICKNESS

Nausea, vomiting or dizziness caused by movement. Examples of motion sickness are sea sickness, car sickness and air sickness.

Motion sickness is caused by irritation of the semicircular canals in the inner ear which sense movement of the body.

a. (1) Sign BOAT — both "cupped" hands are together at chest level and face up. Move both hands forward in a wavy movement indicating waves. (MM)

b. (1) Sign CAR — both "S" hands face each other at chest level and move as if imitating driving a steering wheel. (MM)

c. (1) Sign AIRPLANE — the right "Y" hand faces down and moves slightly in and out a few times. (MM)

(2) The right "claw" hand faces in on the stomach. Move the hand in a circular movement. (MM)

* *The facial expression should reflect sickness.*

(3) Sign SICK — the middle finger of the right "eight" hand touches the forehead and the middle finger of the left "eight" hand touches the stomach. Twist both hands slightly. (SM)

* *Choose the appropriate sign BOAT, CAR, or AIRPLANE, whichever applies then sign (2) and (3).*

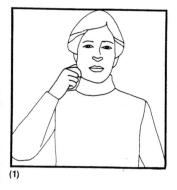
(1)

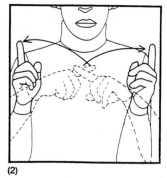
(2)

MOTTLED

A part of the body being covered with spots or places with a color different than the area around it.

When a person has a rash, the skin is mottled red.

(1) Sign SKIN — the index finger and thumb of the right hand grab the right cheek. (SM)
(2) Sign DIFFERENT — both "one" hands face out at chest level, crossing. Move both hands out to the sides. (SM)

(Continued on next page)

MOTTLED, *continued*

(3) Sign COLOR — the right "five" hand faces in at the chin and the fingers wiggle. (MM)
(4) The right "C" hand faces out at the area of the mottled skin. (SM)

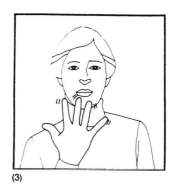
(3)

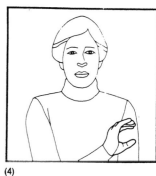
(4)

MOUTH

The opening in the face which contains the teeth and tongue and which leads to the throat.
See Figure 1

(1) The index finger of the right "one" hand circles around the mouth. (SM)

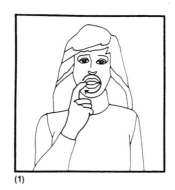
(1)

MOUTH-TO-MOUTH RESUSCITATION

A way to get air to the lungs of a person who has stopped breathing; a form of artificial respiration. The person giving mouth-to-mouth resuscitation forces air from his lungs into the mouth and lungs of the person who has stopped breathing.

Mouth-to-mouth resuscitation may have to be given to someone who has drowned, been electrocuted, poisoned or had a drug overdose.

(1) The right "H" hand faces up in the palm of the left "flat" hand. (SM)
(2) The index finger of the right "one" hand circles around the mouth. (SM)
(3) Both "C" hands face down and the mouth imitates blowing into something. (MM)

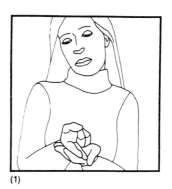
(1)

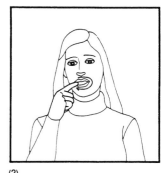
(2)

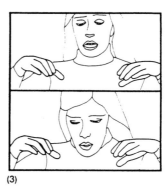
(3)

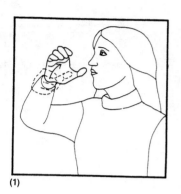
(1)

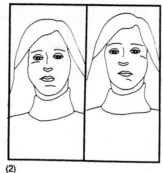
(2)

MOUTHWASH

A liquid, usually flavored, used to clean a person's mouth, to make the breath smell fresh and to destroy germs or bacteria.

A mouthwash will not prevent colds, cavities or gum disease.

(1) Sign DRINK — the right "C" hand moves towards the mouth as if imitating taking a drink. (SM)
(2) Imitate gargling with the cheeks. (MM)

MUCUS

A thick fluid made by certain glands and membranes and used to protect certain parts of the body and keep areas moist and flexible. Mucus can vary in thickness from watery to very thick and stringy.

The salivary glands in the mouth make mucus which is mixed with food as we chew to moisten it and allow it to slip easily down the esophagus when we swallow.

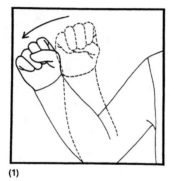
(1)

MULTIPLE SCLEROSIS

A disease of the nervous system which slowly affects a person by causing scars to form on the nerves of the brain and spinal cord; commonly called MS. Multiple Sclerosis usually affects young adults; its symptoms include double vision, slow, difficult speech, and weakness and trembling when trying to do something. The cause of the disease is unknown.

Although Multiple Sclerosis occassionally disappears for no known reason, it more often suddenly becomes much worse.

(1) Fingerspell "M-S".
* *This may need further explanation before signing.*

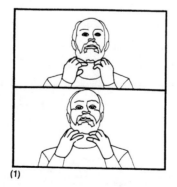
(1)

MUMPS

An infectious disease caused by a virus which causes inflammaiton of the salivary glands. Symptoms of mumps are headache, a fever, pain when moving the jaws and swelling in the salivary glands below and in front of the ears.

Mumps may spread to the ovaries and testes and cause inflammation which may lead to sterility.

(1) Both "claw" hands are at the sides of the neck. Open both hands slightly and at the same time, the cheeks should puff out. (SM)

MURMUR

In medicine, an abnormal, soft blowing sound which may be heard when listening to the heart or the large blood vessels around it, caused by movements of the blood through the heart and large blood vessels. Murmurs may be caused by a valve in the heart not working correctly, an abnormal narrowing or enlargement of one of the vessels near the heart, or openings in the heart where they shouldn't be.

Different kinds of murmurs make their own sounds and can tell a doctor of any problems or abnormalities.

MUSCLE

A type of tissue made up of special cells which can contract and cause movement of an organ or a part of the body. Different types of muscles do different kinds of work. A few of the places muscles are found are the walls of blood vessels, the walls of structures or passages that must change size like the bladder or stomach, the walls of the intestine, the heart, and attached to the skeleton to move the body.

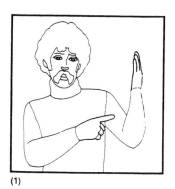

(1)

(1) The index finger of the right "one" hand touches the left upper arm. (SM)

MUSCLE STRAIN

Severe pain caused by working a muscle too hard.

Heavy objects must be lifted in the right way because it is easy to get muscle strain in the lower back muscles.

(1) The index finger of the right "one" hand touches the left upper arm. (SM)
(2) Sign PAIN — both "one" hands point to each other and twist in opposite directions a few times. (MM)

* *The facial expression should reflect pain.*

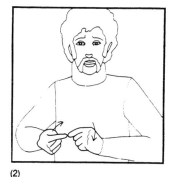

(1)　　　　　　　　(2)

MUSCULAR DYSTROPHY

A hereditary disease that causes the muscles to become wasted away and lose their strength. The disease, which affects males more often than females, usually starts at an early age. Along with damage to the muscles, there is usually deformation of the body, infections of the airways and heart failure.

The cause of Muscular dystrophy·is thought to be a mistake in the way muscles use nutrients; there is no cure.

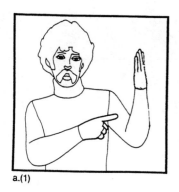
a.(1)

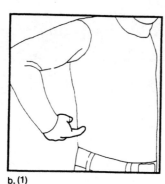
b.(1)

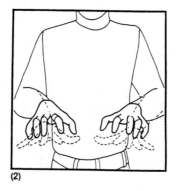
(2)

MUSCULAR PARALYSIS

Loss of a muscle's ability to contract, causing a person or a part to be unable to move.

Muscular paralysis can be caused by a problem in the way a muscle is working, by a problem in the nerve controlling the muscle's movement or a problem in the brain or spinal cord.

a. (1) The index finger of the right "one" hand touches the left upper arm. (SM)

b. (1) The index finger of the right "one" hand points to the back. (SM)

* These are just examples, the right index finger should point to the area affected.

(2) Sign FREEZE — both "five" hands face down at chest level. Move both hands up slightly into "claw" hands. (SM)

MUSCLE SYSTEM

The total muscle tissue in the body that moves bones of the skeleton or holds them in a certain position. The muscle system also helps to give shape to the body. *See Figure 4 or 5*

MUSLIN BINDER

A broad bandage used to go around someone's abdomen or chest to give support or to cover a large wound. A muslin binder is usually of sturdy cotton cloth but can be any other large, clean piece of material.

When a muslin binder is put around the chest, it should not be so tight that it makes breathing difficult.

(1) Sign BODY — the fingers of both "flat" hands touch the chest and then the stomach. (SM)

(2) Sign BANDAGE — the left "B" hand faces in at chest level. The right "B" hand moves around the left hand as if imitating wrapping a bandage. (MM)

(3) The right "flat" hand faces down at shoulder level and the left "flat" hand faces up at stomach level. (SM)

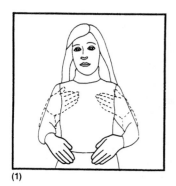
(1)

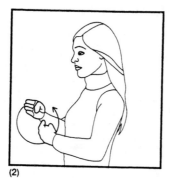
(2)

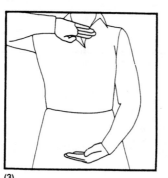
(3)

MUTATION

A change; also any inherited change of genes or chromosomes in a person or animal.

Mutations can occur due to exposure to radioactive substances, or naturally, such as in animals who have changed with the environment.

MUTE

Not able to speak.

Some severe forms of mental disorders can cause a person to become mute.

(1) Sign CAN'T — the left "one" hand faces down at chest level. The right "one" hand moves down to strike the left index finger. (SM)
(2) Sign TALK — the index finger of the right "one" hand touches the mouth then moves out from the mouth in small repeated circular movements. (MM)

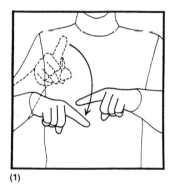
(1)

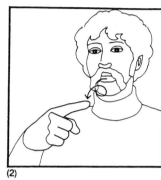
(2)

MYOCARDIAL INFARCTION

The dying of a part of the heart muscle because the blood flow through an artery bringing fresh blood to the heart is decreased or stopped; commonly called heart attack. The person will have a severe squeezing pain in the chest, irregular heartbeats, may go into shock and the heart may stop beating.

A person who may have a myocardial infarction should be taken to a hospital as quickly as possible because a dead area in the heart may cause the heart to suddenly quit beating.

(1) Sign HEART — the middle finger of the right "eight" hand taps the chest a few times.
(2) Sign ATTACK — the left "flat" hand faces right at chest level. The right "S" hand moves down to sharply hit the left palm. (SM)

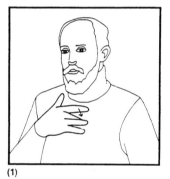
(1)

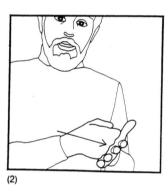
(2)

MYOCARDIUM

The muscular middle layer of the heart that makes up most of the heart. It contracts and pumps the blood through the body. There are several layers in the heart wall. The inside layer is the endocardium, just a thin membrane; then there is the myocardium, the thick muscular layer; and covering the outside of the heart is the epicardium, also a thin membrane. *See Figure 16*

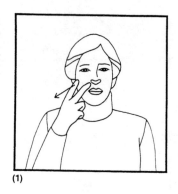
(1)

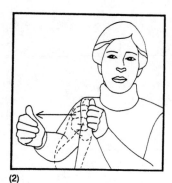
(2)

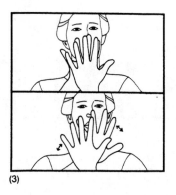
(3)

MYOPIA

The vision abnormality in which close things are seen clearly while things at a distance are blurred; also called nearsightedness.

Myopia is caused by the eye being too long and the light rays not being focused on the retina, resulting in what we see being out of focus.

(1) Sign SEE — the right "V" hand faces in and moves out from the eyes. (SM)
(2) Sign FAR — both "A" hands are together at chest level. Move the right hand out forward. (SM)
(3) Both "five" hands are together at eye level, the right hand behind the left. Move both hands alternately from left to right a few times. (MM)

382

n

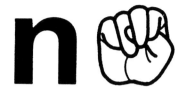

NAIL

The hard, flat structures on top of the ends of the fingers and toes made by special cells in the skin (at the root of the nail).

Because growth and shape of the nails are affected by disease and nutrition as well as age and season, a doctor will often check them when doing an examination.

(1) The right index finger taps the left thumbnail. (SM)

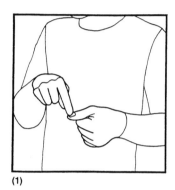

NAPE

The back of the neck. *See Figure 3*

(1) The index finger of the right "one" hand moves down the back of the neck. (SM)

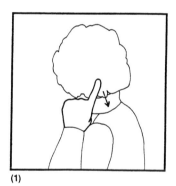

NARCISSISM

The mental condition of being abnormally in love with oneself.

A person with narcissism will get sexual pleasure from looking at his or her own body.

NARCOLEPSY

A problem in which a person has sudden uncontrollable attacks of tiredness and sleep. A person with narcolepsy will fall asleep suddenly during the day, even in the middle of some activity.

The cause of narcolepsy is not known but it can be treated with stimulants like amphetamines.

(Continued on next page)

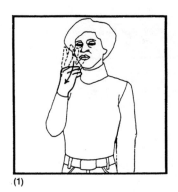

(1)

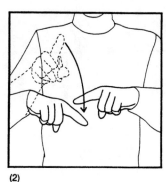

(2)

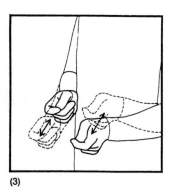

(3)

NARCOLEPSY, *continued*

(1) Sign SLEEP — the right "five" hand faces in at face level. Move the hand down slightly into a "flat-O" hand. At the same time, the eyes should close. (SM)

(2) Sign CAN'T — the left "one" hand faces down with the index finger pointing out. The index finger of the right "one" hand strikes down the left index finger. (SM)

(3) Sign CONTROL — both "modified-A" hands face each other and move alternately forward and back a few times at chest level. (MM)

NARCOTICS

A group of drugs which calm a person, relieve pain and cause sleep by lowering the activity of the nervous system. Examples of narcotics are opium, heroin, morphine, cocaine, paregoric, dilaudid, meperidine (Demerol), and methadone (Dolophine).

Narcotics should be used carefully because most can cause addiction if they are used for a long time.

NASAL

Referring to the nose.

Nasal sinuses are the spaces in the bones of the skull around the nose.

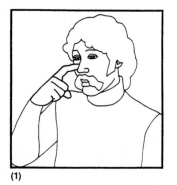

(1)

(1) The index finger of the right "one" hand taps the nose. (SM)

NATURAL

Not artificial or man-made. In medicine, natural can be used to mean normal.

By brushing the teeth regularly, using dental floss, not eating a lot of sweets, eating well balanced meals and going to the dentist regularly, we can keep our natural teeth for our entire lives, instead of having them replaced with dentures.

(Continued on next page)

(1) The left "S" hand faces down at chest level. The right "N" hand makes a small counterclockwise circle above the left hand then touches the back of the left hand. (SM)

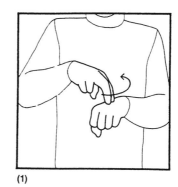

(1)

NATURAL CHILDBIRTH

Delivery of a baby without using drugs or surgical procedures.

Natural childbirth involves education, training and mental preparation of the mother for the baby's birth.

(1) Sign NATURAL — the left "S" hand faces down at chest level. The right "N" hand makes a small counterclockwise circle above the left hand then touches the back of the left hand. (SM)

(2) Sign BABY — the right hand and forearm face up, resting on the left hand and forearm which also face upwards. Both are then rocked back and forth a few times as if holding a baby. (MM)

(3) Sign DELIVER — both "five" hands face up at left chest level. Move both hands in towards the body. (SM)

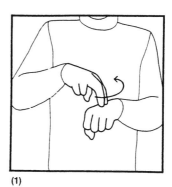

(1)

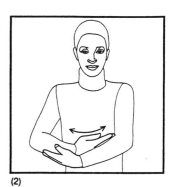

(2)

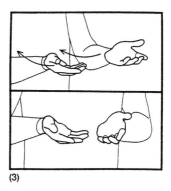

(3)

NATUROPATHY

A system which treats problems or diseases using natural procedures or remedies instead of drugs.

Some of the things that may be used in naturopathy to treat disease are sunlight, water, heat, massage, diet and herbs.

(1) Sign SPECIALIZE — the left "B" hand faces right at chest level. The right "B" hand faces left on top of the left hand. Move the right hand straight out on the left index finger. (SM)

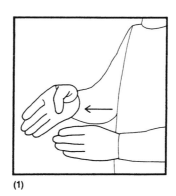

(1)

(Continued on next page)

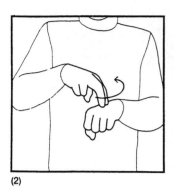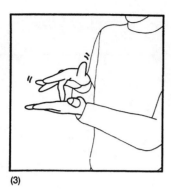

(2)   (3)

(2) Sign NATURAL — the left "S" hand faces down at chest level. The right "N" hand makes a small counterclockwise circle above the left hand then moves down to touch the back of the left hand. (SM)

(3) Sign MEDICINE — the left "flat" hand faces up at chest level. The middle finger of the right "eight" hand touches the left palm then pivots slightly from left to right a few times. (MM)

NAUSEA

An upset stomach or a feeling of having to vomit. Some of the causes of nausea are motion sickness, pregnancy, poisoning, and intestinal infections caused by worms, bacteria, and viruses.

There are some drugs which can be taken through the mouth or injected to prevent nausea if it is severe and won't go away.

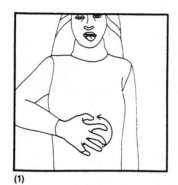

(1)

(1) The right "claw" hand faces in at the stomach and moves in a circular movement. (SM)

* *The facial expression should reflect pain or illness.*

NAVEL

The small scar in the middle of the abdomen; commonly called the belly button. The navel is where the fetus was attached by the umbilical to its mother. *See Figure 1*

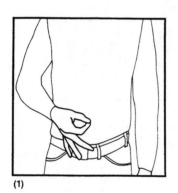

(1)

(1) The right "F" hand faces in at the navel. (SM)

NEARSIGHTEDNESS

The vision abnormality in which close things are seen clearly while things at a distance are blurred; also called "myopia".

Nearsightedness is caused by the eyeball being too long or a mistake in the way the images are focused on the retina, causing what we see to be blurred.

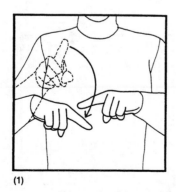

(1)

(1) Sign CAN'T — the left "one" hand faces down at chest level, pointing out. The right "one" hand faces out and moves down to strike the left index finger. (SM)

(Continued on next page)

NEARSIGHTEDNESS, *continued*

(2) Sign SEE — the right "V" hand faces in at eye level and moves out forward. (SM)

(3) Sign FAR — both "A" hands are together at chest level. Move the right hand out forward. (SM)

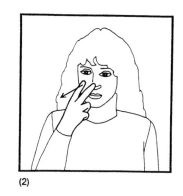
(2)

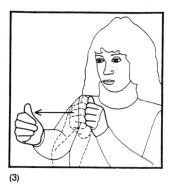
(3)

NECK

The part of the body between the head and shoulders; also the narrowed part of a structure or organ. The neck has the esophagus, trachea, vertebral column and spinal cord and large blood vessels running through it. *See Figure 2*

(1) The fingertips of the right "cupped" hand touch the top then the bottom of the neck. (SM)

* Sign this only if referring to the neck as a part of the body.

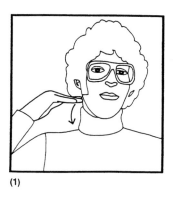
(1)

NECROSIS

The death of an area of the body. Necrosis can be caused by the blood supply to an area being stopped or slowed by damage to the arteries, by poisons from bacteria, or by chemicals destroying the tissue in an area.

> When a part of the body undergoes *necrosis,* the dead tissues must be removed before healing can occur.

(1) The right "one" hand points to the left hand. (SM)

* In this example, the hand is pointed to. You should point to the area referred to.

(2) Sign DEAD — the left "flat" hand faces up at chest level and the right "flat" hand faces down at chest level. Turn both hands over so that the left hand faces down and the right hand faces up. (SM)

(3) The left hand grabs the right wrist. Shake the right hand slightly. (MM)

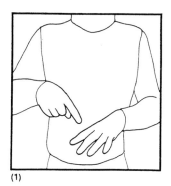
(1)

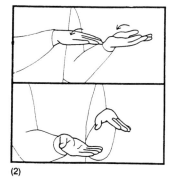
(2)

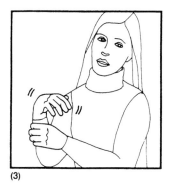
(3)

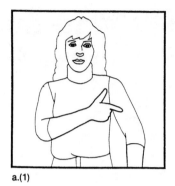
a.(1)

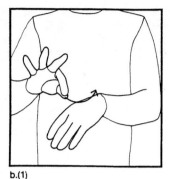
b.(1)

NEEDLE

There are two main kinds of needles used in medicine. One, the hypodermic needle, is straight, thin and hollow and is attached to a tube or syringe with a drug in it which is injected under the skin. The other, the surgical needle, is used during surgery with a special kind of thread to sew up incisions or cuts.

*The **needles** used by doctors are very sharp so they pass through the skin easily.*

a. (1) The index finger of the right "L" hand touches the left upper arm. (SM)

* Use this sign if referring to a hypodermic syringe.

b. (1) The left "flat" hand faces down at chest level. The right "F" hand imitates sewing on the back of the left hand. (SM)

* Use this sign if referring to a surgical needle for stitching.

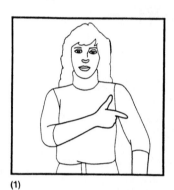
(1)

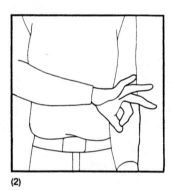
(2)

NEEDLE MARKS

The small red or blue marks that are left on the skin after a person has had an injection.

*Drug addicts will often have a series of **needle marks**, called "tracks", in the place they inject the drug.*

(1) Sign INJECTION — the index finger of the right "L" hand touches the left upper arm. (SM)

(2) The right "F" hand faces out on the left arm and touches it a few times as if imitating needle marks. (MM)

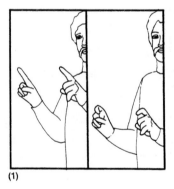
(1)

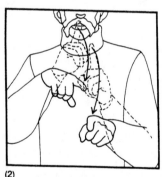
(2)

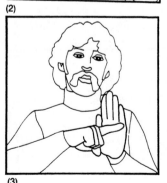
(3)

NEGATIVE

In medicine, the term used when a substance, bacteria, virus or some other thing being checked for is not found.

*If the results of a pregnancy test are **negative**, it means the woman is not pregnant or it is too soon to tell.*

(1) Sign TEST — both "one" hands face out at chest level, both pointing up. Move both hands down slightly and at the same time, bend and straighten both index fingers. Repeat this movement three times until the hands end at waist level. (MM)

(2) Sign RESULTS — both "one" hands face each other with the fingers pointing up and the right index finger touching the mouth. Drop both hands down so the palms are facing down. (SM)

(3) The left "flat" hand faces out at chest level. The index finger of the right "one" hand points to the left on the left palm, indicating the negative sign. (SM)

NEMBUTAL®

The name pentobarbital, a barbiturate, is sold under.

Nembutal is often used during labor, to control convulsions and before a person is given an anesthetic.

NEOPLASM

A new abnormal growth on the body; a tumor. A neoplasm may be benign (not cancerous) and cause no problems or it may be malignant (cancerous) and spread.

*Any **neoplasm** should be examined by a doctor to make sure it is not malignant.*

(1) The right "O" hand touches the left forearm, then opens slightly into a "claw" hand. At the same time, the cheeks should puff out. (SM)

* *This could be signed at the area of the neoplasm.*

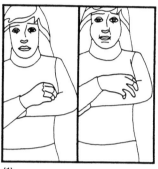

(1)

NEPHRITIS

Inflammation of the kidneys. It may be caused by a form of bacteria (streptococci), diptheria or toxic drugs such as mercury, arsenic or alcohol.

*Symptoms of **nephritis** may be fever, a dull pain in the lower back, edema, rapid pulse, vomiting and discoloration of the urine.*

NERVE

A bundle of nerve cells. Nerves contain the special kind of cell which carries small electrical messages between the brain or spinal cord and other parts of the body. In the body, a nerve looks like a white, shiny thread.

*If a **nerve** is damaged or cut, we cannot sense things or move the part which the **nerve** goes to.*

(1) Fingerspell "N-E-R-V-E".

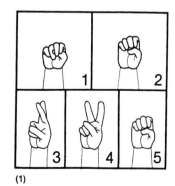

(1)

389

NERVE CELL

The special kind of cell found in the brain, spinal cor, nerves, and sensory organs (like the eyes or ears); also called a neuron. The nerve cells carry information about our environment to the brain, and then are used to carry messages from the brain to other parts of the body so we can react to our environment. The nerve cell receives information through long, thin structures called "dendrites"; these signals are processed in a small round structure called the "body"; and finally a signal is sent out on a long thin cord called the "axon". All the messages are transmitted with electrical impulses.

Nerve cells are so specialized that they don't divide or reproduce, so if they are damaged badly, they won't grow back or be replaced and paralysis may result.

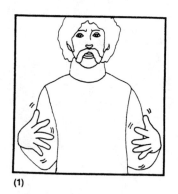

(1)

NERVOUS

The state of being very excited and unable to rest.

If a person is very nervous all the time, a doctor may prescribe Valium to calm him down, but it should be used carefully because it may cause addiction.

(1) Both "five" hands face in at the sides of the body and shake slightly. (SM)
* *The facial expression should reflect nervousness.*

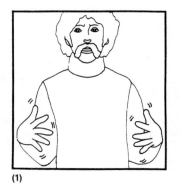

(1)

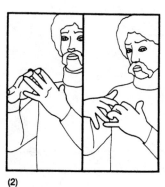

(2)

NERVOUS BREAKDOWN

A mental or emotional disorder in which the person is tired, has no energy, loses his memory and doesn't feel good about himself; nervous exhaustion.

*When someone has what is called a **nervous breakdown**, there is either a disease which needs treatment or a mental condition which needs psychiatric care.*

(1) Sign NERVOUS — both "five" hands face in at the sides of the body and shake slightly. (SM)
(2) Sign BREAKDOWN — the fingertips of both "five" hands form a peak. Drop both hands as if imitating the peak collapsing. (SM)

NERVOUS EXHAUSTION

See NERVOUS BREAKDOWN

NERVOUS SYSTEM

The system in the body made up of nerve cells, including the brain, spinal cord and all the nerves in the body. It controls the body and receives and reacts to information which comes in from a person's surroundings. The nervous system is divided into two parts, the Central Nervous System and the Peripheral Nervous System. The Central nervous system is made up of the brain and spinal cord which process information and cause action. The Peripheral nervous system consists of all the nerves and sense organs outside the Central nervous system; it connects all the parts of the body with the brain and spinal cord. *See Figure 8*

NEUROLOGIST

A doctor who specializes in treating diseases of the nerves and nervous system.

If a person shows symptoms of a nerve disorder, he should see a neurologist.

(1) Sign DOCTOR — the right "M" hand taps the left inside wrist. (DM)
(2) Sign SPECIALIZE — the left "B" hand faces right at chest level. The right "B" hand faces left on top of the left hand. Move the right hand straight out on the left index finger. (SM)
(3) Fingerspell "N-E-R-V-E".

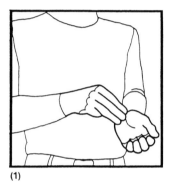
(1)

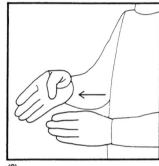
(2)

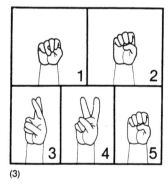
(3)

NEUROLOGY

The area of medicine which studies and treats diseases of the nerves and nervous system.

Neuritis (inflammation of a nerve) is one kind of disorder that would be studied by a doctor of neurology.

(1) Sign SPECIALIZE — the left "B" hand faces right at chest level. The right "B" hand faces left on top of the left hand. Move the right hand straight out on the left index finger. (SM)
(2) Fingerspell "N-E-R-V-E".

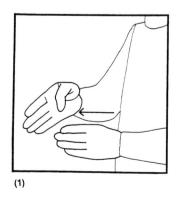
(1)

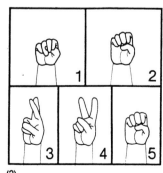
(2)

NEURON

See NERVE CELL

NEUROSIS

A mental or emotional disorder caused by stress or conflict. There are several different kinds of neurosis. Depending on the kind, the person may be tired, nervous, afraid, depressed, hysterical or very worried about his or her health. He may also have nausea, a fast heart beat, diarrhea and may shake. A person with a neurosis is said to be neurotic.

A neurosis usually affects a person's personality and is treated with therapy, tranquilizers and sedatives.

NEUROSURGERY

Surgery on the nervous system.

A neurectomy (cutting or removal of a nerve) is a form of neurosurgery.

NEUROTIC

A person with a neurosis or nervous disorder.

If a person becomes neurotic, his personality may change.

NEUTRALIZE

In medicine, to make ineffective.

In first-aid treatment for poisoning, a person should try to neutralize the poison as quickly as possible, sometimes by causing vomiting.

(1) Both "one" hands cross at chest level. (SM)
(2) Both "flat-O" hands face up at chest level. While moving the hands down sideways, brush the thumbs across the other fingers, ending in "A" hands. (SM)

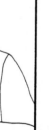

NEWBORN

A baby that has just been born.

A baby is a newborn between birth and one month of age.

(1) Sign NEW — the left "flat" hand faces up at chest level. The back of the right "flat" hand brushes up the left palm. (SM)
(2) Sign BABY — the right hand and forearm face up, resting on the left hand and forearm which also face upwards. Both are then rocked back and forth a few times as if holding a baby. (MM)

NIACIN

A vitamin found in yeast, liver, grains, green vegetables, fish and lean meats. Niacin is part of a substance which is important in cell metabolism and in preventing pellagra, a disease causing nervous system disorders, nausea, diarrhea and inflammation of the skin and mouth.

(1) Sign VITAMIN — the right "V" hand faces out at chest level and shakes slightly from left to right a few times. (MM)

(2) Fingerspell "N-I-A-C-I-N".

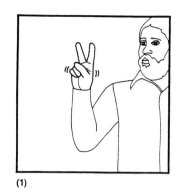

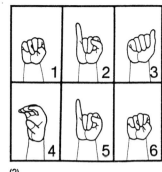

(1)   (2)

NICOTINE

A very poisonous substance found in all parts of the tobacco plant, especially the leaves. Whenever a person smokes or chews tobacco, his body absorbs some of the nicotine.

Symptoms of severe nicotine poisoning may include excitement, restlessness, confusion, weakness, nausea and vomiting, abdominal cramps and diarrhea, increased saliva, rapid and irregular pulse, and rapid breathing.

(1) Sign POISON — both "bent-V" hands face in and cross at chest level. (SM)

(2) Sign IN — the right "flat-O" hand moves into the left "O" hand. (SM)

(3) The fingertips of the right "cupped" hand touch the right cheek and pivot slightly from side to side a few times. (MM)

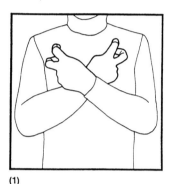

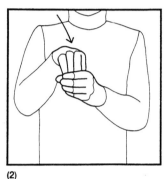

(1)   (2)

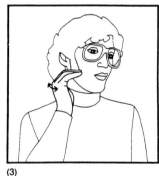
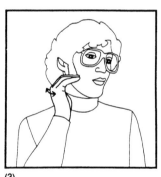

(3)

NIGHT BLINDNESS

The inability to see well or at all in the dark. Night blindness is caused by not having a certain substance in the rods in the retina of the eye or by the substance being abnormal.

Night blindness may be caused by not getting enough vitamin A, which helps make up the substance in the rods of the eyes.

(1) Sign NIGHT — the left "flat" hand faces down, the arm bent at the elbow. The heel of the right "cupped" hand touches the back of the left hand. (SM)

(2) Sign BLIND — the right "bent-V" hand faces in at eye level and moves in slightly. (SM)

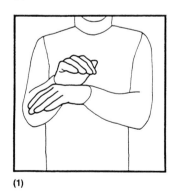

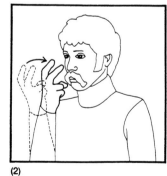

(1)   (2)

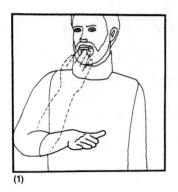

(1)

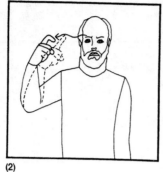

(2)

NIGHTMARE

A very unpleasant or scary dream.

During a nightmare, a person may feel like he cannot breathe.

(1) Sign BAD — the fingertips of the right "flat" hand touch the mouth. Turn the hand out then move it down, the palm ends facing down. (SM)

(2) Sign DREAM — the index finger of the right "one" hand touches the forehead then moves out towards the side, with the index finger moving in a wavy motion. (SM)

* The facial expression should reflect unpleasantness.

NIGHT WALKING

See SLEEPWALKING

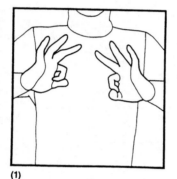

(1)

NIPPLE

The small bump at the center of the breast containing the outlets of the milk duct. *See Figure 1*

(1) Both "F" hands face out at the nipples. (SM)

NITROGEN

An element which is a colorless, odorless gas, and makes up a large amount of the air we breathe. Nitrogen is found in proteins, along with carbon, hydrogen and oxygen.

Nitrogen is needed by both plants and animals to build body parts.

NITROGLYCERIN

A heavy, oily liquid.

Nitroglycerin is used to dilate blood vessels and to treat angina pectoris.

NITROUS OXIDE

A colorless, pleasant-smelling gas used as a light anesthetic to make a person relax or become unconscious; also called "laughing gas." Dentists use nitrous oxide often when doing minor surgery and filling teeth.

Nitrous oxide is good for minor surgery because the effects wear off quickly when someone stops breathing it.

(Continued on next page)

(1) Sign LAUGH — both "L" hands move up the sides of the face from the mouth. The signer should smile at the same time.
(2) Fingerspell "G-A-S".

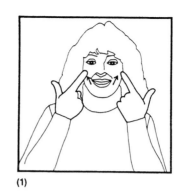
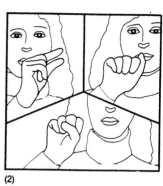

(1)   (2)

NOCTURNAL EMISSION

The release of semen from a man's penis when he is asleep; also called a wet dream.

A nocturnal emission usually occurs during a sexually exciting dream.

(1) Sign WET — the fingertips of the right "flat" hand touch the mouth. Then open and close both "flat-O" hands a few times. (MM)
(2) Sign DREAM — the index finger of the right "one" hand touches the forehead then moves out towards the side, with the index finger moving in a wavy motion. (SM)

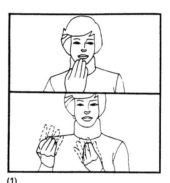
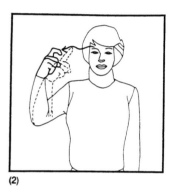

(1)   (2)

NODE

A small, round structure, organ or growth.

A node can be a normal part of the body, such as a lymph node, or it can be an abnormal growth, such as a tumor.

NORMAL

Something which is regular, natural or working properly.

A fever is the normal reaction of the body to an infection.

(1) Sign NATURAL — the left "S" hand faces down at chest level. The right "N" hand makes a small counterclockwise circle above the left hand then moves down to touch the back of the left hand. (SM)

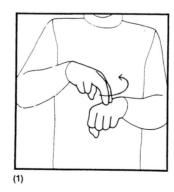

(1)

395

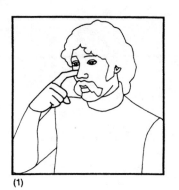
(1)

NOSE

The structure in the middle of the face which we breathe through and can smell with. The nose also warms, moistens and filters the air we inhale to prepare it for the lungs. *See Figure 1*
(1) The index finger of the right "one" hand touches the nose. (SM)

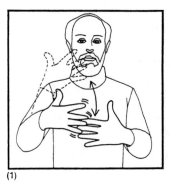
(1)

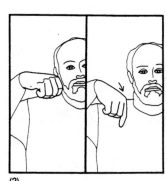
(2)

NOSEBLEED

Blood coming from a person's nose. Injury to the nose, sneezing, high altitudes, picking the nose and some diseases can cause nosebleeds.

A nosebleed is caused by the small blood vessels lining the inside of the nose being broken.

(1) Sign BLOOD — the left "five" hand is at chest level with the palm towards the body. The palm of the right "five" hand is towards the body with the middle fingertips touching the mouth. Move the right hand down the back of the left hand. Wiggle the fingers of the right hand as if moves. (MM)
* *This movement should be short, repeated and somewhat restrained.*
(2) The right "S" hand faces down at the nose. Flick the index finger down. (SM)

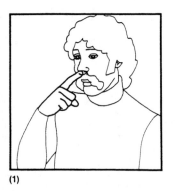
(1)

NOSTRIL

One of the two openings in the lower end of the nose which allow air into and out of the lungs. *See Figure 10*
(1) The index finger of the right "one" hand touches both nostrils. (SM)

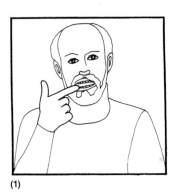
(1)

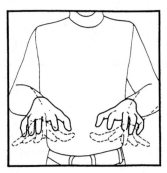
(2)

NOVOCAINE®

The name under which procaine hydrochloride is sold; novocaine is used primarily in dentistry as a local anesthetic.

Dentists use novocaine as a local anesthetic to prevent pain in an area while they do dental work.

(1) Sign INJECTION — the index finger of the right "L" hand touches the mouth. (SM)
(2) Sign FREEZE — both "five" hands face down at chest level. Move both hands slightly up into "claw" hands. (SM)

NOXIOUS

Harmful or dangerous.

Chlorine is a noxious gas because it can irritate and destroy the linings of the respiratory tract.

a. (1) Sign DANGEROUS — the index finger of the right "bent-three" hand hooks over the nose. (SM)

b. (1) Sign DANGEROUS — the left "A" hand faces in at chest level. The thumb of the right "A" hand brushes up and out in a circular movement on the back of the left hand. (SM)

* The facial expression should reflect something bad.

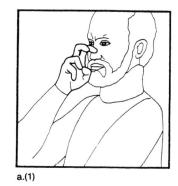 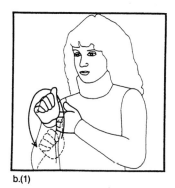

a.(1)   b.(1)

NUCLEUS

The center part of a cell which controls the activities of the cell, including growth, chemical reactions, and reproduction.

The nucleus of a cell contains the chromosomes, which direct the development of the cell.

NUMB

Being unable to feel things or sense things.

When a part of the body has an anesthetic injected into it or when a part of the body becomes cold, it will become numb.

(1) Sign FREEZE — both "five" hands face down chest level. Move both hands up slightly into "claw" hands. (SM)

(2) Sign CAN'T — the left "one" hand is palm down at chest level. The index finger of the right "one" hand strikes down on the left index finger. (SM)

(3) Sign FEEL — the middle finger of the right "eight" hand moves up the chest. (SM)

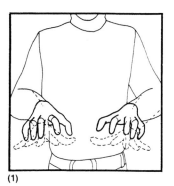 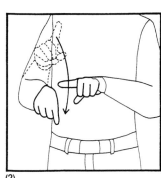

(1)   (2)

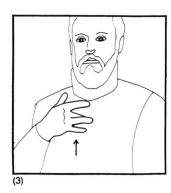

(3)

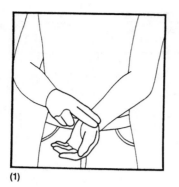
(1)

NURSE

A person trained to take care, under the direction of a doctor, of sick or injured people. A nurse may do anything from simple patient care to very expert care or procedures needed in the treatment of very sick people.

The amount and type of work a nurse does depends on on the amount of training she has had.

(1) The right "N" hand taps the left inside wrist. (DM)

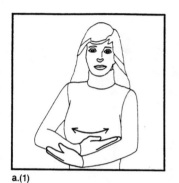
a.(1)

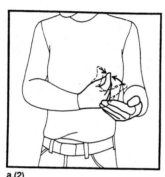
a.(2)

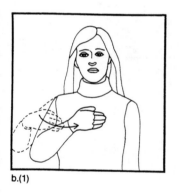
b.(1)

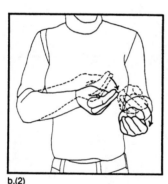
b.(2)

NURSE/NURSING

To feed a baby with mother's milk from the breast.

A baby should be allowed to nurse if possible because no formula is able to provide the nutrients and antibodies that are present in mother's milk.

a. (1) Sign BABY — the right hand and forearm face up, resting on the left hand and forearm which also face upwards. Both are then rocked back and forth as if holding a baby. (MM)

(2) Sign FEED — the left "cupped" hand faces up at the left breast. The right "flat-O" hand also faces up at the left breast and open and closes a few times. (MM)

b. (1) Sign BREAST — the fingertips of the right "cupped" hand touches the right then the left chest areas. (SM)

(2) Sign FEED — both "flat-O" hands face up at the left breast. Drop both hands slightly. (SM)

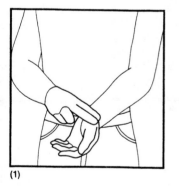
(1)

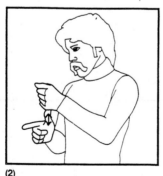
(2)

NURSE'S AIDE

A person who helps a nurse by doing things which don't need special training.

A nurse's aide may feed and bathe patients and take temperature, pulse and respiration measurements.

(1) Sign NURSE — the right "N" hand taps the left inside wrist. (DM)

(2) Sign HELPER — the left "A" hand faces right at chest level. The thumb of the right "L" hand is inside the left fist, the palm facing left. Move both hands up and down a few times. (MM)

NURSING HOME

A building specially equipped to take care of older people or people who need special care while they recover from an injury or disease.

A nursing home may also be called a convalescent center or rest home.

(1) Sign NURSE — the right "N" hand taps the left inside wrist. (DM)
(2) Sign HOME — the fingertips of the right "cupped" hand touch the chin then the right cheek. (SM)

* This is borrowed order from English. The idea of "home for sick" or "home for the aged" should be explained.

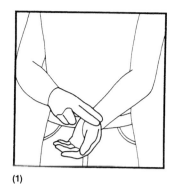
(1)

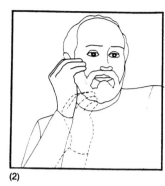
(2)

NUTRIENT

A food that gives the body energy or materials needed to carry on body activities and build body parts.

Nutrients that supply energy are carbohydrates, fats and proteins and nutrients needed for body activities are water, vitamins and minerals.

NUTRITION

The total process by which a person takes in food and uses it to grow, carry on body activities and replace worn-out body parts.

Nutrition involves eating the food, digesting it, absorbing it, and then changing it into a form which can be used by the cells for energy.

(1) Sign EAT — the right "flat-O" hand moves towards the mouth. (SM)
(2) The fingertips of the right "U" hand touch the right then the left side of the chin. (SM)

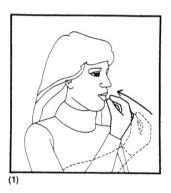
(1)

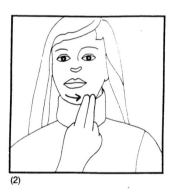
(2)

NYSTAGMUS

Repeated, uncontrollable, fast movement of the eye.

Nystagmus may be caused by irritation in the inner ear, working in darkness for a long time, a brain problem, or looking at things regularly passing by, like telephone poles when one is in a car driving past them.

(1) Both "F" hands face out at the eyes and shake slightly. (MM)

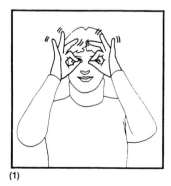
(1)

399

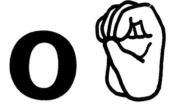

O

OBESE
Very fat.

Obese people are more likely to get diabetes and diseases which affect the heart.

(1) The left "flat" hand faces up at waist level. The right "Y" hand faces down in the left palm. Pivot the right hand from side to side a few times and at the same time, the cheeks should puff out. (MM)

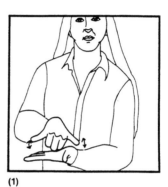

(1)

OBESITY
The condition of being abnormally fat.

Obesity can be caused by eating too much and then not getting enough exercise, or by a problem with the way the body uses food.

(1) The left "flat" hand faces up at waist level. The right "Y" hand faces down in the left palm. Pivot the right hand from side to side a few times and at the same time, the cheeks should puff out. (MM)

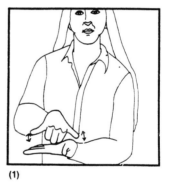

(1)

OBSESSION
An uncontrollable desire to do a certain thing or to think continually about something.

Sometimes normal people will have an obsession, but if it lasts a long time or becomes worse, it may lead to a mental problem or may be a sign of a mental disease.

(1) The index finger of the right "one" hand touches the forehead. (SM)
(2) The left "flat" hand faces down at chest level. The middle finger of the right "eight" hand touches the back of the left hand. Move both hands out and around in a circular movement. (SM)

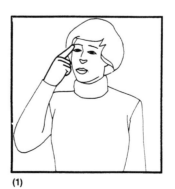

(1)

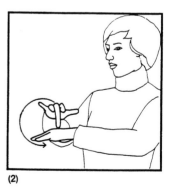

(2)

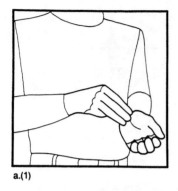

a.(1)

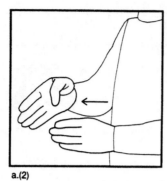

a.(2)

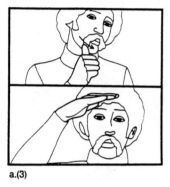

a.(3)

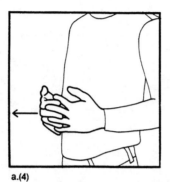

a.(4)

OBSTETRICIAN

A doctor who specializes in treating and caring for women during pregnancy and childbirth.

*It is important that a woman start seeing an **obstetrician** as soon as she knows she is pregnant so he can prevent any problems.*

a. (1) Sign DOCTOR — the right "M" hand taps the left inside wrist. (DM)

(2) Sign SPECIALIZE — the left "B" hand faces right at chest level. The right "B" hand faces left on top of the left hand. Move the right hand straight out on the left index finger. (SM)

(3) Sign WOMAN — the thumb of the right "A" hand moves down the right cheek then to a "flat" hand facing down at the forehead. (SM)

(4) Sign PREGNANT — both "five" hands face in and mesh together at stomach level. Move both hands out slightly. (SM)

b. (1) Fingerspell "O-B".

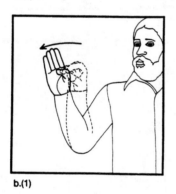

b.(1)

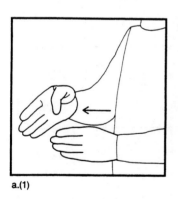

a.(1)

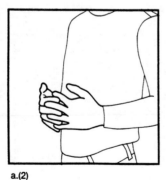

a.(2)

OBSTETRICS

The area of medicine which treats and cares for women during pregnancy, birth and the time right after birth.

*Midwives are becoming more important in natural childbirths and **obstetrics**.*

a. (1) Sign SPECIALIZE — the left "B" hand faces right at chest level. The right "B" hand faces left on top of the left hand. Move the right hand straight out on the left index finger. (SM)

(2) Sign PREGNANT — both "five" hands face in and mesh together at stomach level. Move both hands out slightly. (SM)

(Continued on next page)

402

b. (1) Fingerspell "O-B".

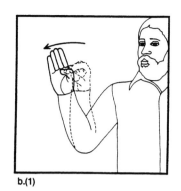

b.(1)

OBSTRUCTION
The blocking of a structure or closing off of a passage.

An obstruction will not allow the movement of materials and will prevent the area from working normally.

(1) Sign BLOCK — both "flat" hands cross and move out slightly at chest level. (SM)

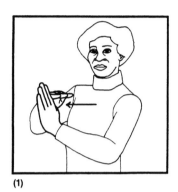

(1)

OCCIPITAL
Referring to the back of the head.

There is a bump on the skull in the occipital region that, on a man's skull, is larger than on a woman's.

(1) The right "one" hand points to the back of the head. (SM)

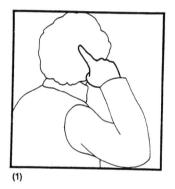

(1)

OCCLUSION
The closing off of a passage.

In dentistry, occlusion refers to the bite, that is, the fitting together of the teeth when the jaws are closed.

(1) The index finger of the right "one" hand points to the teeth. (SM)

(2) The left "flat" hand faces right at shoulder level. The right "cupped" hand faces down and moves from the inside of the left hand, to touching the fingertips, then moving to the outside of the left hand. (SM)

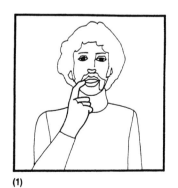

(1)

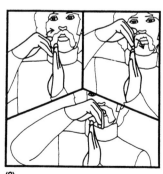

(2)

403

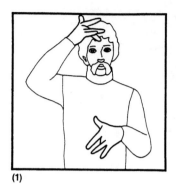

(1)

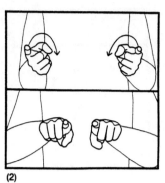

(2)

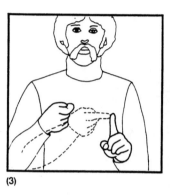

(3)

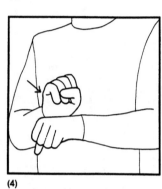

(4)

OCCUPATIONAL DISEASE

A disease a person gets from working around dangerous materials or doing hazardous things.

Some examples of occupational diseases are black lung disease in coal miners, emphysema in people who work in dusty environments, some kinds of cancer caused by working with asbestos, and hemorrhoids in people who sit for long periods of time.

(1) Sign DISEASE — the middle finger of the right "eight" hand touches the forehead and the middle finger of the left "eight" hand touches the stomach. (SM)

(2) Sign HAPPEN — both "one" hands face up at chest level, pointing out. Turn both hands over so that the palms end facing down. (SM)

(3) Sign FROM — the left "one" hand points up at chest level. The index finger of the right "one" hand touches the left index finger. Move the right hand back towards the body and at the same time, bend the index finger in. (SM)

(4) Sign WORK — the left "S" hand faces down at chest level. The right "S" hand faces out and touches the left hand. (SM)

OCCUPATIONAL THERAPY

The treatment of a person who has a physical or mental problem by having him do activities that will help him recover. In occupational therapy, a person will usually be taught to do something productive or creative.

A doctor may want to start a patient, who has been badly injured, in occupational therapy to help him gain confidence and learn new skills.

OCULAR

Having to do with the eye or vision.

An ocular is also the eyepiece of a microscope.

(1) The index finger of the right "one" hand points to both eyes. (SM)

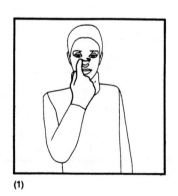

(1)

OCULTIST

A doctor who specializes in treating diseases of the eye.

Ocultist is an old term for ophthalmologist; and members of the profession would presently rather be called ophthalmologists.

(Continued on next page)

404

(1) Sign DOCTOR — the right "M" hand taps the left inside wrist. (DM)

(2) Sign SPECIALIZE — the left "B" hand faces right at chest level. The right "B" hand faces left on top of the left hand. Move the right hand straight out on the left index finger. (SM)

(3) Sign EYES — the index finger of the right "one" hand points to both eyes. (SM)

(4) Sign DISEASE — the middle finger of the right "eight" hand touches the forehead and the middle finger of the left "eight" hand touches the stomach. (SM)

* *The facial expression should reflect sickness.*

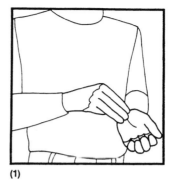
(1)

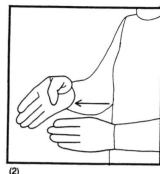
(2)

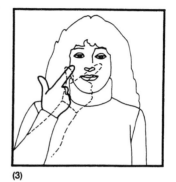
(3)

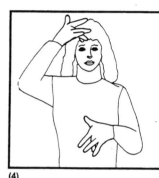
(4)

ODOR

A smell.

> *Odors are detected by special cells and nerves lining the inner parts of the nose.*

(1) Sign SMELL — the fingertips of the right "flat" hand brush up the nose a few times. (MM)

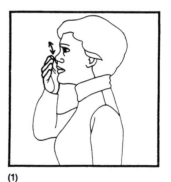
(1)

OEDIPUS COMPLEX

An abnormally strong love of a child for the parent of the opposite sex. A person with an Oedipal complex is usually jealous of the parent of the same sex and the extreme feelings may cause guilt and emotional problems.

> *In psychoanalysis, the Oedipus complex, though not widely used, refers to the strong love of a son for his mother.*

OINTMENT

A salve, paste or soft substance which can be spread over a part of the body to help a wound heal.

> *Ointments are usually made out of petroleum jelly or lanolin and may have an antibiotic or other medicine added to them.*

(Continued on next page)

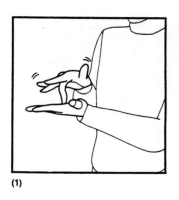
(1)

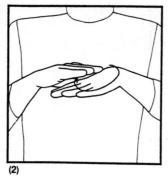
(2)

OINTMENT, *continued*

(1) Sign MEDICINE — the left "flat" hand faces up at chest level. The middle finger of the right "eight" hand touches the left palm and pivots slightly from left to right a few times. (Mm)
(2) Sign RUB ON — the left "flat" hand faces down at chest level. The right "flat" hand rubs the back of the left hand in circular movements. (MM)
This could be signed at the area that the ointment is being applied.

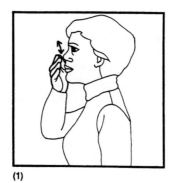
(1)

OLFACTORY

Having to do with smell.

> *The nose is the **olfactory** organ.*

(1) Sign SMELL — the fingertips of the right "flat" hand brush up the nose a few times. (MM)

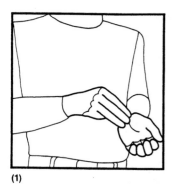
(1)

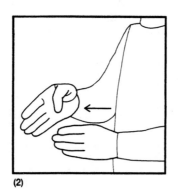
(2)

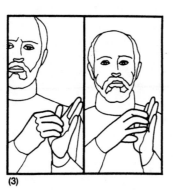
(3)

ONCOLOGIST

A doctor who specializes in the study and treatment of tumors.

> *An **oncologist** treats conditions such as oncosis (the development of tumors).*

(1) Sign DOCTOR — the right "M" hand taps the left inside wrist. (DM)
(2) Sign SPECIALIZE — the left "B" hand faces right at chest level. The right "B" hand faces left on top of the left hand. Move the right hand straight out on the left index finger. (SM)
(3) The left "flat" hand faces right at chest level. The fingertips of the right "O" hand touch the left palm. Open the right hand slightly into a "claw" hand and at the same time, the cheeks should puff out. (SM)

OPHTHALMOLOGIST

A doctor who specializes in treating disorders of the eye; also called an ocultist.

*Ophthalmitis or Ophthalmia (inflammations of the eye) are disorders that an **ophthalmologist** would treat.*

(1) Sign DOCTOR — the right "M" hand taps the left inside wrist. (DM)
(2) Sign SPECIALIZE — the left "B" hand faces right at chest level. The right "B" hand faces left on top of the left hand. Move the right hand straight out on the left index finger. (SM)
(3) Sign EYES — the right index finger points to the eyes. (SM)
(4) Sign DISEASE — the middle finger of the right "eight" hand touches the forehead and the middle finger of the left "eight" hand touches the stomach. (SM)

* The facial expression should reflect sickness.

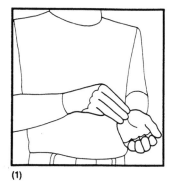
(1)

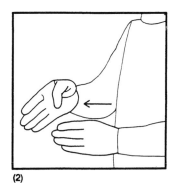
(2)

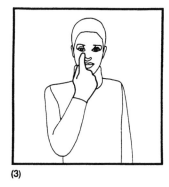
(3)

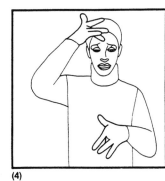
(4)

OPHTHALMOLOGY

The science which studies the eye and its diseases.

*Ophthalmorrhagia (bleeding in the eye) is one disorder studied in **ophthalmology**.*

(1) Sign SPECIALIZE — the left "B" hand faces right at chest level. The right "B" hand faces left on top of the left hand. Move the right hand straight out on the left index finger. (SM)
(2) Sign EYES — the right index finger points to the eyes. (SM)
(3) Sign DISEASE — the middle finger of the right "eight" hand touches the forehead and the middle finger of the left "eight" hand touches the stomach. (SM)

* The facial expression should reflect sickness.

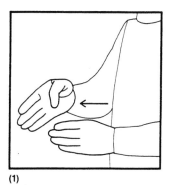
(1)

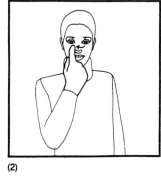
(2)

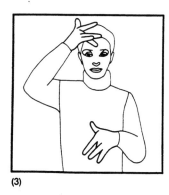
(3)

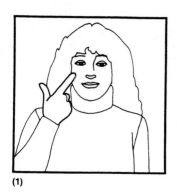
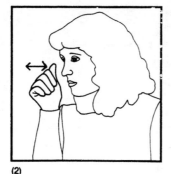

(1)　　　　　　(2)

OPHTHALMOSCOPE

An instrument used to look at the inside of the eye.

An ophthalmoscope has a lens and a light which will light up the inside of the eye so the retina can be examined.

(1) Sign EYES — the right index finger points to the eyes. (SM)

(2) The right "A" hand faces left and moves in and out from the eyes a few times. (MM)

* *The word "O-P-H-T-H-A-L-M-O-S-C-O-P-E" should be fingerspelled before these signs.*

OPIATE

A drug made from opium, used to cause sleep.

The common opiates are opium, morphine, codeine and heroin, and all can cause addiction.

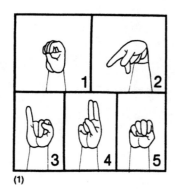

(1)

OPIUM

A drug made by drying the juice of the opium poppy (Papaver somniferum). Opium is a narcotic which may be used as a sedative to cause sleep, to relieve pain, to stop coughing or to slow the heart rate.

Morphine, codeine and heroin are drugs which are found in opium.

(1) Fingerspell "O-P-I-U-M".

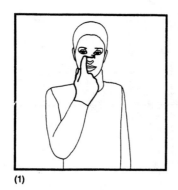

(1)

OPTIC

Referring to the eyes or vision; optical.

The eyes are very fragile, highly developed optic devices which should be protected and well cared for.

(1) Sign EYES — the right index finger points to the eyes. (SM)

408

ONCOLOGY

The area of medicine which studies and treats tumors.

Oncology and cancer research are closely related.

(1) Sign MEDICINE — the left "flat" hand faces up at chest level. The middle finger of the right "eight" hand touches the left palm and pivots slightly from left to right a few times. (MM)

(2) Sign SPECIALIZE — the left "B" hand faces right at chest level. The right "B" hand faces left on top of the left hand. Move the right hand straight out on the left index finger. (SM)

(3) The left "flat" hand faces right at chest level. The fingertips of the right "O" hand touch the left palm. Open the right hand slightly into a "claw" hand and at the same time, the cheeks should puff out. (SM)

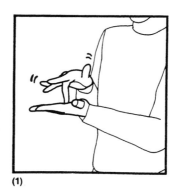
(1)

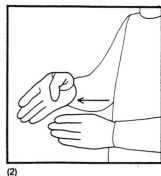
(2)

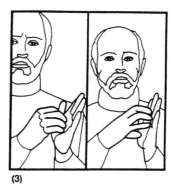
(3)

ONE HALF

See HALF

OOPHORECTOMY

Surgical removal of an ovary.

If a woman has an oophorectomy, she will probably be given hormones to replace those normally made by the ovaries.

(1) Sign WOMAN — the thumb of the right "A" hand moves down the right cheek then to a "flat" hand facing down at the forehead. (SM)

(2) The right "F" hand faces in at the lower right stomach area. (SM)

(3) The thumb is inside the right fist at the lower right stomach area. Flick the thumb out. (SM)

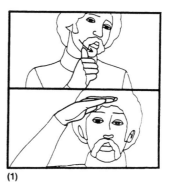
(1)

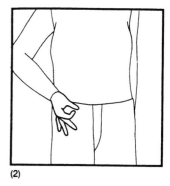
(2)

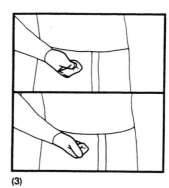
(3)

OOPHOROHYSTERECTOMY

See OVARIOHYSTERECTOMY

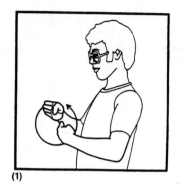
(1)

OPEN OR CLOSED SPIRAL BANDAGE

A temporary bandage wrapped around a part of the body.

In first-aid, an open or closed spiral bandage is used to cover a large burn or to hold a splint in place.

(1) Sign BANDAGE — the left "B" hand faces in at chest level. The right "B" hand faces in and moves around the left hand as if wrapping a bandage. (MM)

* This could be signed at the area the bandage is being applied. "Spiral" could be fingerspelled before signing BANDAGE.

OPEN FRACTURE

See COMPOUND FRACTURE

OPERABLE

A problem which can be cured or made better by surgery.

Some kinds of cancer found early may be operable and the person can be cured.

(1) Sign CAN — both "A" hands face out at chest level. Drop both hands down so that they face down. (SM)

(2) Both "cupped" hands face in and move out slightly. (SM)

(3) Sign OPERATE — the left "flat" hand faces out at chest level. The thumb of the right "A" hand moves down the left palm as if imitating cutting. (SM)

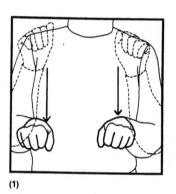
(1)

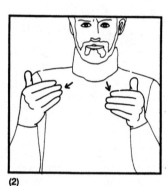
(2)

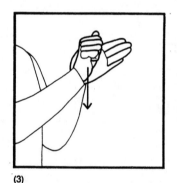
(3)

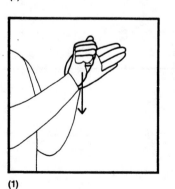
(1)

OPERATION

Any surgical procedure for treating an injury or ailment done with special instruments. An operation usually involves cutting into a part of the body.

Before someone has an operation, the area is shaved, the patient may be given a drug for relaxation and just before the operation, the area is cleaned with antiseptics.

(1) Sign OPERATE — the left "flat" hand faces out at chest level. The thumb of the right "A" hand moves down the left palm as if imitating cutting.

OPTIC DISK

The small area on the retina in the back of the eyeball where the optic nerve leaves the retina; also called the blind spot. No vision can occur at the optic disc because there are no rods or cones in the area. *See Figure 22*

OPTICAL

See OPTIC

OPTICIAN

One who makes optical devices.

An optician is skilled in making glasses and contact lenses.

(1) Sign PERSON — both "flat" hands face each other at chest level. Move both hands down to waist level. (SM)
(2) Sign SPECIALIZE — the left "B" hand faces right at chest level. The right "B" hand faces left on top of the left hand. Move the right hand straight out on the left index finger. (SM)
(3) Sign MAKE — the left "S" hand faces right and the right "S" hand faces left on top of the left hand. Twist both hands slightly so that they both face in. (SM)
(4) Sign GLASSES — both "G" hands face each other at the eyes. Move both hands out slightly to the sides and at the same time, the index fingers and thumbs touch. (SM)

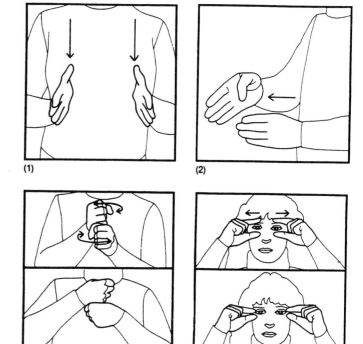

(1)   (2)

(3)   (4)

OPTOMETRIST

One specially trained to test a person's vision and to prescribe glasses to correct vision problems.

An optometrist is a Doctor of Optometry, abbreviated O.D.

(1) Sign DOCTOR — the right "M" hand taps the left inside wrist. (DM)
(2) Sign SPECIALIZE — the left "B" hand faces right at chest level. The right "B" hand faces left on top of the left hand. Move the right hand straight out on the left index finger. (SM)

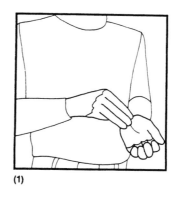

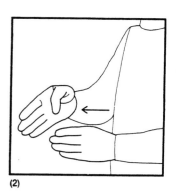

(1)   (2)

(Continued on next page)

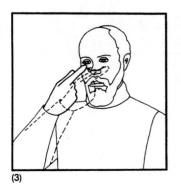
(3)

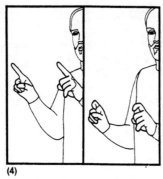
(4)

OPTOMETRIST, *continued*

(3) Sign EYES — the right index finger points to both eyes. (SM)

(4) Sign TEST — both "one" hands face out, the fingers pointing up at chest level. Move both hands down slightly, and at the same time, bend and straighten the index fingers. Repeat this movement three times, the hands ending at waist level. (MM)

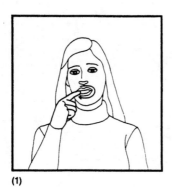
(1)

ORAL

Having to do with the mouth.

> An *oral* medication is a medicine or a drug which is taken through the mouth and swallowed.

(1) The index finger of the right "one" hand circles around the mouth. (SM)

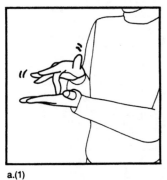
a.(1)

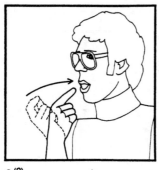
a.(2)

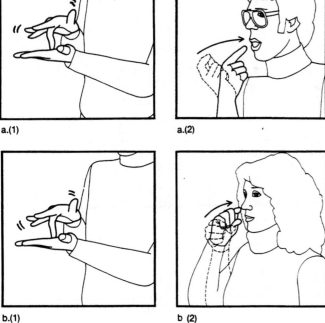
b.(1) b (2)

ORAL MEDICINE

Medicine taken through the mouth and swallowed.

> *Oral medicine is usually taken in the form of a pill or a liquid.*

a. (1) Sign MEDICINE — the left "flat" hand faces up at chest level. The middle finger of the right "eight" hand touches the left palm and pivots slightly from left to right a few times. (MM)

(2) Sign PILL — the thumb and index finger of the right hand touch, the palm faces in. Flick the index finger towards the mouth as if popping a pill into the mouth. (SM)

b. (1) Sign MEDICINE — the left "flat" hand faces up at chest level. The middle finger of the right "eight" hand touches the left palm and pivots slightly from left to right a few times. (MM)

(2) Sign DRINK — the right "modified-C" hand faces in and moves towards the mouth as if imitating taking a drink. (SM)

> * Sign MEDICINE then, PILL or DRINK, whichever applies.

ORALOGY

The study of diseases of the mouth; dental and medical hygiene.

> *Oralogy is also called stomatology.*

(1) Sign SPECIALIZE — the left "B" hand faces right at chest level. The right "B" hand faces left on top of the left hand. Move the right hand straight out on the left index finger. (SM)

(2) Sign MOUTH — the index finger of the right "one" hand circles around the mouth. (SM)

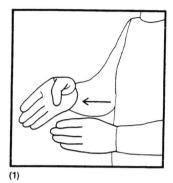 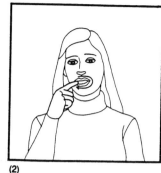

(1)　　　　　　　　　　(2)

ORGAN

In medicine, a bodily structure made up of certain kinds of cells which performs a special action. The heart, liver, lungs, kidneys and brain are all organs.

> *Most organs are paired and work so well that part of an organ can usually be removed without causing any problems.*

* Fingerspell the specific organ.

ORGANIC COMPOUND

Substances made by plants or animals or substances composed of carbon combined with hydrogen, oxygen or nitrogen.

> *Depending on their structure and arrangement, organic compounds can be carbohydrates, fats, or proteins.*

ORGANISM

Any living thing, including plants and animals.

> *An organism may be just one cell, as bacteria or yeast, or it may be many cells, such as man.*

ORGAN TRANSPLANT

The surgical replacement of a diseased organ with a healthy organ from another human. Organs that have been transplanted are the heart, kidneys, liver, lung, some glands, corneas, and even the whole eye.

> *The greatest problem with an organ transplant is the body's recognizing the new organ as being foreign (not a normal part of the body), resulting in the body's defenses attacking and destroying the organ.*

(Continued on next page)

413

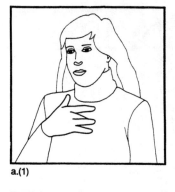

a.(1)

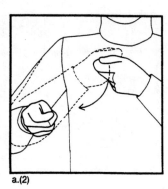

a.(2)

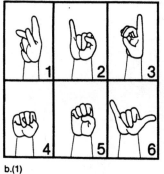

b.(1)

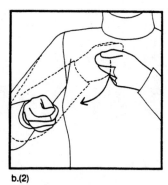

b.(2)

ORGAN TRANSPLANT, *continued*

a. (1) Sign HEART — the middle finger of the right "eight" hand taps the chest a few times.

(2) Sign EXCHANGE — the left "A" hand faces in at chest level. The right "A" hand faces in and moves under the left hand then out forward. (SM)

b. (1) Fingerspell "K-I-D-N-E-Y".

(2) Sign EXCHANGE — the left "A" hand faces in at chest level. The right "A" hand faces in and moves under the left hand then out forward. (SM)

* *These are examples, the specific organ or part should be signed or fingerspelled if known, then sign EXCHANGE.*

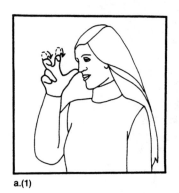

a.(1)

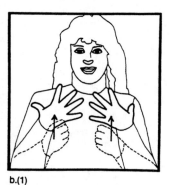

b.(1)

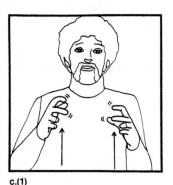

c.(1)

ORGASM

The extreme excitement felt during sexual intercourse; also called climax.

In males, orgasm is usually accompanied by ejaculation of semen.

a. (1) The thumb of the right "three" hand touches the nose. Bend and straighten the index and middle fingers a few times. (MM)

b. (1) Both "S" hands face in at waist level. Move both hands up to chest level, ending in "five" hands. (SM)

c. (1) Both "three" hands face each other at waist level. Move the hands up to chest level and at the same time, bend and straighten the fingers a few times. (MM)

ORTHOPEDICS

The area of medicine which prevents or corrects diseases or disorders of the structures that move the body.

Orthopedics deals mostly with the skeleton, muscles and joints.

ORTHOPEDIST

A doctor who treats diseases or disorders of the structures that move the body, dealing with the skeleton, muscles and joints.

Some treatments used by an orthopedist are manipulation, special devices (braces) and surgery.

ORTHODONTIST

A dentist who prevents or straightens crooked teeth.

It used to be that children were the only people who went to orthodontists and wore braces, but today more and more adults are seeing orthodontists and having their teeth straightened.

(1) Sign DOCTOR — the right "M" hand taps the left inside wrist. (DM)
(2) Sign SPECIALIZE — the left "B" hand faces right at chest level. The right "B" hand faces left on top of left hand. Move the right hand straight out on the left index finger. (SM)
(3) The right "modified-C" hand moves towards the mouth. (SM)

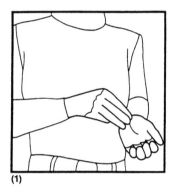
(1)

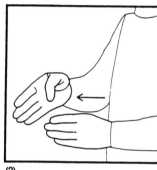
(2)

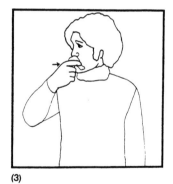
(3)

OSMOSIS

The process in which a liquid moves through a membrane or barrier with very tiny holes when there is a difference in concentration between the two sides. The liquid moves through the membrane but the things dissolved in the liquid will not. The fluid will move to the side with the highest concentration to make it less strong and to make the concentrations on each side equal.

Osmosis is very important in the kidneys, which control the amount of water in the body.

OSSICLE

A small bone.

Ossicle is usually used when talking about the malleus, incus, or stapes, which are small bones located in the middle ear.

OSSIFICATION

Formation and development of bone in tissues or cartilage.

Ossification is also called osteogenesis.

OSTEOPOROSIS

The condition in which bones become soft, brittle and less strong because of removal of the minerals which make the bones hard and strong. The bones of people who have osteoporosis are more likely to break.

Osteoporosis is most often seen in women after menopause, and older people.

(1) Fingerspell "B-O-N-E".
(2) Both "flat-O" hands face in and open and close a few times. (MM)
(3) Sign WEAK — the left "flat" hand faces right at chest level. The fingertips of the right "claw" hand touch the left palm. Keeping the right hand in place, bend and straighten the fingers at the knuckles a few times. (MM)

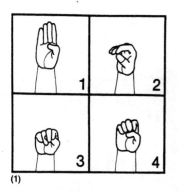
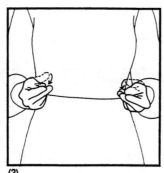
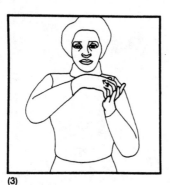

OTITIS

Inflammation of the ear. Symptoms of otitis are dizziness, headache, pain, fever, ringing in the ears and sometimes deafness.

Otitis can be caused by an infection in the ear, another disease like measles, plugging of the eustachian tube stopping pressure equalization, or by something getting into the ear which shouldn't be there.

(1) Sign EAR — the index finger of the right "one" hand points to the right ear. (SM)
(2) Sign INFECTION — the right "I" hand faces out at chest level and shakes slightly from left to right a few times. (MM)

* Mouth the word "infection" while signing.

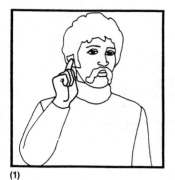
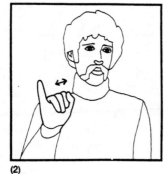

OTOLOGIST

A doctor who specializes in the functions and diseases of the ear.

Another name for an otologist is "aurist."

(1) Sign DOCTOR — the right "M" hand taps the left inside wrist. (DM)

(2) Sign SPECIALIZE — the left "B" hand faces right at chest level. The right "B" hand faces left on top of the left hand. Move the right hand straight out on the left index finger. (SM)

(3) Sign EAR — the index finger of the right "one" hand points to the right ear. (SM)

(4) Sign DISEASE — the middle finger of the right "eight" hand touches the forehead and the middle finger of the left "eight" hand touches the stomach. (SM)

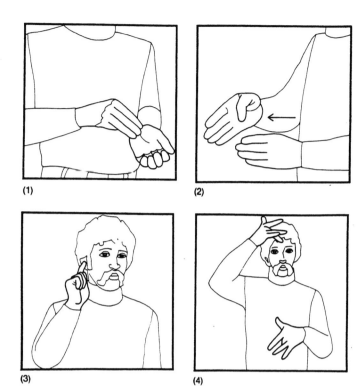

(1) (2) (3) (4)

OTOLOGY

The science dealing with the functions and diseases of the ear.

Otitis is a disorder that is studied in otology.

(1) Sign SPECIALIZE — the left "B" hand faces right at chest level. The right "B" hand faces left on top of the left hand. Move the right hand straight out on the left index finger. (SM)

(2) Sign EAR — the index finger of the right "one" hand points to the right ear. (SM)

(3) Sign DISEASE — the middle finger of the right "eight" hand touches the forehead and the middle finger of the left "eight" hand touches the stomach. (SM)

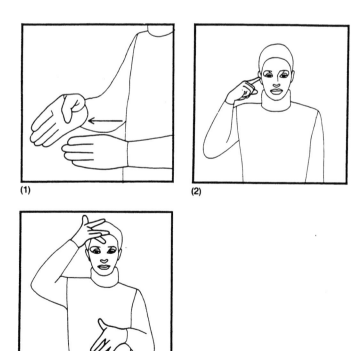

(1) (2) (3)

417

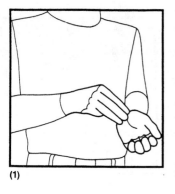
(1)
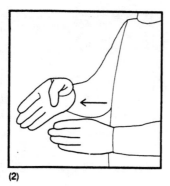
(2)

OTORHINOLARYNGOLOGIST

A doctor who specializes in treating diseases or disorders of the ear, nose or throat.

An otorhinolaryngologist may treat a person with otosclerosis (growth of spongy bone in the inner ear).

(1) Sign DOCTOR — the right "M" hand taps the left inside wrist. (DM)
(2) Sign SPECIALIZE — the left "B" hand faces right at chest level. The right "B" hand faces left on top of the left hand. Move the right hand straight out on the left index finger. (SM)
(3) Sign EAR — the index finger of the right "one" hand points to the right ear. (SM)
(4) Sign NOSE — the index finger of the right "one" hand points to the nose. (SM)
(5) Sign THROAT — the index finger of the right "one" hand points to the throat. (SM)

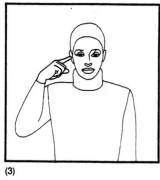
(3)
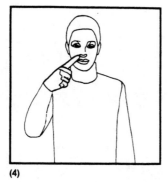
(4)

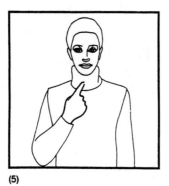
(5)

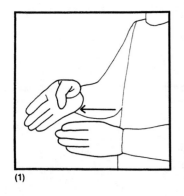
(1)
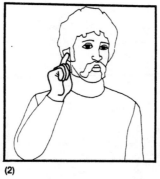
(2)

OTORHINOLARYNGOLOGY

The area of medicine that deals with treating diseases and disorders of the ear, nose or throat.

Otomycosis (a fungal disease of the ear) is one disorder studied in otorhinolaryngology.

(1) Sign SPECIALIZE — the left "B" hand faces right at chest level. The right "B" hand faces left on top of the left hand. Move the right hand straight out on the left index finger. (SM)
(2) Sign EAR — the index finger of the right "one" hand points to the right ear. (SM)

(Continued on next page)

(3) Sign NOSE — the index finger of the right "one" hand points to the nose. (SM)

(4) Sign THROAT — the index finger of the right "one" hand points to the throat. (SM)

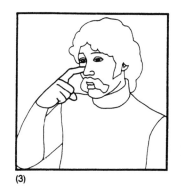
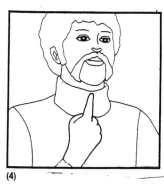

(3) (4)

OTOSCLEROSIS

A disorder in which a person slowly becomes deaf because bone forms around the oval window and stapes. The bone makes it impossible for the stapes to move so the sound waves can't be carried to the inner ear. The cause of otosclerosis is unknown but it may run in families.

> *There are some operations which may be done on peo-ple with otosclerosis which may improve hearing.*

OTOSCOPE

An instrument used to examine the ear; also called auriscope.

> *An otoscope usually has a light and a magnifier to make looking in the ear easier.*

(1) Sign EAR — the index finger of the right "one" hand points to the right ear. (SM)

(2) The right "A" hand faces left and moves in and out a few times from the eyes. (MM)

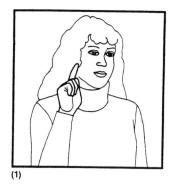
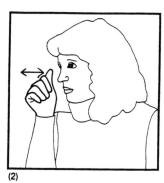

(1) (2)

OUTER EAR

The part of the ear which can be seen and which is designed to funnel sounds into the middle and inner ear, where they are sensed. The outer ear is made up of the ear flap (the pinna or auricle), the canal leading into the head (the external auditory meatus), and then the eardrum or tympanic mem-brane. *See Figure 20*

(1) The index finger of the right "one" hand points to the right ear then moves up and out slightly. (SM)

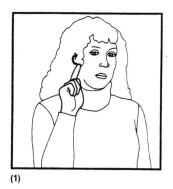

(1)

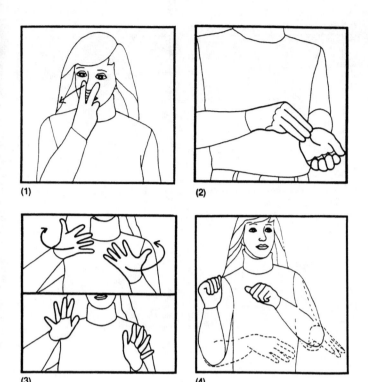

(1)

(2)

(3)

(4)

OUTPATIENT

A person treated at a hospital or clinic without having to stay there.

If it is safe and if the doctor says it is alright, being treated on an outpatient basis can make an operation or procedure less expensive.

(1) Sign SEE — the right "V" hand faces in and moves from the eyes out forward. (SM)

(2) Sign DOCTOR — the right "M" hand taps the left inside wrist. (SM)

(3) Sign FINISH — both "five" hands face up at chest level. Turn both hands so that the face down. (SM)

(4) Sign LEAVE — both "A" hands face down at right chest level. Drop both hands down to left waist level, ending in "five" hands. (SM)

OVAL WINDOW

The oval hole in the cochlea of the inner ear that one of the small bones in the ear, the stapes, fits into. The stapes move so when sound waves hit the eardrum and this movement is passed on through the oval window into the cochlea. The cochlea then turns the movement into small electrical impulses which are sent to the brain and detected as sound. *See Figure 20*

OVARIECTOMY

See OOPHORECTOMY

OVARIES

The two sex organs in a female found in the pelvic region which produce the ova or eggs needed for reproduction. The ovaries also produce hormones responsible for feminine traits and which prepare a woman's body for pregnancy. About once a month, an ovum will mature in the ovary, be released and travel down the fallopian tube to the uterus. *See Figure 12*

(Continued on next page)

(1) Sign WOMAN — the thumb of the right "A" hand moves down the right cheek then to a "flat" hand facing down at the forehead. (SM)
(2) Both "F" hands face in on the lower stomach. (SM)

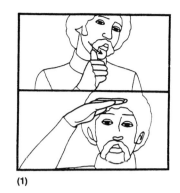

(1)

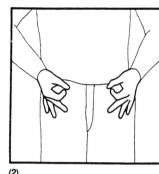

(2)

OVARIOHYSTERECTOMY

Surgical removal of the ovaries and uterus. A woman may have this operation because of cancer.

A woman who has had an ovariohysterectomy will not menstruate and may be given hormones to replace those which are normally made by the ovaries.

(1) Both "F" hands face in on the lower stomach. (SM)
(2) Both "U" hands make the shape of the uterus. (SM)
(3) Sign CUT — the thumb of the right "A" hand moves across the stomach from left to right as if cutting. (SM)
(4) Sign REMOVE — the left "flat" hand faces right at chest level. The right "A" hand touches the left palm then moves down into a "five" hand as if throwing something away. (SM)

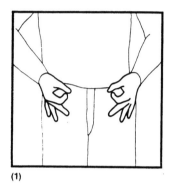

(1)

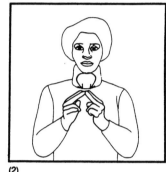

(2)

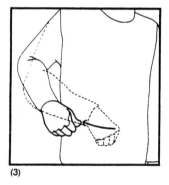

(3)

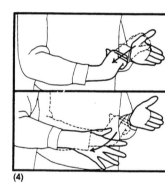

(4)

OVERACTIVE

See HYPERACTIVE

OVERDOSE

Being given or taking too much of a drug either accidentally or on purpose.

Depending on the drug taken, an overdose may cause poisoning with convulsions, unconsciousness, coma or death.

(Continued on next page)

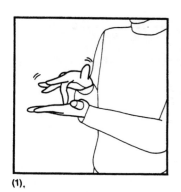
(1).

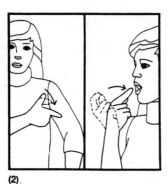
(2).

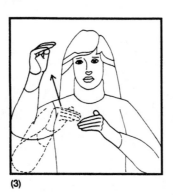
(3)

OVERDOSE, *continued*

(1) Sign MEDICINE — the left "flat" hand faces up at chest level. The middle finger of the right "eight" hand touches the left palm and pivots slightly from left to right a few times. (MM)

(2) Sign INJECTION — the index finger of the right "L" hand touches the left upper arm. Bend the thumb in as if imitating injecting something into the arm. (SM)

Sign PILL — the thumb and index finger of the right hand touch, the palm faces in. Flick the index finger towards the mouth s if popping a pill into the mouth. (SM)

(3) Sign TOO MUCH — both "cupped" hands face down at chest level. Move the right hand up slightly. (SM)

OVERWEIGHT

See OBESITY

OVIDUCT

See FALLOPIAN TUBE

OVULATION

The release of an ovum from the ovary and its movement down the fallopian tube to the uterus. Ovulation usually occurs about two weeks before the beginning of the menstrual period.

Ovulation may be accompanied by a twinge or pain in the abdomen as the ovum is released from the ovary.

(1) Sign EGG — the fingers of both "H" hands cross. Pivot both hands in and out a few times. (MM)

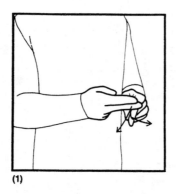
(1)

OVUM

An egg made in the ovary of a woman. When an ovum and sperm join, a baby will begin to develop. The ovum of a human has half the chromosomes needed for the development of a baby, a sperm cell has the other half. (The plural of ovum is ova.)

The ovum from a human is so small that it cannot be seen with the naked eye.

(Continued on next page)

(1) Sign WOMAN — the thumb of the right "A" hand moves down the right cheek then to a "flat" hand facing down at the forehead. (SM)

(2) Both "F" hands face in at the lower stomach. (SM)

(3) Sign EGG — the fingers of both "H" hands cross. Pivot both hands in and out a few times. (MM)

(4) Sign IN — the right "flat-O" hand moves into the left fist a few times. (MM)

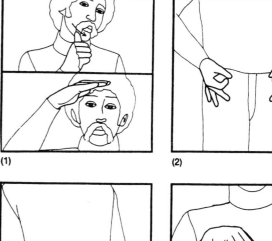

(1)

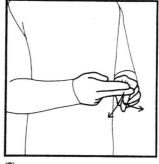

(2)

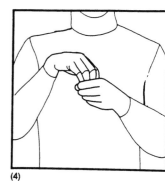

(3)

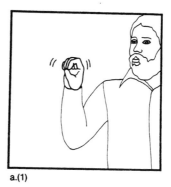

(4)

OXYGEN

A colorless, odorless, tasteless gas found in the air we breathe and which helps make up animals, plants, minerals and water. Oxygen is necessary for breathing Oxygen is absorbed by plants (in the forms of water and carbon dioxide) and then changed into organic substances that are used as food for humans. It is then returned into the air by man in waste products and carbon dioxide.

*In medicine, **oxygen** is used with anesthetics to reduce reactions after surgery and for such conditions as severe anemia, shock, pneumonia, cardiac surgery, intestinal obstructions, radiation therapy of tumors and carbon monoxide poisoning.*

a. (1) The right "O" hand faces out at chest level and shakes slightly. (MM)

b. (1) The right "O" hand faces out at chest level and shakes slightly. (MM)
(2) The right "claw" hand taps over the nose and mouth a few times. (MM)

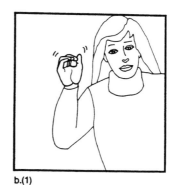

a.(1)

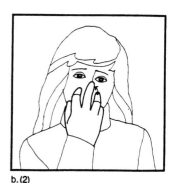

b.(1)

b. (2)

p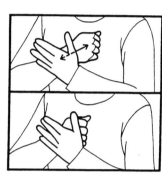

PACEMAKER

A group of cells found in the heart which cause the muscle of the heart to contract. The natural pacemaker in the heart sends a small electrical current through the heart causing the muscle cells to contract and the blood to be pumped. A pacemaker can also be a small man-made device which can control the beating of the heart by giving it small electricl shocks.

*A man-made or artificial **pacemaker** is given to someone when the group of cells in the heart which act as the natural **pacemaker** stop working.*

FOR ARTIFICIAL PACEMAKER
(1) Sign HEART — the middle finger of the right "eight" hand taps the chest a few times. (MM)
(2) Sign BEAT — the left "flat" hand faces in at chest level. The right "A" hand faces in at chest level. The back of the right hand sharply hits the palm of the left hand several times. (MM)
(3) Sign CONTROL — both "modified-A" hands face each other at chest level. Move both hands in and out alternately a few times. (MM)
(4) Sign FALSE — the right "L" hand faces left and brushes past the nose. (SM)
(5) Sign MACHINE — both "five" hands mesh together at chest level and bounce up and down a few tirnes. (MM)

FOR NATURAL PACEMAKER

(1) Sign HEART (See above).
(2) Sign BEAT (See above).
(3) Sign CONTROL (See above).

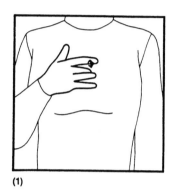

(1)

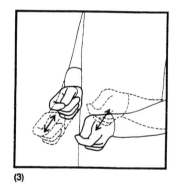

(3)

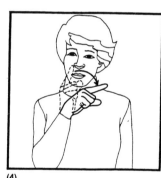

(4)

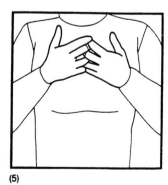

(5)

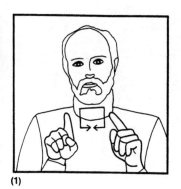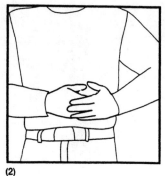

PACK

A wet or dry, hot or cold cloth which is put on a part of the body to treat a disease or injury.

Hot packs are usually put on an area to relax muscles or increase blood flow to the area and cold packs are usually used to prevent swelling and decrease pain.

(1) Both "one" hands outline the shape of a packing.
(2) Both "flat" hands face in with the left hand on top of the right hand.

* This can be signed on any area.

PACKING

Filling a wound or space in the body with gauze or some other material to absorb blood or other fluids. from the area, to allow the area to drain and heal slowly and correctly.

Packing is used to allow the area to drain and heal correctly.

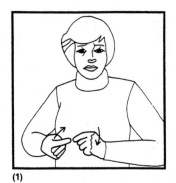

PAIN

A feeling causing a person to be uncomfortable; a hurting or ache in a part of the body.

Pain is usually a symptom of some sort of inflammation or damage.

(1) Both "one" hands point to each other and twist in opposite directions.(MM)

* This can be signed on any area. Facial expression should show pain.

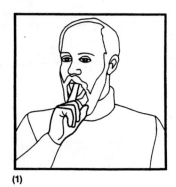

PALATE

The part of the upper mouth which separates the mouth from the nose region. The palate is arched and divided into two halves. The front half, made up of bone, is called the hard palate and the back half, soft and flexible, is called the soft palate.

See Figure 23

(1) The right index finger touches the roof of the mouth.(SM)

426

PALE

Referring to a person's skin color being whitish or lighter than normal.

*A person will become **pale** when the blood vessels in the skin become smaller, when the blood is needed elsewhere, or because it has been lost through a bleeding.*

(1) The right index finger circles around the face.(SM)

(2) Sign WHITE — the right "five" hand touches the chest and moves out ending in a "flat-O" hand.(SM)

(3) The right "flat-O" hand faces in and moves up the face, ending in "five" hand.(SM)

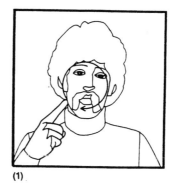
(1)

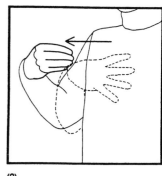
(2)

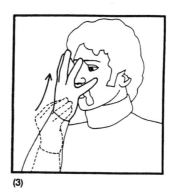
(3)

PALLIATIVE

A treatment, drug or medicine which will not cure a disease or disorder but will lessen the pain, symptoms or suffering caused by the illness.

*A hospice often uses **palliative** treatments for terminal patients.*

(1) Sign MEDICINE — the left "flat" hand faces up at chest level. The middle finger of the right "eight" hand touches the left palm and the hand pivots slightly from left to right.(DM)

(2) Sign SUFFER — the back of the thumb of the right "A" hand touches the mouth and pivots slightly from left to right.(DM)

(3) Sign REDUCE — the left "flat" hand faces up at chest level. The right "flat" hand faces down at shoulder level. Move the right hand down to the left hand.(SM)

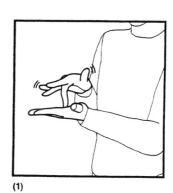
(1)

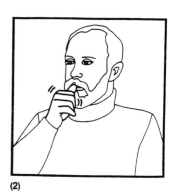
(2)

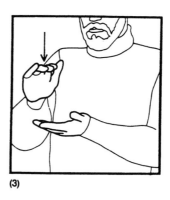
(3)

427

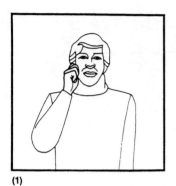
(1)

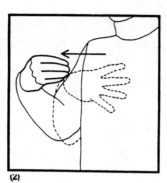
(2)

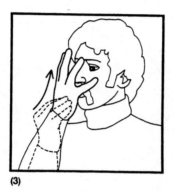
(3)

PALLOR

A lack of color in someone's skin; paleness.

Pallor can be caused by being indoors a lot, anemia, shock, bleeding, poor circulation of blood or tightening of the small blood vessels in the skin.

(1) Sign SKIN — the thumb and index finger of the right fist grab the right cheek. (SM)
(2) Sign WHITE — the right "five" hand touches the chest and moves out ending in a "flat-O" hand. (SM)
(3) The right "flat-O" hand faces in and moves up the face, ending in "five" hand.(SM)

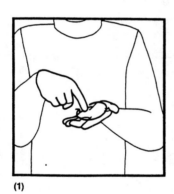
(1)

PALM

The front of the hand between the wrist and fingers. *See Figure 1*

(1) The right index finger circles the left palm.(SM)

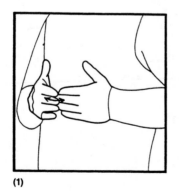
(1)

PALPATE

To examine a part of the body by touching it or feeling it.

When a woman has a pelvic exam, the doctor will palpate her uterus and ovaries to make sure they are normal and in the correct positions.

(1) The left "flat" hand faces in on the body. The right "flat" hand hits the back of the left hand a few times.(MM)

* This can be signed on any area that is being palpated.

428

PALPITATION

A rapid, strong throbbing or movement felt in a part of the body. Palpitation is usually used to describe throbbing of the heart.

Heart palpitations may be caused by excitement, anemia, a heart infection, damage to the heart from an injury, or poor nutrition.

a. (1) Sign HEART — the middle finger of the right "eight" hand taps the chest a few times.
(2) The left "flat" hand faces in at chest level. The right "A" hand faces in at chest level behind the left hand. The right hand sharply hits the palm of left hand a few times. (MM)

* *The facial expression should reflect excitement and the movement should be short and repeated. These should be used when referring to the heart.*

b. (1) Both "claw" hands face in at chest level, the right on top of the left. Open and close both hands a few times. (MM)

* *This should be used when referring to any other general palpitation.*

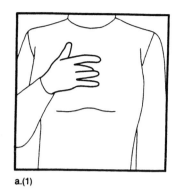

a.(1)

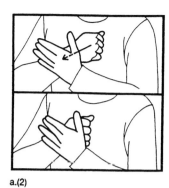

a.(2)

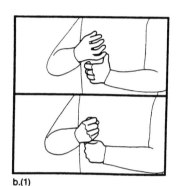

b.(1)

PALSY

The temporary or permanent loss of feeling in a part of the body, the loss of ability to move a part of the body, or the loss of control over a part of the body. Palsy is another word for paralysis.

The word palsy is usually used with another word which will tell what kind of palsy a person has such as Cerebral palsy, shaking palsy or birth palsy.

PANACEA

A medicine which is supposed to cure all illnesses, difficulties or diseases.

In medicine, there is no such thing as a panacea.

PANCREAS

A special gland found near the stomach and connected by a tube to the upper part of the small intestine. The pancreas is special because it makes substances which are put into the digestive tract and substances which are put into the blood stream. The pancreas puts a watery substance into the upper small intestine, when there is food there, which has enzymes in it to help digest the food. The pancreas also makes two hormones, one of which is insulin, which is put into the blood to help the body use carbohydrates and sugars. *See Figure 9*

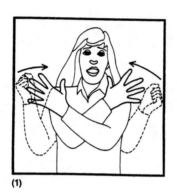
(1)

PANIC

A sudden fright or terror. Panic is usually used when talking about a great fear without reason and which causes one to behave without thinking.

People in deep water sometimes panic from the fear of drowning, and tire themselves out trying to reach safety too quickly.

(1) Both "S" hands face each other at shoulder level. Move both hands towards the center, ending in "five" hands, crossing the arms.(SM)

* Facial expression should show panic.

PANORAMIX X-RAY
See X-RAY

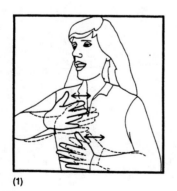
(1)

PANT

To breathe hard, gasp for air.

To pant after working hard physically or after being frightened is normal and does not last long.

(1) Sign BREATHE — both "five" hands move in and out from the chest with quick, short, repeated movements.(MM)

* This sign should be emphasized according to the situation.

PAPILLAE

Small bumps or structures which are slightly raised above the area around it. The word papilla is usually used with another word which describes where or what kind of bump it is.

Dermal papillae are the small ridges in the lower layer of skin which come through the layers of skin and cause fingerprints.

PAP SMEAR/PAP TEST

A test which is done on cells from the vagina or cervix of a woman which will detect cancer early.

To do a pap smear, cells are scraped from the cervix then specially treated and looked at with a microscope to make sure they are normal.

(1) Sign VAGINA — the thumbs and index fingers of both "L" hands touch.(SM)
(2) The left "flat" hand faces out at chest level. The index finger of the right "X" hand scrapes the left palm upwards.(MM)

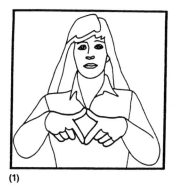
(1)

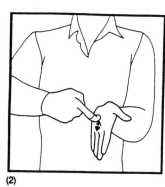
(2)

PARALDEHYDE

A nonbarbiturate drug which acts as a sedative and will make a person relax and sleep.

Paraldehyde is often used to treat a person having hallucinations caused by alcoholism.

(1) Sign MEDICINE — the left "flat" hand faces up at chest level. The middle finger of the right "eight" hand touches the left palm and the hand pivots slightly from left to right.(MM)

(2) Sign HELP — The left "flat" hand faces up at waist level. The right "S" hand faces left on the left palm. Move both hands up to chest level.(SM)

(3) Both "flat" hands face down at chest level. Move both hands down a little.(SM)

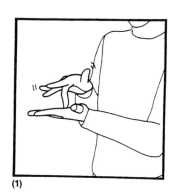
(1)

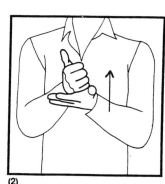
(2)

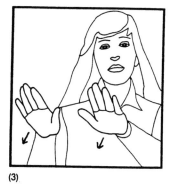
(3)

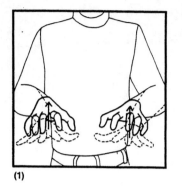
(1)

PARALYSIS

Loss of feeling in a part of the body or when a person loses the ability to move a part of the body; palsy.

The most common cause of paralysis is damage to the brain or nerves going to the muscles which move a part of the body.

(1) Sign FREEZE — both "flat" hands face down at chest level. Move both hands up slightly ending in "claw" hands.(SM)

* *Sign the part referred to.*

PARAMEDIC

A person trained in first aid and emergency medical care who goes to places where people are injured or sick and gives immediate professional care.

Paramedics often ride in ambulances so they can give care to people while they are driven to a hospital.

PARAMEDICAL WORKERS

Highly trained people who work with doctors to treat or cure patients.

Examples of paramedical workers are physical therapists, occupational therapists, speech therapists, pharmacists and social workers.

PARANOIA

A mental disease in which a person thinks other people are treating him badly or bothering him on purpose. A paranoid person will be very sensitive, suspicious, jealous, and stubborn.

A person with paranoia seems to have clear thinking and can logically explain why he thinks others are treating him badly.

(1) Sign SUSPICIOUS — the index finger of the right "one" hand moves up and down the forehead.(MM)

(2) Sign PEOPLE — both "P" hands face down at chest level. Move both hands alternately in small circles forward.(MM)

(3) The left "flat" hand faces right at chest level. Move the right "flat" hand towards the left, so the fingertips touch the left palm.(SM)

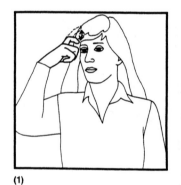
(1)

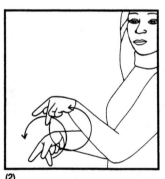
(2)

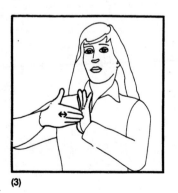
(3)

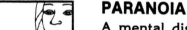

PARAPLEGIC

A person whose legs and lower body are paralyzed, sometimes with problems with some other body functions.

A disease of or damage to the spinal cord usually causes the paraplegic's paralysis.

(1) Both "flat" hands are at waist level, facing down with the left hand on top. Move the right hand down slightly.(SM)

(2) Sign FREEZE — both "five" hands face down at chest level. Move both hands up slightly ending in "claw" hands.(SM)

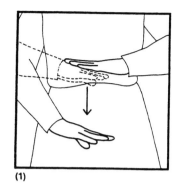
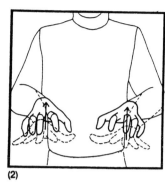

(1)　　　　　(2)

PARASITE

A plant or animal living on or in another plant or animal, doing harm to it. Many different types of animals and plants live in or on each other and don't do any damage, and in some cases, one or both of them may do better because they are living together. A parasite, though, lives by eating parts of the animal it is living on, by taking things which the animal needs to survive, or by injuring the animal.

Examples of parasites are ticks, fleas, tapeworms, pinworms, hookworms, roundworms and any bacteria or virus which causes disease or injury.

PARATYPHOID FEVER

An illness like typhoid but not as severe caused by several different kinds of bacteria infecting the intestines. The person will have symptoms of a fever, upset stomach, diarrhea and perhaps a rash.

A person usually gets paratyphoid fever by eating food which has the bacteria which cause the disease in it.

PAREGORIC

A narcotic drug made from opium.

Paregoric is often used to treat severe diarrhea but it should be used carefully because a person can become addicted to it.

(Continued on next page)

433

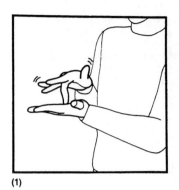
(1)

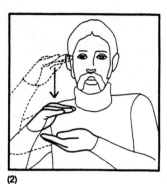
(2)

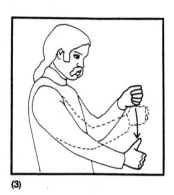
(3)

(1) Sign MEDICINE — the left "flat" hand faces up at chest level. The middle finger of the right "eight" hand touches the left palm and the hand pivots slightly from left to right.(DM)

(2) The left "flat" hand faces up at chest level and the right "flat" hand faces down at shoulder level. Move the right hand down to the left. (SM)

(3) Sign DIARRHEA — the left "S" hand faces right at chest level. The thumb of the right "five" hand is in the fist of the left hand, facing left. Move the right hand down from the left hand several times.(MM)

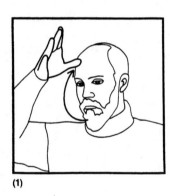
(1)

PARENT

A father or mother.

> *It is often important for a doctor to know a little bit about a person's **parents'** health because some diseases may run in families and can be passed from **parents** to children.*

(1) The right "five" hand faces left, with the thumb touching the chin then moves up to touch the forehead.(SM)

* *The chin position denotes mother and the forehead position denotes father.*

PARESIS

Weakness or slight paralysis of a part of the body.

> *Paresis is also an old name for syphilis.*

PARIETAL

Referring to anything forming the wall of a cavity.

> *The two **parietal** bones form the roof and sides of the skull.*

PARKINSON'S DISEASE

A long term nervous disease causing a slow spreading shaking, weak muscles, a rigid body, slow speech, numbness, and a strange way of walking, becoming faster; also called "shaking palsy."

There are medicines that can help the symptoms of Parkinson's Disease, but there is no cure.

PAROXYSM

A sudden quick, short attack of a disease's symptoms. Paroxysm is another word for a fit or convulsion.

The disease "whooping cough" gets its name from paroxysms of coughing, with deep breaths.

PARTURITION

Childbirth; the process of giving birth to a baby.

When a woman is having her first baby, parturition usually takes about 16 to 18 hours and for later babies it will usually take between 8 to 10 hours.

(1) Fingerspell "L-A-B-O-R"

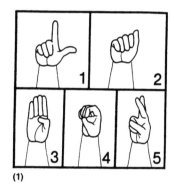
(1)

PASS GAS

See FLATULENCE

PASTEURIZATION

The heating of a liquid to a certain temperature for a period of time to destroy any bacteria which could cause a disease. Pasteurization won't affect the taste or nutritional value of the food.

We are most familiar with the pasteurization of milk in which it is heated to about 150° F and held at that temperature for 30 minutes to kill harmful bacteria.

435

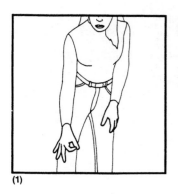

(1)

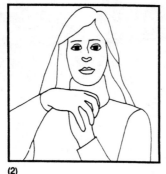

(2)

PATELLA

A small, round bone, found in front of the knee joint, which tendons attach to; also called the "kneecap". *See Figure 26*

(1) The right "F" hand faces in on the right knee. (SM)
(2) The right "claw" hand faces down on the left fist. (SM)

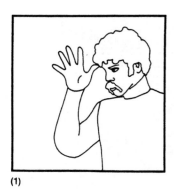

(1)

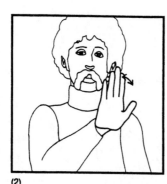

(2)

PATERNAL

Referring to a father.

When an egg is fertilized by a sperm, each parent has provided one half of the chromosomes needed to direct a baby's development and the paternal half is carried to the egg by the sperm.

(1) Sign FATHER — the thumb of the right "five" hand touches the forehead. (SM)
(2) Sign HISSELF — the right "flat" hand faces out at chest level and moves slightly forward a few times. (MM)

PATERNITY TEST

A test of a man's blood to see if he could be the father of a certain child. A paternity test decides the blood type of a man and compares it to that of the child to see if the child's blood type is one that could have been inherited from his mother and the man.

A paternity test cannot be used to prove a man is a child's father; it can only be used to rule out the possibility of a man being a child's father.

PATHOGEN

Something which can cause a disease, especially a living thing like a virus, bacteria or parasite.

The pathogens causing colds are several kinds of virus which attack the lining of the respiratory tract.

436

PATHOLOGICAL CHANGES

The changes in the structure of a part, or in the way it works, caused by a disease.

During an autopsy, the pathologist looks for pathological changes the organs.

PATHOLOGIST

A doctor who studies the cause of a disease, how an organism causes a disease and the changes in structure of an area during a disease.

Pathologists study pieces of tissue removed during surgery or after death to see if a person had a disease and, if so, what kind of disease it was.

(1) Sign DOCTOR — the right "M" hand touches the left inside wrist.(SM)

(2) Sign SPECIALIZE — the left "B" hand faces right at chest level. The right "B" hand faces left on top of the left hand. Move the right hand straight out on the left index finger.(SM)

(3) Sign DISEASE — the middle finger of the right hand touches the forehead and the middle finger of the left hand touches the stomach.(SM)

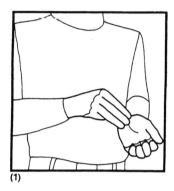
(1)

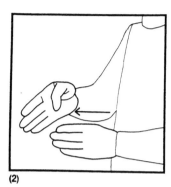
(2)

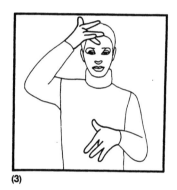
(3)

PATHOLOGY

The part of medicine that studies the causes of diseases and how they affect structures and body activities.

There are different areas in pathology such as cellular pathology, clinical pathology and surgical pathology.

(1) Sign SPECIALIZE — the left "B" hand faces right at chest level. The right "B" hand faces left on top of the left hand. Move the right hand straight out on the left index finger.(SM)

(2) Sign DISEASE — the middle finger of the right hand touches the forehead and the middle finger of the left hand touches the stomach.(SM)

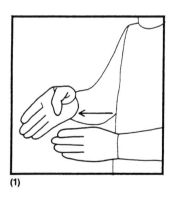
(1)

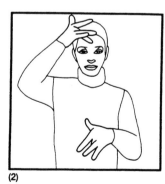
(2)

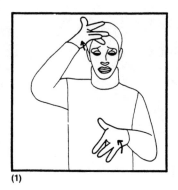
(1)

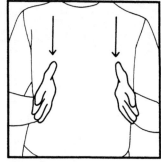
(2)

PATIENT

Someone who is being treated for an illness or injury.

A person is a patient if he is receiving medical care or attention, even if he shows no signs of illness.

(1) Sign SICK — the middle finger of the right "eight" hand touches the forehead and the middle finger of the left "eight" hand touches the stomach. Twist both hands slightly. (SM)

* The facial expression should reflect sickness.

(2) Sign PERSON — both "flat" hands face each other at chest level. Move both hands down to waist level. (SM)

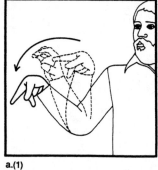
a.(1)

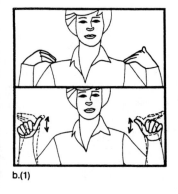
b.(1)

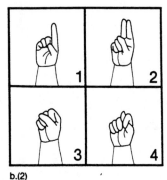
b.(2)

PCP

This is the short name for the drug phencyclidine; also called "angel dust". This powerful drug was originally used by veterinarians as a large animal anesthetic but when people take it, it acts as a hallucinogen. It can cause very strange behavior, fear, an increase in blood pressure and heart rate, muscle contractions, convulsions and perhaps a coma in which the person's eyes stay open. PCP comes in a powder form which is usually smoked.

One of the greatest dangers of PCP is that its effects can take three to four days to appear and then last a long time or, come back again and again.

a. (1) Fingerspell "P-C-P"
b. (1) Sign ANGEL — the fingertips of both "flat" hands touch the shoulders. Turn both hands out away from the shoulders then move the fingers up and down a few times as if showing wings.(MM)
(2) Fingerspell "D-U-S-T"

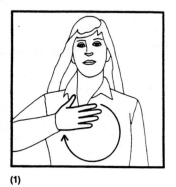
(1)

PECTORAL

Referring to the chest.

The breasts are located in the pectoral region.

(1) The right "five" hand circles the chest.(SM)

438

PECTORALIS MAJOR

One of the muscles on the upper front part of the chest. The pectoralis major is the large, triangular muscle attached to the ribs, sternum and humerous which helps us to breathe and move the arm. *See Figure 4*

PEDIATRICIAN

A doctor who specializes in caring for children and treating their diseases.

*A child should have a regular **pediatrician** who has a complete record of his vaccinations, treatments and past health.*

(1) Sign DOCTOR — the right "M" hand touches the left inside wrist.(MM)

(2) Sign SPECIALIZE — the left "B" hand faces right at chest level. The right "B" hand faces left on top of the left hand. Move the right hand straight out on the left index finger.(SM)

(3) Sign CHILD — the right "flat" hand faces down and imitates patting the head of an imaginary child. (DM)

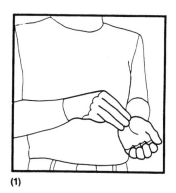
(1)

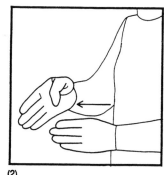
(2)

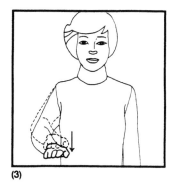
(3)

PEDIATRICS

The area of medicine that deals with the diseases, treatment and care of children.

*Most hospitals have a section or floor totally concerned with **pediatrics**, where children are cared for and treated.*

(1) Sign SPECIALIZE — the left "B" hand faces right at chest level. The right "B" hand faces left on top of the left hand. Move the right hand straight out on the left index finger.(SM)

(2) Sign MEDICINE — the left "flat" hand faces up at chest level. The middle finger of the right "eight" hand touches the left palm and pivots slightly from left to right a few times. (MM)

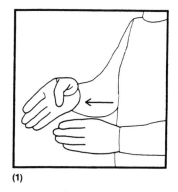
(1)

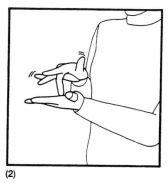
(2)

(Continued on next page)

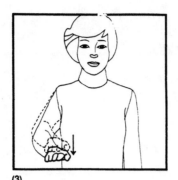
(3)

PEDIATRICS, *continued*

(3) Sign CHILD — the right "flat" hand faces down and imitates patting the head of an imaginary child. (DM)

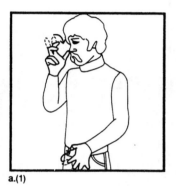
a.(1)

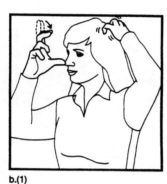
b.(1)

PEDICULOSIS

A condition where a person is infected with a large number of lice (parasite Pediculus); also called "crabs," crab louse or lice. Pediculosis occurs in hair regions, especially the head and genitals. Symptoms may include itching and the formation of pustules, similar to eczema or dermatitis.

Pediculosis can be caught by using an infested person's brush or comb, unclean conditions, or sexual contact with an infested person.

a. (1) The thumb of the right "three" hand touches the nose with the palm facing left. Bend and straighten the fingers of the right hand. At the same time, the left "claw" hand scratches near the pubic area.(MM)

b. (1) The thumb of the right "three" hand touches the nose with the palm facing left. Bend and straighten the fingers of the right hand. At the same time, the left "claw" hand scratches near head.(MM)

* This sign would be used if referring to head lice.

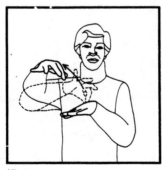
(1)

PEELING

Shedding the outer layer of skin; also called desquamation.

When a person gets a sunburn, his skin may blister and then will begin peeling off.

(1) The left "flat" hand faces down at chest level. The thumb and index finger of the right "F" hand touch the back of the left hand and move out forward as if peeling something off.(MM)

* This can be signed at any area where the skin in peeling.

PELLAGRA

A disease caused by the lack of niacin in the diet. The disease causes a skin rash, digestive and nervous problems, and mental disorders.

Pellagra can be treated with vitamins and minerals.

PELVIC EXAM

An examination of the organs in the pelvic region. Pelvic exams are most often done on women by a gynecologist.

During a pelvic exam, a doctor will check the health and position of a woman's vagina, uterus, cervix and ovaries.

(1) Sign VAGINA — the thumbs and index fingers of both "L" hands touch.(SM)
(2) The left "flat" hand faces right at chest level. The index finger of the right "one" hand moves up the palm of the left hand.(SM)

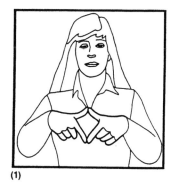
(1)

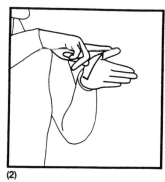
(2)

PELVIC INFLAMMATORY DISEASE

A serious infection in the fallopian tubes, ovaries or uterus; also known as PID. The first symptoms may be vaginal bleeding between menstrual periods and maybe some cramping. If the infection gets worse, there may be severe abdominal pain, nausea, vomiting, vaginal discharge or a fever. It used to be thought that PID was caused by a venereal disease, but research now shows that women who wear IUD's (intrauterine devices) are more likely to develop PID.

If pelvic inflammatory disease is not treated quickly with antibiotics, it can cause sterility and even death.

(1) Fingerspell "P-I-D"

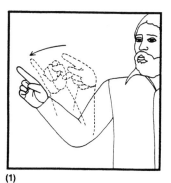
(1)

PELVIS

The large, bony, cup-shaped structure in the lower abdomen that protects some internal organs. Each half of the pelvis is made up of three separate bones which are connected: the ilium, ischium and pubis. *See Figure 26*
(1) The fingertips of both "flat" hands tap the sides of lower stomach. (MM)

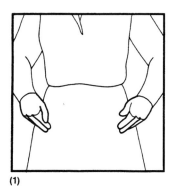
(1)

441

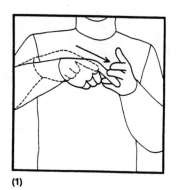

(1)

PENETRATE

To pierce or be forced into.

*The needles and knives used by doctors are very sharp so they can **penetrate** the skin cleanly and easily.*

(1) The index finger of the right "one" hand moves through the fingers of the left "five" hand.(SM)

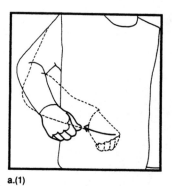

a.(1)

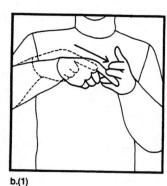

b.(1)

PENETRATING INJURY OR WOUND

A wound which goes through the skin and into an organ or a cavity in the body, usually caused by an object such as glass, pieces of wood or metal, or knives.

*A person with a serious **penetrating injury or wound** should see a doctor immediately to avoid infection and more injury.*

a. (1) Sign CUT — the right "A" hand faces in at waist level. Move the hand across the stomach as if cutting. (SM)

b. (1) Sign PENETRATE — the index finger of the right "one" hand moves through the fingers of the left "flat" hand. (SM)

* The specific thing or area should be signed or indicated first before these signs.

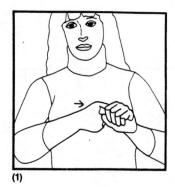

(1)

PENETRATION

The act of entering into something. Penetration is often used to describe insertion of a man's penis into a woman's vagina.

*When pain is felt often or all the time by a man or woman during **penetration**, something is wrong and a doctor should be seen.*

(1) The left "O" hand faces down at chest level. The index finger of the right "one" hand moves into the left fist.(SM)

442

PENICILLINS

A large group of antibiotics, some man-made and some produced by certain bacteria, used to stop infections caused by several other types of bacteria and small parasites. Common forms of this drug are penicillin G, penicillin V, and ampicillin. The penicillins differ in structure and so are effective against different sorts of infections. The penicillins can be injected into a muscle or taken orally. The penicillins are a very widely used group of antibiotics. They are used against some throat infections, gangrene, tetanus, syphilis, and some types of pneumonia and meningitis.

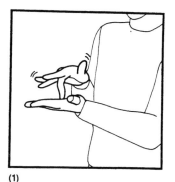
(1)

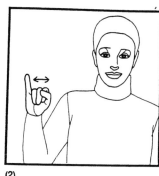
(2)

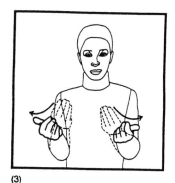
(3)

Because penicillin is used so much, the bacteria it is used against often start to resist its effect and then a different kind of penicillin must be used against that infection.

(1) Sign MEDICINE — the left "flat" hand faces up at chest level. The middle finger of the right "eight" hand touches the left palm and the hand pivots slightly from left to right.(DM)

(2) Sign INFECTION — the right "I" hand faces out at chest level and shakes from side to side a few times. (MM)

* Mouth the word "infection" while signing.

(3) Sign MELT — both "flat-O" hands face up at chest level. Move both hands slightly to the sides and at the same time, the thumbs of both hands rub across the fingers. (SM)

PENIS

The male sex organ, used to place sperm in a woman's vagina and to urinate. The penis is attached to the body where the legs meet. During sexual excitement, blood flow to the penis increases and spaces in the penis fill with blood causing it to become hard and erect. *See Figure 13*

(1) The middle finger of the right "P" hand taps the nose a few times.

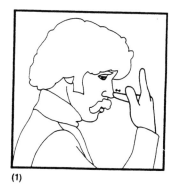
(1)

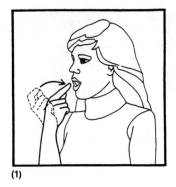
(1)

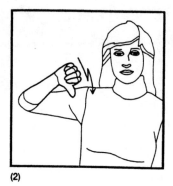
(2)

PENTOBARBITAL

A barbiturate drug which acts as a depressant or sedative and slows down the body's activities, causing relaxation and sleep. Another name for Pentobarbital is Nembutal and the slang name is "yellow jackets"."

Pentobarbital is often used during labor or before someone has an operation.

(1) Sign PILL — the thumb and index finger of the right hand touch, the palm faces the mouth. Flick the index finger towards the mouth as if popping a pill into the mouth.(SM)

(2) Sign DOWNER — the right "A" hand with the thumb pointing down, moves down at shoulder level twice.(DM)

* This is a general sign for depressants ("downers"). The specific type of drug should also be fingerspelled and all side effects explained.

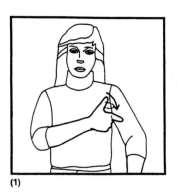
(1)

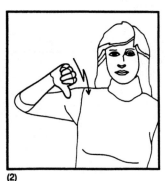
(2)

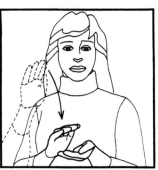
(3)

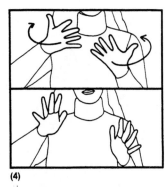
(4)

PENTOTHAL

A barbiturate drug which acts as a sedative and pain killer. Sodium thiopental is another name for pentothal.

When pentothal is injected into a vein, it acts for a very short time.

(1) Sign INJECTION — the right "L" hand faces in with the index finger touching the upper left arm. Move the thumb of the right hand in as if injecting something into the left arm.(SM)

(2) Sign DOWNER — the right "A" hand with the thumb pointing down, moves down at shoulder level twice.(DM)

(3) Sign SHORT — the left "H" hand faces right at chest level. The fingers of the right "H" hand brush out from the left fingers.(SM)

(4) Sign FINISH — both "five" hands face in at chest level. Turn both hands in, ending with palms facing down.(SM)

* This is a general sign for depressants ("downers"). The specific type of drug should also be fingerspelled and all side effects explained.

PEP PILLS

The slang name for amphetamine or benzedrine, a drug that acts as a stimulant and makes a person feel more alert and less tired.

Besides pep pills, other names for amphetamine are "wake-ups," "bennies," and "speed."

(Continued on next page)

PEP PILLS, *Continued*

(1) Sign PILL — the thumb and index finger of the right hand touch, the palm faces the mouth. Flick the index finger towards the mouth as if popping a pill into the mouth.(SM)
(2) Sign UPPERS — the right "A" hand with the thumb pointing up, moves up at shoulder level twice.(DM)

* *This is a general sign for stimulants ("uppers"). The specific type of drug should also be fingerspelled and all side effects explained.*

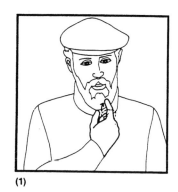
(1)

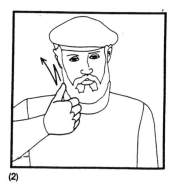
(2)

PEPTIC ULCER

An open sore in the lining and related tissue of the lower end of the esophagus, the stomach or upper small intestine. Symptoms of a peptic ulcer include constant pain, which comes on a couple of hours after eating, in the area just below the chest, and indigestion, heart burn, nausea and vomiting. Peptic ulcers are caused by the digestion of part of the esophagus by acids and enzymes from the stomach.
 They can also be caused by too much digestive juice being made or by digestive juice being made at the wrong time, causing it to digest a part of the stomach or upper intestine.

> *A peptic ulcer may develop from a person worrying, smoking or drinking too much, causing the stomach to make digestive juices when it shouldn't.*

(1) Sign PAIN — both "one" hands are at chest level pointing at each other and twist in opposite directions.(MM)

* *Facial expression should show pain.*

(2) Both "flat" hands touch the stomach area.(SM)

* *This would be signed at area of ulcer.*

(3) Fingerspell "U-L-C-E-R"

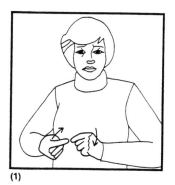
(1)

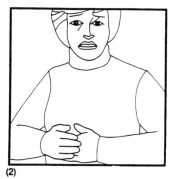
(2)

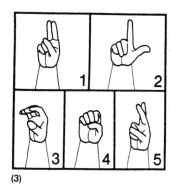
(3)

PERCEPTION

Consciousness or being aware of things around us by using our senses.

> *Some drugs will change our **perception** of the world around us by acting on our nervous systems.*

(Continued on next page)

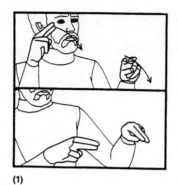

(1)

PERCEPTION, *continued*

(1) Both "V" hands face out and move slightly down. The eyes should follow the movement of the hands. (SM)

PERCUSSION

Light tapping on areas of the body to check an organ or structure. Percussion is done to check the organ's size, position and whether there may be fluid or pus in it.

Some structures that are checked by percussion are the abdomen, bladder, chest, heart, liver, kidneys, ovaries, spleen and uterus.

PERFORATED ULCER

An open sore, caused by acids and enzymes in digestive juices eating into the lining of the lower esophagus, stomach or upper intestine, which breaks through into the abdomen, letting out stomach contents. Symptoms of a perforated ulcer are a sharp pain which spreads over the abdomen, a hard abdomen, vomiting and rapid respirations and pulse.

A perforated ulcer is very dangerous and must be operated on because the material which has gotten into the abdomen from the stomach or intestine can cause an infection known as peritonitis.

PERINEAL BODY
See PERINEUM

PERINEUM

The area of the body between the vulva and anus in a woman or between the scrotum and anus in a man. The perineum is made up of skin, muscle and connective tissue. A woman's perineum can easily be torn during delivery of a baby. *See Figure 12 or 13*

PERIOD

In medicine, "period" usually refers to the menstrual period or menstruation.

During their period, some women may have pain, abdominal cramping or mood changes like depression.

(1) Sign MENSTRUATION — The knuckles of the right "A" hand tap the right cheek a few times.(MM)

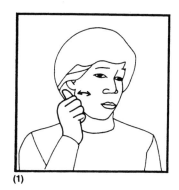

(1)

PERIODONTAL

Referring to the area or structures around the teeth.

Periodontal is also called "peridental".

(1) Fingerspell "G-U-M"
(2) The right index finger circles the gums.(SM)

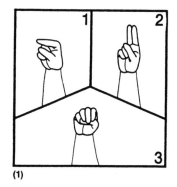

(1)

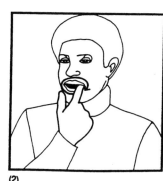

(2)

PERIODONTAL ATTACHMENT

The point where the gum attaches to the tooth. The periodontal attachment is not where the gum can be seen to meet the tooth but slightly below that point. *See Figure 25*

PERIODONTAL DISEASE

Inflammation of the gums and structures around the teeth, usually caused by poor care of the teeth; also called Pyorrhea or periodontitis. In periodontal disease, the gums will pull away from the teeth, the teeth will become loose, pus will be made because of infection and the teeth may fall out.

A person can prevent most kinds of periodontal disease by brushing the teeth after eating, using dental floss, not eating sweets and by seeing a dentist regularly.

(1) Fingerspell "G-U-M"
(2) The right index finger circles the gums.(SM)

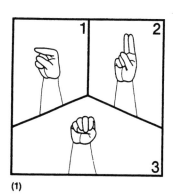

(1)

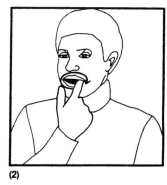

(2)

(Continued on next page)

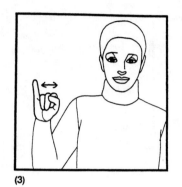
(3)

(3) Sign INFECTION — the right "I" hand faces out at chest level and shakes from side to side a few times. (MM)

* *Mouth the word "infection" while signing.*

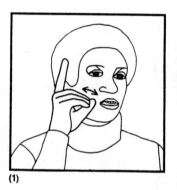
(1)

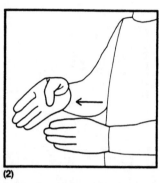
(2)

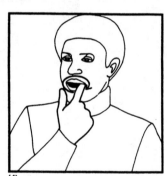
(3)

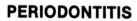

(4)

PERIODONTIST

A dentist specializing in treating diseases of the tissues around the teeth.

> *If your regular dentist finds problems with your gums, he may refer you to a periodontist, who can specially treat them.*

(1) The right "D" hand taps the right side of the mouth a few times.(MM)

* *Newer sign.*

(2) Sign SPECIALIZE — the left "B" hand faces right at chest level. The right "B" hand faces left on top of the left hand. Move the right hand straight out on the left index finger.(SM)

(3) Fingerspell "G-U-M"

(4) The right index finger circles the gums.(SM)

PERIODONTITIS

See PERIODONTAL DISEASE

PERIPHERAL VISION

Vision which allows us to see things we aren't looking directly at.

> *Peripheral vision is not as clear as direct vision because there aren't as many rods and cones on the outer edges of the retina to detect the images.*

(1) Sign SEE — the right "V" hand faces in and moves from the eyes out.(SM)

(2) Both "flat" hands face each other. Move both hands out to the sides in a V direction.(SM)

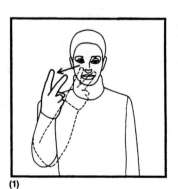
(1)

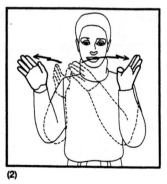
(2)

448

PERISTALSIS

The wave-like movement, caused by muscles contracting in succession, that occurs in most tubes of the body and moves materials through these tubes. We cannot control peristalsis; it occurs as a reflex when something is in the tube.

Peristalsis is often used to describe the contraction of muscles in the digestive tract, which serves to mix the food and move it through the body.

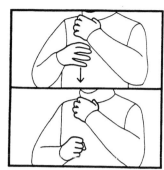
(1)

(1) Both "claw" hands face in at chest level, the right hand above the left. Move both hands down slightly and at the same time, close the hands to "S" hands. (SM)

* *This could be signed at the area where the peristalsis occurs.*

PERITONEUM

The thin membrane which lines the inner part of the abdominal cavity and lies over the organs in the abdomen. The peritoneum helps to prevent friction between the organs in the abdomen and helps hold organs in place. *See Figure 9*

PERITONITIS

Inflammation of the peritoneum, the thin membrane lining the abdominal cavity and lying over the organs in the abdomen. The inflammation is caused by an infection, due to bacteria which get into the abdominal cavity. These bacteria enter through an incision or wound in the abdomen, a perforated ulcer, the bloodstream, or a ruptured appendix.

Symptoms of peritonitis are a fever, severe pain in the abdomen, vomiting and swelling of the abdomen. Peritonitis is very dangerous and, if not treated quickly, may cause death.

Peritonitis can be treated with rest, antibiotics, and surgery to clean out or repair any damage of the abdomen.

PERMANENT

Something which stays or doesn't change.

*Some viruses become a **permanent** part of the body by living in certain cells.*

(1) The thumb of the right "A" hand presses against the thumbnail of the left "A" hand. Move both forward.(SM)

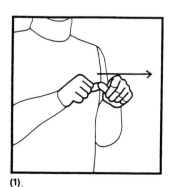
(1).

449

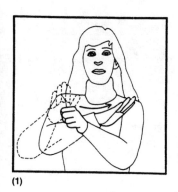

(1)

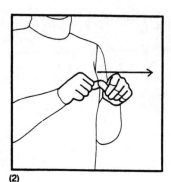

(2)

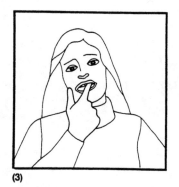

(3)

PERMANENT TEETH

The teeth that replace the baby teeth or deciduous teeth starting at about 6 years of age. The average adult has 32 permanent teeth. *See Figures 24*

*A person's **permanent** teeth should last an entire lifetime if one protects them and gives them good care.*

(1) Sign FULL — the left "S" hand faces right at chest level. The right "flat" hand faces down and brushes back towards the body on the left fist.(SM)
(2) Sign PERMANENT — the thumb of the right "A" hand is on top of the thumb of the left "A" hand, both facing down. Move both hands out forward. (SM)
(3) Sign TEETH — the right index finger moves from left to right on the teeth.(SM)

PERNICIOUS ANEMIA

A severe form of blood disease resulting in the decrease of red blood corpuscles, muscular weakness, and gastrointestinal and nerve problems.

*If **pernicious anemia** is not treated quickly, it can cause death.*

PERSONALITY

The ways a person behaves, acts and thinks that make him different from other people. Personality is all the mental characteristics that help make a person what he is.

*Mental disease often causes changes in the person's **personality**.*

(1) The right "P" hand circles once at the left chest. (SM)

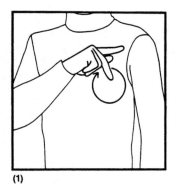

(1)

PERSPIRATION

The salty fluid made by special glands in the skin to remove heat from the body; also called "sweat". Once perspiration reaches the skin, body heat is used to evaporate it. Perspiration increases when it gets warmer, when we exercise, are excited or nervous, and when we are in pain or are feeling nauseous.

(Continued on next page)

Perspiration is made up mostly of salt and water, so when we are perspiring a lot, we need to drink fluids to replace the lost salt.

(1) The left "five" hand is at chest level with the fingers pointing down. The right "five" hand is at the head with the fingers pointing down. Move the right hand down to the left hand as if showing sweat coming down.(SM)

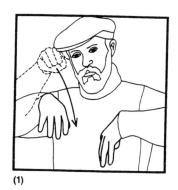
(1)

PERTUSSIS
See WHOOPING COUGH

PEST

A plant or animal that is mildly dangerous or that bothers people.

The word pest is most often used for destructive insects.

(1) Sign INSECT — the thumb of the right "three" hand touches the nose and the fingers bend up and down a few times.(MM)

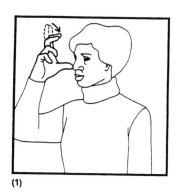
(1)

PESTICIDE

A substance used to kill pests, usually a chemical used to kill rodents or insects.

A pesticide can be dangerous because it may stay on fruits or vegetables which people eat or it may stay in the environment and poison other plants and animals.

(1) The right "modified-X" hand faces out and imitates spraying something.

(2) Sign KILL — the left "flat" hand faces right at chest level. The index finger of the right "one" hand moves down the palm of the left hand.(SM)

(3) Sign INSECT — the thumb of the right "three" hand touches the nose and the fingers bend up and down a few times.(MM)

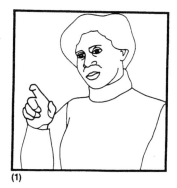
(1)

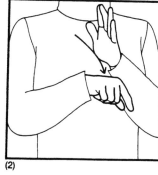
(2)

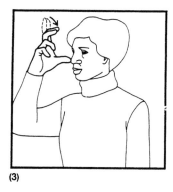
(3)

PETIT MAL SEIZURE

A mild epileptic attack in which a person loses consciousness or just stops what he is doing and stares straight ahead.

There is seldom falling or convulsions in a petit mal seizure.

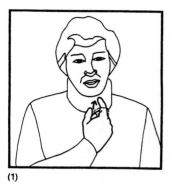 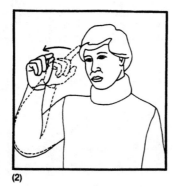

PEYOTE

A hallucinogenic drug made from a certain kind of cactus, also called "mescaline".

Peyote, made from the mescal cactus, can be very poisonous.

(1) Sign PILL — the thumb and index finger of the right hand touch, the palm faces the mouth. Flick the index finger towards the mouth as if popping a pill into the mouth.(SM)

(2) The index finger of the right "one" hand touches the forehead and moves out forward, ending with the index finger and thumb touching.(SM)

PHALANGES

The bones that make up a finger or toe.
See Figure 26

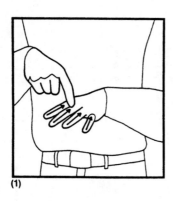

(1) The right index finger moves up the fingers of the left hand.(MM)

PHARMACIST

A person trained and licensed to prepare and sell drugs; also called a druggist.

A pharmacist cannot sell most drugs without a prescription from a doctor.

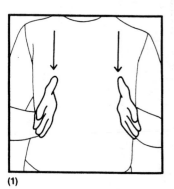 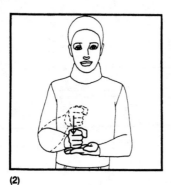

(1) Sign PERSON — both "flat" hands face each other at chest level. Move both hands down to waist level. (SM)

(2) Sign CERTIFY — the left "flat" hand faces up at chest level. The right "S" hand faces right and moves down to rest in the left palm. (SM)

(Continued on next page)

(3) Sign STORE — both "flat-O" hands face down at chest level and move slightly from side to side a few times. (MM)

(4) Sign MEDICINE — the left "flat" hand faces up at chest level. The middle finger of the right "eight" hand touches the left palm and pivots slightly from left to right a few times. (MM)

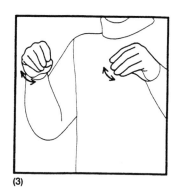
(3)

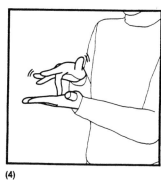
(4)

PHARMACOLOGIST

A person who studies drugs, where they come from, how they are made, how they are used, and what they do to people.

Pharmacologists often study pharmacogenics, the side effects of drugs on people.

PHARMACY

A place where medicines are prepared and sold to people; also called a drugstore.

When a doctor prescribes a drug for a person to take, the person must go to a pharmacy to get the drug.

(1) Sign STORE — both "flat-O" hands point down at chest level. Shake both hands from left to right a few times.(MM)

(2) Sign BUY — the left "flat" hand faces up at chest level. The right "flat-O" hand faces up in the left palm and moves out forward.(SM)

(3) Sign MEDICINE — the left "flat" hand faces up at chest level. The middle finger of the right "eight" hand touches the left palm and the hand pivots slightly from left to right.(MM)

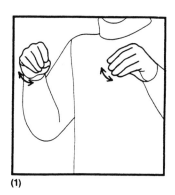
(1)

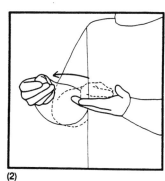
(2)

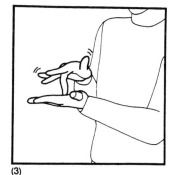
(3)

PHARYNX

A tube-shaped area behind the mouth that is part of the digestive and respiratory systems. The pharynx runs from the base of the skull to about half way down the neck. The pharynx has the eustachian tube, the back of the nose, the mouth, esophagus and larynx opening on it. The pharynx is important in swallowing and breathing. *See Figure 10*

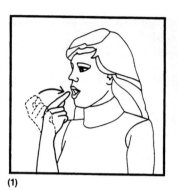
(1)

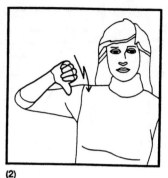
(2)

PHENOBARBITAL

A long-lasting barbiturate drug which acts as a sedative by slowing down the body's activities, causing the person to relax and sleep. Some slang names for phenobarbital are "barbs", "sleepers", "downers", "bennies", and "goofballs".

Phenobarbital is often used to treat convulsions like those in epilepsy or fevers.

(1) Sign PILL — the thumb and index finger of the right hand touch, the palm faces the mouth. Flick the index finger towards the mouth as if popping a pill into the mouth.(SM)

(2) Sign DOWNER — the right "A" hand with the thumb pointing down, moves down at shoulder level twice.(DM)

* This is a general sign for depressants ("downers"). The specific type of drug should also be fingerspelled and all side effects explained.

PHENOTHIAZINE

A drug used to make insecticides, worm medicine for animals and tranquilizers. Drugs made from phenothiazine are used to calm and quiet patients with mental diseases, to relax people before surgery and to stop nausea and vomiting.

Phenothiazine should be used carefully because it can lower a person's blood pressure and cause dizziness.

PHLEBITIS

Inflammation of a vein. Symptoms of phlebitis are pain along the vein, swelling below the inflammation and a change in color of the skin.

Phlebitis can be very dangerous because the inflammation of the vein can cause a clot to form which may be carried to some other part of the body and plug an artery.

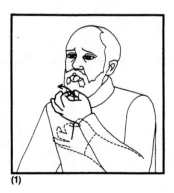
(1)

PHLEGM

The very thick, slippery mucus which may be coughed up from the trachea and bronchi.

Phlegm is made in larger amounts when a person has a cold or respiratory infection, and when the respiratory tract is irritated by something like smoke.

(1) The right "C" hand faces in and moves from chest level up the throat up and out forward.(SM)

PHOBIA

An abnormal fear of something.

A phobia is often caused by a mental problem or something that happened to the person in the past.

(1) Fingerspell "P-H-O-B-I-A"
(2) Sign FEAR — both "S" hands face each other at the sides. Move both hands in ending in "five" hands.(SM)

* The facial expression should reflect fear. If the exact type of phobia is known, it should be signed or fingerspelled before these signs.

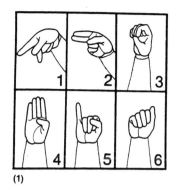

(1)

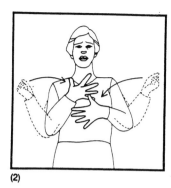

(2)

PHOROPTER

The large instrument used by an optometrist or ophthalmologist which a person looks through and which measures how bad the defect is in a person's vision. Sometimes, for some reason, light rays aren't focused directly on the retina of the eye, causing what is seen to be out of focus. A phoropter measures how badly out of focus the images may be so glasses can be made to correct the error and make vision clear.

A phoropter has many different lenses which a doctor can switch around to see which ones make a person's vision better.

(1) Sign EYES — the right index finger points to both eyes.(SM)
(2) Sign MACHINE — both "five" hands mesh together at chest level and bounce up and down a few times.(MM)
(3) Both "C" hands face out in front of the eyes. Twist both hands out to the sides.(SM)

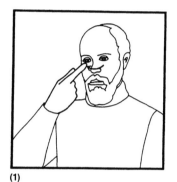

(1)

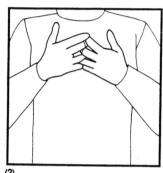

(2)

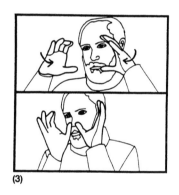

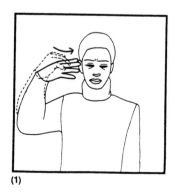

(3)

PHOTOPHOBIA

An abnormal sensitivity to light. When a person has photophobia, light will cause the eyes to hurt.

Photophobia may be caused by measles, meningitis, an eye infection, or migraine headaches.

(1) Sign LIGHT — the right "flat-O" hand faces down with the fingers pointing towards the head. Move the right hand towards the head ending in "five" hands.(SM)
(2) Sign EYES — the right index finger points to both eyes.(SM)

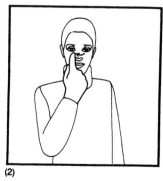

(1)

(2)

(Continued on next page)

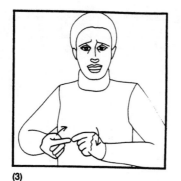
(3)

PHOTOPHOBIA, *continued*

(3) Sign PAIN — both "one" hands are at chest level pointing at each other and twist in opposite directions.(MM)

* *Facial expression should show pain.*

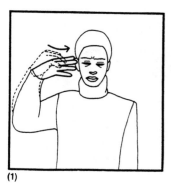
(1)

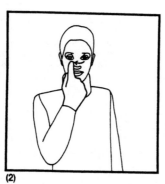
(2)

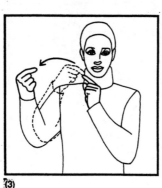
(3)

PHOTOSENSITIVITY

Being very sensitive or allergic to light, especially sunlight. A person can be photosensitive because of taking drugs like phenothiazine or sulfa, because of hormones or because of poisoning with some metals.

Photosensitivity is often an allergic reaction to substances formed when the sun's rays change chemicals in the skin.

(1) Sign LIGHT — the right "flat-O" hand faces down with the fingers pointing towards the head. Move the right hand towards the head ending in "five" hand.(SM)

(2) Sign EYES — the right index finger points to both eyes.(SM)

(3) The right "one" hand faces out and the left "one" hand faces in at waist level with the index fingers almost touching. Move the right hand away from the left hand.(SM)

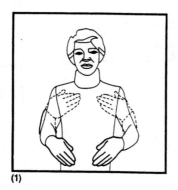
(1)

PHYSICAL

In medicine, having to do with the body.

A person's mental well being is very closely tied to his physical health.

(1) Sign BODY — both "flat" hands face in. The fingertips of both hands touch the chest and then the stomach.(SM)

PHYSICAL DEPENDENCE

The body's need for a certain drug. Regular usage of some drugs causes change in the body such that the drug becomes a physical necessity. Generally, the amount used must be increased to meet the body's increasing tolerance to the substance.

Most narcotics, like opium, morphine, codeine, methodone or Demerol can cause physical dependence or psychological dependence.

(1) Sign BODY — both "flat" hands face in. The fingertips of both hands touch the chest and then the stomach.(SM)

(2) The right index finger hooks the right corner of the mouth and pulls it back.(SM)

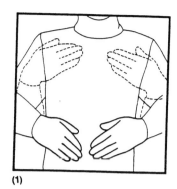
(1)

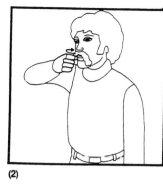
(2)

PHYSICAL THERAPY

Special treatment or therapy using physical means rather than drugs; physiotherapy.

Physical therapy uses heat, light, water, electricity, massage, exercise, and radiation.

(1) Sign BODY — both "flat" hands face in. The fingertips of both hands touch the chest and then the stomach.(SM)

(2) Sign THERAPY — the left "flat" hand faces up at waist level. The right "T" hand faces left on top of the left palm. Move both hands up to chest level.(SM)

* This is a newer English version and may need some explanation before using.

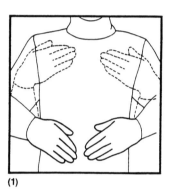
(1)

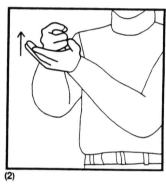
(2)

PHYSICIAN

A person who has completed medical school and is licensed to practice medicine.

Physician is another name for doctor.

(1) Sign DOCTOR — the right "M" hand touches the left inside wrist.(DM)

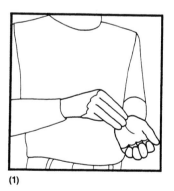
(1)

PHYSIOLOGICAL

Having to do with normal body activities and functions.

A physiological salt solution is the combination of salt and water, in the amounts found in the body, and is sometimes used in enemas to treat dehydration.

PHYSIOLOGY

The study of the activities of cells, tissues and organs of the entire body.

A physiologist is one who studies physiology.

PHYSIOTHERAPY

See PHYSICAL THERAPY

PID

See PELVIC INFLAMMATORY DISEASE

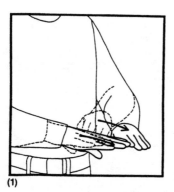

PIGEON-TOED

Referring to walking with the toes turned inward.

Pigeon-toed may also be called pes varus.

(1) Both "flat" hands face down at waist level. Move both hands forward alternately with the fingers pointing in towards each other.(MM)

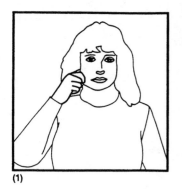
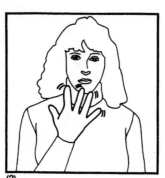

PIGMENT

A substance that gives color to things. In medicine, it is a natural coloring substance found in the body.

An example of pigment is melanin, which gives color to the skin and hair.

(1) Sign SKIN — the index finger and thumb of the right hand pinch the right cheek.(SM)

(2) Sign COLOR — the right "five" hand faces in under the chin with the fingers pointing up. Wiggle the fingers.(SM)

PILES

See HEMORRHOIDS

PILL

Medicine put or made into small, hard round or oval shapes. A pill is a way of giving someone a drug so that he can chew or swallow it. The contraceptive pill containing hormones taken by women to prevent pregnancy is called "the pill".

A pill may have a coating on it to make it taste better or be easier to swallow.

(Continued on next page)

(1) Sign PILL — the thumb and index finger of the right hand touch, the palm faces the mouth. Flick the index finger towards the mouth as if popping a pill into the mouth.(SM)

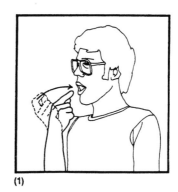

(1)

PILLOW SPLINT

An emergency splint made from a pillow used to hold an arm or leg still when it may be broken.

> Along with *pillow splints,* other emergency splints can be made with blankets, boards, sticks and rolled-up newspapers.

PIMPLE

A small bump on the skin in which pus collects. Pimples are caused by a small inflammation at the base of a hair in the skin. (Young adults, whose bodies and metabolism are changing rapidly, often get pimples in patches on their bodies.)

> *Pimples* should not be picked at or scratched because scarring or an infection may result.

(1) The right index finger touches the right cheek several times as if pointing to pimples.(MM)

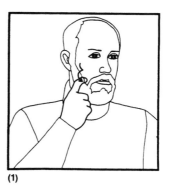

(1)

PINKEYE

An inflammation of the thin membrane covering the eye, called the conjunctiva. In pinkeye, a person's A very common, small parasitic worm which lives in a person's intestines and rectum. Pinworms get their name because they are small and slender, with pointed tails. Most of the problems caused by pin-worms are due to females leaving the body through the anus to lay eggs on the skin; this activity causes severe itching. A person with pinworms may be nervous, lose his appetite, have nightmares, lose weight and be unable to sleep. There are several drugs which are very effective in getting rid of pin-worms.

> *Pinkeye* gets its name from the red or pinkish color of the eye caused by tiny blood vessels in the conjunctiva of the eye becoming larger and letting more blood into the area.

(Continued on next page)

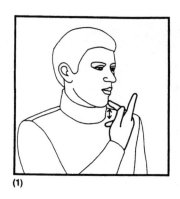
(1)

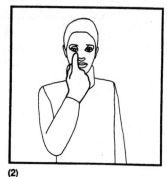
(2)

PINK EYE, continued

(1) Sign PINK — the middle finger of the right "P" hand brushes the chin a few times.(MM)

(2) Sign EYE — the right index finger points to the right eye.(SM)

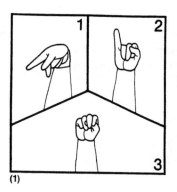
(1)

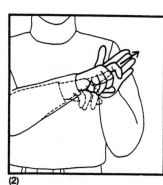
(2)

PINWORM

A very common, small parasitic worm which lives in a person's intestines and rectum. Pinworms get their name because they are small and slender, with pointed tails. They may be from 1/8 to 1/2 inch in length. Most of the problems caused by pinworms are due to females leaving the body through the anus to lay eggs on the skin; this activity causes severe itching." A person with pinworms may be nervous, lose his appetite, have nightmares, lose weight and be very unable to sleep. There are several drugs which are very effective in getting rid of pinworms.

Pinworms, the most common worm parasite of people, are found in all areas of the world.

(1) Fingerspell "P-I-N"

(2) Sign WORM — the "flat" hand faces right at chest level. The index finger of the right "one" hand wiggles in and out on the left palm.(MM)

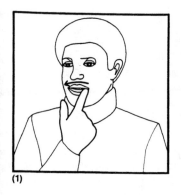
(1)

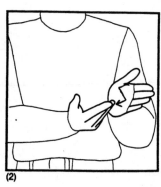
(2)

PIT

A small hollow or dent in a structure. In dentistry, it is a dent in the enamel of a tooth.

Along with fissures, a pit is usually found in the development of a tooth.

(1) Sign TOOTH — the right index finger points to the teeth.(SM)

(2) Sign CRACKED — the left "flat" hand faces right at chest level. The right "flat" hand makes an "S" shape on the left palm.(SM)

PITUITARY GLAND

A small, round gland attached to the base of the brain. The pituitary gland produces several very important hormones. These hormones are chemicals which travel through the blood to affect other organs and structures. The pituitary gland hormones affect the thyroid gland, the breasts, the testicles, the ovaries, the adrenal glands and the uterus. The pituitary gland helps control growth, reproduction and how the body uses some nutrients. The pituitary gland itself is controlled by the part of the brain just above it called the hypothalamus. The pituitary gland is also called the master gland because it controls so many body activities. *See Figure 18*

PLACEBO

A substance which is not a drug or medicine and has no chemical effect on a person. A placebo is a fake medicine given to someone who thinks he is getting a medicine.

When studying the effects of a new drug, a ***placebo*** *is often given to one group of patients and the real drug to another group, and then the results are compared.*

PLACENTA

The oval structure attached to the inside of the uterus during pregnancy. The placenta has the umbilical cord attached to the center of it which carries fresh blood with food and oxygen in it to the baby and carries wastes away. The placenta normally comes out of the uterus after the baby is born and is called "the afterbirth".

The ***placenta*** *acts as a connection between the mother's and child's bloodstreams.*

a. (1) The left "flat" hand faces down at chest level. The right "flat" hand faces left and moves out and over the back of the left hand.(SM)

(2) Sign BIRTH — the left "flat" hand faces in at chest level. The right "flat" hand is behind the left hand and moves down and out forward.(SM)

(3) Both "five" hands face up at chest level. Move both hands out and up ending with the palms facing each other.(SM)

(Continued on next page)

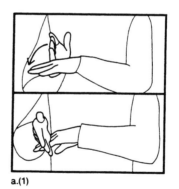

a.(1)

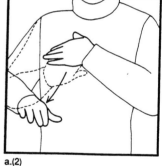

a.(2)

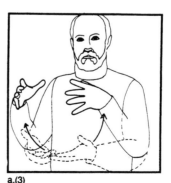

a.(3)

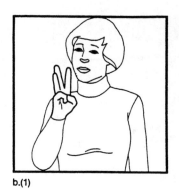
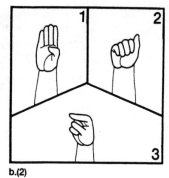

b.(1)   b.(2)

PLACENTA, *continued*

b. (1) Sign WATER — the right "W" hand faces left and taps against the right side of the mouth a few times.(MM)
   (2) Fingerspell "B-A-G"

PLACIDYL®

The name under which the drug ethchlorvynol is sold. Placidyl is a sedative drug used to lessen tensions and help a person relax or to help them sleep.

Severe withdrawal symptoms like a loss of coordination, nervousness, shaking, hallucinations, delirium and perhaps convulsions, can occur if someone has been taking placidyl for a long time.

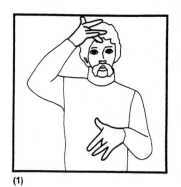
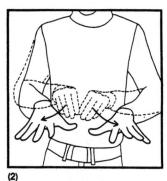

(1)   (2)

PLAGUE

A word that use to be used for any contagious disease affecting and killing many people all at once. Now the word is used for a disease caused by bacteria (yersinia pestis) which are spread by fleas or which are breathed in from an infected person. The bacteria causing the disease are widely found in rats, squirrels and other rodents, and if fleas from these animals bite a person, they may pass plague to the person. The symptoms of plague are a high fever, confusion, shock, coma, and very swollen lymph nodes. If the bacteria gets into the bloodstream, they will kill the person quickly.

Antibiotics like tetracyclines, chloramphenocol and streptomycins can be effective against plague if used early enough.

(1) Sign SICK — the middle finger of the eight hand touches the forehead and the middle finger of the left hand touches the stomach. Twist both hands slightly.(SM)
(2) Sign SPREAD — both "flat-O" hands face down together at waist level. Move both hands out forward ending in "five" hands.(SM)

462

PLANTAR WART

A wart which is on the sole of the foot. (See WART)

Plantar warts are usually very painful because of the pressure put on them when walking.

(1) Fingerspell "W-A-R-T"

(2) Fingerspell "F-O-O-T".

(3) The right "F" hand faces out on the left palm. (SM)

* This could be signed at the area of the wart.

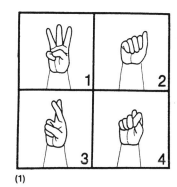

(1)

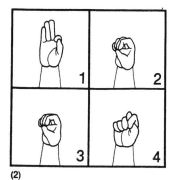

(2)

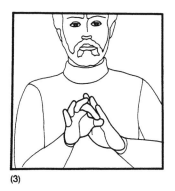

(3)

PLAQUE

In medicine, a small, flat, abnormal area or patch on the body, usually diseased. A plaque can form on the inside of arteries and interfere with circulation, as in arteriosclerosis. In dentistry, a sticky combination of bacteria formed on teeth.

Dental plaque, which helps to cause cavities and gum disease, can be prevented by flossing and brushing the teeth daily.

PLASMA

The thin and clear, or slightly yellow, liquid part of blood and lymph. The red and white blood cells float in the plasma. It carries materials like gases, glucose, proteins, fats, minerals, hormones, vitamins and antibodies to all parts of the body and also carries wastes away.

Blood serum is plasma with the proteins and substances needed for clotting removed.

(1) Sign BLOOD — the left "five" hand is at chest level with the palm toward the body. The palm of the right "five" hand is toward the body with the middle fingertips touching the mouth. Move the right hand down the back of the left hand. Wiggle the fingers of the eight hand as it moves.

* This movement should be short, repeated and somewhat restrained.(MM)

(2) Fingerspell "P-L-A-S-M-A".

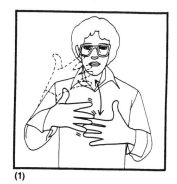

(1)

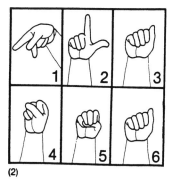

(2)

463

PLASTER OF PARIS

A powder mixed with water to make a thick paste which becomes hard very quickly, used to make casts.

*Often, **plaster of paris** is put on bandages which are dipped in water and then wrapped around a part with a broken bone, to make a cast.*

PLASTIC SURGERY

An operation to repair damage to someone's body or correct a deformity. Sometimes bone, skin or other tissue is taken from another part of the person's body and used to repair the damaged part.

*Cosmetic surgery is a kind of **plastic surgery** done to make someone look better.*

PLATE

A flat substance or part.

*In dentistry, a **plate** is a structure which holds false teeth, a denture.*

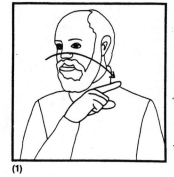

(1) Sign FALSE — the right "one" hand faces left and brushes past the nose.(SM)
(2) Sign TEETH — the right index finger moves from left to right on the teeth.(SM)
(3) The thumb of the right "A" hand moves up to touch the roof of the mouth.(SM)

(1)

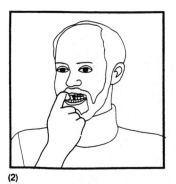
(2)

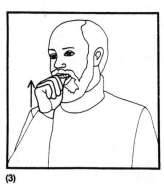
(3)

PLATELETS

Very small, round disks found in blood which are important in forming clots and stopping bleeding. Platelets are smaller than red blood cells, they don't have hemoglobin in them and they are made by special cells in bone marrow.

*When there is an injury to a blood vessel, **platelets** will be attracted to the area, stick to each other and to the edges of the wound and form a plug to stop the blood flow.*

PLEURISY

Inflammation of the thin membrane covering the outside of the lungs, the inside of the chest and the top of the diaphragm. There are several different kinds of pleurisy but the symptoms are usually a temperature, painful breathing and maybe a collection of pus, blood or clear fluid in the chest. Pleurisy may be caused by an ordinary cold, pneumonia or tuberculosis.

When someone has pleurisy, rest is very important and the person should not move much or do anything that will increase breathing.

PNEUMONIA

An infection in the lungs caused by a virus, bacteria, fungus or chemical irritating the lungs. Several different types of bacteria and viruses can cause pneumonia; pneumococci, staphylococci, streptococci or bacilli. The most common symptoms of pneumonia are a high fever, chest pain, a cough which brings up blood or pus, vomiting and weakness. The infection or irritation in the lungs causes blood and fluids to pour out from the tissues, which takes up lung space, making it hard to get air into the lungs and oxygen into the blood. Because of this, the person must often be given oxygen. A person with pneumonia is given antibiotics to kill the bacteria causing it, or if it is caused by something other than bacteria, the antibiotics will prevent bacteria from infecting the lungs and making the disease worse. Depending on the cause of the pneumonia, some of the antibiotics used are penicillin, sulfa drugs, erythromycin and tetracycline.

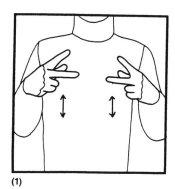
(1)

Pneumonia often attacks people, especially older people or very young children, when they are weak from fighting off another disease such as a cold, strep throat, flu or tuberculosis.

(1) Both "P" hands face in and move from chest level down.(SM)

465

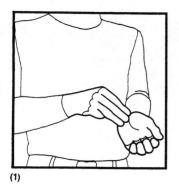
(1)

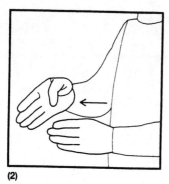
(2)

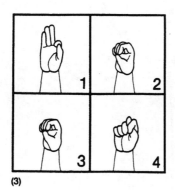
(3)

PODIATRIST

A doctor who treats foot disorders; also called a chiropodist.

A person usually sees a podiatrist for problems like bunions, corns, fallen arches and toenail problems.

(1) Sign DOCTOR — the right "M" hand touches the left inside wrist.(MM)

(2) Sign SPECIALIZE — the left "B" hand faces right at chest level. The right "B" hand faces left on top of the left hand. Move the right hand straight out on the left index finger.(SM)

(3) Fingerspell "F-O-O-T".

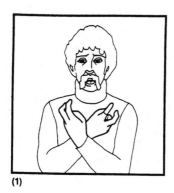
(1)

POISON

A substance which, when is taken into the body in some way, will cause damage, stop normal body activities or cause death. Almost anything taken into the body in large enough amounts can act as a poison.

People don't think of aspirin as a poison but this drug, taken in large amounts, kills more children every year than any other dangerous substance.

(1) Both bent "V" hands cross at the wrists and face in at chest level.(SM)

POISONING

The result of taking in a substance that will harm the body.

In a case of poisoning, a doctor or poison control center should be contacted immediately and the poison container should be kept to help identify the poison.

POISON IVY OR OAK

Climbing, vine-like plants (Ivy - Rhus toxicodendron, Oak - Rhus radicans or diversiloba) both containing an extremely irritating oily substance (urushiol). When poison ivy or oak are touched, they cause a severe skin reaction or form of dermatitis. Symptoms can occur from after a few hours to several days, depending on the skin's condition and how sensitive it is.

Touching poison ivy or poison oak can cause itching or burning, followed by small blisters that break and release serum or pus, and later crust over.

(1) Sign PLANT — the left "O" hand faces in at chest level. The right "flat-O" hand moves up through the left fist ending in "five" hand.(MM)
(2) Sign POISON — both bent "V" hands cross at the wrists and face in at chest level.(SM)

   a. (3) Fingerspell "I-V-Y".
   b. (3) Fingerspell "O-A-K".

* Sign PLANT and POISON, then fingerspell "I-V-Y" or "O-A-K", whichever applies.

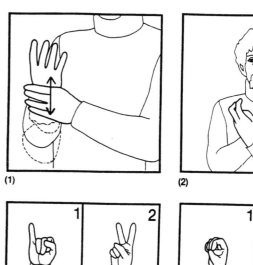
(1)   (2)

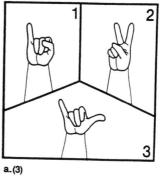
a.(3)

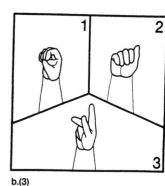
b.(3)

POLIO

See POLIOMYELITIS

POLIOMYELITIS

A severe infectious disease usually affecting children, caused by a virus which may affect several parts of the body; also called polio or infantile paralysis. Symptoms of poliomyelitis may include a fever, headache, sore throat, stiff neck, upset stomach and possible paralysis of one or more muscles. Severe forms of poliomyelitis (acute anterior or bulbar) can affect parts of the spinal cord and cause a person to be unable to swallow, become paralyzed and have respiratory failure, leading to death.

There is a very effective oral vaccine to prevent poliomyelitis, and babies should start getting the vaccine at two months of age, before starting school and every two to three years after that.

POLLEN

A powder made up of very tiny pieces of materials which comes from the male part of flowers. A pollen grain is needed to fertilize the egg cell so a seed will form.

Pollen carried by the wind may be inhaled by a person who is allergic to the pollen, causing hay fever.

467

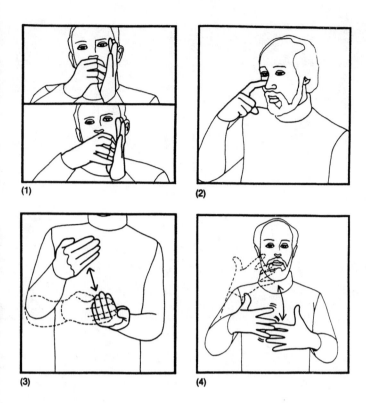

(1)

(2)

(3)

(4)

POLYP

A tumor that easily bleeds and is commonly found in organs such as the nose, uterus and rectum.

A polyp should be checked to see if it is malignant and if so, should be removed surgically.

(1) Sign GROWTH — the left "flat" hand faces right at shoulder level. The right "claw" hand faces left against the left palm. Open the right hand fingers a little.(SM)

(2) The right index finger points to the nose.(SM)

* Point to the appropriate location of the polyp.

(3) Sign EASY — the left cupped "flat" hand faces up at chest level. The fingertips of the right cupped "flat" hand brush up the fingers of the left hand twice.(DM)

(4) Sign BLEED — the left "five" hand is at chest level with the palm towards the body. The palm of the right "five" hand is towards the body with the middle fingertips touching the mouth. Move the right hand down the back of the left hand. Wiggle the fingers of the right hand as it moves.(SM)

* This movement should be longer and slower.

PONS

A part of the brain found on the lower front part of the brain just above the medulla oblongata. The pons connects different parts of the brain to each other and helps control breathing and some muscles. *See Figure 18*

POPLITEAL ARTERY

The large artery behind the knee region which carries fresh blood to the lower leg. The femoral artery becomes the popliteal artery in the knee region. *See Figure 6*

PORCELAIN

A hard, glass-like tooth-colored material used to make artificial teeth. Porcelain is made up of special clays and other materials heated to very high temperatures.

Crowns made of porcelain are usually used on front teeth, while gold and silver crowns are put on back teeth.

PORE

A very tiny opening on the skin which is the outlet of a sweat gland.

*A **pore** has very tiny muscles around it which allow it to become smaller in the cold and open up in the heat.*

POSITION

The place a thing is put into or the way something is arranged.

*In an accident, if a person's body or part of the body is in an unnatural or strange **position**, the person should be handled carefully because there may be broken bones or dislocations.*

POSITIVE

In medicine, the term used for the results of a test in which a substance being checked for is found in a sample.

*If a pregnancy test turns out **positive**, it means the woman is pregnant.*

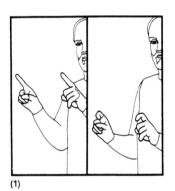
(1)

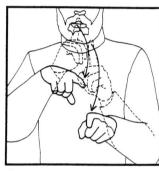
(2)

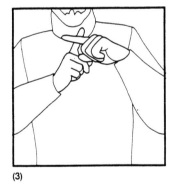
(3)

(1) Sign TEST — both "one" hands face out at chest level, pointing up. Move both hands down and at the same time, bend and straighten both index fingers. Repeat this movement three times until the hands end at waist level. (MM)
(2) Sign RESULTS — both "one" hands face each other with the fingers pointing up and the right index finger touching the mouth. Drop both hands down so the palms are facing down.(SM)
(3) Sign POSITIVE — the index fingers of both "one" hands cross at chest level.(SM)

POSTERIOR

Referring to a structure or thing at the back or towards the rear of something. The kidneys are in the posterior part of the abdominal cavity. *See Figure 3*

POSTERIOR TIBIAL ARTERY

A large artery in the back of the lower leg which carries fresh blood to the foot. The popliteal artery branches below the knee to form the posterior and anterior tibial arteries. *See Figure 6*

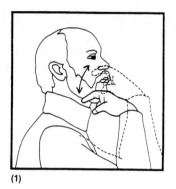
(1)

POSTNASAL DRIP

Constant dripping of mucus made by the sinuses down the back of the throat instead of out the nose. Postnasal drip may be caused by allergies, a sinus infection, cold and damp climates or smoking.

Postnasal drip may cause a cough.

(1) The right "X" hand moves down several times on the right side of the head.(MM)

POSTURAL DRAINAGE

Draining fluids or other materials from the lungs or airways by having a person get in positions which will allow the material to flow out. Postural drainage will make a person cough.

Postural drainage may be used if a person has problems breathing because of pneumonia, bronchitis, whooping cough and some other lung infections.

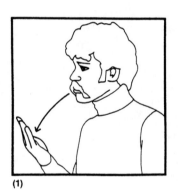
(1)

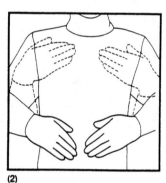
(2)

POSTURE

The position of the body.

To have good posture a person must stand straight, draw in the abdomen, square the shoulders, keep the chin in and keep the weight even on the feet.

(1) Sign GOOD — the right "flat" hand faces in with the fingers touching the mouth and moves out and down forward.(SM)

(2) Sign BODY — both "flat" hands face in. The fingertips of both hands touch the chest and then the stomach.(SM)

* The body should be straight while signing BODY.

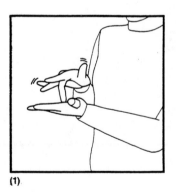
(1)

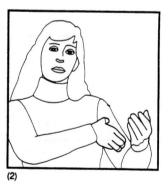
(2)

POTENCY

The strength or power of something; also the ability of a male to perform sexual intercourse.

Two people given a drug of the same potency may be affected by it in different ways because their bodies may use the drug differently.

(1) Sign MEDICINE — the left "flat" hand faces up at chest level. The middle finger of the right "eight" hand touches the left palm and the hand pivots slightly from left to right.(DM)

(2) Sign STRENGTH — the left arm is slightly bent at the elbow. The right "C" hand touches the left upper arm then the inside elbow.(SM)

POTENTIATE

To increase the strength or action of something.

*When taking a drug, a person should be careful about taking any other drug or chemical because one may **potentiate** the effects of the other, as alcohol and barbiturates.*

(1) Sign STRENGTH — the left arm is slightly bent at the elbow. The right "C" hand touches the left upper arm then the inside elbow.(SM)

(2) Sign INCREASE — the left "H" hand faces down at chest level. The right "H" hand faces up at chest level.   Move the right hand up and over in an arch ending on top of the fingers of the left hand.(SM)

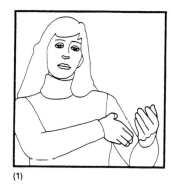
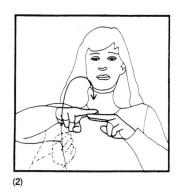

POTION

A liquid dose of medicine or poison.

In medicine today, the term "potion" is rarely used.

(1) Sign MEDICINE — the left "flat" hand faces up at chest level. The middle finger of the right "eight" hand touches the left palm and the hand pivots slightly from left to right.(DM)

(2) Sign SMALL DRINK — the thumb and index finger of the right fist from a small "C". The hand faces left and moves towards the mouth as if drinking a small amount.(SM)

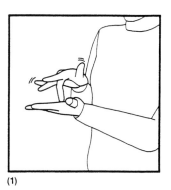
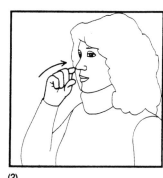

POULTICE

A soft, moist mass made from some material mixed with water and wrapped in a cloth. A poultice is usually hot and is applied to a part of the body to relieve pain and help circulation in the area.

*A **poultice** may be made from bread, mustard, clay, linseed, or herbs.*

(1) Both "one" hands outline the shape of a packing.
(2) Both "flat" hands face in with the left hand on top of the right hand.

* This can be signed on any area.

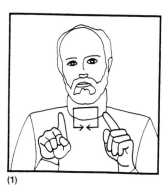
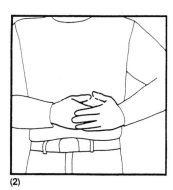

POX

A contagious disease causing eruptive sores containing pus.

*Examples of **pox** are chickenpox and smallpox.*

(Continued on next page)

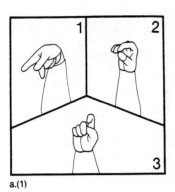

a.(1)

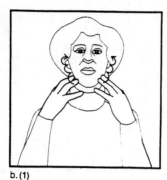

b.(1)

a. (1) Fingerspell "P-O-X"
b. (1) Both "five" hands move up the sides of the face several times.(MM)

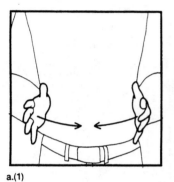

a.(1)

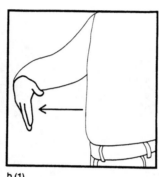

b.(1)

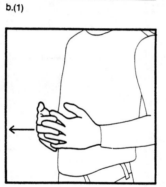

c.(1)

PREGNANCY

The time in which a woman is carrying a developing baby in her uterus. Some of the changes in a woman's body during pregnancy are stopping of menstruation, perhaps nausea, darkening of the nipples and enlarging of the abdomen as the baby grows. Pregnancy lasts about 280 days in humans.

Pregnancy can be very hard on a woman's body so she should take good care of herself, eat correctly and see an obstetrician to make sure she and her baby stay in good health.

a. (1) Sign CONCEIVE — both "five" hands face each other at the sides. Move both hands in ending with the fingers interlocking.(SM)
b. (1) Both "five" hands mesh together at waist level. Move both hands out forward from the body as if showing the stomach growing.(SM)
c. (1) The right "flat" hand faces the body and moves straight out forward.(SM)

PREMATURE

Happening before the usual or normal time.

The more premature a baby is, the less likely it is to survive.

(1) Sign BABY — the right hand and forearm face up, resting on the left hand and forearm which also face upwards. Both are then rocked back and forth as if holding a baby.(SM)

(2) Sign DELIVER — the left "flat" hand faces in at chest level. The right "flat" hand faces in behind the left hand. Move the right hand down under the left hand then out forward. (SM)

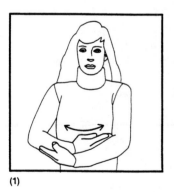

(1)

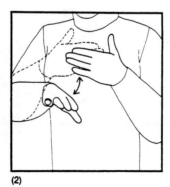

(2)

(Continued on next page)

472

(3) Sign EARLY — the left "flat" hand touches the right inside elbow. The right "flat" hand faces up.
(4) Sign NOT YET — the right "flat" hand faces back and moves back from the body. (SM)
(5) Sign FULL — the left "S" hand faces down at chest level. The right "flat" hand faces down and brushes out on the left fist. (SM)
(6) Sign DEVELOP — the left "flat" hand faces right at chest level. The right "D" hand touches the bottom then top of the left palm. (SM)

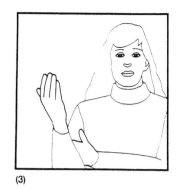
(3)

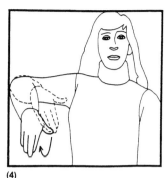
(4)

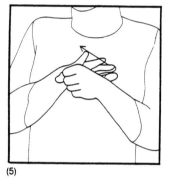
(5)

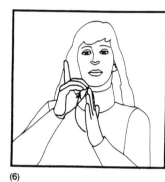
(6)

PREMENSTRUAL TENSION

A condition happening usually one week to 10 days before menstruation and ending after the menstrual flow begins.

Premenstrual tension may include nervousness, mood changes and grumpiness, headaches and maybe depression.

PREMOLAR

See BICUSPID

PRENATAL CARE

The care given to a woman during pregnancy. Prenatal care includes regular examinations to check her weight, blood pressure, changes in the size of her uterus and the condition of the baby.

Good prenatal care can include a woman's seeing a doctor regularly, taking good care of herself, not smoking, not drinking a lot of alcohol and checking with her doctor before taking any drugs.

(1) Sign PREGNANT — both "five" hands face in at the stomach with the fingers meshed together. Move both hands out forward as if showing the stomach growing. (SM)

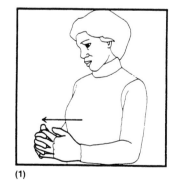
(1)

(Continued on next page)

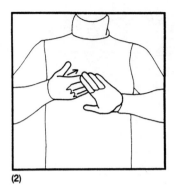
(2)

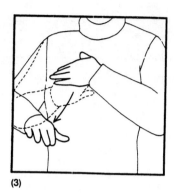
(3)

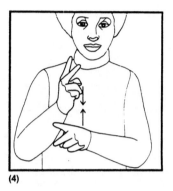
(4)

(2) Sign BEFORE — the left "flat" hand faces out at chest level. The right "flat" hand faces in with the fingers touching. Move the right hand back towards the body. (SM)

(3) Sign BIRTH — the left "flat" hand faces in at chest level. The right "flat" hand faces in behind the left hand and moves down under the left hand then out forward. (SM)

(4) Sign CARE — the right "K" hand faces left and the left "K" hand faces right, both at chest level. Tap the hands together a few times. (MM)

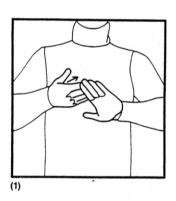
(1)

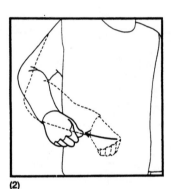
(2)

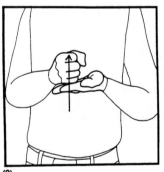
(3)

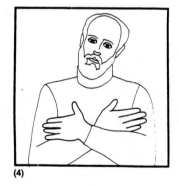
(4)

PREOPERATIVE SEDATIVE

A calming, tranquilizing substance given before any surgery.

> *Preoperative sedatives can be in the form of local or general anesthetics, nitrous oxide gas, or enemas.*

(1) Sign BEFORE — the left "flat" hand faces out at chest level. The right "flat" hand faces in with the fingers touching. Move the right hand back towards the body.(SM)

(2) Sign OPERATE — the right "A" hand faces in at waist level. Move the hand right across the stomach as if cutting.(SM)

(3) Sign HELP — the left "flat" hand faces up at waist level. The right "S" hand faces left on the left palm. Move both hands up to chest level.(SM)

(4) Sign RELAX — both "flat" hands cross on the chest.(SM)

* *The type of sedative used should be signed first if known such as gas, an injection or oral medication.*

PREPUCE
See FORESKIN

PRESBYOPIA

A problem with vision that usually comes on between 40 and 45 years of age; farsightedness. In presbyopia, a person will see things which are far away more clearly than things which are close.

Presbyopia is caused by the lens of the eye becoming less flexible making it hard to focus on things which are close.

(1) Sign EYES — the right index finger points to both eyes.(SM)
(2) Sign DETERIORATE — both "A" hands with thumbs extended up, face in at chest level. Move both hands down the sides in wavy motions.(SM)
(3) Sign CAN'T — the left "one" hand is palm down at waist level. The right index finger strikes the left index finger.(SM)
(4) Sign SEE — the right "V" hand faces in and moves from the eyes out forward.(SM)
(5) The right "flat" hand faces in and moves in towards the eyes. (SM)

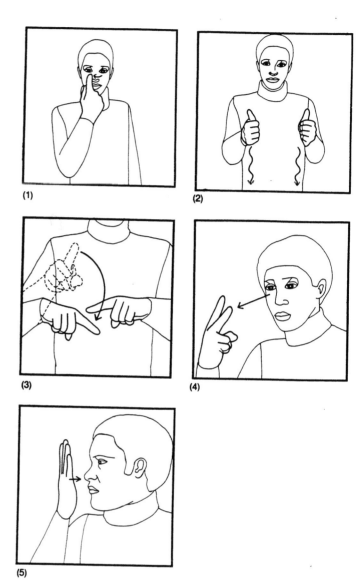

(1)   (2)   (3)   (4)   (5)

PRESCRIBE

To give directions for taking a medicine or treatment to a person to cure a disease or injury.

*A doctor may **prescribe** an antibiotic if a person has a virus-caused illness like influenza.*

(1) Both "one" hands face each other with the fingers pointing up and the right index finger touching the mouth. Drop both hands down so the palms are facing down.(SM)
(2) Sign MEDICINE — the left "flat" hand faces up at chest level. The middle finger of the right "eight" hand touches the left palm and the hand pivots slightly from left to right.(DM)

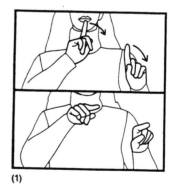

(1)

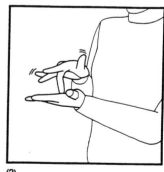

(2)

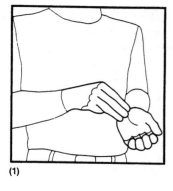
(1)

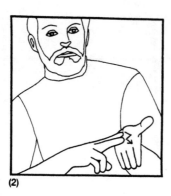
(2)

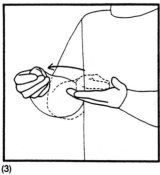
(3)

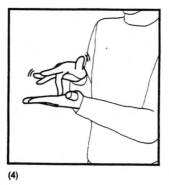
(4)

PRESCRIPTION

Written instruction given to a person by a doctor to buy a certain drug. A prescription, signed by a doctor, is needed to get a drug from a drugstore or pharmacy. When someone gets a prescription for a drug, the person should know exactly why the drug is being prescribed and what it will do; they should know the name of the drug including the possible side effects of the drug and what effects other drugs the person may be taking will have on the new drug.

A person should never use another person's prescription because it may affect them differently.

(1) Sign DOCTOR — the right "M" hand taps the left inside wrist twice. (DM)
(2) The fingertips of the right "U" hand moves down the left "flat" palm as if imitating writing on it. (SM)
(3) Sign BUY — the left "flat" hand faces up at chest level. The right "flat-O" hand faces up in the left palm and moves out forward. (SM)
(4) Sign MEDICINE — teh left "flat" hand faces up at chest level. The middle finger of the right "eight" hand touches the left palm and pivots slightly from left to right a few times. (MM)

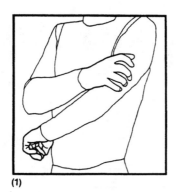
(1)

PRESSURE

A continuous force or pushing against something.

Direct pressure over a wound with a hand or bandage will slow bleeding.

(1) The right hand grabs the left upper arm as if applying pressure to it.(SM)

* This can be signed on any area that pressure is being applied.

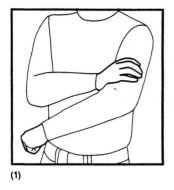
(1)

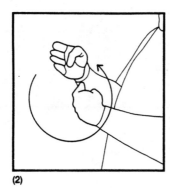
(2)

PRESSURE BANDAGE

A bandage used to apply pressure to a wound to stop bleeding.

A pressure bandage is used to press the bleeding vessels against bone or uninjured tissues, which will help control bleeding.

(1) Sign PRESSURE — the right hand grabs the left upper arm as if applying pressure to it.(SM)

* This can be signed at the area where pressure is being applied.

(2) Sign BANDAGE — the right "B" hand circles around the left "B" hand in front of the body. The right hand fingers point left and the left hand fingers point right.(MM)

* This can be signed at the area where the bandage is being applied.

476

PRESSURE POINT

Areas of the body which can be pressed on to stop bleeding. Major pressure points are temporal, facial, radial, ulnar, iliac, femoral, popliteal, and the anterior and posterior tibial arteries.

Pressure points are areas where an artery passes over a bone or hard area and by pressing there, blood flow through the artery is cut off, slowing bleeding.

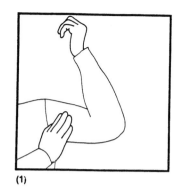
(1)

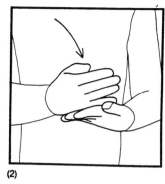
(2)

(1) The fingertips of the right "flat" hand press on the left upper arm.(SM)

* This can be signed at the area of the wound or injury.

(2) Sign STOP — the left "flat" hand is palm up at chest level. The right "flat" hand faces left and moves down to sharply hit the left palm.(SM)

(3) Sign BLEED — the left "five" hand is at chest level with the palm towards the body. The palm of the right "five" hand is towards the body with the middle fingertips touching the mouth. Move the right hand down the back of the left hand. Wiggle the fingers of the right hand as if it moves.(SM)

* This movement should be longer and slower.

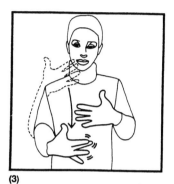
(3)

PREVENT

To keep someone from doing something; to keep from happening.

A good way to help prevent lung disease is to not smoke.

(1) Both "flat" hands cross at chest level and move out forward.(SM)

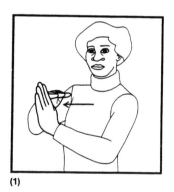
(1)

PREVENTIVE MEDICINE

The area of medicine which tries to prevent mental or physical diseases.

Education, exercise, nutrition, stress, and vaccinations are some things that preventive medicine are concerned with.

PRICKLY HEAT

The formation of small red bumps on the skin which itch and tingle.

Prickly heat is usually seen in hot weather and is caused by inflammation of the skin around sweat glands.

PRIMARY LESION

The first or original lesion from which a second one occurs.

Examples of primary lesions are lesions from syphilis or a chancre.

PROBE

A blunt, thin instrument used to find out the depth and direction of a wound or cavity in the body.

A doctor will use a probe to gently push around in a wound to see how much damage has been done.

PROBLEM

Referring to a difficult situation or person.

A person with mental problems may not be able to deal with other people or situations.

a. (1) Sign DIFFICULTY — the fingers of both "V" hands are bent and touching knuckles to knuckles. The left palm is up and the right palm is down. Twist the hands so that the palms face the opposite directions as from the beginning. (MM)

b. (1) Sign DIFFICULTY — the fingers of both "V" hands are bent with the palms facing in. The right hand is at chest level and the left hand is at waist level. Hit the knuckles together while changing the levels of the hands.(MM)

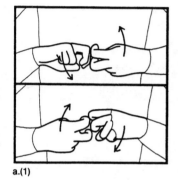
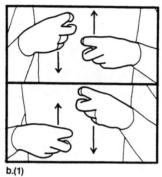

a.(1)   b.(1)

PROCAINE

A drug which acts as an anesthetic to prevent pain in an area. Procaine is sold under the name of Novocaine®.

Dentists often inject procaine into the gums to deaden nerves and prevent pain.

(1) Sign INJECT — the right "L" hand faces in with the index finger touching the side of the mouth. Move the thumb in as if injecting someting into the mouth.(SM)

(2) Sign FREEZE — both "five" hands face down at chest level. Move both hands up slightly ending in "claw" hands.(SM)

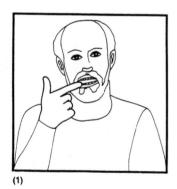
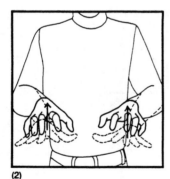

(1)   (2)

PROCESS

In medicine, a structure that sticks out from or grows out of a part. "Process" is most often used for a part of a bone that sticks out from the rest of the bone.

The scapula or shoulder blade has two processes on it, one of which attaches to the clavicle or collarbone.

PROCTOSCOPE

An instrument used to examine the rectum.

If there is pain or bleeding in the rectum, a doctor will use a proctoscope to see if there is any illness or injury.

PROGESTERONE

A hormone made in a woman's ovaries or the placenta. Progesterone helps cause the monthly changes in the uterus which help it get ready to receive a fertilized egg; progesterone also helps in the development of the breasts.

Progesterone, very important in keeping a pregnancy going, may be used to prevent miscarriages and to treat some menstrual problems.

PROGNOSIS

The results or the outcome of a disease or illness.

A doctor's prognosis may include the possible course of a disease, the length of the illness and what condition it will leave a person in.

(1) Sign DOCTOR — the right "M" hand touches the left inside wrist.(SM)

(2) The right "flat" hand faces out and moves out slightly.(SM)

(3) Sign OPINION — the right "O" hand faces out at the right side of the head and shakes a little.

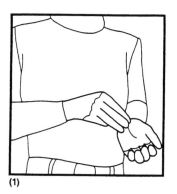
(1)

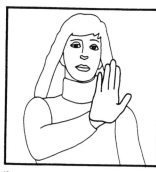
(2)

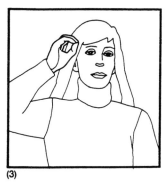
(3)

PROGRESSIVE

Going on or advancing.

A progressive disease would be one which goes from bad to worse.

(Continued on next page)

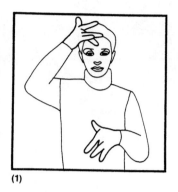
(1)

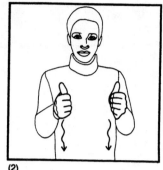
(2)

(1) Sign DISEASE — the middle finger of the right "eight" hand touches the forehead and the middle finger of the left "eight" hand touches the stomach. (SM)

(2) Sign DETERIORATE — both "A" hands with thumbs extended up, face in at chest level. Move both hands down the sides in wavy motions.(SM)

PROLAPSE

The movement of an organ or inner part of the body from its usual position by dropping down or out of the body.

The most common kinds of prolapse are of the vagina, where the organs may be seen pushing out through the vaginal opening, or of the rectum, where they push out through the anus.

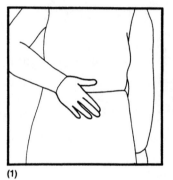
(1)

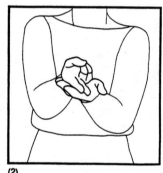
(2)

PRONE

Lying flat on one's stomach, with the face downward.

Prone is the opposite of supine.

(1) Sign STOMACH — the right "flat" hand touches the stomach area.(SM)

(2) Sign LIE DOWN — the left "flat" hand faces up at chest level and the right "H" hand faces up on the left palm.

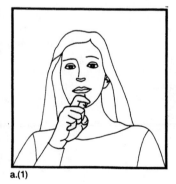
a.(1)

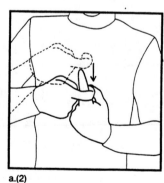
a.(2)

PROPHYLACTIC

A substance or device used to prevent disease, especially a rubber sheath used during sexual intercourse to prevent venereal disease.

The condom or "rubber" is both a contraceptive and a prophylactic.

a. (1) Sign RUBBER — the right "X" hand is at the right side of the face, palm out. Tap the chin downward twice.(MM)

(2) The left "one" hand faces in at chest level with the index finger pointing up. The right "X" hand hooks down over the left finger.(SM)

(Continued on next page)

b. (1) Sign RUBBER — the right "X" hand is at the right side of the face, palm out. Tap the face downward twice.(DM)

* *This can also be signed by tapping the chin downward twice.*

(2) The left "one" hand faces in at chest level with the index finger pointing up. The right "one" hand faces out behind the left hand. Move the right index finger up and over the left index finger.(SM)

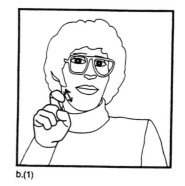

b.(1)

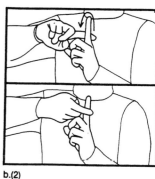

b.(2)

PROPHYLAXIS

Following certain rules in order to prevent disease. In dentistry, cleaning the surface of the teeth.

*When we go to a dentist for a **prophylaxis**, he will polish the surface of the teeth to remove material that brushing and flossing can't get off.*

(1) Sign SPECIALIZE — the left "B" hand faces right at chest level. The right "B" hand faces left on top of the left hand. Move the right hand straight out on the left index finger.(SM)

(2) Sign CLEAN — the left "flat" hand is face up at chest level. The right "flat" hand brushes across the palm of the left hand to the fingertips.(SM)

(3) Sign TEETH — the index finger of the right "one" hand brushes up and down the teeth.(MM)

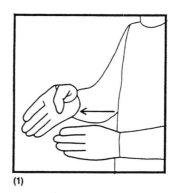

(1)

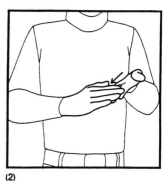

(2)

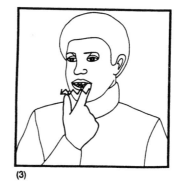

(3)

PROSTATE

A gland found in men which surrounds the lower bladder and beginning of the urethra. The prostate gland makes a milky fluid which is put into the urethra during ejaculation and helps to make up the semen. The prostate may become inflamed in infections of the urinary tract, such as gonorrhea. After middle age, the prostate may become enlarged, making it difficult to urinate. *See Figure 13*

(1) Fingerspell "P-R-O-S-T-A-T-E G-L-A-N-D"

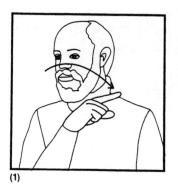
(1)

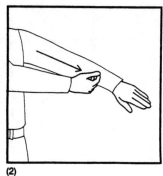
(2)

PROSTHESIS

An artificial organ or part used to replace a damaged or missing structure or to help a part of the body do its job, such as a hearing aid.

A person who has had an amputation of an arm or leg will usually be fitted with a prosthesis or artificial limb.

(1) Sign FALSE — the right "L" hand faces left and brushes past the nose.(SM)

(2) Sign ARM — the right "flat" hand brushes down the left arm.(SM)

* This is an example. Sign the part referred to.

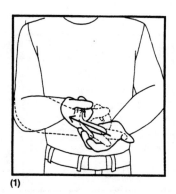
(1)

PROSTRATION

Total exhaustion; extremely weakened.

Prostration could be caused by physical or mental activity.

(1) Sign EXHAUSTED — the left "flat" hand is at waist level with the palm up. The right "V" hand is on top of the left palm, facing up. Move the right hand back towards the body about 2 inches.(SM)

* Facial expression should show exhaustion.

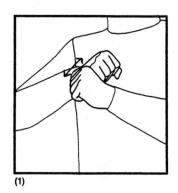
(1)

PROTECT

To keep from harm or injury; to guard or cover.

Wounds should be cleaned and covered with a bandage to protect them from infections.

(1) The right "S" hand is against the left "S" hand at chest level. The palms are down. Move the hands abruptly forward.(SM)

PROTEIN

A group of substances made up mostly of carbon, hydrogen, oxygen and nitrogen arranged in certain ways. Proteins are needed by the body to make new tissue and to repair old and damaged structures. Proteins also provide energy and heat to the body. Proteins are taken into the body in food, broken down in the stomach into amino acids which are absorbed and then rearranged into new proteins.

Some sources of proteins are meats, fish, eggs, cheese, milk and vegetables such as soy beans.

PROTOZOA

A one-celled, microscopic organism; the smallest form of animal life; ameba. A protozoa is asexual (without sex) and reproduces by fission (splitting in half).

*Some diseases which occur from a **protozoa** are malaria, leishmaniasis and amebic dysentary.*

PROTRUDE

To stick out or push out.

*A woman's abdomen will start to **protrude** after about the fifth month in a pregnancy.*

(1) The right "claw" hand is placed at the sight of a protrusion and moves outward slightly.(SM)

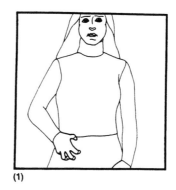

(1)

PSILOCYBIN

A hallucinogenic substance found in certain mushrooms. Psilocybin causes mood changes including extreme anxiety and extreme pleasure; it causes hyper-awareness of colors, body functions and speech; it also causes illusions and delusions, strange behavior, changes in the perception of time and space, and recall of old memories.

*Psychological effects from **psilobybin** may include strong emotional feelings of joy and peace, a feeling of creativity, changes in senses (sounds are seen, ordinary things are beautiful and colors seem to be heard), awareness of religion, feelings of oneness with the world, and extreme self-awareness.*

(1) Sign MUSHROOM — the left "one" hand points up at chest level and the right "claw" hand faces down on the left index finger.(SM)

(2) Sign EAT — the fingertips of the right "flat-O" hand tap the mouth a few times. (MM)

(3) The index finger of the right "one" hand touches the forehead and moves out forward ending with the index finger and thumb touching.(SM)

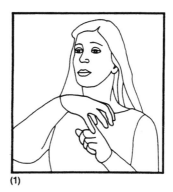

(1)

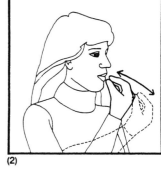

(2)

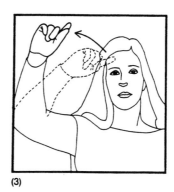

(3)

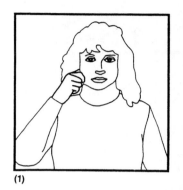
(1)

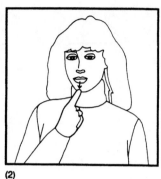
(2)

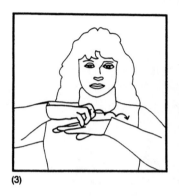
(3)

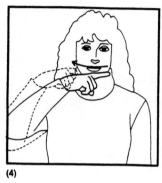
(4)

PSORIASIS

A non-contagious skin irritation which usually lasts a long time. Symptoms of psoriasis are red bumps and patches with a dry, scaly surface. The bumps can be on any part of the body, but the knees and elbows are the usual sites.

Although the cause of psoriasis is unknown and there is no cure, there are treatments to control the disease and make the person more comfortable.

(1) Sign SKIN — the right index finger and thumb pinch the right cheek.(SM)
(2) Sign RED — the index finger of the right "one" hand brushes down the chin a few times.(DM)
(3) The fingertips of the right "claw" hand move up the back of the left "flat" hand.(MM)
(4) Sign DRY — the right "one" hand points to the left under the mouth, palm down. Move the hand to the right ending in a "X" hand.(SM)

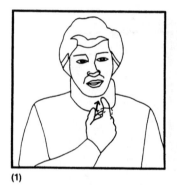
(1)

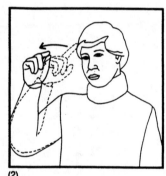
(2)

PSYCHEDELIC

Referring to hallucinogenic drugs which make a person's mind wander and cause him to hear, see, taste, feel and smell things that are not there.

LSD and mescaline are examples of psychedelics.

(1) Sign PILL — the thumb and index finger of the right hand touch, the palm faces the mouth. Flick the index finger towards the mouth as if popping a pill into the mouth.(SM)
(2) Sign MIND FADE — the index finger of the right "one" hand touches the forehead and moves out forward ending with the index finger and thumb touching.(SM)

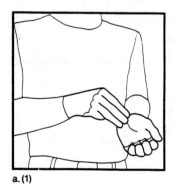
a.(1)

PSYCHIATRIST

A doctor who specializes in studying, preventing and treating mental or emotional diseases. A psychiatrist is a physician who has had several years of special training in his field and also a doctor's usual training.

A psychiatrist can prescribe drugs, do surgery and counsel people.

a. (1) Sign DOCTOR — the right "M" hand touches the left inside wrist. (DM)

(Continued on next page)

PSYCHIATRIST, *continued*

a. (2) Sign SPECIALIZE — the left "B" hand faces right at chest level. The right "B" hand faces left on top of the left hand. Move the right hand straight out on the left index finger. (SM)
(3) Sign MIND — the right index finger touches the forehead.
(4) Sign ANALYZE — both "bent-V" hands face down at chest level. Drop both hands down slightly and at the same time, move the hands down to waist level. (MM)

b. (1) The middle finger of the right "P" hand taps the left inside wrist. (DM)

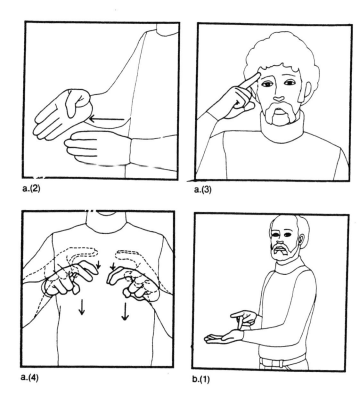

a.(2)   a.(3)

a.(4)   b.(1)

PSYCHIATRY

The area of medicine which studies, prevents and treats mental or emotional diseases.

Psychiatry studies phobias such as acrophobia (fear of heights) and claustrophobia (fear of being in small places).

a. (1) Sign SPECIALIZE — the left "B" hand faces right at chest level. The right "B" hand faces left on top of the left hand. Move the right hand straight out on the left index finger. (SM)
(2) Sign MIND — the right index finger touches the forehead. (SM)
(3) Sign ANALYZE — both "bent-V" hands face down at chest level. Drop both hands down slightly and at the same time, move both hands down to waist level. (MM)

b. (1) Sign SPECIALIZE — the left "B" hand faces right at chest level. The right "B" hand faces left on top of the left hand. Move the right hand straight out on the left index finger. (SM)

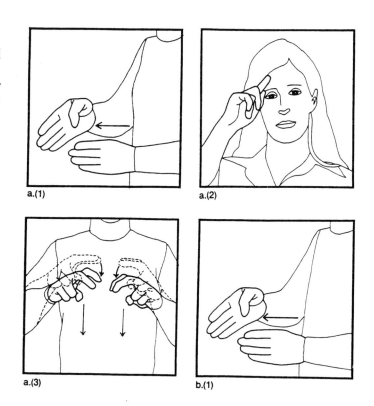

a.(1)   a.(2)

a.(3)   b.(1)

(Continued on next page)

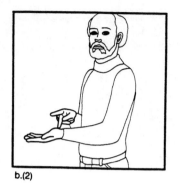

b.(2)

b. (2) The middle finger of the right "P" hand taps the left inside wrist. (DM)

PSYCHOANALYSIS

A way of curing mental problems by having a person remember past emotional experiences; often called analysis. In psychoanalysis, it is thought that abnormal emotions and behavior are caused by a person's refusing to remember or recognize painful experiences. These experiences have been apparently forgotten but they are still in the mind and have an effect on the unconscious, causing dreams, slips of the tongue, tension, anger and other problems.

By making a person aware of a problem, the cause of it and how he is expressing the problem, psychoanalysis can lessen or get rid of mental or emotional problems.

PSYCHOLOGIST

A person who studies normal and abnormal mental activities and how they affect a person's total behavior.

An animals' psychologist is one who studies animal's behaviors.

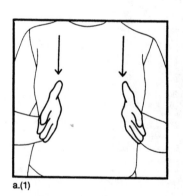

a.(1)

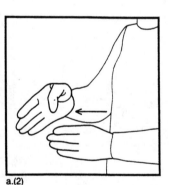

a.(2)

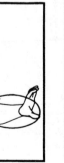

a.(3)

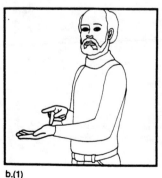

b.(1)

a. (1) Sign PERSON — both "flat" fhands face each other at chest level. Move both hands straight down to waist level. (SM)
(2) Sign SPECIALIZE — the left "flat" hand faces right at chest level. The right "flat" hand faces left on top of the left hand. Move the right hand straight out on the left index finger. (SM)
(3) Sign BEHAVIOR — both "C" hands face out at chest level. At the same time, the left hand moves in counterclockwise circles and the right hand moves in clockwise circles a few times. (MM)
b. (1) The middle finger of the right "P" hand taps the left inside wrist. (DM)

b. (2) Sign PERSON — both "flat" hands face each other at chest level. Move both hands down to waist level. (SM)

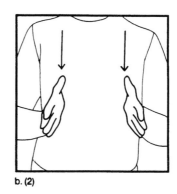

b. (2)

PSYCHOLOGY

The science that studies emotions and mental activities and how they affect behavior.

There are several different types of psychology; each has its own theory to explain people's behavior.

(1) Sign SPECIALIZE — the left "B" hand faces right at chest level. The right "B" hand faces left on top of the left hand. Move the right hand straight out on the left index finger.(SM)

(2) Sign BEHAVIOR — both "C" hands face out at chest level. At the same time, the left hand moves in counterclockwise circles and the right hand moves in clockwise circles a few times. (MM)

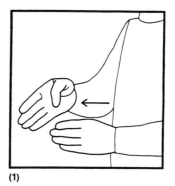

(1)

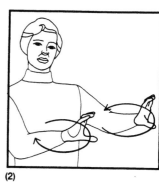

(2)

PSYCHOPATH

A person with a mental disorder causing his personality to change.

A psychopath's behavior is often aggressive against people and things in society.

(1)Sign MIND — the right index finger points to the right temple.(SM)

(2) The left "flat" hand faces up at chest level. The right "flat" hand faces left on the left hand. Move the right hand out along the edge of the left hand and curve left as it follows the shape of the fingers.(SM)

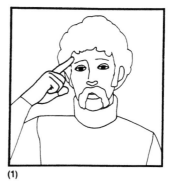

(1)

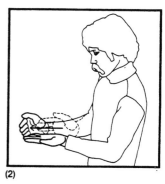

(2)

PSYCHOSIS

A mental disorder in which a person's personality changes a great deal and he loses contact with reality.

A person with psychosis will have delusions, hallucinations and abnormal, antisocial or strange behavior and may have to be hospitalized.

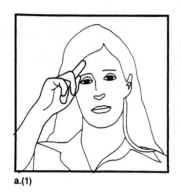
a.(1)

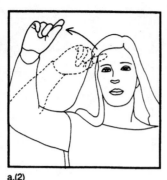
a.(2)

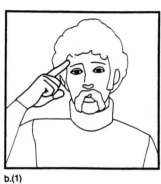
b.(1)

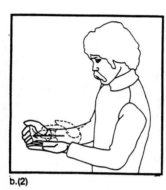
b.(2)

a. (1) Sign MIND — the right index finger touches the forehead. (SM)
(2) The index finger of the right "one" hand touches the forehead and moves out forward ending with the index finger and thumb touching. (SM)
b. (1) Sign MIND — the right index finger touches the forehead. (SM)
(2) The left "flat" hand faces up at chest level. The right "flat" hand faces left on the left hand. Move the right hand out along the edge of the left hand and curve left as it follows the shape of the fingers. (SM)

PSYCHOSOMATIC

Referring to the relationship and effects of mental and body functions. "Psychosomatic" usually refers to symptoms or illnesses that are emotional or in the mind.

*Hypochondriacs often have **psychosomatic** illnesses.*

PSYCHOTIC

A person having a mental disorder, psychosis.

*A **psychotic** person's personality will change greatly and he may lose contact with reality.*

(1) Sign MIND — the right index finger touches the forehead. (SM)
(2) The left "flat" hand faces right at chest level. The right "cupped" hand makes a "S" movement in the left palm. (SM)

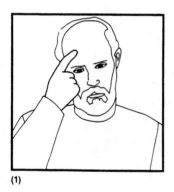
(1)

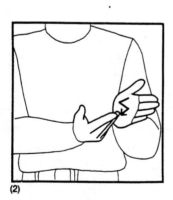
(2)

PTOMAINE POISONING

The old name for food poisoning caused by eating food containing bacteria.

***Ptomaine poisoning** got its name from a poisonous substance called ptomaine made by some bacteria when they break down proteins.*

(Continued on next page)

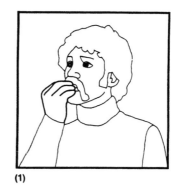
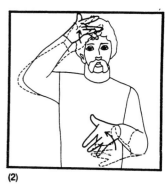

(1) Sign FOOD — the fingers of the right "flat-O" hand touch the mouth a few times.(MM)

(2) Sign SICK — the middle finger of the right "eight" hand touches the forehead and the middle finger of the left "eight" hand touches the stomach. Twist both hands slightly.(SM)

* *The facial expression should show sickness or pain.*

(1)   **(2)**

PUBERTY

The stage of development when a person of either sex becomes able to reproduce.

> *Puberty,* *occuring between the ages of 13-15 in boys and 9-16 in girls, is a time of rapid physical changes.*

PULMONARY

Having to do with the lungs.

> The *pulmonary* arteries and *pulmonary* veins are the large blood vessels which carry blood between the heart and the lungs.

(1) The fingertips of both "flat" hands brush up and down on the chest.(DM)

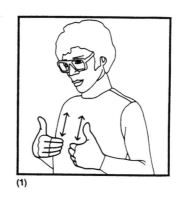

(1)

PULMONARY EDEMA

The collection of serum-like fluids in the airspaces and tissues of the lungs. A person with pulmonary edema will have a lot of difficulty breathing, will cough up a frothy bloody material, they will have cold limbs and be bluish.

> *Pulmonary edema* can be caused by the heart not pumping blood well or by going up to high altitudes quickly and then doing hard work.

PULP

In dentistry, the soft, inner part of a tooth which has blood vessels and nerves running through it. *See Figure 25*

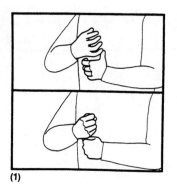
(1)

PULSATION

A regular throbbing or rhythmic beating.

*The heart has regular **pulsations** running through it because of the contraction of the heart muscle, and the large arteries have regular **pulsations** to them because of the movement of blood through them.*

(1) Both "claw" hands face in at chest level, the right hand on top of the left hand. Close both hands to "O" hands a few times. (MM)

* This can be signed at any area where taking a pulse.

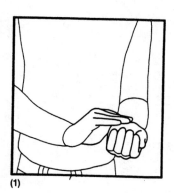
(1)

PULSE

The regular enlargement and shrinking of arteries caused by the movement of blood in them. The pulse rate is the same as the heart rate because as the heart contracts, it pushes a large amount of blood all at once through an artery, causing it to expand. After the contraction ends and the heart is filling, the artery will narrow down a little because the blood flow through it is less. The normal pulse rate in an adult is 70-80 beats per minute.

*There are several places on the body where a large artery is close enough to the surface of the body to take a **pulse**, the most common being in the wrist and in the neck.*

(1) Sign PULSE — the fingertips of the right "flat" hand touch the left inside wrist.(SM)

* This can be signed at any area where taking a pulse.

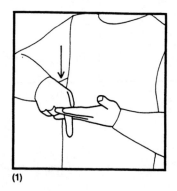
(1)

PUNCTURE

To make a hole in something with a sharp pointed instrument.

*In some conditions, a doctor may **puncture** the spinal membranes around the spinal cord with a needle by going through the back and between two vertebrae to get a sample of cerebrospinal fluid.*

(1) The left "flat" hand faces up at chest level. The index finger of the right "one" hand moves down through the fingers of the left hand as if puncturing it.(SM)

* This can be signed at the area of the puncture.

PUNCTURE WOUND

A deep, narrow wound caused by a sharp object going into the body.

Puncture wounds can easily become infected because they may not bleed much. they are hard to clean and because bacteria may be pushed deep into the body by the object.

(1) Sign PUNCTURE — the left "flat" hand faces up at chest level. The index finger of the right "one" hand moves down through the fingers of the left hand as if puncturing it.(SM)

(2) The right "F" hand faces down and touches the left arm.(SM)

* This can be signed at the area of the wound.

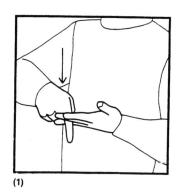 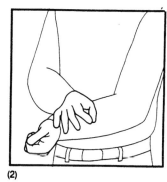

(1) (2)

PUNGENT

Sharp or bitter smelling or tasting.

Pungent medicines which have to be eaten are often put in capsules so they can't be smelled or tasted, or they are disguised with sweet smells or tastes.

(1) Sign SMELL — the right "flat" hand brushes up the nose a few times.(MM)

(2) Sign TASTE — the middle finger of the right hand touches the tongue or chin.(SM)

(3) Both "S" hands face in at chest level. Move both hands down slightly.(SM)

* Facial expression should show bad smells or taste.

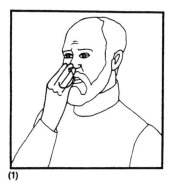 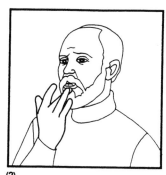

(1) (2)

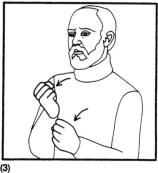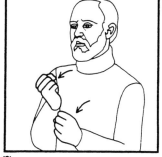

(3)

PUPIL

In medicine, the dark opening in the center of the colored part of the eye which allows light rays into the eyeball, where they strike the retina. The pupil light getting into the eye and it can dilate in dim light to let in as much light as possible.

there isn't much light to let in as much light as possible. *See Figure 21*

(1) Sign BLACK — the index finger of the right "one" hand moves across the forehead from left to right.(SM)

(2) The thumb and index finger of the right "F" hand make a small circle in front of the right eye.(SM)

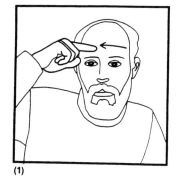 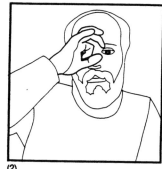

(1) (2)

491

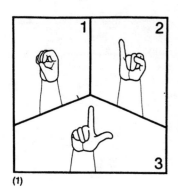

(1)

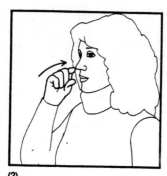

(2)

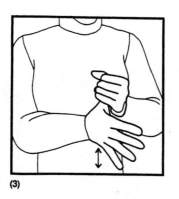

(3)

PURGATIVE

A substance that causes a person to empty the intestines by having a lot of watery bowel movements.

A purgative, such as castor oil or mineral oil, may be used to relieve constipation or to empty the intestinal tract before surgery or X-ray.

(1) Fingerspell "O-I-L"
(2) Sign SMALL DRINK — the index finger and thumb of the right fist form a small "C". The hand faces left and moves towards the mouth as if drinking a small amount.(SM)
(3) Sign DIARRHEA — the left "S" hand faces right at chest level. The thumb of the right "five" hand is in the fist of the left hand, facing left. Move the right hand down from the left hand several times.(MM)

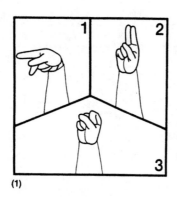

(1)

PURULENT

Containing or producing pus.

Pyorrhea, a gum disease, often causes the gums to become purulent.

(1) Fingerspell "P-U-S"

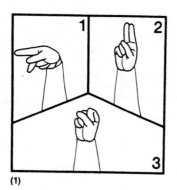

(1)

PUS

A thick, yellowish liquid made in areas of inflammation, made up of serum body cells, bacteria and white blood cells. Pus is made when bacteria get into an area of the body and cause an infection. White blood cells are sent to the area to destroy the bacteria and stop the infection. When white blood cells are also destroyed or damaged, they collect in the area, forming pus.

The presence of pus is a sign of infection, so once it has been drained from the body, it should be gotten rid of carefully because it still contains harmful bacteria which may still cause more infection.

(1) Fingerspell "P-U-S"

492

PUSTULE

A small bump of skin filled with pus or lymph.

Pustules often occur in eczema, dermatitis, syphilis or smallpox.

PYOMETRA

A condition where pus is held in the uterine cavity and can't go out through the cervix.

Pyometra may be caused by a malignancy or an opening that is abnormally closed.

PYORRHEA

A discharge of pus or pus-containing fluids from the gums or area around the teeth; also, infection and inflammation of the gums and the bone around them; periodontal disease.

When the gums are affected with pyorrhea, they will pull back from the teeth, the bone of the teeth may start to be absorbed, the teeth may become loose and fall out, and the breath will smell bad.

(1) Fingerspell "P-U-S."

(2) The right index finger circles the gums.(SM)

(3) Sign INFECTION — the right "I" hand faces out at chest level and shakes slightly from side to side a few times. (MM)

* *Mouth the word "infection" while signing.*

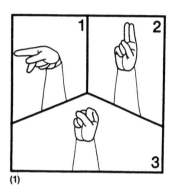
(1)

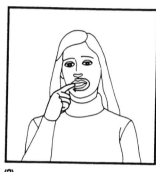
(2)

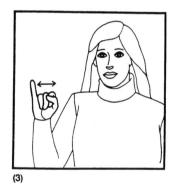
(3)

PYRIDOXINE

See VITAMIN B COMPLEX

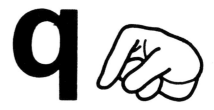

QUAALUDE®

The name under which methoqualone is sold. It is used to calm a person or to help him sleep.
sleep.

Because **quaaludes** *can cause addiction, they shouldn't be taken regularly.*

(1) Sign PILL — the thumb and index finger of the right hand touch, the palm faces the mouth. Flick the index finger towards the mouth as if popping a pill into the mouth.(SM)

(2) Sign DOWNER — the right "A" hand with the thumb pointing down, moves down at shoulder level twice.(DM)

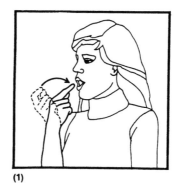

(1)

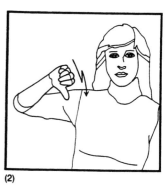

(2)

* This is a general sign for depressants ("downers"). The specific type of drug should also be fingerspelled and all side effects explained.

QUADRICEPS FEMORIS

The large muscle on the front of the thigh, consisting of four muscles: rectus femoris, vastus lateralis, vastus medialis and vastus intermedius. *See Figure 4*

QUADRIPLEGIC

A person whose arms and legs are paralyzed.

A person may become a **quadriplegic** *if the spinal cord is cut, damaged or diseased in the neck region so that the brain doesn't get nerve impulses to the muscles in those areas.*

(1) Sign PERSON — both "flat" hands face each other at chest level. Move both hands straight down ending at waist level.(SM)

(2) Sign ARMS — the right "flat" hand brushes down the left arm and then the left "flat" hand brushes down the right arm. (SM)

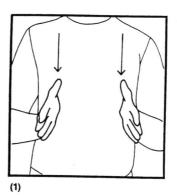

(1)

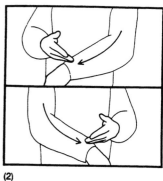

(2)

(Continued on next page)

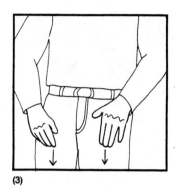

(3)

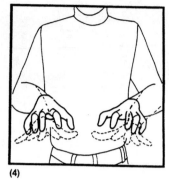

(4)

(3) Sign LEGS — both "flat" hands brush down both legs.(SM)
(4) Sign FREEZE — both "five" hands face down at chest level. Move both hands up slightly ending in "claw" hands.(SM)

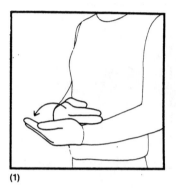

(1)

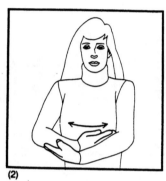

(2)

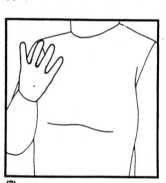

(3)

QUADRUPLETS

Four children given birth to by a woman in one pregnancy.

> *When a woman has quadruplets, it is usually because she has taken a pill to help her become pregnant by allowing the release of several ova all at once, instead of just one.*

(1) Sign BORN — the left "flat" hand faces in at chest level. The right "flat" hand is behind the left hand and moves down and out forward.(SM)
(2) Sign BABY — the right hand and forearm face up, resting on the left hand and forearm which also face upwards. Both are then rocked back and forth as if holding a baby.(SM)
(3) Sign FOUR — the right "four" hand faces in at chest level.

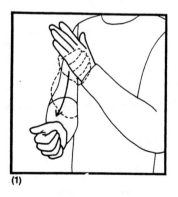

(1)

QUALIFIED

Being able or specially conditioned.

> *Paramedics are qualified to give medical treatment to injured people.*

(1) The left "flat" hand faces right at chest level. The right hand grabs the little finger side of the left hand then moves down into an "A" hand.(SM)

* This is a general sign for skilled, as proficient. The word "qualified" should be mouthed while making the sign.

QUARANTINE

The period of time that a person with a contagious disease or one who has been exposed to a person with a contagious disease is kept away from other healthy people. People are quarantined to prevent the spread of a disease.

*People exposed to a contagious disease, who seem healthy, are usually kept in **quarantine** for a period of time equal to the longest possible time it takes the disease to develop.*

(1) The right index finger points to the left "one" hand.(SM)

(2) Sign SICK — the middle finger of the right "eight" hand touches the forehead and the middle finger of the left "eight" hand touches the stomach. Twist both hands slightly.(SM)

(3) Sign ALONE — the right "one" hand points up and faces out at chest level. Turn the hand to the left down and around in a circle, ending with the hand facing in. (SM)

(4) Sign PREVENT — both "flat" hands cross at chest level and move out forward.(SM)

(5) Sign SPREAD — both "flat-O" hands face down at chest level. Move both hands forward and out to the sides, ending in "five" hands.(SM)

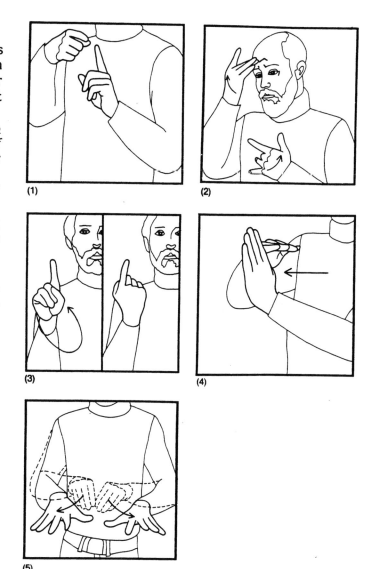

QUICKENING

The first movements a woman feels of a baby in her uterus.

Quickening usually occurs four and one half to five months after conception.

(1) Sign PREGNANT — the right "flat" hand faces in at waist level and moves out forward as if showing the stomach growing.(SM)

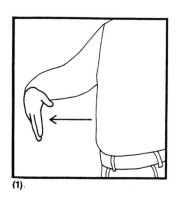

(Continued on next page)

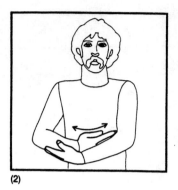 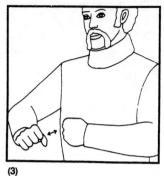

(2)

(3)

(2) Sign BABY — the right hand and forearm face up, resting on the left hand and forearm which also face upwards. Both are then rocked back and forth as if holding a baby.(MM)

(3) Both "S" hands face down at the stomach. Move the right hand in and out from the body a few times as if imitating the movement of a baby in the womb. (MM)

QUIESCENT

Not active or not causing any symptoms.

Some viral diseases, such as genital herpes, chicken-pox, cold sores or fever blisters become **quiescent** *in the nerve cells until something causes them to come out and attack the skin again.*

QUININE

A bitter drug made from the bark of the cinchona tree. Quinine is used to relieve pain, to lower fevers, and especially to treat malaria.

Today, **quinine** *has been replaced in the treatment of malaria by other drugs which are more effective and have fewer side-effects.*

QUINTUPLETS

Five children given birth to by a woman in the same pregnancy.

When a woman has quadruplets or **quintuplets,** *they are usually born prematurely because there is not enough room in the uterus for all of them to develop normally.*

(1) Sign BORN — the left "flat" hand faces in at chest level. The right "flat" hand is behind the left hand and moves down and out forward.(SM)

(2) Sign BABY — the right hand and forearm face up, resting on the left hand and forearm which also face upwards. Both are then rocked back and forth as if holding a baby.(SM)

(3) Sign FIVE — the right "five" hand faces out at chest level.(SM)

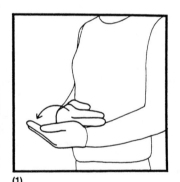 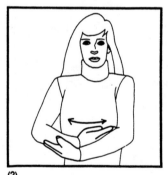 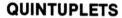

(1)

(2)

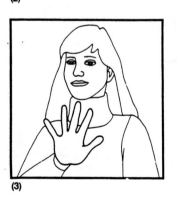

(3)

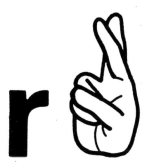

r

RABID
Having rabies. (See RABIES)

RABIES
An infectious disease caused by a virus which attacks the whole body, especially the nervous system, and almost always causes death if not treated; also called hydrophobia. Although rabies virus can affect all warm-blooded animals, dogs, cats, skunks, foxes and bats are most commonly infected. Humans usually get rabies by being bitten by an infected animal. If someone is bitten or scratched by an animal, the wounds should be cleaned well and the animal should be caught and watched for 10 days to see if it starts to show signs of illness. If the animal gets a fever, has a sudden change in temperament, becomes restless, nervous, is very sensitive to light or sound, has convulsions, paralysis, goes into a coma or dies, then it should be reported to the local health department. The person may then have to have shots to immunize him against the disease. A person with rabies will first have a headache, nausea, sore throat, fever, nervousness and fear and may salivate and perspire more than normal. After a few days, if not treated, the person will have convulsions or go into a coma and die.

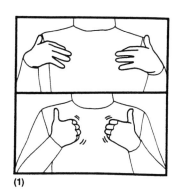
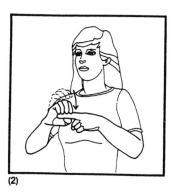

(1)   (2)

Rabies is best controlled by destroying stray animals and by immunizing cats every year against rabies and dogs every two or three years.

(1) Sign ANIMAL — the fingertips of both "five" hands touch the chest. Keeping the fingertips in place, bend and straighten the fingers at the knuckles a few times. (MM)

(2) Sign BITE — the left "one" hand faces down at chest level, pointing out. The right "C" hand moves down as if biting the left index finger. (SM)

(Continued on next page)

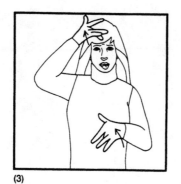
(3)

RABIES, *continued*

(3) Sign SICK — the middle finger of the right "eight" hand touches the forehead and the middle finger of the left "eight" hand touches the stomach. Twist both hands slightly. (SM)

* *The facial expression should reflect sickness.*

RADIAL ARTERY

The large artery which carries fresh blood to the front or thumb side of the lower arm. The radial artery is often used to take a person's pulse. Below the elbow, the brachial artery branches into the radial artery and ulnar artery. *See Figure 6*

RADIATION

Energy given off from an object in the form of small particles or waves. Light, heat, sound and radioactivity are all forms of radiation. Radiation is most often used for the very tiny particles given off from certain substances, such as radium, uranium and plutonium and nuclear bombs when they explode. These particles have a great deal of energy so they may be able to pass through things. Nuclear radiation can be dangerous to living things because as these small particles pass through them, they may cause changes in the structure of molecules. This is especially important with chromosomes.

Carefully controlled radiation is used to take X-rays by having the particles pass through the body and then imprint on a special kind of film.

RADIATION BURNS

Injury to the skin caused by being exposed to radioactive substances like radium and plutonium.

People with radiation burns may have some of the substance, which caused the burns, still on them so they should be handled carefully and taken to a place with special equipment needed to care for them.

RADIATION SICKNESS

Illness caused by exposing the body to radioactive substances. There are different degrees of radiation sickness depending on the amount of exposure. Some of the symptoms are a headache, nausea, vomiting and diarrhea. After a period of time, there may be bleeding without reason, loss of hair and teeth, a lowering of the number of red and white blood cells, sterility, changes in the chromosomes of the reproductive cells causing birth defects and cancers and perhaps death.

Radiation sickness is also called Radiation Syndrome.

RADIOACTIVITY

The giving off of very tiny particles which have a great deal of energy and travel very fast. The particles are called alpha, beta or gamma particles or rays, depending on their size and energy. Some particles which are given off by a radioactive substance have enough energy or speed to go through solid material. When these particles go through a person's body, they can cause changes in the shapes of molecules, which affects how the body works.

A person should be protected against radioactivity because even in small amounts, it can cause changes in or damage to chromosomes resulting in cancer or birth defects.

RADIOLOGY

The area of medicine that deals with radioactive substances to help in preventing, diagnosing and treating diseases.

Some things used in radiology are X-rays, radioactive isotopes (chemical elements) and different forms of radiation.

RADIUM

A rare, bright radioactive substance. (A metallic element having 13 isotopes, the mass numbers between 213 and 230, having the atomic weight of 226 and half life of 1,622 years.

Radium is used in radium therapy for treating cancer.

RADIUM THERAPY

The treatment of diseases using radium (metallic element); also called radiotherapy.

Radium therapy may be used to help treat tumors and kill cancer cells.

RADIUS

One of the two bones in the forearm, running between the elbow and wrist; the shorter bone on the same side as the thumb. *See Figure 26*

RAGWEED

A kind of weed whose pollen is the most common cause of hay fever.

The pollen from ragweed is made from the middle of August until the middle of October, the first hard frost.

(1) Sign GROW — the right "flat-O" hand moves up through the left fist into a "five" hand. (SM)
(2) Sign CAUSE — both "A" hands face up at chest level. Drop both hands down to the left, ending in "five" hands facing up. (SM)
(3) The right index finger touches the nose. (SM)
(4) Both "one" hands point to each other at chest level. Move the right hand away from the left. (SM)

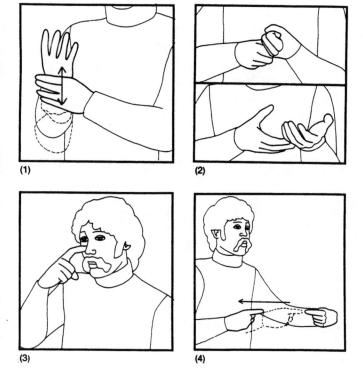

(1) (2)

(3) (4)

RANCID

Having a sour smell or taste because the substance has become rotten; most often used to describe fats or oils which have begun to break down.

Butter will become rancid more quickly than margarine because the oils in the margarine have been chemically treated to make them more stable and less likely to become rotten.

(1) Both "X" hands face each other at chest level, the right hand slightly above the left. Move the right hand forward. (SM)

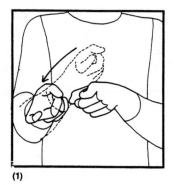

(1)

(Continued on next page)

RANCID, *continued*

(2) Sign SMELL — the fingertips of the right "flat" hand brush up the nose. (MM)

(3) Sign TASTE — the middle finger of the right "eight" hand taps the chin a few times.

* *The facial expression should reflect bad tasting or smelling.*

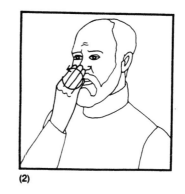
(2)

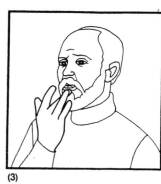
(3)

RAPE

Sexual intercourse between two people in which one of them does not want to have sexual intercourse and is forced or tricked into it by the other. Rape is most often performed by a man on a woman. When one of the people is below a certain age, which varies from state to state, or is not intelligent enough to agree to sexual intercourse and know what is involved, it is also called rape. Rape is an illegal act of violence committed by one person against another. This crime can be physically and emotionally very damaging to the person who is raped and the people close to them.

There are now many support groups in the country who can aid a victim of rape by giving knowledgeable advice, going with the victim to the police, being on hand while the victim is examined by a doctor, staying with the victim during police questioning about what happened, providing legal advice and support during a trial and by giving long term counseling.

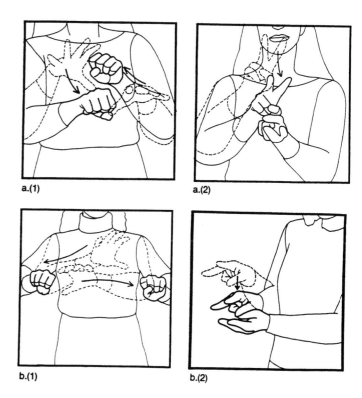
a.(1)   a.(2)

b.(1)   b.(2)

a. (1) Both "five" hands face down, the left hand in front of the right. Move both hands towards each other, ending in "S" hands. (SM)

(2) The left "V" hand faces up at chest level. The right "V" hand faces down and moves down to the left hand. (SM)

b. (1) Both "five" hands face out and cross at the wrists. Move both hands to the sides ending in "S" hands. (SM)

(2) The left "V" hand faces up at chest level. The right "V" hand faces down and moves down to the left hand. (SM)

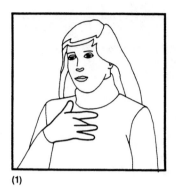

(1)

(2)

RAPID PULSE

A faster pulse than normal (usually over 150 beats per minute); also called "accelerated pulse." A rapid pulse is a common symptom of fever or inflammation.

A rapid pulse may occur from heart disease, a tumor, meningitis, shock, disease of the ovary and uterus, or using certain drugs such as belladonna or alcohol.

(1) Sign HEART — the middle finger of the right "eight" hand taps the chest a few times.

(2) Sign BEAT — the left "flat" hand faces in at chest level. The right "S" hand hits the left palm a few times. (MM)

* *The movement should be short and repeated.*

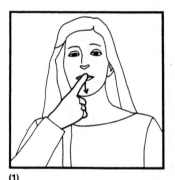

(1)

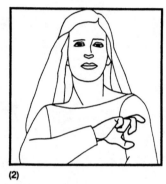

(2)

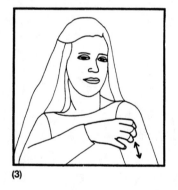

(3)

RASH

Redness or patches of red on the skin, sometimes with bumps.

A rash will usually last a short time and may be caused by a virus or bacteria attacking the skin, by an allergy, or by irritation.

(1) Sign RED — the index finger of the right "one" hand brushes down the chin a few times. (MM)

(2) The right "C" hand faces out on the left upper arm. (SM)

* *This could be signed at the area of the rash.*

(3) Sign SCRATCH — the fingertips of the right "claw" hand scratch up and down on the left upper arm a few times. (MM)

* *This could be signed at the area of the rash.*

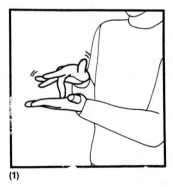

(1)

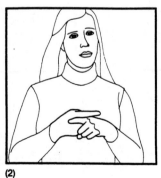

(2)

REACTION

The response of a living thing to something which has happened to it, been given to it or done to it.

Many people have allergic reactions to pollen, dust, or certain foods.

(1) Sign MEDICINE — the left "flat" hand faces up at chest level. The middle finger of the right "eight" hand touches the left palm and pivots slightly from left to right a few times. (MM)

(2) Sign CONFLICT — both "one" hands cross at chest level. (SM)

(Continued on next page)

(3) Sign ANSWER — both "R" hands face out, the right hand touches the mouth. Drop both hands down slightly. (SM)

(4) Sign POSITIVE — the index fingers of both "one" hands cross indicating the positive sign. (SM)

(5) Sign NEGATIVE — the left "flat" hand faces out at chest level. The index finger of the right "one" hand points to the left and touches the left palm indicating the negative sign. (SM)

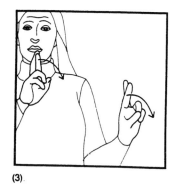

(3)

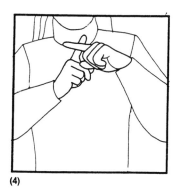

(4)

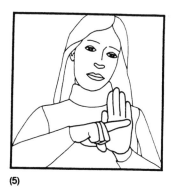

(5)

RECESSION OF GUMS

Pulling away of the gums from the teeth. Along with recessions of the gums, there is often inflammation, destruction of the root of the tooth and loosening of the tooth.

Recession of the gums is a sign of gum or tooth disease and a dentist should be seen.

RECIPIENT

A person who receives or gets something. In medicine, recipient is used for someone getting blood, tissues or organs from a donor.

In an organ transplant, the recipient of the organ is often given drugs to make the body's immune system less effective so the organ will not be recognized as foreign to the body and destroyed.

(1) Sign PERSON — both "flat" hands face each other at chest level. Move both hands down to waist level. (SM)

(2) Sign RECEIVE — the thumbs of both "five" hands touch the chest. Close both hands to "flat-O" hands. (SM)

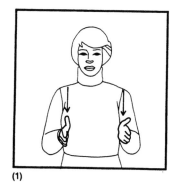

(1)

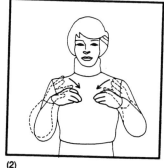

(2)

(Continued on next page)

505

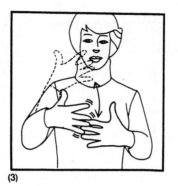

RECIPIENT, *continued*

(3) Sign BLOOD — the left "five" hand is at chest level with the palm toward the body. The palm of the right "five" hand is toward the body with the middle fingers touching the mouth. Move the right hand down the back of the left hand. Wiggle the fingers of the right hand as it moves. (MM)

* *This movement should be short, repeated and somewhat restrained. BLOOD is just an example. Sign or fingerspell the specific thing if known.*

(3)

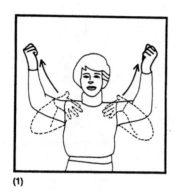

RECOVER

To get better or become healthy after a disease or injury.

> *The more damage done by an injury or the more severe the disease, the longer it will take a person to recover.*

(1) Sign HEALTH — both "five" hands touch the chest then move up to "S" hands. (SM)

(1)

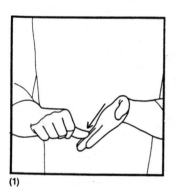

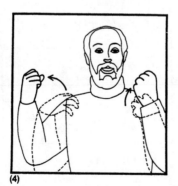

RECOVERY ROOM

An area in a hospital with special equipment and nurses where patients who have just had surgery are cared for.

> *Patients are kept in a recovery room until they become conscious and are not drowsy or affected by the anesthetic anymore.*

(1) Sign OPERATE — the left "flat" hand faces up at chest level. The thumb of the right "A" hand moves down the left palm as if cutting. (SM)
(2) Sign FINISH — both "five" hands face up at chest level. Turn both hands over so that they face down. (SM)
(3) Sign BRING — both "flat" hands face up at the left chest level. Move both hands to the right side. (SM)
(4) Sign HEALTH — both "five" hands touch the chest, then move up to "S" hands. (SM)

(1)   (2)   (3)   (4)

(Continued on next page)

(5) Both "flat" hands face each other at chest level. Move both hands towards the center, both hands facing in and the right hand in front of the left hand. (SM)

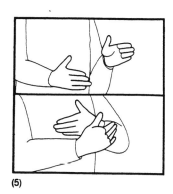

(5)

RECTAL THERMOMETER

A thermometer inserted through the anus into the rectum, used for taking a person's body temperature.

A rectal thermometer would be used instead of an oral thermometer on children or people with face or head injuries.

(1) The index finger of the right "one" hand is inside the left "S" hand. Move the right hand down out of the left fist and shake it slightly as if shaking down a thermometer. (SM)

(2) The index finger of the right "one" hand points to the anus. (SM)

(3) The left "S" hand faces in at chest level. The thumb of the right "A" hand moves up into the left fist. (SM)

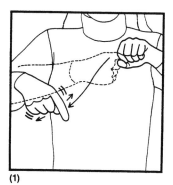

(1)

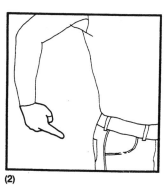

(2)

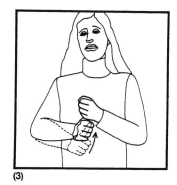

(3)

RECTUM

The lower part of the colon or large intestines where feces are held until we have a bowel movement. The rectum is about five inches long, ending at the anus. *See Figure 12 or 13*

(1) The index finger of the right "one" hand points to the anus. (SM)

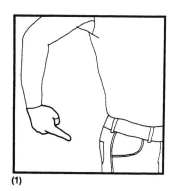

(1)

RECTUS ABDOMINUS

The outermost muscle of the abdomen, attached to the ribs and the lower front part of the pelvis. The rectus abdominus is used to flatten the abdomen, bend the backbone and increase the pressure in the abdomen. *See Figure 4*

RECUPERATE

See RECOVER

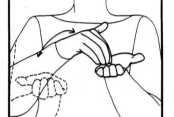
(1)

RECURRENT

Returning from time to time.

The major symptoms of malaria are recurrent chills, fever and sweats.

(1) Sign AGAIN — the left "flat" hand faces up at chest level. The right "cupped" hand faces up. Turn the right hand up and over so that the fingertips touch the left palm a few times. (MM)

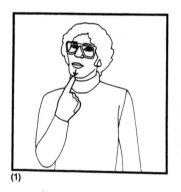
(1)

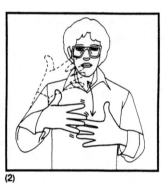
(2)

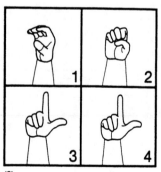
(3)

RED BLOOD CELLS

One of the very small, round, indented, red cells found in the blood. They contain hemoglobin which is the substance which can pick up oxygen at the lungs and release it at the tissues. Red blood cells are made in the bone marrow, last about 120 days and, when they become old or damaged, are taken out of circulation by the liver or spleen, where they are broken down and some parts are recycled and some parts are used to make bile. Red blood cells are also called erythrocytes.

There are about 35 trillion red blood cells in a person's body.

(1) Sign RED — the index finger of the right "one" hand brushes down the chin a few times. (MM)

(2) Sign BLOOD — the left "five" hand is at chest level with the palm towards the body. The palm of the right "five" hand is toward the body with the middle fingertips touching the mouth. Move the right hand down the back of the left hand. Wiggle the fingers of the right hand as it moves. (MM)

* *This movement should be short, repeated and somewhat restrained.*

(3) Fingerspell "C-E-L-L".

RED CROSS

An international organization that helps wounded, sick or homeless people during wartime or natural disasters.

When large numbers of people are injured, such as during a flood or hurricanes the Red Cross will be there.

(1) The right "G" hand makes a cross in the air. (SM)

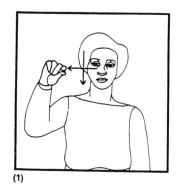

(1)

RED DEVILS

See SECOBARBITAL

REDNESS

Referring to the abnormal red color of an area on the skin, usually the result of inflammation.

Some allergies can irritate the skin, causing a rash and redness.

(1) The index finger of the right "one" hand makes a small circle on the back of the left "S" hand. (SM)
* *This could be signed at the area of the redness.*

(2) Sign RED — the index finger of the right "one" hand brushes down the chin a few times. (MM)

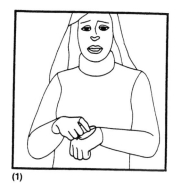

(1)

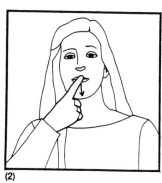

(2)

REDUCE

To lessen or weaken; also to return structures or parts to their normal position or relationship. The ends of a bone can be reduced when the fracture is set, and a hernia or dislocation can be reduced by pushing the part which is out of position to where it belongs.

A person giving first aid should not try to reduce a fracture or dislocation; only a doctor should do this.

(1) The left "cupped" hand faces up at chest level and the right "cupped" hand faces down at shoulder level. Move the right hand down to the left hand. (SM)

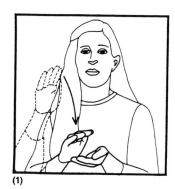

(1)

509

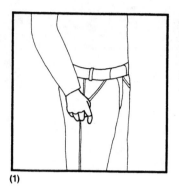
(1)

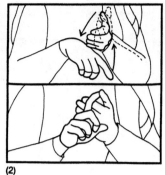
(2)

REFLEX

A movement or action which occurs without conscious control or thought. Reflexes are responses which, in a healthy, normal person, will occur in a certain predictable way. Reflexes are actions which usually serve a purpose and help us survive or help the body work better. Reflexes involve chains of nerves which go from the site where something happened into the spinal cord, perhaps up to the brain and then out of the spinal cord to the part of the body that is going to respond in some way. We don't have to think about the response or decide to do it, it just happens. Reflexes allow the body to function without our having to think about controlling it. The heartbeat, breathing, vomiting, the movement of food through the intestine, bowel movements, contraction of the pupil, and blinking when something comes near the eye are all reflexes.

When a doctor takes his hammer and taps the tendon below the knee, he is checking a certain reflex to see if our nervous system is healthy and normal.

(1) The index finger of the right "one" points to the area. (SM)

(2) The right "one" hand faces down and the left "flat" hand faces in on top of the back of the right hand. Move the right hand up at the wrist, keeping the left hand in place. (SM)

REFRACTION

In medicine, measuring vision errors of an eye so it can be corrected by contact lenses or glasses. Refraction is also the bending of light rays as they pass from one substance to another.

Images are focused on the retina of the eye by refraction of light rays as they hit the cornea and lens of the eye.

REFRACTIVE ERROR

A defect in the shape of the eye, the cornea or lens in the eye causing images to be out of focus on the retina.

An optometrist can measure the refractive error with special instruments and prescribe lenses to correct the vision.

REFRACTURE

Breaking a bone again which was broken and has not healed correctly.

(Continued on next page)

A doctor will **refracture** *a bone that has not been set correctly or which has healed in a wrong position.*

(1) Sign BREAK — both "S" hands are together and face down at chest level. Turn both hands up so that they face each other, as if imitating breaking something. (SM)

(2) Sign AGAIN — the left "flat" hand faces up at chest level. The right "cupped" hand faces up. Turn the right hand up and over so that the fingertips touch the left palm once. (SM)

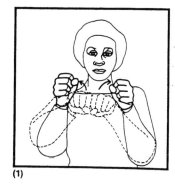 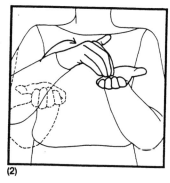

(1) (2)

REGENERATION

The repair or growing back of a damaged, diseased or missing part.

Regeneration of nerve cells is possible if they are only slightly damaged.

(1) Sign NEW — the left "flat" hand faces up at chest level. The right "cupped" hand faces up and brushes up the left palm. (SM)

(2) Sign GROW — the right "flat-O" hand moves up through the left fist. (SM)

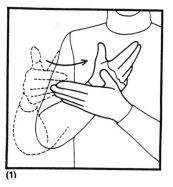 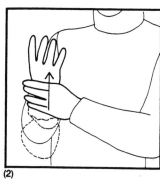

(1) (2)

REGION

Referring to a particular area or space.

The abdominal **region** *contains all structures in the area of the abdomen.*

(1) The fingertips of the right "flat" hand rub the left upper arm. (SM)

* This could be signed at the area referred to.

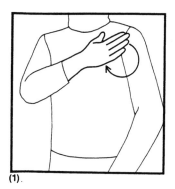

(1).

REGRESS

The return of a disease or its symptoms.

A person's illness may **regress** *due to a mental disorder such as schizophrenia, severe fatigue or frustration.*

(1) Sign DECLINE — both "A" hands face each other at chest level with the thumbs extended. Move both hands down to waist level in a wavy movement. (SM)

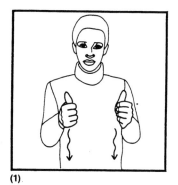

(1).

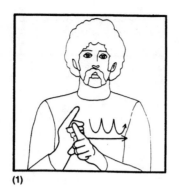
(1)

REGULAR

In medicine, happening at evenly spaced times, steady or constant.

A person's bowel movements or a woman's menstrual periods are usually regular.

(1) The right "one" hand faces left on top of the left "one" hand which faces right. Tap the hands together in a circular movement a few times and at the same time, move both hands to the left side. (MM)

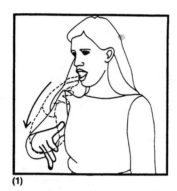
(1)

REGURGITATION

A backward flow of materials. Regurgitation is most often used to mean the returning of food into the mouth from the stomach.

Vomiting is slightly different from regurgitation in that regurgitation doesn't involve the physical effort that vomiting does.

(1) The index finger of the right "five" touches the mouth. Move the hand down forward. (SM)

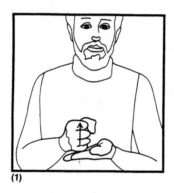
(1)

REHABILITATE

Returning a person who has been ill, injured or is handicapped to a full and normal life.

People who have been affected by problems like blindness, heart disease, deafness, amputation, or paralysis may need to be rehabilitated by re-education and retraining.

(1) Sign HELP — the left "flat" hand faces up at waist level. The right "S" hand rests on the left palm. Move both hands up to chest level. (SM)

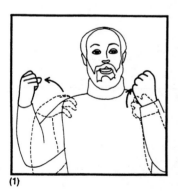
(1)

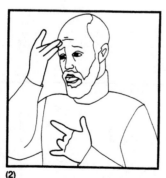
(2)

RELAPSE

The return of a disease or its symptoms after a person seemed to get over it.

After even a minor illness like the flu, a person should take good care of himself because the body is weakened and he may suffer a relapse.

(1) Sign HEALTHY — both "five" hands touch the chest, then move up to "S" hands. (SM)
(2) Sign DISEASE — the middle finger of the right "eight" hand touches the forehead and the middle finger of the left "eight" hand touches the stomach. (SM)

(Continued on next page)

(3) Sign AGAIN — the left "flat" hand faces up at chest level. The right "cupped" hand faces up. Turn the right hand up and over so that the fingertips touch the left palm once. (SM)

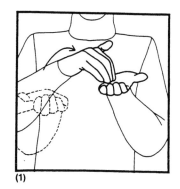

(1)

RELAX

To become restful and calm, lessening the amount of strain, anxiety, and tension.

It is good for a person's physical and mental health to totally relax every now and then if he is under stress.

a. (1) Both "flat" hands cross on the chest. (SM)

* *The facial expression should reflect relaxation.*

b. (1) Both "five" hands face out at chest level. Drop both hands down so that they face down. (SM)

* *The facial expression should reflect relaxation.*

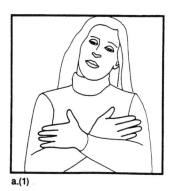
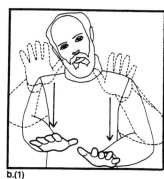

a.(1)   b.(1)

RELAXANT

Any substance or drug used to make a person less tense or active.

A relaxant can relieve mental, emotional, or muscular tension.

(1) Sign MEDICINE — the left "flat" hand faces up at chest level. The middle finger of the right "eight" hand touches the left palm and pivots slightly from left to right a few times. (MM)

(2) Sign RELAX — both "five" hands face out at chest level. Drop both hands down so that they face down. (SM)

* *The facial expression should reflect relaxation.*

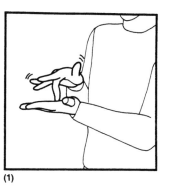
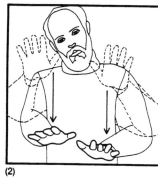

(1)   (2)

RELIEVE

To free from or remove discomfort or pain.

Some drugs may help relieve the symptoms of the common cold.

(1) Sign FEEL — the middle finger of the right "eight" hand brushes the chest in small circular movements a few times. (MM)

(2) Sign IMPROVE — the right "flat" hand faces in and moves up the left arm, touching several times. (MM)

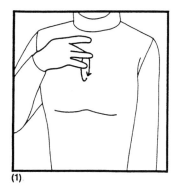
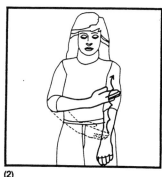

(1)   (2)

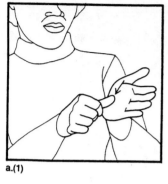

a.(1)

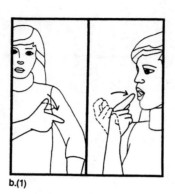

b.(1)

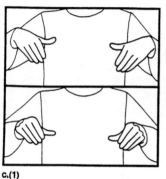

c.(1)

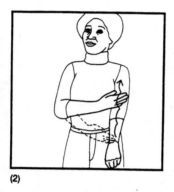

(2)

REMEDY

Something that prevents, relieves or cures a disease.

Because cancer is such a frightening disease, people who have it may do anything or try any remedy to cure it even though the remedy has not been shown to work and may be dangerous.

a. (1) Sign OPERATE — the left "flat" hand faces in at chest level. The thumb of the right "A" hand moves down the left palm as if cutting. (SM)

b. (1) Sign SHOT — the index finger of the right "L" hand touches the left upper arm. Bend the thumb in as if imitating injecting something into the arm. (SM)

Sign PILL — the thumb and index finger of the right hand touch, the palm faces in. Flick the index finger towards the mouth as if popping a pill into the mouth. (SM)

c. (1) Sign MASSAGE — both "flat" hands face down and imitate massaging. (SM)

* *Sign OPERATE, SHOT, PILL, or MASSAGE if the specific is known.*

(2) Sign IMPROVE — the right "flat" hand moves up the left arm, touching several times. (MM)

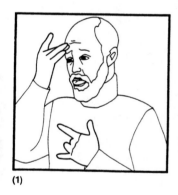

(1)

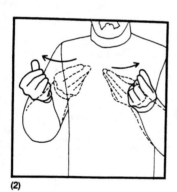

(2)

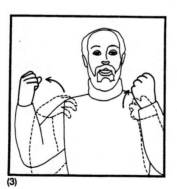

(3)

REMISSION

The lessening or going away of the symptoms of a disease.

When a remission occurs in a disease, it doesn't always mean a person is cured of the disease.

(1) Sign DISEASE — the middle finger of the right "eight" hand touches the forehead and the middle finger of the left "eight" hand touches the stomach. (SM)

(2) Both "flat-O" hands face up at chest level. Move both hands to the sides and at the same time, slide the thumbs across the fingers. (SM)

(3) Sign HEALTH — both "five" hands touch the chest, then move up to "S" hands. (SM)

REMOVABLE PARTIAL DENTURE

A set of artificial teeth which replace one or more but not all of a person's natural teeth and which can be easily put into or taken out of the mouth by the person wearing them.

A removable partial denture is held in place by the natural teeth around it and the gums.

(1) Sign FALSE — the right "L" hand faces left and brushes past the nose. (SM)
(2) Sign TEETH — the index finger of the right "one" moves across the teeth from left to right. (SM)
(3) The right "modified-C" hand moves away from the mouth. (SM)

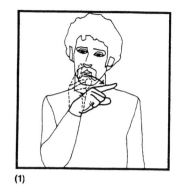
(1)

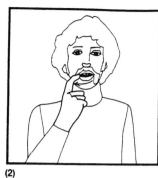
(2)

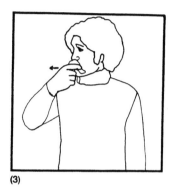
(3)

REMOVE

To take away or get rid of something.

Doctors don't remove people's tonsils now as much as they used to because the tonsils are important in protecting against other infections.

a. (1) The right fist faces left at chest level with the thumb inside the fist. Flick the thumb out. (SM)
b. (1) The left "flat" hand faces up at chest level. The right "A" hand with the thumb inside the fist touches the left palm. Move the right hand out and at the same time, flick the thumb out. (SM)

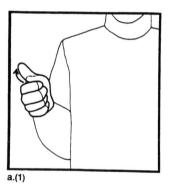
a.(1)

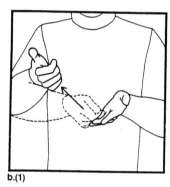
b.(1)

REPRODUCTION

The process by which animals or humans make babies.

Reproduction begins when a male reproductive cell (the sperm) joins with and fertilizes a female reproductive cell (the ovum).

(1) Fingerspell "S-P-E-R-M".
(2) Sign EGG — the fingers of both "H" hands cross at chest level. Pivot both hands out slightly a few times. (MM)

(Continued on next page)

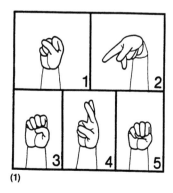
(1)

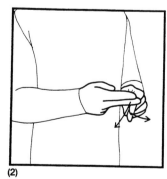
(2)

515

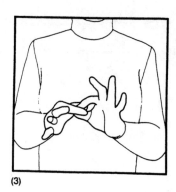
(3)

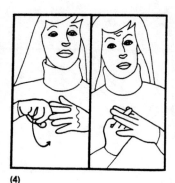
(4)

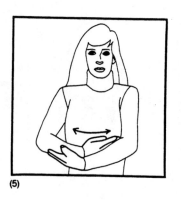
(5)

REPRODUCTION, *continued*

(3) Sign JOIN — both "F" hands join at chest level. (SM)

(4) Sign BEGIN — the left "five" hand faces right at chest level. The index finger of the right "one" hand moves through the left index and middle fingers, then twists slightly. (SM)

(5) Sign BABY — the right hand and forearm face up, resting on the left hand and forearm which also face upwards. Both are then rocked back and forth as if holding a baby. (MM)

REPRODUCTIVE ORGANS
See REPRODUCTIVE SYSTEM

REPRODUCTIVE SYSTEM

The two different sets of organs and structures in the male and female which make, transport and care for the ovum and sperm. The reproductive system causes fertilization to occur and, in the female, nourishes and protects the offspring. In the male, the major parts of the reproductive system are the testes, vas deferens, prostate gland, penis and urethra. In the female, they are the ovaries, fallopian tubes, uterus and vagina. *See Figure 12 or 13*

RESERPINE

A tranquilizing drug which calms and relaxes a person, used to treat people with mental diseases or high blood pressure.

Reserpine does not cause addiction but it can cause mental depression and too much can cause respiratory failure.

(Continued on next page)

a. (1) Sign MEDICINE — the left "flat" hand faces up at chest level. The middle finger of the right "eight" hand touches the left palm and pivots slightly from left to right a few times. (MM)
(2) Sign RELAX — both "flat" hands cross on the chest. (SM)

b. (1) Sign MEDICINE — the left "flat" hand faces up at chest level. The middle finger of the right "eight" hand touches the left palm and pivots slightly from left to right a few times. (MM)
(2) Sign RELAX — both "five" hands face out at chest level. Drop both hands down so that they face down. (SM)

* *The facial expression should reflect relaxation.*

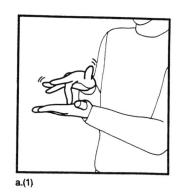
a.(1)

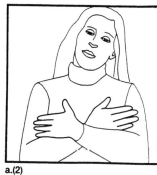
a.(2)

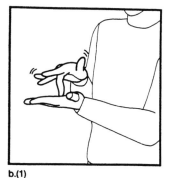
b.(1)

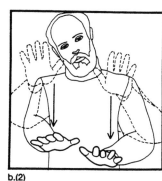
b.(2)

RESIDUE

Something left behind after a part of it has been removed. In medicine, whatever remains in a space or organ after some or most of the substance has been removed.

In some conditions, like digestive problems, a doctor may have a person go on a low roughage diet, which leaves little residue in the intestine, making it easy to handle.

(1) Sign LEAVE — both "five" hands face each other at chest level. Drop both hands down slightly. (SM)

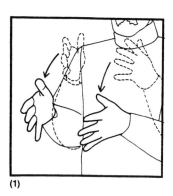
(1)

RESISTANCE

In medicine, the ability of the body to fight off or prevent infections. Resistance to infections is provided by the body's activities and structures which prevent infection and damage caused by organisms getting into the body that shouldn't. Immunity is a kind of resistance which protects the body against a specific infection.

A very young or old or weak person will be more likely to get a disease because his resistance may be lower than normal.

(1) Sign RESIST — the right "S" hand faces down at chest level and moves in and out slightly a few times. (MM)

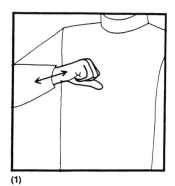
(1)

517

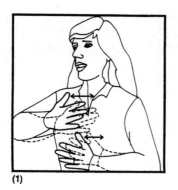
(1)

RESPIRATION

The act of breathing; inhalation and exhalation. Respiration is also the process in which the body takes in oxygen, uses it in the cells and then gives off carbon dioxide.

The rate of respiration is automatically controlled by special areas in the pons and medulla oblongata of the brain and can also be consciously controlled by the cerebrum.

(1) Sign BREATHE — both "flat" hands move in and out from the chest a few times as if imitating breathing. (MM)

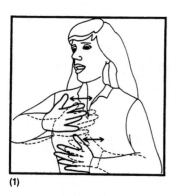
(1)

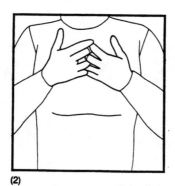
(2)

RESPIRATOR

A machine used to help a person who is having problems breathing normally.

A respirator may also be used to clean, warm or add medicine to the air passing through into the person's lungs.

(1) Sign BREATHE — both "flat" hands move in and out from the chest a few times as if imitating breathing. (MM)
(2) Sign MACHINE — both "five" hands mesh together and face in at chest level. Bounce the hands slightly a few times. (MM)

RESPIRATORY

Something which has to do with respiration or breathing.

The respiratory center in the medulla oblongata deals with respiratory movements.

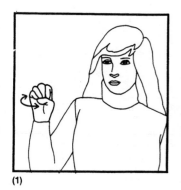
(1)

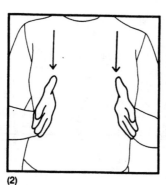
(2)

RESPIRATORY EMERGENCY

A situation in which a person has stopped breathing or isn't breathing well enough to get air into the lungs.

A respiratory emergency may be caused by electrocution, drowning, shock, heart disease, strangulation or depressant drugs such as narcotics.

(1) Sign EMERGENCY — the right "E" hand faces out at chest level and twists from side to side a few times. (MM)
(2) Sign PERSON — both "flat" hands face each other at chest level and move down to waist level. (SM)

(Continued on next page)

(3) Sign BREATHE — both "flat" hands face in and move in and out from the chest a few times as if imitating breathing. (MM)

(4) Sign STOP — the left "flat" hand faces up at chest level. The right "flat" hand faces left and moves down to sharply hit the left palm. (SM)

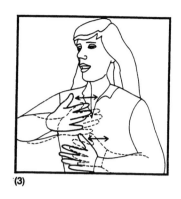
(3)

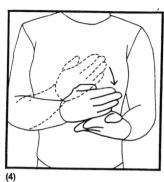
(4)

RESPIRATORY FAILURE

Any failure of the lungs to work and to get oxygen into the blood.

Respiratory failure can be caused by an object blocking the airways, narrowing of the airways, something stopping the chest muscles which inflate the lungs from working, a collapsed lung, or filling of the lungs with a fluid which keeps the oxygen from reaching the lungs, as in drowning.

(1) Sign BREATHE — both "flat" hands face in and move in and out from the chest a few times as if imitating breathing. (MM)

(2) Sign STOP — the left "flat" hand faces up at chest level. The right "flat" hand faces left and moves down to sharply hit the left palm. (SM)

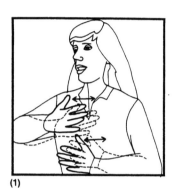
(1)

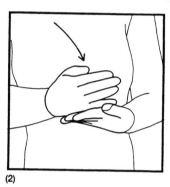
(2)

RESPIRATORY SYSTEM

The structures and airways which get air from outside of the body into the lungs; this includes the lungs, pleura, bronchi, pharynx, larynx, tonsils and the nose. The respiratory system helps get oxygen to the bloodstream and also removes carbon dioxide, which has left the blood and entered the lungs, of the body. The respiratory system works very closely with the circulatory system to get oxygen to the cells and to carry carbon dioxide away from the cells and out of the body. *See Figure 10*

RESPONSE

A reaction to something which has happened. Response can also mean how a person is doing under a certain treatment or drug.

*A common **response** of the body to infection is a fever, caused by extreme heat being given off by the cells as they become more active in trying to fight off the infection.*

519

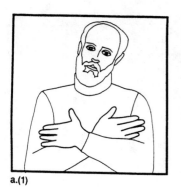
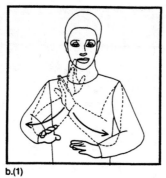

a.(1)　　　　b.(1)

REST

To be either mentally or physically quiet; not active.

Sleep allows the brain and body to rest.

a. (1) Sign RELAX — both "flat" hands cross on the chest. (SM)

* *The facial expression should reflect relaxation.*

b. (1) Sign RELAX — both "flat" hands cross at the wrists at chest level and move down to the sides. (SM)

* *The facial expression should reflect relaxation.*

REST HOME

See NURSING HOME

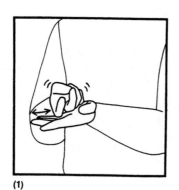

(1)

RESTLESS

Not able to relax or be still.

Smoking cigarettes or drinking caffeine before going to sleep will cause a person to be restless.

(1) The left "flat" hand faces up at chest level. The right "X" hand faces up in the left palm and shakes from side to side a few times. (MM)

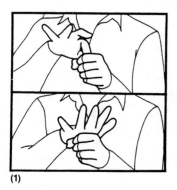
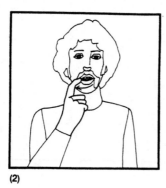

(1)　　　　(2)

RESTORATION

In dentistry, the process of filling or repairing a tooth which is decayed or contains a cavity.

The type of material a dentist uses for restorations depends on which tooth is decayed and the size of the cavity.

(1) The left "S" hand faces right at chest level. The index finger of the right hand is inside the left fist. Pull the index finger out,then change the hand to a "five" hand and sharply hit the left fist. (SM)

(2) Sign TEETH — the index finger of the right "one" hand moves across the teeth from the left to the right. (SM)

RESTORATIVE

Something that helps a person become healthy or get his strength back.

Not getting enough of a vitamin can make a person unhealthy but getting large amounts of the vitamin can act as a restorative.

(1) Sign HELP — the left "flat" hand faces up at waist level. The right "S" hand faces left on the left palm. Move both hands up to chest level. (SM)
(2) Sign BECOME — both "flat" hands face each other, the right hand faces out and the left hand faces in. Twist both hands so that the right hand faces in and the left hand faces out. (SM)
(3) Sign HEALTHY — both "five" hands touch the chest, then move up to "S" hands. (SM)

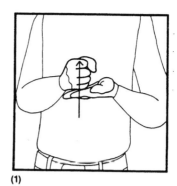
(1)

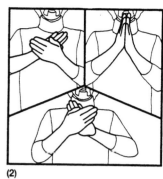
(2)

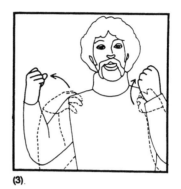
(3)

RESTRICT

To hold back or limit.

People with high blood pressure should restrict the amount of salt in their diet.

(1) Sign LIMIT — both "cupped" hands face each other, the right hand slightly higher than the left. Move both hands out forward. (SM)

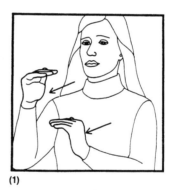
(1)

RESUSCITATION

Bringing someone back to consciousness after they have collapsed or seem dead.

Cardiopulmonary resuscitation is a kind of resuscitation in which someone's breathing and heartbeat are kept going artificially after they have stopped, helping the person to stay alive.

(1) Sign HELP — the left "flat" hand faces up at waist level. The right "S" hand faces left on the left palm. Move both hands up to chest level. (SM)
(2) Sign BREATHE — both "flat" hands move in and out from the chest a few times as if imitating breathing. (MM)

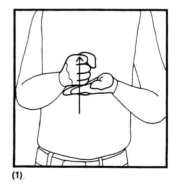
(1)

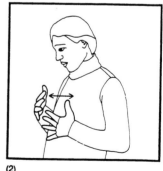
(2)

521

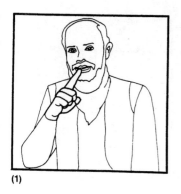
(1)

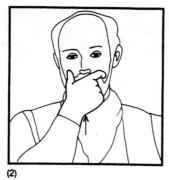
(2)

RETAINER

In dentistry, a device worn in a person's mouth to hold teeth in place after having worn braces.

A retainer may also be called a retaining appliance.
(1) Sign TEETH — the index finger of the right "one" hand points to the teeth. (SM)
(2) The right "modified-C" hand moves towards the mouth. (SM)

RETARDATION

The slowing down or delay of mental or physical activities.

If a splint or cast is not placed on a broken bone, there may be retardation of the healing process.

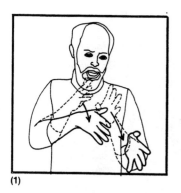
(1)

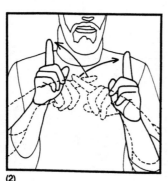
(2)

RETCH

Uncontrollably trying to vomit.

When someone retches, he doesn't actually produce anything, he just has the feeling and muscle action which goes with vomiting.

(1) Sign VOMIT — both "five" hands face each other at the mouth. Drop both hands down. (SM)
(2) Sign BUT — both "one" hands cross at the index fingers at chest level. Move both hands slightly out to the sides. (SM)
(3) Sign NOTHING — the right "A" hand faces out under the chin. Drop the hand down into a "five" hand facing down. (SM)
(4) The right "one" hand points out. (SM)

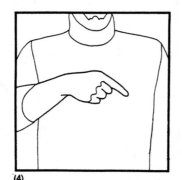
(3)

(4)

RETENTION

In medicine, holding something in the body which does not belong there or which should normally be gotten rid of. Things which may be retained in the body are urine, feces or the material made by a gland.

During a woman's menstrual period, she may have some puffiness or water retention.

(Continued on next page)

RETENTION, *continued*

(1) Sign WATER — the index finger of the right "W" hand taps the mouth a few times. (MM)
(2) The right "S" hand makes a small counterclockwise circle at chest level. (SM)

* These signs refer to "water retention". Sign the specific URINE, FECES, etc. if known.

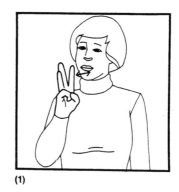 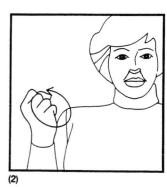

(1)　　　　　　　　　(2)

RETINA

The inside layer of the eyeball, made up of special nerve cells called rods and cones. The rods and cones are able to detect light and colors and are connected to the optic nerve which carries impulses to the brain. The lens of the eye focuses images on the retina, where the rods and cones sense. The retina has the macula lutea, fovea centralis and optic disk in it. *See Figure 22*

RETINAL DETATCHMENT

The separation of the inner (sensory) layer of the retina and the outer pigment (epithelium) layer, causing loss of function.

Retinal detachment may be caused by a hole or break in the inner sensory layer which then allows fluid to collect between the two layers.

RETINITIS

Inflammation of the retina.

A person with retinitis will not be able to see well nor be able to stand light.

RETINITIS PIGMENTOSA

A disease that causes the retina to work less and less until the person becomes blind. In retinitis pigmentosa, the cells in the retina, especially the rods, quit working, and the optic nerve shrinks and quits working. Early signs of the disease are poor night vision and being able to see less area with an eye.

The cause of retinitis pigmentosa is unknown but it tends to be hereditary.

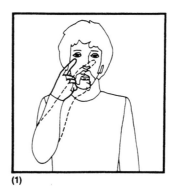 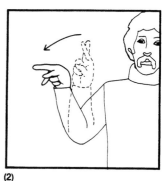

(1)　　　　　　　　　(2)

(1) Sign EYES — the index finger of the right "one" hand points to both eyes. (SM)
(2) Fingerspell "R-P".

* This may need further explanation before signing.

523

RETINOPATHY

Any disease or disorder of the retina.

Retinopathy may be caused by high blood pressure, looking directly at the sun, arteriosclerosis or diabetes.

RETROLENTAL FIBROPLASIA

A condition where a membrane of fibers grows on the surface of the lens of the eye.

Retrolental fibroplasia usually occurs in premature babies who have been in incubators for a long time and exposed to high oxygen levels.

Rh BLOOD GROUP

A special blood group. People who are Rh positive have a certain kind of protein in their red blood cells that Rh negative people don't have. If a person with Rh negative blood gets Rh positive blood in a transfusion, the body will recognize the new protein as not belonging in the body and make antibodies against it to destroy the foreign protein and blood cells. If a woman who is Rh negative has an Rh positive baby, the baby's blood may get into her blood during childbirth. The woman's body will then make antibodies against Rh positive blood. This won't affect the baby she just had. If she becomes pregnant again and the baby has Rh positive blood, then the antibodies in her blood may get into the baby's blood and destroy its red blood cells. They may cause an abortion or the birth of a baby who is very anemic and unhealthy because it had many red blood cells destroyed.

A woman who is pregnant should know her Rh blood group because if she is Rh negative and the father of a baby she is carrying is Rh positive, there may be problems with later pregnancies which can be prevented if her doctor is told.

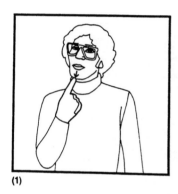
(1)

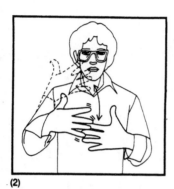
(2)

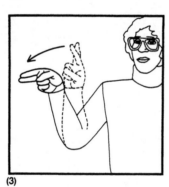
(3)

(1) Sign RED — the index finger of the right "one" hand brushes down the chin a few times. (MM)

(2) Sign BLOOD — the left "five" hand is at chest level with the palm towards the body. The palm of the right "five" hand is toward the body with the middle fingertips touching the mouth. Move the right hand down the back of the left hand. Wiggle the fingers of the right hand as it moves. (MM)

* *This movement should be short, repeated and somewhat restrained.*

(3) Fingerspell "R-H".

524

RHEUMATIC FEVER

A disease which attacks people who have just had an infection caused by a certain kind of streptococcus bacteria. This infection is in the throat and usually called strep throat or streptococcal sore throat. Rheumatic fever can result if the infection is not treated with antibiotics. The person will suddenly have joint pain and fever and inflammation of the heart may occur. The valves of the heart are commonly damaged, leading to pain and weakness of the heart. Kidney damage may also be caused by rheumatic fever.

When someone has a bad sore throat with a fever, he should go to a doctor to see if it is caused by this kind of bacteria because antibiotics can be given to cure the infection and prevent Rheumatic fever.

RHEUMATISM

The general name for a group of diseases which affect the special tissues of the body which hold things together. The diseases usually affect the muscles, tendons, joints, bones or nerves. When someone has rheumatism, there will usually be pain, stiffness and swelling of muscles and joints.

Some of the specific diseases people may have when they say they have rheumatism are rheumatic fever, rheumatoid arthritis, osteoarthritis, gout and bursitis.

RHEUMATOID ARTHRITIS

A kind of arthritis in which a person has inflamed and swollen joints, stiffness and pain. The disease usually stays with a person for a long time and usually leads to deformities and crippling. The cause in unknown but it may be due to a condition caused by antibodies from a person's immune system damaging the joints. The disease often goes away suddenly.

There is no specific cure for rheumatoid arthritis but people are treated with rest, aspirin and heat applications for the pain, physical therapy and splints on the inflamed joints.

RHINITIS

Inflammation of the mucus membrane in the nose.

There is no special treatment for Rhinitis but a doctor may suggest rest, plenty of fluids and a well-balanced diet to help relieve the symptoms.

RHYTHM

A movement or activity which happens regularly or with the same amount of time between strong and weak elements; also a method of contraception in which a woman keeps track of her menstrual period and figures out when she is ovulating and might become pregnant. A woman may also take the temperature of her vagina and test the mucus from her cervix to see when she should not have sexual intercourse.

The rhythm method of contraception is the least effective form of birth control and a woman is more likely to become pregnant using it than using any of the other methods.

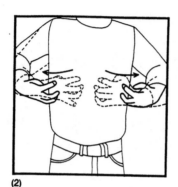
(1)

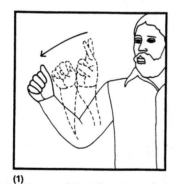
(2)

RIB

One of the 24 narrow, long, curved bones which make up the chest and which protect the lungs and heart. The ribs are attached to the 12 thoracic vertebrae in the back and some are connected directly to the sternum at the front. The five lower pairs are attached to the sternum by cartilage. *See Figure 26*

(1) Fingerspell "B-O-N-E".

(2) The fingertips of both "claw" hands touch the rib area and move slightly to the sides. (SM)

RIBOFLAVIN

See VITAMIN B COMPLEX

RIBONUCLEIC ACID (RNA)

An important substance (of large molecular weight) found in the nucleus of a cell; commonly called RNA. Some viruses may contain a strand of RNA.

Ribonucleic acid plays an important roll in protein synthesis and metabolism within the cells.

(1) Fingerspell "R-N-A".

* *This may need further explanation before signing.*

RICKETS

A softening and degeneration of the bones, often in children, caused by a lack of calcium and phosphorus being put into their forming bones. Rickets results when someone doesn't get enough vitamin D, needed to absorb the minerals used to make bone.

(Continued on next page)

A person with rickets will perspire on the head, have soreness throughout the body, an enlarged liver and spleen, badly formed teeth, curvature of the spine, and the long bones in the body may be curved and brittle.

(1) Sign CHILD — the right "flat" hand faces down at waist level and imitates patting the head of an imaginary child. (DM)

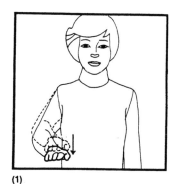
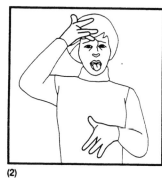

(2) Sign SICK — the middle finger of the right "eight" hand touches the forehead and the middle finger of the left "eight" hand touches the stomach. (SM)

* *The facial expression should reflect illness.*

(3) Fingerspell "B-O-N-E".
(4) Sign SOFT — both "flat-O" hands face up at chest level and open and close a few times. (MM)

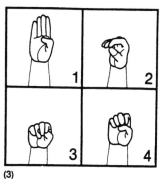
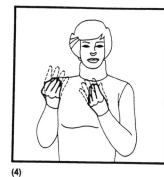

RIGID

Stiff or hard, unable to bend.

After death, the body becomes rigid due to rigor mortis.

(1) Sign STIFF — the left "flat" hand faces in at chest level. The right hand grabs the fingers of the left hand and shakes a few times. (MM)

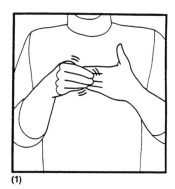

RIGOR MORTIS

The stiffness seen in a body after death. Rigor mortis usually sets in around five to six hours after death.

It actually takes energy for the muscles to relax after they contract, so when someone dies, this energy is no longer made and rigor mortis sets in as the muscles contract and cannot relax.

(1) Sign DEAD — the left "flat" hand faces up at chest level and the right "flat" hand faces down. Turn both hands over so that the left hand ends facing down and the right hand ends facing up. (SM)

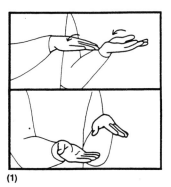

(Continued on next page)

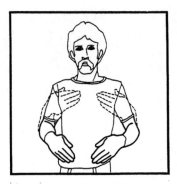

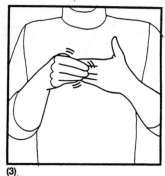

RIGOR MORTIS, *continued*

(2) Sign BODY — both "flat" hands touch the chest, then the stomach. (SM)
(3) Sign STIFF — the left "flat" hand faces in at chest level. The right hand grabs the fingers of the left hand and shake a few times. (MM)

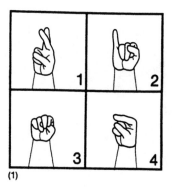

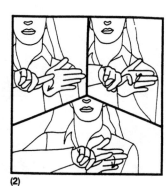

RINGWORM

A skin disease caused by a fungus which usually attacks children; also called tinea. Symptoms of the disease are a round spot where hair falls out, with redness, scaling and itching. Ringworm is treated with oral antibiotics and by putting chemicals on the sore to kill the fungus.

Ringworm is spread by coming into contact with hair or skin scales from an infected person or by contact with a sore on a dog or cat.

(1) Fingerspell "R-I-N-G".
(2) Sign WORM — the left "flat" hand faces right at chest level. The right "one" hand faces down on the left palm. Move the right hand out along the left palm and at the same time, bend and straighten the index finger a few times. (MM)

RITALIN

See METHYLPHENIDATE

ROCKY MOUNTAIN SPOTTED FEVER

An infectious disease caused by a parasite, carried by wood ticks; also called "tick fever." Symptoms are a fever, pain in the bones and muscles, and reddish spots especially on the wrists, ankles, feet and bottoms of the feet.

Quick diagnosis and treatment of Rocky Mountain Spotted Fever can prevent a person from dying from the disease.

ROD

One of the special kinds of cells which makes up the retina of the eye. Along with the cones, the rods detect light and color and send small electrical impulses to the brain so we can see. Rods help us to see dark and light and are important in helping us to see in dim light. *See Figure 22*

ROOT

In dentistry, the part of a tooth below the gums and inside the bone of the jaw. Depending on the kind of tooth, there may be one to four roots. The root of the tooth has a substance around it which attaches it to its socket and holds the whole tooth in place. *See Figure 25*

ROOT CANAL

This is the center area of a tooth root containing blood vessels and nerves. *See Figure 25*

ROOT CANAL THERAPY

In dentistry, removing the nerve in a root canal because of disease or inflammation. Root canal therapy may be done if a cavity is very deep or if the tooth has been injured or broken so that the nerve is exposed.

> *After **root canal therapy**, the tooth should be capped because that tooth is now dead and could break easily.*

ROOT CURETTAGE

In dentistry, scraping and smoothing of the surface of a tooth's root to get rid of substances that shouldn't be there.

> *A **root curettage** may be done in certain gum diseases so the gum can reattach to the root of the tooth and return to normal health.*

ROOT RESECTION

See APICOECTOMY

ROT

To decay, degenerate or fall apart.

> *When an area is cut off from its blood supply, it may get gangrene and rot.*

(1) Sign DECAY — both "A" hands face in at chest level. Drop both hands down into "five" hands facing up. (SM)

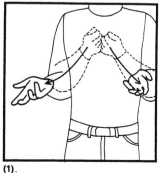

(1).

ROUGHAGE

A name for coarse fibers in foods which can't be digested by humans. Fruits, vegetables and grains are foods with a lot of roughage in them. Roughage in the diet adds bulk to the material in the intestines because it can't be broken down or absorbed and this helps the muscular action of the intestinal tract.

A diet with plenty of roughage in it will prevent constipation.

ROUNDWORM

A general name for worms which are parasites and live in the bodies of animals, including man. They are round, usually white and usually not very large.

When talking about roundworms, a person is usually also talking about ascarids or whipworms, the worms that cause trichinosis, hookworms, strongyles and pinworms.

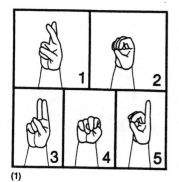
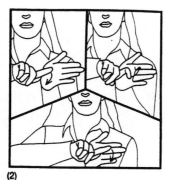

(1) Fingerspell "R-O-U-N-D".
(2) Sign WORM — the left "flat" hand faces right at chest level. The right "one" hand faces down on the left palm. Move the right hand out along the left hand and at the same time, bend and straighten the right index finger a few times. (MM)

RUBELLA

See GERMAN MEASLES

RUBEOLA

See MEASLES

RUPTURE

A break or tear in something, often used for a hernia.

During labor, the membranes surrounding the fetus will normally rupture and cause the sudden release from the uterus of some fluid, called breaking the bag of water.

a. (1) The right "F" hand faces out on the stomach. (SM)

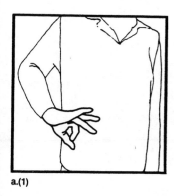
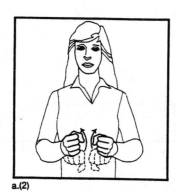

* *This is just an example, the specific area or thing should be indicated or signed first.*

(2) Sign BREAK — both "S" hands face down at chest level. Turn both hands up so that they face each other, as if imitating breaking something. (SM)

* *This should be signed only if referring to something breaking.*

(Continued on next page)

RUPTURE, *continued*

b. (1) Fingerspell "S-P-L-E-E-N".

This is just an example, the specific area or thing should be indicated or signed first.

(2) Sign TEAR — both "A" hands face down at chest level. Move both hands away from each other as if imitating tearing something. (SM)

This should be signed only if referring to something tearing.

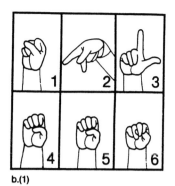

b.(1)

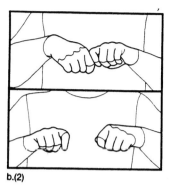

b.(2)

531

S

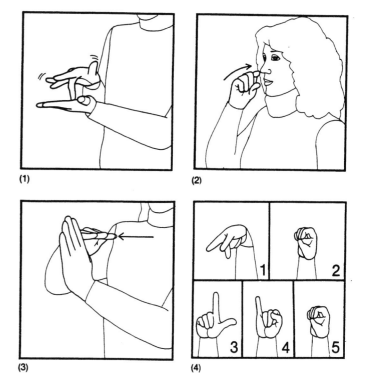

SABIN VACCINE

An oral vaccine given to make someone immune to polio. There was another popular vaccine used against polio called the Salk vaccine but because the dose of medicine in the Sabin vaccine is more like the real disease, it gives better protection.

Children should be immunized against polio with the Sabin vaccine starting at two months and should get three other vaccinations after that, and then a booster when they start school.

(1) Sign MEDICINE — the left "flat" hand faces up at chest level. The middle finger of the right "eight" hand touches the left palm and pivots slightly from side to side a few times. (MM)
(2) Sign DRINK — the right "modified-C" hand faces left and moves towards the mouth as if imitating taking a drink. (SM)
(3) Sign PREVENT — both "flat" hands cross at chest level and move slightly forward. (SM)
(4) Fingerspell "P-O-L-I-O".

(1)

(2)

(3)

(4)

SAC

A bag-like cavity or pouch.

A sac sometimes contains fluid, such as the amniotic sac which holds the developing embryo.

(1) Both "five" hands face up at waist level. Move both hands up and around as if imitating the shape of a sac. The cheeks should also puff out slightly. (SM)

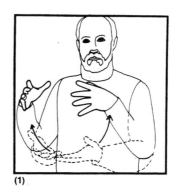

(1)

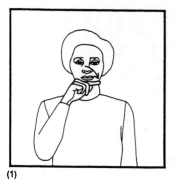 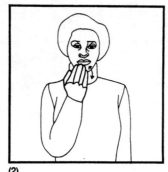

(1)   (2)

SACCHARIN

A man-made sweet, white powder made from coal tar.

Saccharin is a calorie free, artificial sweetener that is 300-500 times sweeter than sugar.

(1) Sign FALSE — the right "L" hand faces left and brushes past the nose. (SM)
(2) Sign SWEET — the fingertips of the right "flat" hand brush down the chin a few times. (MM)

SACRAL

Having to do with the five vertebrae which grow together to form the sacrum and help make up the back part of the pelvis.

The sacral region of the body is the lower back, above the buttocks.

SACRAL VERTEBRAE

The five vertebrae which grow together to form one bone called the sacrum. The sacral vertebrae are found in the lower back and help to make up part of the pelvis. *See Figure 26*

SACROILIAC

Referring to the sacrum and iliac bones or the joint formed by them.

Sacroiliitis is inflammation of sacroiliac joint.

SACRUM

The triangular shaped bone made up of five vertebrae which join together to form one bone. The sacrum forms the base of the backbone and helps to make up the back of the pelvis. (The sacrum of a man is narrower than that of a woman.)
See Figure 26

SADISM

The abnormal sexual pleasure or excitement received by mentally or physically hurting another person.

Sadism is a mental disorder and should be treated.

534

SADIST

A person who gets sexual pleasure or excitement by mentally or physically hurting another person.

A sadist *may also be called algolagnist or masochist.*

SALINE

Containing or having to do with salt.

A saline *solution is a solution which has the same concentration of salt in it as the body does, so when it is used on or in the body, it doesn't have a great effect.*

(1) Sign SALT — the left "V" hand faces down at chest level. The fingers of the right "V" hand alternately tap the top of the left hand fingers a few times. (MM)

(2) Sign MIX — both "claw" hands face each other at chest level. Move both hands alternately in circular movements a few times as if indicating mixing something. (MM)

(3) Sign WITH — both "A" hands are together at chest level.

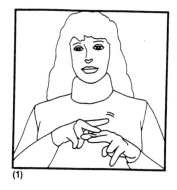
(1)

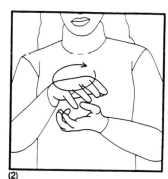
(2)

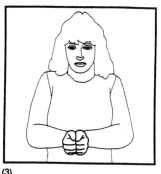
(3)

SALIVA

The clear, tasteless fluid, made by the salivary glands, which is made up of water, proteins and enzymes. In large amounts, saliva helps to keep the mucus membranes lining the mouth moist and flexible, helps moisten food so it can be swallowed, allows us to taste things and, since it contains enzymes, helps us start digesting our food in the mouth.

A person makes about three pints of saliva *in 24 hours.*

(1) Sign WATER — the index finger of the right "W" hand taps the mouth a few times. (MM)

(2) Sign IN — the right "flat-O" hand moves into the left fist. (SM)

(3) The index finger of the right "one" hand circles the mouth. (SM)

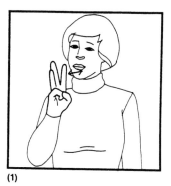
(1)

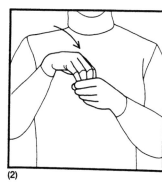
(2)

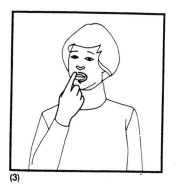
(3)

SALIVARY GLAND

The five glands around the mouth that make the clear fluid called saliva. There is one below each ear on each side of the face, another two lie just inside the lower jawbone on either side and another lies just under the tongue.

The virus that causes mumps has a tendency to infect the salivary glands and cause them to swell painfully.

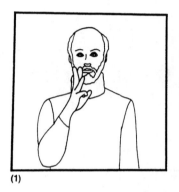

(1)

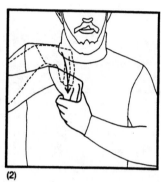

(2)

SALIVATION

The putting out of saliva from the salivary glands.

Salivation is controlled by the nervous system and may be brought on by food being in the mouth, seeing food or smelling food.

(1) Sign WATER — the index finger of the right "W" hand taps the mouth a few times. (MM)
(2) Sign IN — the right "flat-O" hand moves into the left fist. (SM)
(3) The index finger of the right "one" hand circles the mouth. (SM)

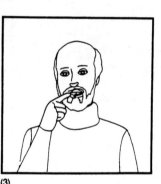

(3)

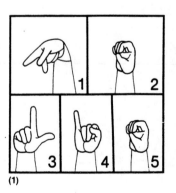

(1)

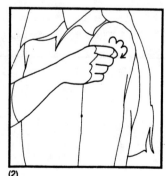

(2)

SALK VACCINE

This was the first vaccine against polio which worked. The Salk vaccine has three kinds of dead polio viruses in it.

The older Salk vaccine has been replaced by the newer Sabin vaccine, which provides better immunity against polio.

(1) Fingerspell "P-O-L-I-O."
(2) The right index finger taps the left upper arm a few times. (MM)

SALMONELLA

Food poisoning caused from a form of bacteria (Enterobacteriaceae).

There are three forms of salmonella in man, ranging from mild gastric problems to possible death.

(1) Sign EAT — the fingertips of the right "flat-O" hand tap the mouth. (SM)
(2) Sign SICK — the middle finger of the right "eight" hand touches the forehead and the middle finger of the left "eight" hand touches the stomach. (SM)

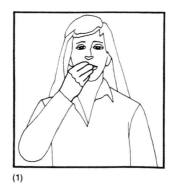
(1)
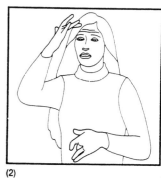
(2)

SALVE

A soft, jelly-like material made of petroleum, fat or lanolin with a medicine in it; also called ointment.

A salve is put on wounds or sores to clear up or prevent an infection, to help healing and to protect the wound from the air.

(1) Sign MEDICINE — the left "flat" hand faces up at chest level. The middle finger of the right "eight" hand touches the left palm and pivots slightly from side to side a few times. (MM)
(2) The fingers of the right "flat" hand rub in a small circular movement on the back of the left "flat" hand. (SM)

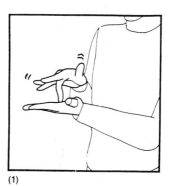
(1)
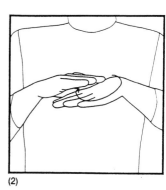
(2)

SANATORIUM

A private place where people who aren't very sick or who have long-term diseases go to be treated; also spelled sanatarium. Sanatoriums often deal with preventing diseases along with treating them.

People may go to a sanatorium to be treated for tuberculosis, mental disorders, drug or alcohol addiction or to get medical attention while they recover from a disease.

(1) Sign HOSPITAL — the fingertips of the right "H" hand make a cross on the left upper arm. (SM)

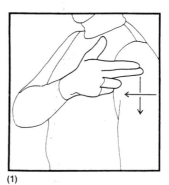
(1)

SANE

Mentally normal, the mind working right.

Sane is the opposite of insane.

(1) Sign MIND — the index finger of the right "one" hand touches the forehead. (SM)
(2) Sign STRAIGHT — the left "B" hand faces right at chest level. The right "B" hand faces left and moves out along the left index finger. (SM)

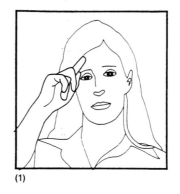
(1)
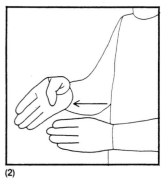
(2)

SANITARY

Having to do with health; also clean, free of germs.

Conditions in this country are usually kept very sanitary.

(1) Sign CLEAN — the left "flat" hand faces up at chest level. The right "flat" hand brushes out on the left palm. (SM)

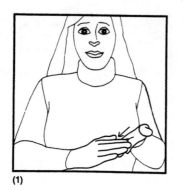

SANITARY NAPKIN

A pad worn over the genital region or against the body, especially between the legs, to absorb fluids from the body.

A sanitary napkin is most often used by women to absorb menstrual fluid.

(1) Sign MENSTRUATE — the right "A" hand taps the right cheek a few times. (MM)
(2) Both "G" hands imitate the shape of a sanitary napkin. (SM)

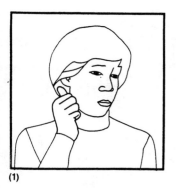
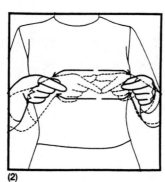

SANITIZE

To clean or to make free of germs; to sterilize.

When people have a contagious, dangerous disease, care should be taken to sanitize everything they use or come into contact with.

(1) Sign CLEAN — the left "flat" hand faces up at chest level. The right "flat" hand brushes back and forth on the left palm a few times. (MM)

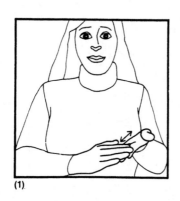

SANITY

The normal, healthy state of mind.

The term "mental health" is commonly used when referring to a person's sanity.

(1) Sign MIND — the index finger of the right "one" hand touches the forehead. (SM)

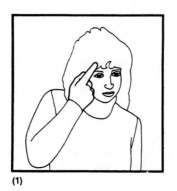

(Continued on next page)

(2) Sign STRAIGHT — the left "flat" hand faces right at chest level. The right "flat" hand faces left and moves out along the left index finger. (SM)
(3) Sign HEALTHY — both "claw" hands touch the chest, then move up to "S" hands. (SM)

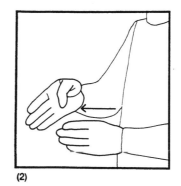
(2)

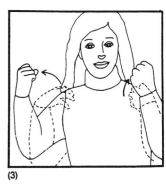
(3)

SARCOMA

A type of cancer in which a tumor is formed in one of the types of tissue which holds the body together, such as the bones, muscles or cartilage. This type of tumor is very dangerous and tends to grow and spread quickly.

Sarcomas tend to attack children and young adults most often and may affect the bladder, kidney, liver, lungs, salivary glands and spleen as well as bones, muscles, and cartilage.

SARTORIUS

A long, thin, flat muscle in the thigh which helps bend the knee. The sartorius is the longest muscle in the body. *See Figure 4*

SATISFACTORY CONDITION

In medicine, referring to a pleasing or acceptable physical condition.

A satisfactory condition is not good or bad, but "OK" or adequate.

(1) Sign HEALTHY — both "claw" hands touch the chest, then move up to "S" hands. (SM)
(2) Sign GOOD — the fingertips of the right "flat" hand touch the mouth, then drop the hand slightly down. (SM)
(3) Sign ENOUGH — the left "S" hand faces right at chest level. The right "flat" hand brushes out on the left fist. (SM)

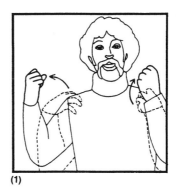
(1)

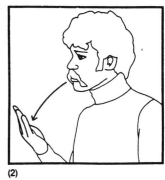
(2)

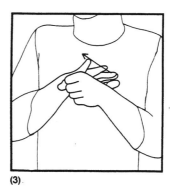
(3)

539

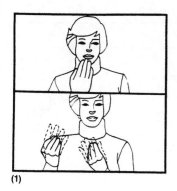
(1)

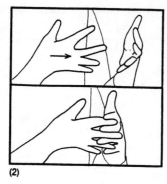
(2)

SATURATE

To soak, fill completely or more; absorb.

When a bandage is saturated with blood from a wound, it is important to leave it in place and add a new bandage on top of it.

(1) Sign WET — the fingertips of the right "flat" hand touch the mouth. Then, both "flat-O" hands face up at chest level and open and close a few times. (MM)
(2) The right "five" hand faces in and moves into the fingers of the left "five" hand. Both are at chest level. (SM)

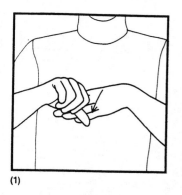
(1)

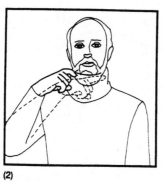
(2)

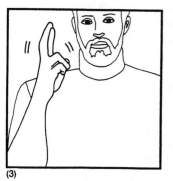
(3)

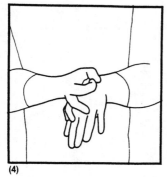
(4)

SCAB

The dried crust that forms over an open sore or wound.

A scab is formed from the serum and other fluids that escape from the wound and acts to protect the healing skin underneath.

(1) Sign CUT — the left "flat" hand faces in at chest level. The thumb of the right "A" hand moves down the back of the left hand as if imitating cutting. (SM)
(2) Sign DRY — the right "one" hand faces down at the chin. Move the hand to the right and at the same time, bend the index finger. (SM)
(3) The right "R" hand shakes, and twists slightly from side to side a few times. (MM)
(4) The right "F" hand faces down on the area of the scab.

SCABIES

A very contagious skin disease caused by a small insect, the itch mite. This insect burrows beneath the skin and causes severe itching, bumps and eczema. The skin between the fingers and toes, the armpits, the inner thighs, genitals and the area around the breasts are the most commonly affected places.

The insect which causes scabies can be gotten rid of by repeatedly using a special salve, a form of insecticide.

(Continued on next page)

(1) Sign INSECT — the thumb of the right "three" hand touches the nose. Bend and straighten the index and middle fingers a few times. (MM)

(2) Sign SCRATCH — both "claw" hands move up and down on the chest as if imitating scratching. (MM)

* This could be signed at the area of the scabies. The facial expression should reflect unpleasantness.

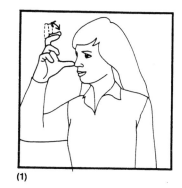
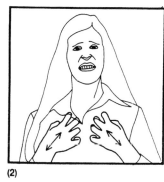

(1)　　　(2)

SCALD

A burn caused by a hot liquid or steam. Cold water should be applied to a scald immediately to reduce pain and help healing.

Because a scald is a deeper burn than a burn caused by a dry source of heat, it may damage more tissue, take longer to heal and leave a worse scar.

(1) Sign HOT — the right "claw" hand faces in at the face. Turn the hand to the right, then down, so that the palm faces down. (SM)

(2) Sign WATER — the index finger of the right "W" hand taps the mouth a few times. (MM)

(3) The right "C" hand faces out and moves towards the left arm as if imitating pouring something on it. (SM)

(4) Fingerspell "B-U-R-N" at the area of the burn.

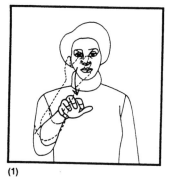
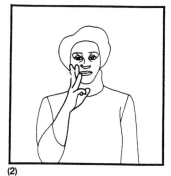

(1)　　　(2)

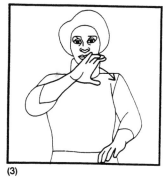
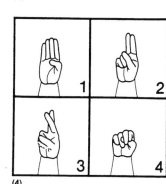

(3)　　　(4)

SCALE

A small, thin, dry piece of dead tissue shed from the upper layers of skin.

Shedding scales in small amounts is normal but large amounts could be the result of eczema, psoriasis, syphilis or seborrhea.

(1) Sign SKIN — the index finger and thumb of the right hand grab the right cheek. (SM)

(2) Sign PEEL — the left "flat" hand faces down at chest level. The index finger and thumb of the right "F" hand touch the back of the left hand, then move up and out as if imitating peeling something off it.

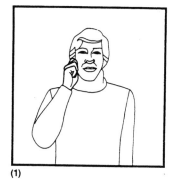
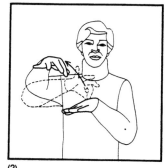

(1)　　　(2)

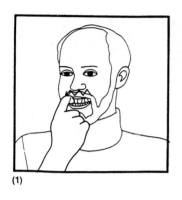
(1)
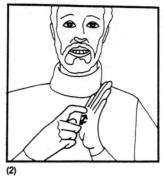
(2)

SCALING

In dentistry, the removal of substances on the teeth to prevent decay.

Scaling is done to remove such substances as tartar, plaque and heavy stains.

(1) The index finger of the right "one" hand moves up and down on the teeth. (MM)
(2) The left "flat" hand faces right at chest level. The index finger of the right "one" hand moves down the left palm as if imitating scraping it. (MM)

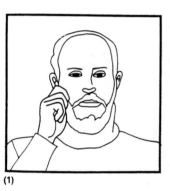
(1)
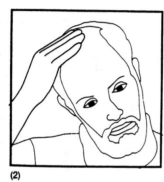
(2)

SCALP

The skin that covers the top of the head.

See Figure 1

(1) Sign SKIN — the index finger and thumb of the right hand grab the right ckeek. (SM)
(2) The right "flat" hand touches the top of the head. (SM)

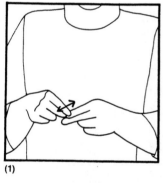
(1)
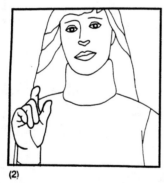
(2)
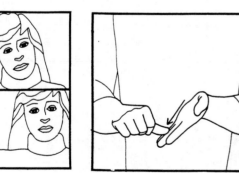
(3)   (4)

SCALPEL

A small knife with a thin, curved, very sharp blade used by a surgeon to cut into the body and to cut structures in the body.

A surgeon's scalpel is kept sterile and the blade is changed between each operation.

(1) Sign KNIFE — the left "H" hand faces right at chest level. The fingers of the right "H" hand move up and down on the fingers of the left hand a few times. (MM)
(2) Sign SMALL — the right "G" hand faces out at chest level indicating something small. (SM)
(3) Sign FOR — the index finger of the right "one" hand touches the forehead. Turn the hand to the right so that it points out forward. (SM)
(4) Sign OPERATE — the left "flat" hand faces right at chest level. The thumb of the right "A" hand moves down the left palm as if imitating cutting. (SM)

SCAPULA

The large, flat bone found on the back, upper part of the shoulder; also called the shoulder blade. The scapula serves as a place for the attachment of many muscles. *See Figure 26*

SCAR

The mark left on the skin or tissue after a wound, sore or injury has healed.

A scar results because the tissue that replaces the injured tissue is of a different type and is tough and fibrous.

(1) Fingerspell "S-C-A-R".

* *Point to the area of the scar after fingerspelling.*

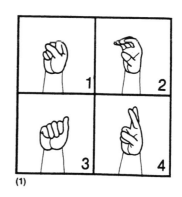
(1)

SCARLET FEVER

A disease caused by a certain kind of bacteria (streptococcus). The disease usually comes on very quickly and starts with a sore, red throat, fever and vomiting. A day later the person will get a red rash.

A person who may have scarlet fever should get antibiotics, most likely penicillin, for at least 10 days to fight off the infection and prevent the development of other diseases such as rheumatic fever or kidney disease.

SCAR TISSUE

An overgrowth of tissue over a scar, inside or outside the body, due to an injury or surgical incision; also called keloid.

Scar tissue will appear red, raised, hard and thick, and may grow for a long time.

SCHIZOPHRENIA

A type of mental illness which affects a person's personality. The person will be out of touch with the real world, may have hallucinations and mood changes, be withdrawn and paranoid and have strange behavior.

A person with schizophrenia may be hospitalized and treated with drugs and psychological therapy.

(1) Sign MIND — the index finger of the right "one" hand touches the forehead. (SM)

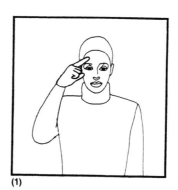
(1)

(Continued on next page)

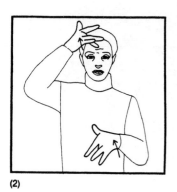
(2)

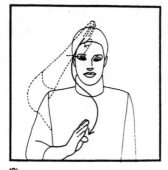
(3)

SCHIZOPHRENIA, *continued*

(2) Sign SICK — the middle finger of the right "eight" hand touches the forehead and the middle finger of the left "eight" hand touches the stomach. Twist both hands slightly. (SM)

* *The facial expression should reflect illness.*

(3) The right "four" hand faces left at the head. Move the hand down in an "S" movement to chest level. (SM)

SCIATICA

Severe pain in the back of the thigh along the length of the large sciatic nerve running down the leg, caused by inflammation or damage to the nerve. Symptoms of sciatica are a sharp pain running down the back of the thigh, numbness and tingling.

> *Sciatica may be treated with surgery, rest, applications of heat, drugs to lessen the pain and a good diet.*

SCIATIC NERVE

The largest nerve in the body. It runs from the hip down the back of the thigh, passing under the buttocks and dividing at the knee into the tibial and peroneal nerves. *See Figure 8*

SCLERA

The tough, white tissue which makes up what is called the white of the eye. The sclera covers the entire eye except the very front, where the cornea is, and where the optic nerve leaves the eye.
See Figure 22

SCLEROSIS

The hardening of an organ or area caused by the growth of fiber tissue.

> *The most common kinds of sclerosis are those affecting the brain and spinal cord, like multiple sclerosis, or hardening in the walls of the arteries, called arteriosclerosis.*

SCOLIOSIS

Any abnormal sideways curvature of the spine. There are usually two curves in the spine forming an "S" shaped spine. Scoliosis may be caused by bad posture, disease of the vertebrae, hip disease, a birth defect of the spine or weakness in the muscles of the spine. Sometimes the curve can be straightened or kept from getting worse by wearing a special brace or by keeping the muscles in the back strong by exercising.

Scoliosis is more common in girls than boys and many schools are now checking the backs of their students to catch the disorder early.

(1) Sign BACK — the right "flat" hand pats the back. (SM)
(2) The left "F" hand faces down at waist level. The right "F" hand faces down and moves from waist level to head level in an "S" movement. (SM)

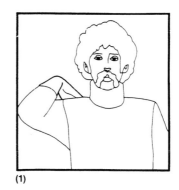
(1)

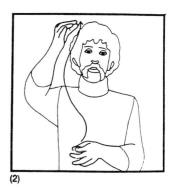
(2)

SCOTOMA

A blind spot or area of darkness in a person's field of vision.

Scotoma can occur because of migraine headaches, damage or a defect in the retina, or missing rods and cones in an area of the retina.

(1) Sign SEE — the right "V" hand faces in at eye level and moves out forward. (SM)
(2) Sign BLACK — the index finger of the right "one" hand moves across the forehead from left to right. (SM)
(3) The right "F" hand faces out at head level indicating a spot. (SM)

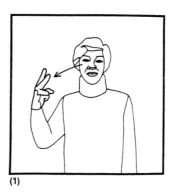
(1)

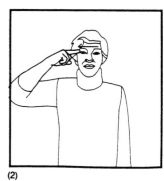
(2)

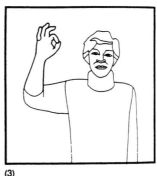
(3)

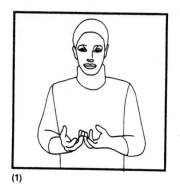
(1)

SCROTUM

The sac holding the testicles in males, found below the penis. *See Figure 13*

(1) Sign TESTICLES — both "claw" hands face up at waist level and bounce slightly. (SM)

* *It may be more clear to fingerspell "S-A-C" after the sign.*

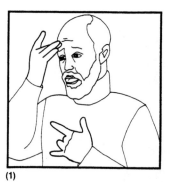
(1)

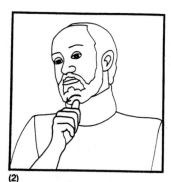
(2)

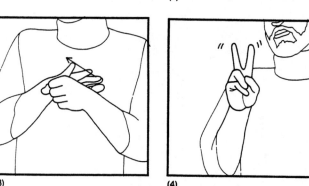
(3)   (4)

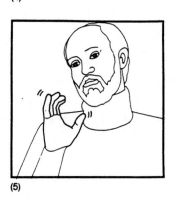
(5)

SCURVY

A disease caused by not getting enough vitamin C. A person with scurvy will be tired, have pain in the limbs and joints and loosening of the teeth, be anemic and bleed very easily, especially from the gums.

Since fresh fruits and vegetables have vitamin C in them, a person can prevent getting scurvy by eating plenty of them.

(1) Sign DISEASE — the middle finger of the right "eight" hand touches the forehead and the middle finger of the left "eight" hand touches the stomach. (SM)

(2) Sign NOT — the thumb of the right "A" hand touches under the chin. Move the hand straight out. (SM)

(3) Sign ENOUGH — the left "S" hand faces right at chest level. The right "flat" hand faces down and brushes out forward over the left fist. (SM)

(4) Sign VITAMIN — the right "V" hand faces out at chest level and shakes slightly from side to side a few times. (MM)

(5) Sign "C" — the right "C" hand faces out at chest level and shakes slightly from side to side a few times. (MM)

SEASICKNESS

See MOTION SICKNESS

546

SEBACEOUS GLANDS

A small gland in the skin which makes and puts out oil to help keep the skin soft and flexible.

*Most **sebaceous glands** open into the shaft of a small hair on the skin and if the opening of the gland becomes plugged, a pimple forms.*

SEBORRHEA

A disease in which small glands in the skin called sebaceous glands, which make oil, start working abnormally. They start putting out more oil than normal, causing the skin on different parts of the body to become greasy.

*A person with **seborrhea** is more likely to have acne, scaly skin and baldness.*

SECONAL®

The name under which the drug secobarbital is often sold, which acts as a sedative.

Seconal is often used to help a person sleep, to get a person ready for an anesthetic, to control convulsions and to calm someone who is very upset.

(1) Sign PILL — the right thumb and index finger touch, the palm faces in. Flick the index finger towards the mouth as if imitating popping a pill in the mouth. (SM)

(2) Sign DOWNER — the right "A" hand with the thumb extended faces out at shoulder level and moves down twice. (DM)

This is a general sign for depressants ("downers"). The specific type of drug should also be fingerspelled and all side effects explained.

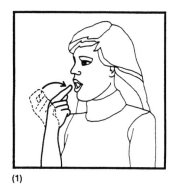

(1)

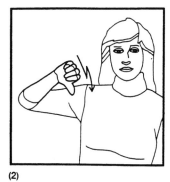

(2)

SECOBARBITAL

A barbiturate drug which acts as a depressant or sedative; also known as "red-devils" and sold under the name of seconal® . Secobarbital slows down body activities and nervous system activities, causing relaxation and sleep.

Secobarbital may be used to help people sleep, to control convulsions or to calm a person with violent behavior.

(1) Sign PILL — the right thumb and index finger touch, the palm faces in. Flick the index finger towards the mouth as if imitating popping a pill in the mouth. (SM)

(2) Sign DOWNER — the right "A" hand with the thumb extended faces out at shoulder level and moves down twice. (DM)

* *This is a general sign for depressants ("downers"). The specific type of drug should also be fingerspelled and all side effects explained.*

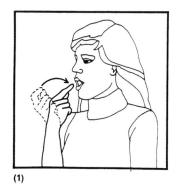

(1)

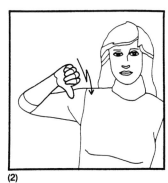

(2)

547

SECOND DEGREE BURN

Burns which damage both layers of the skin, the epidermis and the dermis. The skin of a person with second degree burns will be red and have blisters on it but the damage is not so bad that the skin won't heal. A second degree burn is worse than a first degree burn but not as bad as a third degree burn.

A second degree burn may be caused by a very deep sunburn, by getting hot liquids on the skin or by being burned with things like gasoline and kerosene.

SECRETE

To make and put out a substance. A structure or gland must take the material it is going to secrete from the blood, perhaps change the substance, and then put it back into the blood or carry it through a duct to where it will be used.

Endocrine glands secrete the hormones they make directly into the blood.

SECRETION

The substance made in a gland or structure which is put into the blood, digestive tract or the outside of the body. Examples of secretions are saliva, digestive juices, perspiration, urine and bile.

Hormones are the very important secretions of special glands, such as the pituitary gland, testes, ovaries and pancreas, which are put directly into the blood, circulate, and have effects on distant structures.

SECTION

A small, thin piece taken for microscopic examination; the act of cutting an organ or structure. ture.

A Cesarean section is the incision through the abdominal and uterine walls to deliver a baby.

SEDATIVE

A drug or substance which will calm, quiet or make the whole person or a part of the body less active. Barbiturates are the most important group of sedatives.

Drugs which act as sedatives work by affecting the activity of the nervous system.

(1) Sign MEDICINE — the left "flat" hand faces up at chest level. The middle finger of the right "eight" hand touches the left palm and pivots slightly from side to side a few times. (MM)

(2) Sign CALM — both "flat" hands face down at chest level and move down slightly. (SM)

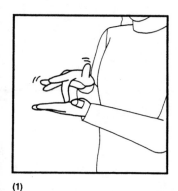
(1)

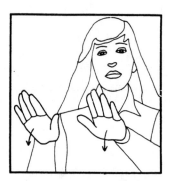
(2)

SEIZURE

A sudden attack or onset of a disease's symptoms.
Seizure is also used for an epileptic attack.

A seizure caused by epilepsy may range from a sudden stopping of what a person is doing and instead staring straight ahead for a few seconds to convulsions and unconsciousness.

SELF-ADMINISTER

Doing something to oneself.

Diabetics often must self-administer injections of insulin.

(1) Sign MYSELF — the right "A" hand faces left and taps the chest. (DM)

a. (1) Sign PILL — the right thumb and index finger touch, the palm faces in. Flick the index finger towards the mouth as if imitating popping a pill in the mouth. (SM)

b. (1) Sign INJECTION — the index finger of the right "L" hand touches the left upper arm. Bend the thumb in as if imitating injecting something into the arm. (SM)

c. (1) Sign DRINK — the right "C" hand faces left and moves up to the mouth as if imitating taking a drink. (SM)

* Sign MYSELF, then PILL, INJECTION, or DRINK, whichever applies.

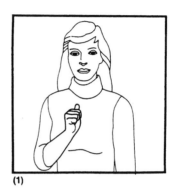
(1)

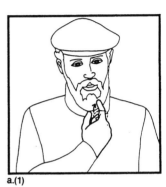
a.(1)

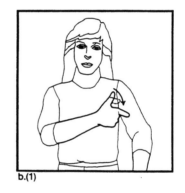
b.(1)

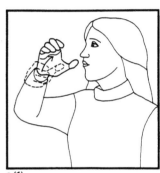
c.(1)

SELF EXAMINATION OF BREASTS

See BREAST SELF EXAMINATION

SEMEN

The thick, milky fluid put out by the penis of a male during orgasm, containing the male reproductive cells called sperm. Semen is made up of fluids made by several glands near the penis and testicles, such as the prostate.

Sperm are not able to survive on their own for very long but the semen supports and nourishes them while they are being stored before and just after being released from a man's body.

(1) Sign PENIS — the middle finger of the right "P" hand taps the nose a few times.

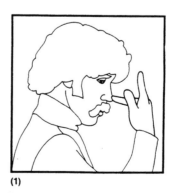
(1)

(Continued on next page)

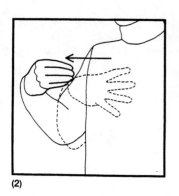

(2)

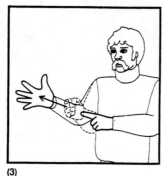

(3)

SEMEN, *continued*

(2) Sign WHITE — the fingertips of the right "five" hand touch the chest. Move the hand out to a "flat-O" hand. (SM)

(3) Sign EJACULATE — the right "S" hand faces left at chest level. The index finger of the left "one" hand touches the right wrist. Keeping the left hand in place, move the right hand slightly out to a "five" hand. (SM)

SEMICIRCULAR CANALS

The three loops found in the inner ear which help us keep our balance and sense the body's position in space. The semicircular canals are filled with a fluid and movement of the head causes this fluid to move around the canal. This movement is picked up by special nerves and carried to the brain. The semicircular canals are arranged in such a way that movement in any direction is picked up. *See Figure 20*

SEMINAL VESICLES

Two sac-like structures in the male, behind the bladder and connected to the deferens on each side. The seminal vesicles put out a thick fluid which forms part of the semen. *See Figure 13*

SENESCENSE

See SENILE

SENILE

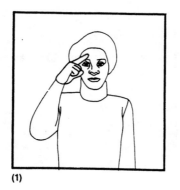

(1)

Having to do with growing old. Senile alone is often used for the mental disorders, loss of memory, and confusion that sometimes affects older people.

The most obvious senile changes seen in the body as one grows older are those in the eyes, skin, bones and joints.

(1) Sign MIND — the index finger of the right "one" hand touches the forehead. (SM)

(Continued on next page)

(2) Sign OLD — the right "S" hand faces left and touches the chin. Move the hand down in a wavy movement. (SM)

(3) Sign DETERIORATE — the right "cupped" hand faces down at shoulder level. Move the hand down in front of the body. (SM)

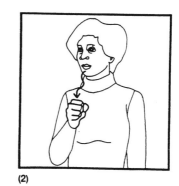
(2)

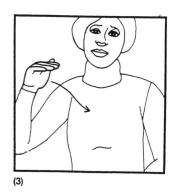
(3)

SENILITY

The mental or physical weakness or deterioration seen in old age. Symptoms of senility are parts of the body not working as well as they once did, resulting in poorer eyesight, getting tired easily, weakened bones, loss of memory, confusion and having less resistance to diseases.

Not all older people are affected by senility; some remain healthy, active, productive and happy for their entire lives.

(1) Sign MIND — the index finger of the right "one" hand touches the forehead. (SM)

(2) Sign OLD — the right "S" hand faces left and touches the chin. Move the hand down in a wavy movement. (SM)

(3) Sign DETERIORATE — the right "cupped" hand faces down at shoulder level. Move the hand down in front of the body. (SM)

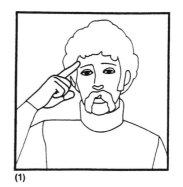
(1)

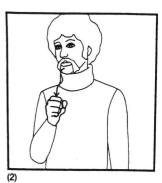
(2)

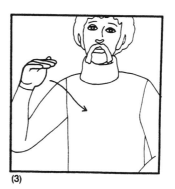
(3)

SENSATION

A feeling or awareness of something going on inside or around the body.

A sensation is the result of nerve cells picking up changes inside or outside the body and carrying small electrical impulses to the brain, where they are sensed.

(1) Sign FEEL — the middle finger of the right "eight" hand moves up and down the chest a few times. (MM)

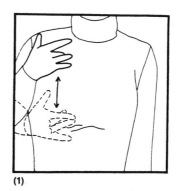
(1)

551

SENSE ORGANS

The structures and organs made up of highly specialized and developed nerves which allow us to pick up special activities or changes going on around us.

*The eyes, ears, nose and tastebuds are highly developed **sense organs**; special areas in the brain take information from them and allow us to be aware of what is going on around us.*

SENSES

Any functions of hearing, seeing, smelling, touching and tasting.

*When a person stops smoking, his **senses** of taste and smell will become sharper.*

(1) Sign HEAR — the index finger of the right "one" hand points to the ear. (SM)

* *Mouth the word "hear" while signing.*

(2) Sign TASTE — the middle finger of the right "eight" hand taps the chin or tongue. (SM)

(3) Sign SEE — the right "V" hand faces in at eye level. Move the hand out slightly. (SM)

(4) Sign SMELL — the right "flat" hand brushes up the nose. (SM)

(5) Sign TOUCH — the middle finger of the right "eight" hand touches the back of the left "flat" hand. (SM)

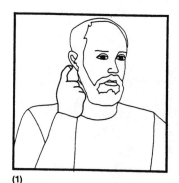
(1)

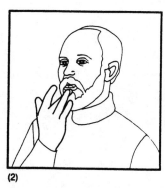
(2)

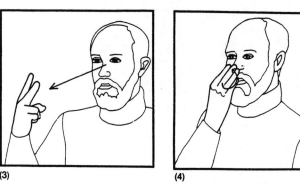
(3)

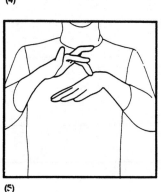
(4)

(5)

SENSORY

Having to do with sensations.

*The nervous system has **sensory** nerve cells which carry information about sensations to the brain and motor nerve cells which allow the brain to control other parts of the body by sending messages out to them.*

SENSITIVE

Something which is easily bothered or changed. Sensitive is often used for being badly affected very easily by a drug or substance.

An allergy occurs because someone is very sensitive to certain substances, usually proteins which have gotten into his body.

(1) Sign FEEL — the middle finger of the right "eight" hand moves up the chest, then out. At the same time, grit the teeth. (SM)

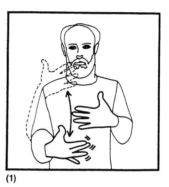
(1)

SEPSIS

A condition of having microorganisms or poisonous substances in the bloodstream.

Sepsis may also be called blood poisoning.

(1) Sign BLOOD — the left "five" hand is at chest level with the palm toward the body. The palm of the right "five" hand is toward the body with the middle fingertips touching the mouth. Move the right hand down the back of the left hand. Wiggle the fingers of the right hand as it moves. (MM)
* This movement should be short, repeated and somewhat restrained.

(2) Sign DISEASE — the middle finger of the right "eight" hand taps the forehead and the middle finger of the left "eight" hand taps the stomach. (SM)

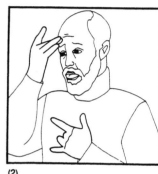

(1)   (2)

SEPTIC

Having to do with disease-causing bacteria or the illness or injury they cause; not clean.

A septic wound is one that has bacteria growing in it and causing damage.

(1) Sign NOT — the thumb of the right "A" hand touches under the chin. Move the hand straight out. (SM)

(2) Sign CLEAN — the left "flat" hand faces up at chest level. The right "flat" hand brushes out on the left palm. (SM)

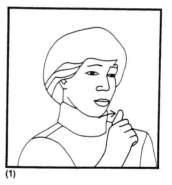
(1)

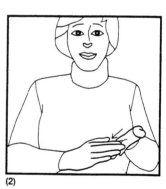
(2)

SEPTUM

A thin wall between two spaces or areas.

The septum which divides the right half of the heart from the left allows blood to be pumped easily to where it should go.

SERRATUS MAGNUS

A muscle which attaches to the shoulder blade and then fans out and attaches to the top of the ribs. The serratus magnus helps hold the scapula or shoulder blade in place against the ribs.
See Figure 4

SERUM

The clear, slightly yellow fluid that is left when the white blood cells, red blood cells and chemicals and proteins needed for blood to clot have been removed. Serum is also used for the fluid part of the blood of an animal which has been infected with a virus, bacteria or poison. The animal makes proteins called antibodies to destroy what was injected into it and these proteins are in the animal's blood.

The serum from an animal can be injected into a person who has a disease and the antibodies in it will quickly destroy the disease.

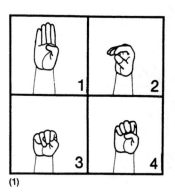
(1)

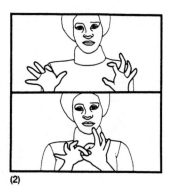
(2)

SET

To put a bone in the correct position and hold it there.

Only a doctor who has taken X-rays of a broken bone should try to set the fracture.

(1) Fingerspell "B-O-N-E".
(2) Both "F" hands join together at chest level. (SM)
* Point to the area referred to after these signs.

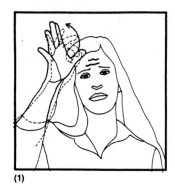
(1)

SEVERE

Very painful, sharp or extreme.

A migraine is a severe headache.

(1) The right "eight" hand faces left at the forehead. Shake the hand slightly twice, then flick the middle finger out. (SM)
* The facial expression should reflect pain.

SEX

The physical and mental characteristics that make a person male or female; also, sexual intercourse.

A certain chromosome, being carried by a man's sperm, will determine a baby's sex at the moment of fertilization.

(1) The right "X" hand faces out and touches the head at eye level, then at the chin. (SM)

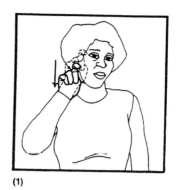

(1)

SEXUAL INTERCOURSE

The action of putting a man's penis in a woman's vagina and releasing sperm.

Sexual intercourse is another word for coitus, copulation, making love or mating.

a. (1) Sign INTERCOURSE — the left "V" hand faces up at chest level. The right "V" hand faces down and moves down to touch the left hand. (SM)

b. (1) Sign SEX — the right "X" hand faces out and touches the head at eye level, then at the chin. (SM)

c. (1) Fingerspell "I-C".

* *These could be signed alone or together for clarification.*

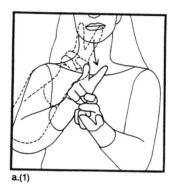

a.(1)

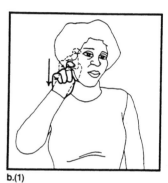

b.(1)

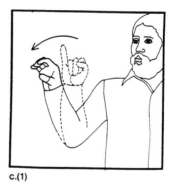

c.(1)

SHARP

Not dull. Having a thin or fine edge for cutting.

Surgeon's knives are very sharp to cut the skin easily.

(1) The left "flat" hand faces in at chest level. The middle finger of the right "eight" hand brushes up the back of the left hand. At the same time, grit the teeth. (SM)

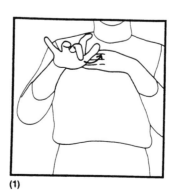

(1)

555

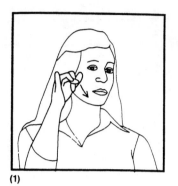
(1)

SHAVE

To cut or remove body hair.

Many times before surgery, the area to be operated on will be shaved.

(1) The thumb of the right "Y" hand moves down the right cheek as if imitating shaving. (SM)

SHIGELLA

A bacteria (Enterobacteriaceae) causing various forms of dysentary, an intestinal disorder.

Shigella can cause digestive disorders ranging from mild diarrhea to severe and often fatal dysentary.

SHIGELLOSIS

A form of dysentary caused by the Shigella bacteria. (See SHIGELLA).

Symptoms of shigellosis may include pain, fever, and severe diarrhea containg blood or mucus.

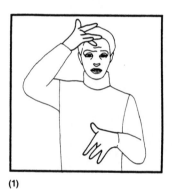
(1)
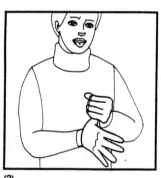
(2)

(1) Sign SICK — the middle finger of the right "eight" hand taps the forehead and the middle finger of the left "eight" hand taps the stomach. (SM)

(2) Sign DIARRHEA — the left "S" hand faces right at chest level. The thumb of the right "five" hand is inside the left fist. Move the right hand down several times. (MM)

SHIN

The front part of the lower leg.

The shin is a hard area of the tibia, the large bone in the lower leg, and is covered only by some skin.

SHIN BONE

See TIBIA

SHINGLES

A skin disease caused by a virus (varicella), the same that causes chickenpox. Shingles start with pain in the area of skin which the nerve goes to and later, bumps like those in chickenpox appear on the skin in one place, usually on one side of the head. The disease is more common in adults and only a person who has had chickenpox at some time in his life has a chance of getting shingles.

Herpes Zoster is another name for shingles.

SHIVER

An uncontrollable trembling or shaking caused by the muscles contracting.

A person will automatically start to shiver if he gets cold enough and this physical activity will cause heat to be made in the muscles, that helps keep the body warm.

(1) The left "bent-V" hand faces up at chest level. The right "bent-V" hand faces out on the left palm. Shake the right hand slightly from side to side as if imitating shivering. At the same time, grit the teeth. (MM)

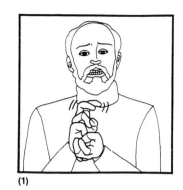

(1)

SHOCK

A condition in which the body's activities are slowed down because the amount of blood going to the tissues is decreased. The blood may be lost from the body through bleeding, it may collect in an area of the body, usually the abdominal organs, or the amount of blood may be lowered because a lot of fluids have been lost from the body. Symptoms of shock are paleness, bluish lips and fingers, a weak and fast heartbeat, rapid breathing, a very low blood pressure and thirst. Shock may be caused by burns, bleeding, an infection, poisoning, a heart attack or a severe allergic reation. Shock is also used for the passing of electricity through the body.

The injured person should be watched closely for signs of shock because untreated, it often leads to death.

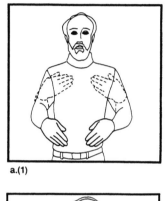

a.(1)

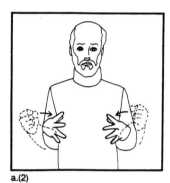

a.(2)

a. (1) Sign BODY — both "flat" hands touch the chest, then the stomach. (SM)
(2) Sign SHOCK — both "S" hands face each other at chest level. Move both hands in towards the center, ending in "five" hands. (SM)

* The facial expression should reflect shock.

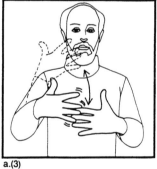

a.(3)

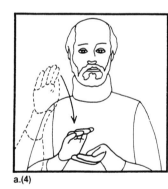

a.(4)

(3) Sign BLOOD — the left "five" hand is at chest level with the palm toward the body. The palm of the right "five" hand is toward the body with the middle fingertips touching the mouth. Move the right hand down the back of the left hand. Wiggle the fingers of the right hand as it moves. (MM)
(4) Sign REDUCE — the left "cupped" hand faces up at chest level. The right "cupped" hand faces down at shoulder level. Move the right hand down to the left hand. (SM)

(Continued on next page)

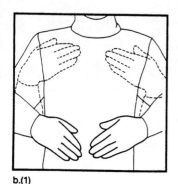

b.(1)

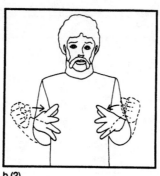

b.(2)

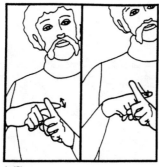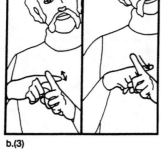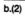

b.(3)

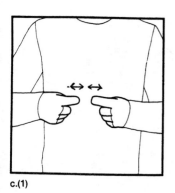

c.(1)

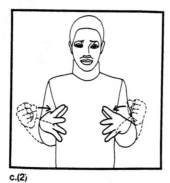

c.(2)

SHOCK, *continued*

b. (1) Sign BODY — both "flat" hands touch the chest, then the stomach. (SM)
(2) Sign SHOCK — both "S" hands face each other at chest level. Move both hands towards the center, ending in "five" hands. (SM)
* *The facial expression should reflect shock.*

(3) Sign TEMPERATURE LOW — the left "one" hand points up at chest level. The index finger of the right "one" hand moves up and down the left index finger a few times, then stops down low as if indicating low. (SM)

c. (1) Sign ELECTRIC — both "X" hands face in at chest level. Taps the knuckles together a few times. (MM)
(2) Sign SHOCK — both "S" hands face each other at chest level. Move both hands in towards the center, ending in "five" hands. (SM)
* *The facial expression should reflect shock.*

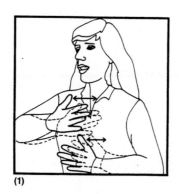

(1)

SHORTNESS OF BREATH

Deep, fast and difficult breathing which may be painful. Shortness of breath is caused by the cells needing more oxygen for some reason or there being too much carbon dioxide in the blood.

When a person exercises hard, some shortness of breath is normal.

(1) Sign BREATHE — both "flat" hands move in and out from the chest in short, quick, repeated movements. (MM)
* *The facial expression should reflect difficulty of breathing.*

SHOT

In medicine, an injection by which a drug or medication is placed under the skin, into a muscle or a vein. A hollow needle attached to a tube containing the drug or medication is placed under the skin and the substance is pushed from the tube into the body.

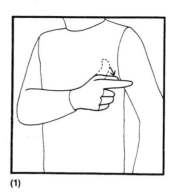
(1)

A person may be given a substance in a shot instead of through the mouth when the drug would be destroyed in the stomach or intestine, when it must start working quickly or when its effects are needed only in a small area.

(1) Sign INJECTION — the index finger of the right "L" hand touches the left upper arm. Bend the thumb in as if imitating injecting something into the arm. (SM)

* This could be signed at the area where the injection is to be given.

SHOULDER

The area where the arm meets the trunk or body. *See Figure 1*

(1) The right "one" hand points to the shoulder. (SM)

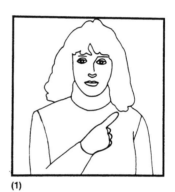
(1)

SHOULDER BLADE

One of the flat, triangular shaped bones in the upper back on either side; the scapula. *See Figure 3*

(1) The fingers of the right "flat" hand rub up and down on the shoulder blade. (MM)

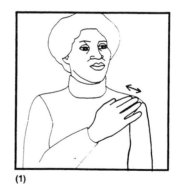
(1)

SIAMESE TWINS

Twin babies whose bodies are joined together at some place. Siamese twins may be attached to each other at their heads, hips or sides and they may share an organ between them.

With careful surgery, a surgeon may be able to separate some siamese twins and cause no damage to either.

(Continued on next page)

559

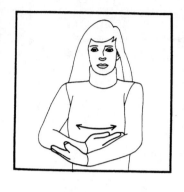
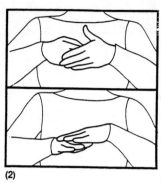
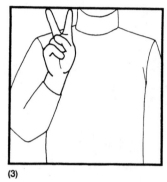
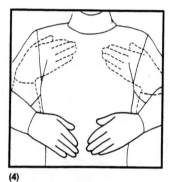
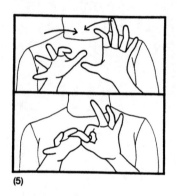

(2)

(3)

(4)

(5)

(1) Sign BABY — the right hand and forearm face up, resting on the left hand and forearm which also face up. Both are then rocked back and forth as if holding a baby. (MM)

(2) Sign BORN — the left "flat" hand faces in at chest level. The right "flat" hand faces in behind the left hand. Move the right hand down under the left, then out forward. (SM)

(3) Sign TWO — the right "V" hand faces out at chest level. (SM)

(4) Sign BODY — both "flat" hands touch the chest, then the stomach. (SM)

(5) Sign CONNECTED — both "F" hands join at chest level. (SM)

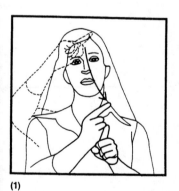
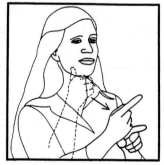

(1)

(2)

SIBLING

A person's brother or sister.

People who are siblings have the same parents.

(1) Sign BROTHER — the left "one" hand points out at chest level, the palm facing right. The right "one" hand faces down at the forehead, then moves down to tap the left hand. (SM)

(2) Sign SISTER — the left "one" hand points out at chest level, the palm facing right. The thumb of the right "A" hand moves down the right cheek. Change the right hand to a "one" hand and tap the left hand. (SM)

560

SICK

Not well, physically or mentally unhealthy.

A person who is sick with a disease that can be passed to other people will be doing other people a favor by staying home and not exposing them to the disease.

(1) The middle finger of the right "eight" hand taps the forehead and the middle finger of the left "eight" hand taps the stomach. (SM)

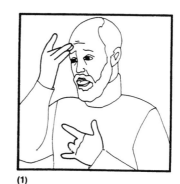

(1)

SICKLE CELL ANEMIA

A disease in which a person's red blood cells are shaped abnormally, causing them to be weak and destroyed more quickly. Because these red blood cells are destroyed more quickly than normal, the person may become anemic. Sickle cell anemia is caused by a person's red blood cells having an abnormal type of hemoglobin in them which makes the cell curve into an abnormal shape. The disease is found only in blacks and is hereditary.

The type of hemoglobin which causes a person to have sickle cell anemia will make that person more resistant to malaria than a person with normal hemoglobin and normal red blood cells.

SIDE EFFECT

A result of or action caused by a drug or treatment which is not wanted or expected.

Many drugs have well known side effects which may be felt by a person taking them, and that person should always be told about the side effects or ask if there are any.

(1) Sign OTHER — the right "A" hand, with the thumb extended, faces down at chest level. Turn the hand up so that the palm faces left. (SM)
(2) Sign EFFECT — the left "flat" hand faces down at chest level. The right "flat-O" hand is on top of the left hand. Move the right hand out over the left into a "five" hand. (SM)

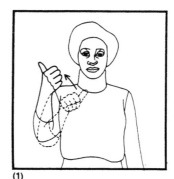

(1)

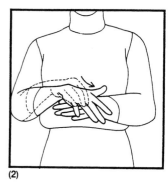

(2)

SIDS

See SUDDEN INFANT DEATH SYNDROME

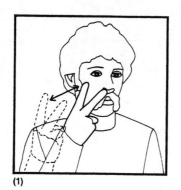
(1)

SIGHT

The power or ability to see things.

The eyes are the organs of sight.

(1) Sign SEE — the right "V" hand faces in at eye level and moves out slightly. (SM)

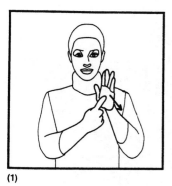
(1)

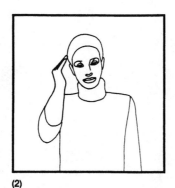
(2)

SIGN

A result or effect of a disease which can be seen or picked up by a doctor.

Signs and symptoms are not the same because a symptom is what is felt by a person with a disease, while a sign is observed and points to a certain disease.

(1) The index finger of the right "one" hand touches the palm of the left "flat" hand. Move both hands forward slightly. (SM)

(2) Sign KNOW — the fingertips of the right "cupped" hand touch the forehead. (SM)

SILICOSIS

Fibrous tissue in the lungs caused by breathing in dust from minerals such as quartz, sand, glass and concrete.

Silicosis may cause long-term shortness of breath.

SILVER NITRATE

A colorless, poisonous substance that turns grayish-black when exposed to light.

Silver nitrate is used in photography, for making mirrors, hair dyes and some external medicines.

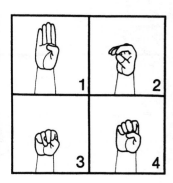

1 2 3 4

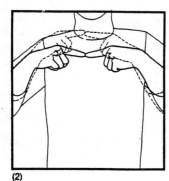
(2)

SIMPLE FRACTURE

A broken bone in which the tissue or area around the break isn't injured.

Most simple fractures occur from an accident or fall and should be splinted before moving the injured person.

(1) Fingerspell "B-O-N-E".

(2) Both index fingers touch, the palms facing down, at chest level. Drop both hands slightly. (SM)

SINUS

A space or cavity which has a narrow opening into it. Sinus is most often used for the nasal sinuses, which are spaces in the bones of the head.

A person who has a cold or allergy may have the **sinuses** *filled with mucus, causing a runny nose and headache.*

(1) Fingerspell "S-I-N-U-S".
(2) The index fingers of both "one" hands move up the nose and around the forehead as if imitating the outline of the sinuses. (SM)

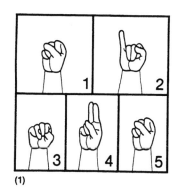

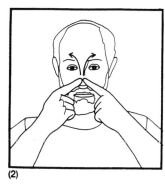

SINUSITIS

Inflammation of a sinus membrane in the nose.

Some causes of **sinusitis** *are viruses, bacteria and allergies.*

SISTER

A female having the same parents as another child.

A **sister** *is a female sibling.*

(1) The thumb of the right "A" hand moves down the right cheek. The right hand changes to a "one" hand and touches the left "one" hand at chest level. (SM)

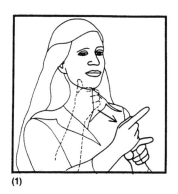

SITZ BATH

A bath that a person sits in, with the water coming up to the hips.

A person usually takes a **sitz bath** *with hot water to treat a disorder in the anal or genital regions.*

(1) Sign BATHE — both "A" hands move in circular movements on the chest as if imitating bathing. (MM)
(2) Sign WATER — the index finger of the right "three" hand taps the mouth. (MM)
(3) Both "modified-C" hands face out at chest level and move to the sides, indicating the tub. (SM)
(4) Sign SIT IN — the right "bent-V" hand faces down at chest level and moves slightly down, indicating sitting in the tub. (SM)

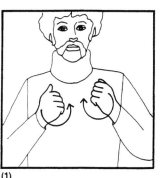

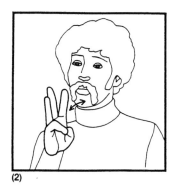

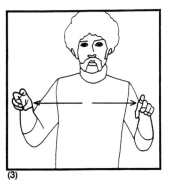

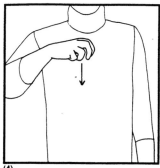

563

SKELETAL SYSTEM

All of the bones in the body along with the cartilage and joints which hold them together. The skeletal system acts as a frame to support the body and its parts and also protects some organs. *See Figure 26*

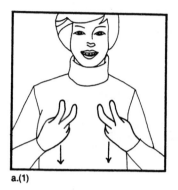 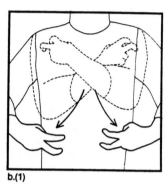

a.(1)   b.(1)

SKELETON

The frame made up of 206 bones which holds up and protects the softer parts of the body.

The skeleton of a man is different from the skeleton of a woman in that the pelvis is shaped differently and the bones are usually larger and heavier.

a. (1) Both "bent-V" hands face in at chest level and move down the body. (SM)

b. (1) Both "bent-V" hands face in and cross at the chest. Move both hands down to the sides. (SM)

SKIN

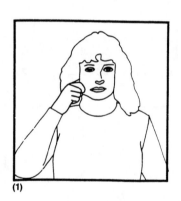

(1)

The tissue which covers the body. The skin is divided into two layers: the outer layer, the epidermis, made up of dead cells, and the inner one, the dermis, made up of live cells with nerves, blood vessels, glands and fat.

The skin is very important in protecting us against injuries and infection, keeping water in the body, helping control body temperature and in getting rid of some body wastes.

(1) The index finger and thumb of the right fist grab the right cheek. (SM)

SKIN GRAFTING

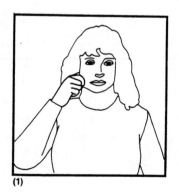

(1)

An operation in which healthy skin from one part of the body is removed and used to cover an area of the body where the skin was so badly damaged that it wouldn't grow back normally.

Skin grafting is often used in third degree burns because the inner layer of the skin is so badly burned that the area won't heal normally.

(1) Sign SKIN — the index finger and thumb of the right fist grab the right cheek. (SM)

(Continued on next page)

(2) Sign CUT — the thumb of the right "A" hand moves down the left upper arm as if imitating cutting. (SM)

(3) The right "claw" hand touches the left upper arm, then moves down to touch the right upper leg. (SM)

* *This could be signed at the area of the skin graft.*

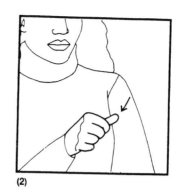
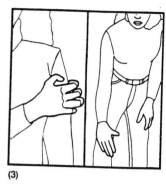

(2)   (3)

SKULL

The bones that make up the head; the cranium. The skull is made up of 22 bones which are closely connected to each other and which act to protect the brain and fragile structures like the eyes and ears. *See Figure 26*

SLEEP

The time during which body activities are stopped or slowed down and the person seems to be almost unconscious. When someone sleeps, the brain's activities are lessened to allow it to rest.

Sleep is so important to health that without it, a person becomes easily upset, clumsy and may collapse or fall asleep after two or three days.

a. (1) The right "five" hand faces in at the face. Move the right hand down to an "A" hand on top of the left "A" hand. At the same time, the eyes should close. (SM)

b. (1) The right "five" hand faces in at the face. Move the hand down slightly into a "flat-O" hand. At the same time, the eyes should close. (SM)

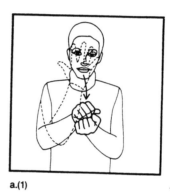
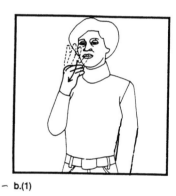

a.(1)   — b.(1)

SLEEPING PILLS

Drugs used to put people to sleep or to relax them so that they can sleep. Barbiturates such as chloralhydrate, paraldehyde, chlordiazepoxide and diazepam are examples of drugs used to make sleeping pills.

Any sleeping pills should be used very carefully because they may cause addiction and then the person would always need pills to sleep.

(1) Sign PILL — the right thumb and index finger touch, the palm faces in. Flick the index finger towards the mouth as if imitating popping a pill in the mouth. (SM)

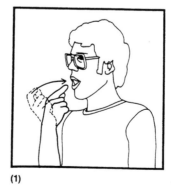

(1)

(Continued on next page)

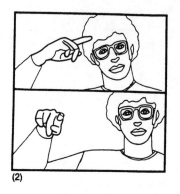

(2)

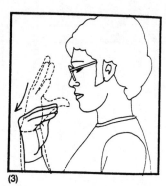

(3)

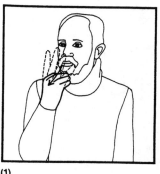

(1)

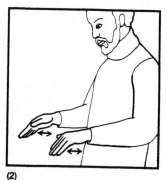

(2)

(2) Sign FOR — the index finger of the right "one" hand touches the forehead. Turn the hand to the right so that it points out forward. (SM)

(3) Sign SLEEP — the right "five" hand faces in at the face. Move the hand slightly down into a "flat-O" hand. At the same time, the eyes should close. (SM)

SLEEP WALKING

Walking around while asleep; nightwalking; somnambulism.

A person found sleep walking should be gently led back to bed and not wakened because it can be very frightening.

(1) Sign SLEEP — the right "five" hand faces in at the face. Move the hand slightly down into a "flat-O" hand. At the same time, the eyes should close. (SM)

(2) Sign WALK — both "flat" hands face down at chest level. Move both hands alternately in and out a few times as if imitating walking. At the same time, the eyes should close. (MM)

SLING

A bandage used to support an injured arm and hold it still.

In first-aid, a person who may have a broken collarbone, shoulder blade, arm, wrist or hand should have the arm put in a sling.

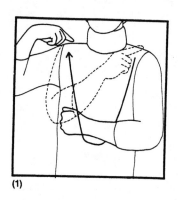

(1)

(1) The left arm is bent at the elbow. The index finger of the right "one" hand touches the left shoulder, moves down under the left arm, then moves up to touch the right shoulder as if imitating the shape of a sling. (SM)

SLIPPED DISK

Damage of the cartilage disks between the vertebrae of the backbone due to too much pressure put on it. The cartilage disks have a center made up of a jelly-like material which helps the disk act as a shock absorber. When pressure is put on the backbone, as when you stand up, the disks flatten and spread out. If severe pressure is put on a disk suddenly, the disk may break open or be moved from its correct position.

(Continued on next page)

A slipped disk will not be able to act as a cushion and may cause severe pain because of pressure on nerves running between the vertebrae.

(1) Sign BACK — the right "flat" hand taps the back. (MM)

(2) Both "F" hands face down at waist level. Move the right hand up to chest level as if imitating the shape of the backbone. (SM)

(3) Both "bent-V" hands face in with the left hand on top of the right hand. Alternately change the positions of the hands as they slightly move up, indicating the disks in the backbone. (MM)

(4) Both "F" hands face down at chest level, the right hand on top of the left. Move the right hand out forward slightly. (SM)

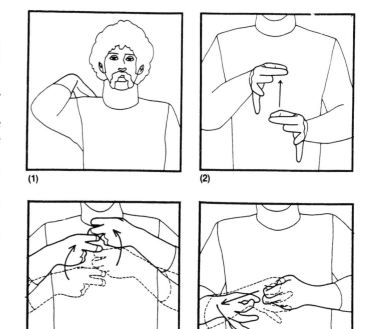

(1) (2) (3) (4)

SLUR

To speak unclearly; not pronouncing words so they can be understood.

Overdoses of many different kinds of drugs will cause a person to slur his speech.

(1) The index finger of the right "five" hand touches the mouth. Move the hand out slightly and at the same time, wiggle the fingers. (SM)

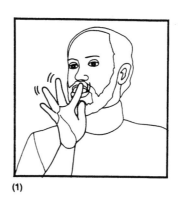

(1)

SMALL INTESTINE

The part of the digestive tract which goes from the stomach to the start of the colon or large intestine. The small intestine is divided into three parts: the duodenum, the jejunum and the ileum. The small intestine takes the food from the stomach, adds a lot of digestive juices to it, mixes the food and does most of the breaking down and absorbing of the food. *See Figure 9*

(1) The right "F" hand faces down at stomach level and moves down in a wavy motion as if indicating the shape of the intestines. (SM)

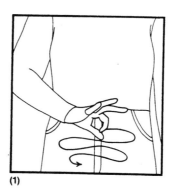

(1)

SMALLPOX

A severe disease caused by a virus which attacks the whole body; also called variola. The most obvious symptom is a rash of large bumps which can cause scarring. Symptoms of smallpox come on quickly, with chills, a headache, fever, vomiting and, after the third or fourth day, bumps appearing. These start out as red bumps which fill with pus and fluid, dry up and crust over; then the crust falls off, leaving a small pit in the skin. These bumps are caused by the virus attacking the skin and reproducing in the bumps. A severe case of smallpox is almost always fatal.

Children in the U.S. are not automatically vaccinated to prevent smallpox anymore because there hasn't been a case here since 1949 but a smallpox vaccination may be needed if traveling to another country.

SMEGMA

Thick, bad-smelling secretions from sebaceous glands.

Smegma is found under the foreskin of the penis (prepuce) and the labias of the vulva.

(1) The right "flat" hand taps the groin area. (SM)
(2) Sign SMELL — the right "flat" hand brushes up the nose. (SM)
(3) Sign BAD — the fingers of the right "flat" hand touch the mouth. Turn the hand out and move it down, the palm faces down. (SM)

* The facial expression should reflect bad smelling.

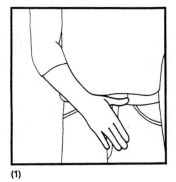
(1)

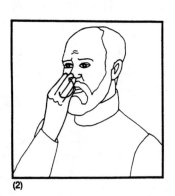
(2)

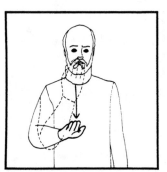
(3)

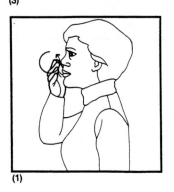
(1)

SMELL

The sense which allows us to detect odors.

Membranes with special nerves cells deep in the nose allow us to smell things.

(1) The right "flat" hand brushes up the nose. (MM)

568

SMOKE

Referring to inhaling any substance such as cigarettes, cigars, or drugs like marijuana or hashish.

A doctor may ask a patient if he smokes in order to help diagnose an illness.

(1) Sign SMOKE — the right "V" hand faces in at the mouth and moves out slightly. (SM)
  a. (2) Sign CIGAR — the right "R" hand faces down at the mouth. (SM)
  b. (2) Sign PIPE — the right "Y" hand faces down at the mouth. (SM)
  c. (2) Sign CIGARETTE — the left "one" hand faces down at chest level. The index and little fingers of the right hand tap the left index finger. (MM)
  d. (2) Sign MARIJUANA — the index finger and thumb of the right "F" hand tap the mouth. (MM)

* *Sign SMOKE, then sign CIGAR, PIPE, CIGARETTE, or MARIJUANA, whichever applies.*

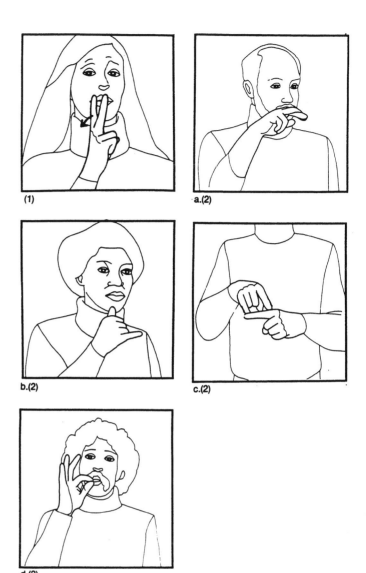

(1)   a.(2)

b.(2)   c.(2)

d.(2)

SNEEZE

To force air out of the nose and mouth very rapidly. Sneezing is a reflex which is caused by something irritating the inner lining of the nose. To sneeze, a person first inhales and then the muscles which help us breathe out contract suddenly, forcing air out quickly to try to get rid of the irritation.

During a sneeze, the speed of the air traveling out of the mouth or nose may reach 200 miles per hour.

(1) The index finger of the right "one" hand touches under the nose, then imitate sneezing. (SM)

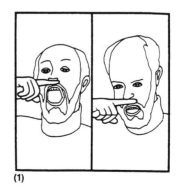

(1)

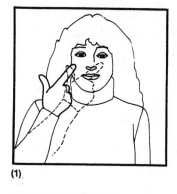

(1)

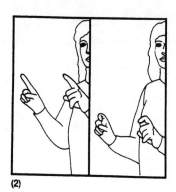

(2)

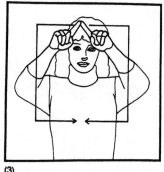

(3)

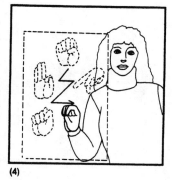

(4)

SNELLEN'S CHART

A piece of paper which has lines of black letters of different sizes on it, used to see how good a person's vision is.

On a Snellen chart, each line of letters is labeled with the distance in feet at which the line could be read by a person with normal vision.

(1) Sign EYES — the index finger of the right "one" hand points to both eyes. (SM)
(2) Sign TEST — both "one" hands point up at chest level, the palms face out. Move both hands down slightly and, at the same time, bend and straighten both index fingers. Repeat this movement three times until the hands end at waist level. (MM)
(3) Sign CHART — the index fingers of both "one" hands make the outline of a chart. (SM)
(4) Fingerspell "E-F-P-O-Z".

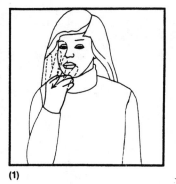

(1)

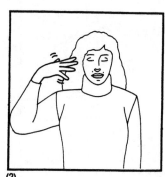

(2)

SNORE

Noisy breathing during sleep.

Snoring is caused by vibration of the back part of the mouth, the soft palate, when someone is completely relaxed.

(1) Sign SLEEP — the right "five" hand faces in at the face. Move the hand down slightly into a "flat-O" hand. At the same time, the eyes should close. (SM)
(2) The right "five" hand faces down at the right ear and shakes slightly as if indicating ringing in the ear. (MM)

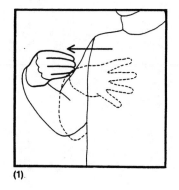

(1)

SNOW BLINDNESS

Irritation of the eyes or temporary blindness caused by sun being reflected off snow. Symptoms of snow blindness in addition to blindness are pain when light hits the eye, squinting and redness of the eye.

Sunglasses which reflect the sun's rays can be worn to prevent snow blindness when skiing or hiking on snow.

(1) Sign WHITE — the fingertips of the right "five" hand touch the chest. Move the hand out into a "flat-O" hand. (SM)

(Continued on next page)

(2) Sign SNOW — both "five" hands face down at chest level. Move both hands down slightly and at the same time, wiggle the fingers. (SM)

(3) The right "flat-O" hand faces down at shoulder level. Drop the hand down to an open "flat-O" hand, then it moves up to the face as if indicating something reflecting in the face. (SM)

(4) Sign CAN'T — the left "one" hand faces down at chest level. The right "one" hand moves down to strike the left index finger. (SM)

(5) Sign SEE — the right "V" hand faces in at eye level and moves out forward slightly. (SM)

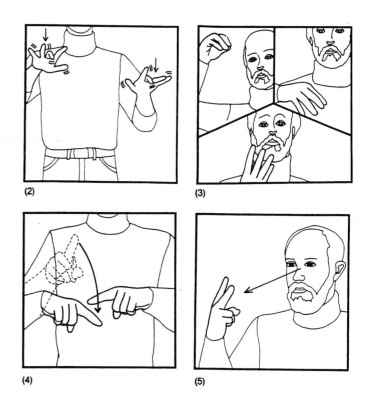

SOAK

Placing something in water for a length of time to treat a problem.

Cold water is used to soak a part of the body to lessen pain, swelling and inflammation, while hot water is used to soak a part of the body to help increase blood flow to the area and to speed healing.

(1) Sign IN — the fingers of the right "flat-O" hand move into the left fist. (SM)

(2) Sign WATER — the index finger of the right "three" hand taps the mouth. (MM)

(3) Sign LEAVE — both "five" hands face in at chest level and move down to waist level. (SM)

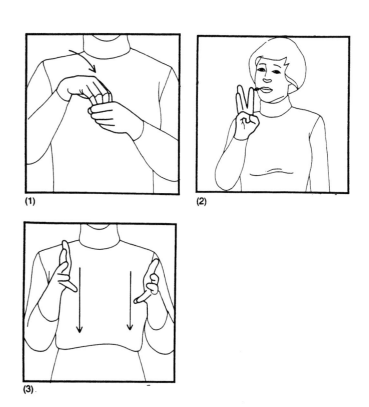

571

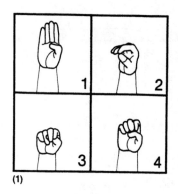

(1)

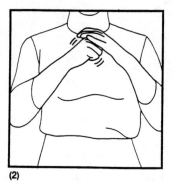

(2)

SOCKET

A hollow space in a bone which surrounds and holds a part of another bone or an organ.

The eyeball fits into a socket in the skull and the roots of each tooth fit into a socket in the jawbone.

(1) Fingerspell "B-O-N-E".

(2) The right "S" hand pivots slightly a few times under the left "flat" hand. (MM)

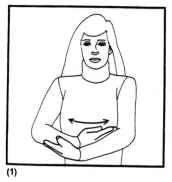

(1)

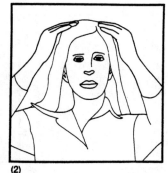

(2)

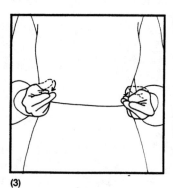

(3)

SOFT SPOTS

The soft spaces between the bones that make up the skull on a baby's head; also called the fontanelles. The bones have not grown together in these places yet and the brain is only covered by the meninges and scalp.

Usually, the soft spots have grown together by the time the baby is two years old.

(1) Sign BABY — the right hand and forearm face up, resting on the left hand and forearm which also face up. Both are then rocked back and forth as if holding a baby. (MM)

(2) The fingers of both "flat" hands touch the head. (SM)

(3) Sign SOFT — both "flat-O" hands face up. Open and close both hands a few times. (MM)

SOLAR PLEXUS

The large nerves and ganglia behind the stomach. The solar plexus supplies nerves to the structures in the abdomen area.

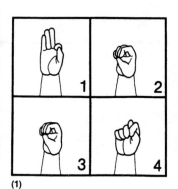

(1)

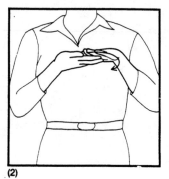

(2)

SOLE

The underside of the foot.

The sole of the foot is protected by calluses made of many layers of dead skin cells.

(1) Fingerspell "F-O-O-T".

(2) The left "flat" hand faces down at chest level. The right "flat" hand faces up and rubs the left palm in a circular movement, indicating the underside. (MM)

SOLEUS

A flat, wide muscle in the back of the lower leg which helps to make up the calf. The soleus helps to extend the foot and point the toe. *See Figure 5*

SOLID

Something which is not a gas or a liquid; something which is hard and will not flow.

*A drug can be given in the form of a gas which is inhaled, a liquid which can be injected or a **solid** which can be taken in the form of a pill and swallowed.*

(1) Sign HARD — the knuckles of the right "bent-V" hand tap the top of the left "bent-V" hand. (MM)

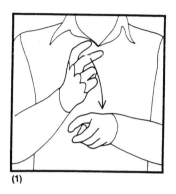
(1)

SOLUTION

A liquid which has something dissolved in it.

*The liquid part of the blood, plasma, is a very complex **solution** which transports dissolved substances through the body..*

SOMNAMBULISM

See SLEEP WALKING

SORE

An open wound or area of the skin.

*A **sore** on the genitals caused by a venereal disease is caused by the virus or bacteria reproducing in the area and damaging cells.*

(1) Fingerspell "S-O-R-E".
(2) The right "modified-C" hand faces out on the left upper arm.

* This could be signed at the area of the sore.

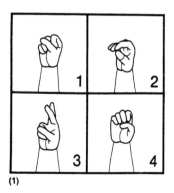
(1)

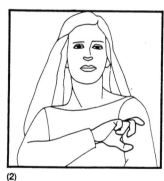
(2)

SORENESS

Painful or tender.

*Sometimes an inflammed hair follicle can cause **soreness** of the skin around it.*

(1) Sign PAIN — both "one" hands point to each other and twist in opposite directions a few times. (MM)

* This could be signed at the area of the soreness. The facial expression should reflect pain.

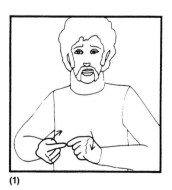
(1)

SOUND

Air vibrations picked up with the ear; noise.

The loudness of a sound is measured in decibels.

(1) Sign HEAR — the index finger of the right "one" hand points to the right ear. (SM)

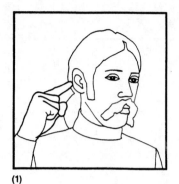

(1)

SPASM

A sudden, uncontrollable movement or muscle contraction.

A strong, painful spasm is called a cramp.

(1) Both "claw" hands face in at chest level. Shake both hands slightly. (MM)

* *The facial expression should reflect spasm.*

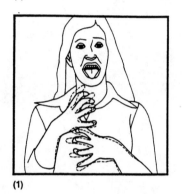

(1)

SPEAKING PERSON

See HEARING PERSON

SPECIALIST

A doctor who has had training in any particular area of medicine after getting out of medical school and who practices in that area of medicine.

A pediatrician is a doctor who is a specialist in the care and treatment of diseases in children.

(1) Sign SPECIALIZE — the left "B" hand faces right at chest level. The right "B" hand faces left and moves out along the left index finger. (SM)

(2) Sign PERSON — both "flat" hands face each other at chest level and move down to waist level. (SM)

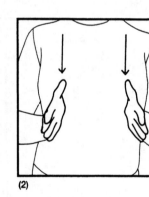

(1)

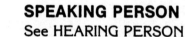
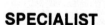
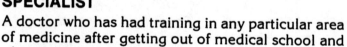

(2)

SPECIALIZE

To train or study in a special activity.

A chiropodist specializes in the treatment of foot disorders.

(1) The left "B" hand faces right at chest level. The right "B" hand faces left and moves out along the left index finger. (SM)

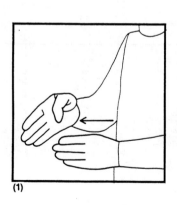

(1)

574

SPECIMEN

A sample of something or a small part of something which is taken to be examined.

A routine part of a physical examination is giving the doctor a specimen of urine so he can see if the kidneys are working normally and if the person may have diabetes.

(1) Sign CUT — the thumb of the right "A" hand moves down the palm of the left "flat" hand as if cutting. (SM)

(2) Sign REMOVE — the left "flat" hand faces right at chest level. The right "A" hand touches the left palm. Move the right hand down into a "five" hand as if imitating throwing something away. (SM)

(3) Sign ANALYZE — both "bent-V" hands face down at chest level. Drop both hands slightly and, at the same time, move both hands down to waist level. (SM)

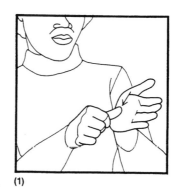
(1)

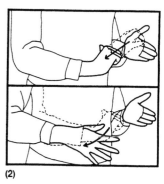
(2)

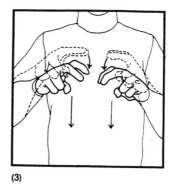
(3)

SPECTACLES

See GLASSES

SPECULUM

An instrument used to examine canals.

A speculum is used to check the canals in the ears, eyes or vagina.

SPEECH

Words or sounds which come from a person's throat and mouth.

The larynx, mouth, lips, chest and abdominal muscles are controlled by the brain and make speech possible.

(1) Sign TALK — the right "five" hand faces left at the mouth. Wiggle the fingers. (SM)

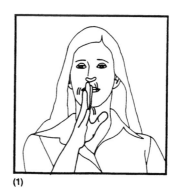
(1)

SPEED

The slang name for methedrine or methamphetamine, a drug which acts as a stimulant and will make a person feel alert.

If speed, or crystal as it is sometimes known, is used for a long time, a person could become addicted to it.

(Continued on next page)

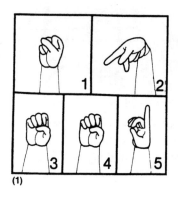
(1)

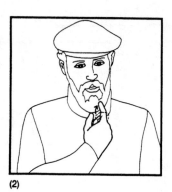
(2)

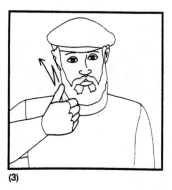
(3)

SPEED, *continued*

(1) Fingerspell "S-P-E-E-D".
(2) Sign PILL — the right thumb and index finger touch, the palm faces in. Flick the index finger towards the mouth as if imitating popping a pill in the mouth. (SM)
(3) Sign UPPER — the right "A" hand with the thumb extended, faces in at shoulder level and moves up twice. (DM)

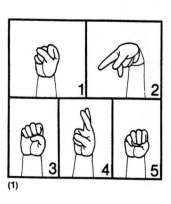
(1)

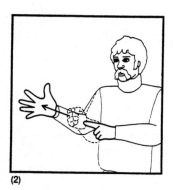
(2)

SPERM

The short name for spermatozoan, a male reproductive cell. Sperm are made in a man's testicles and when they are fully developed, they are released in the semen during ejaculation. Sperm look like tadpoles with very long tails; they are only about 1/500 of an inch long. The head of a sperm contains the DNA or chromosomes which carry one half of the information needed to direct the development of a new person. The long tail of the sperm moves it through fluids and allows sperm deposited in a woman's vagina to swim up through the cervix and uterus to where an ovum may be.

When a single sperm joins with an ovum, fertilization occurs and the development of a new person begins.

(1) Fingerspell "S-P-E-R-M".
(2) Sign EJACULATE — the right "S" hand faces left at chest level. The index finger of the left "one" hand touches the right wrist. Keeping the left hand in place, move the right hand slightly out to a "five" hand. (SM)

SPERMATOZOAN

See SPERM

SPHINCTER

A circular muscle which goes around a tube or opening. When it tightens, it closes the hole in the tube or opening.

The anus is a sphincter which controls the release of feces from the rectum.

(1) Fingerspell "H-O-L-E".
(2) Open and close the right "S" hand a few times. (MM)

* Point to the buttocks before these signs to clarify if necessary.

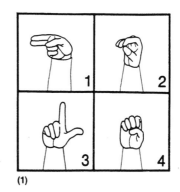

(1)

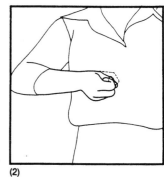

(2)

SPHYGMOMANOMETER

An instrument used to measure blood pressure in the arteries. The sphygmomanometer is wrapped around a person's upper arm and inflated, cutting off the blood flow.

By reading a gauge on the sphygmomanometer and listening through a stethoscope, the doctor can tell when the blood starts flowing again; this is the blood pressure.

(1) Sign BLOOD — the left "five" hand is at chest level with the palm toward the body. The palm of the right "five" hand is toward the body with the middle fingertips touching the mouth. Move the right hand down the back of the left hand. Wiggle the fingers of the right hand as it moves. (MM)

* This movement should be short, repeated and somewhat restrained.

(2) The right hand grabs the left upper arm. (SM)
(3) Sign MACHINE — both "five" hands face in at chest level with the fingers meshed together. Bounce both hands slightly a few times. (MM)

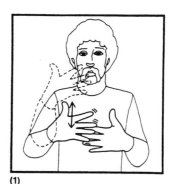

(1)

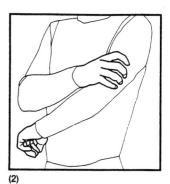

(2)

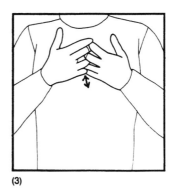

(3)

SPINAL

Referring to the spine or spinal cord.

Spinalgia is pain in the vertebra of the spinal column.

SPINAL CANAL

The space which runs down the center of the backbone. The spinal canal is made up of a series of spaces in the vertebrae stacked on top of one another.

The spinal canal in the vertebrae is the space that a person's spinal cord runs through.

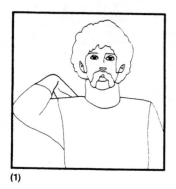

(1)

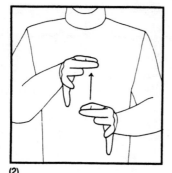

(2)

SPINAL COLUMN

The series of bones which run from the skull to the pelvic bone; the vertebral column, spine, or backbone. The spinal column is made up of a series of 33 bones, called vertebrae, which are stacked on top of one another. The vertebrae have a hole in them which makes a canal for the spinal cord to run through. The major functions of the spinal column are to support the head, neck, trunk and arms and to protect the spinal cord. *See Figure 26*

(1) Sign BACK — the right "flat" hand taps the back. (MM)

(2) Both "F" hands face down at waist level. Move the right hand up to chest level as if imitating the shape of backbone. (SM)

SPINAL CORD

The long collection of nerves which runs down the center of the spinal column. The spinal cord begins at the base of the brain where there is a hole in the skull that it passes through, and it ends around the second lumbar vertebrae. The spinal cord carries the nerves which connect the brain with the limbs and trunk. These nerves leave the spinal cord at special spaces between the vertebrae. The spinal cord, like the brain, is surrounded by special membranes called meninges. *See Figure 8*

SPINAL MENINGITIS

See MENINGITIS

SPINE

See SPINAL COLUMN

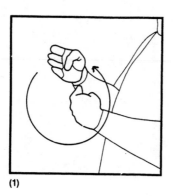

(1)

SPIRAL BANDAGE

A long narrow bandage which is put on by wrapping it around the part many times.

A spiral bandage may be used to hold a splint in place or to hold a large pad over a wound on an arm or leg.

(1) Sign BANDAGE — the left "B" hand faces in at chest level. The right "B" hand faces in and moves around the left hand as if imitating wrapping a bandage. (SM)

* This could be signed at the area where the bandage is being applied.

SPLEEN

A gland-like organ found below the diaphragm in the upper left side of the abdomen. The spleen is about five inches long and is oval in shape. The spleen helps to make, store, and filter the blood to take out worn out red blood cells and bacteria. (The spleen is not necessary for life -- it can be removed and the person will survive.)

See Figure 9

(1) Fingerspell "S-P-L-E-E-N".

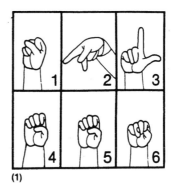

(1)

SPLINT

A stiff device made of wood, metal or plaster of Paris to protect or hold an injured part of the body still.

In an emergency, a splint can be made out of almost anything that will hold a possible dislocation or fracture still until the person can be taken to a hospital.

(1) The left "flat" hand faces down, the arm is bent. The right "flat" hand touches the top of the left arm, then turns over to touch the underside. (SM)

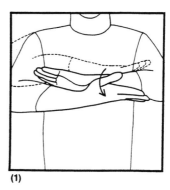

(1)

SPLINTING

Placing a splint on a possible dislocation or fracture to hold it still.

By splinting an injured part of the body, pain can be lessened and additional injury can be prevented while the person can be transported to a hospital.

(1) Sign WOOD — the left "flat" hand faces down at chest level. The right "flat" hand faces left and moves back and forth a few times on the top of the left hand as if imitating sawing wood. (MM)

(2) Sign SPLINT — the left "flat" hand faces down, the arm is bent. The right "flat" hand touches the top of the left arm, then turns over to touch the underside. (SM)

(3) Sign BANDAGE — the left "B" hand faces in at chest level. The right "B" hand faces in and moves around the left hand as if imitating wrapping a bandage. (SM)

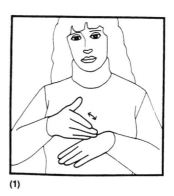

(1)

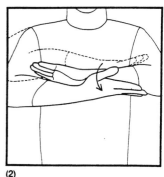

(2)

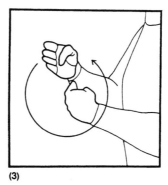

(3)

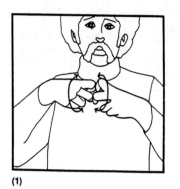
(1)

SPRAIN

An injury to a joint caused by bending it in ways it shouldn't be bent, tearing the ligaments or tendons around it. Symptoms of a sprain are pain, swelling around the joint and perhaps a change in the color of the skin in the area.

In a sprain, there is not a dislocation of the joint or a fracture to any bones, only damage to the tissues around the joint.

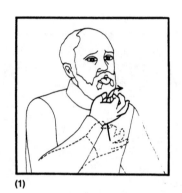
(1)

SPUTUM

The thick, slippery fluid which is coughed up, produced when the throat is cleared. Sputum comes from the airways and is mostly made up of mucus but there may also be blood, pus, dead cells and or germs.

Sputum is not the same as saliva, which is made by special glands around the mouth, but sputum may contain saliva.

(1) The right "C" hand faces in at chest level. Move the hand up to the mouth, then out. (SM)

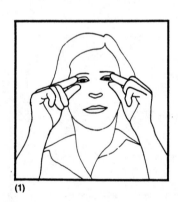
(1)

SQUINT

Having the eyes partly closed.

If a person has strabismus, an eye disorder, it may cause him to have a form of permanent squint.

(1) Both "G" hands face each other at the sides of the eyes. The eyes should squint. (SM)

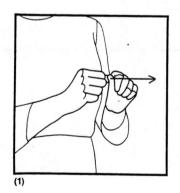
(1)

STABLE

Steady or not changing.

A sick or injured person who is not getting any better or worse is said to be in stable condition.

(1) Sign CONTINUE — the thumb of the right "A" hand is on top of the thumb of the left "A" hand. Move both hands out forward. (SM)

(Continued on next page)

STABLE, *continued*

(2) Sign NOT — the thumb of the right "A" hand touches the under the chin. Move the hand out forward. (SM)

(3) Sign CHANGE — the right "A" hand faces down on top of the left "A" hand which faces up. Twist both hands so that the right hand ends on the bottom facing up and the left hand is on top facing down. (SM)

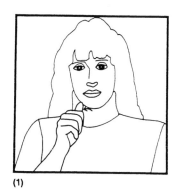

(1)

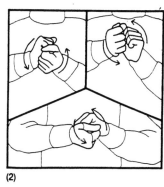

(2)

STAMMERING

A disorder causing hesitant, stumbling, repeating speech.

Stammering may also be called stuttering.

(1) The right "five" hand faces left at the mouth. Move the hand down in a jerky movement and at the same time, wiggle the fingers. (SM)

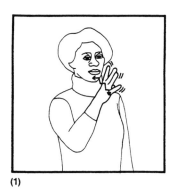

(1)

STAPES

One of the three small bones in the middle ear which moves and helps carry sound waves from the eardrum to the inner ear, where the movement is picked up as sound. The stapes, the innermost bone of the three, fits into the oval window and its movement causes the fluid in the cochlea to move. The stapes is also called the stirrup. *See Figure 20*

STARVATION

The condition of being without food for a long period of time. If the only thing a person takes in for a long time is water, the person will be hungry, lose weight, use up excess body fat, be dizzy and perhaps nauseous. Starvation is also used for not getting enough of a specific food in the diet, causing a disease.

It is not a good idea to lose weight by starvation because it is very hard on the body and can make a person ill.

(1) Sign HUNGER — the right "C" hand faces in at chest level and moves down to waist level. (SM)

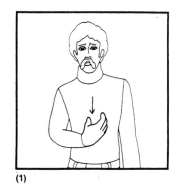

(1)

581

STENOSIS

Narrowing of an opening or passage.

Stenosis in the large blood vessels near the heart or in the passages of the heart will lessen the amount of blood sent to the tissues and cause a murmur which can be heard with a stethescope.

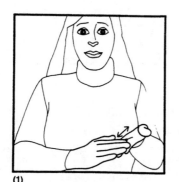
(1)

STERILE

Being free of disease causing organisms; also being unfertile or unable to reproduce.

The skin, the doctor's hands, the instruments used and the clothes worn in any surgical procedure are made as sterile as possible.

(1) Sign CLEAN — the left "flat" hand faces up at chest level. The right "flat" hand faces down and rubs back and forth on the left palm a few times. (MM)

Use this sign only if referring to sterile as being clean. See STERILITY, female and STERILITY, male if referring to sterile as being unable to reproduce.

STERILITY, female

The condition of not being able to become pregnant.

Sterility in a woman may be caused by damage or disease to the ovaries, fallopian tubes, uterus, cervix or vagina.

(1) Sign WOMAN — the thumb of the right "A" hand moves down the right cheek. Move the hand to a "flat" hand facing down at the forehead. (SM)
(2) Sign PREGNANT — both "five" hands face in at stomach level with the fingers meshed together. Move both hands out slightly as if imitating the stomach growing. (SM)
(3) Sign CAN'T — the left "one" hand faces down at chest level. The right "one" hand moves down to strike the left index finger. (SM)

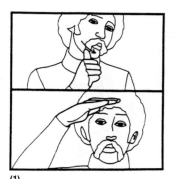
(1)

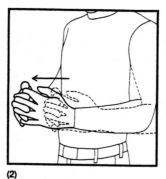
(2)

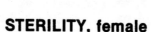

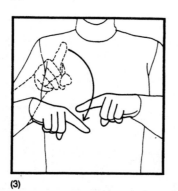
(3)

STERILITY, male

The condition of not being able to make a woman pregnant.

Sterility in a man may be caused by there not being enough sperm, the sperm produced being unhealthy or abnormal, blockage of the ducts carrying the sperm out of the body, disease of the testicles, or abnormal testicles.

(Continued on next page)

STERILITY, male, *continued*

(1) Sign MAN — the right open "flat-O" hand faces down at the forehead. Close the hand and move it out slightly. (SM)

(2) The right "flat" hand faces down at the forehead and moves out slightly. (SM)

(3) Sign EJACULATE — the right "S" hand faces left at chest level. The index finger of the left "one" hand touches the right wrist. Keeping the left hand in place, move the right hand slightly out to a "five" hand. (SM)

(4) Sign PREGNANT — both "five" hands face in at stomach level with the fingers meshed together. Move both hands out forward as if imitating the stomach growing. (SM)

(5) Sign CAN'T — the left "one" hand faces down at chest level. The right "one" hand moves down to strike the left index finger. (SM)

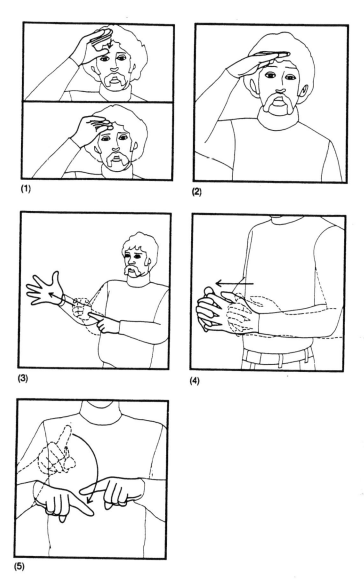

(1)

(2)

(3)

(4)

(5)

STERILIZATION

The process of getting rid of the germs on something; also, the procedure in which a man or woman is made unable to reproduce.

Sterilization can be done by removing the testicles (castration) or ovaries (ovariectomy) but usually in a man it is done by a vasectomy and in a woman by a hysterectomy or tubal ligation.

a. (1) Sign CLEAN — the left "flat" hand faces up at chest level. The right "flat" hand faces down and rubs out on the left palm. (SM)

* Use this sign if referring to cleaning something.

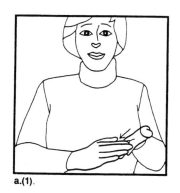

a.(1).

(Continued on next page)

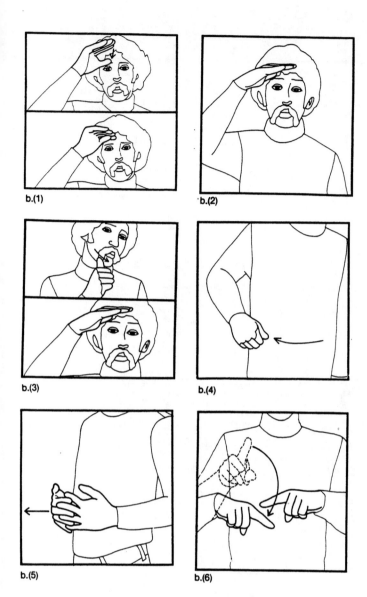

b.(1)

b.(2)

b.(3)

b.(4)

b.(5)

b.(6)

b. (1) Sign MAN — the right open "flat-O" hand faces down at the forehead. Close the hand and move it out slightly. (SM)
(2) The right "flat" hand faces down at the forehead and moves out slightly. (SM)
(3) Sign WOMAN — the thumb of the right "A" hand moves down the right cheek. The right hand changes to a "flat" hand facing down at the forehead and moves out slightly. (SM)
(4) Sign OPERATE — the thumb of the right "A" hand moves across the stomach from left to right as if imitating cutting. (SM)
(5) Sign PREGNANT — both "five" hands face in at stomach level with the fingers meshed together. Move both hands out forward as if imitating the stomach growing. (SM)
(6) Sign CAN'T — the left "one" hand faces down at chest level. The right "one" hand moves down to strike the left index finger. (SM)

* *Use these signs if referring to the operation of sterilization.*

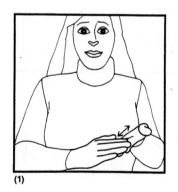

(1)

STERILIZE
To make something free of germs.

To prevent infection, it is important to sterilize anything which is put into the body as much as possible.

(1) Sign CLEAN — the left "flat" hand faces up at chest level. The right "flat" hand faces down and rubs back and forth on the left palm a few times. (MM)

STERNOCLEIDOMASTOID

A muscle which runs from the sternum and clavicle (the breastbone and collarbone) to the mastoid process of the head, the bony bump behind and below the ear. The sternocleidomastoid helps turn the head and bend it towards the shoulder.

See Figure 5

STERNUM

The narrow, flat bone at the center front of the chest which the clavicle (collar bone) and the front part of the ribs attach to. The sternum is also called the breastbone. *See Figure 26*

STETHOSCOPE

An instrument used to listen to sounds made within the body.

A stethoscope is made up of a Y-shaped rubber tube with earpieces and a special device on one end to pick up sounds.

(1) The thumbs and index fingers of both hands touch the ears. Move both hands down to chest level with the thumbs and index fingers touching. (SM)

(2) The fingertips of the right "flat-O" hand touch the chest several times. (MM)

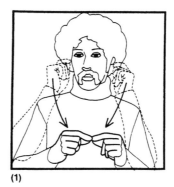
(1)

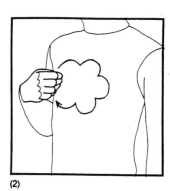
(2)

STIFF

Firm, rigid, not flexible.

After death, the body becomes stiff due to rigor mortis.

(1) The right hand grabs the fingers of the left "flat" hand. Wiggle the right hand. (MM)

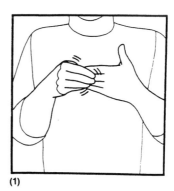
(1)

STIGMATISM

The correct focussing of rays of light on the retina of the eye.

Stigmatism is the normal, healthy state of the eye.

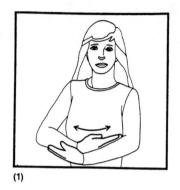

(1)

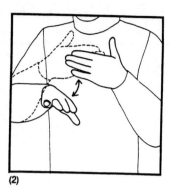

(2)

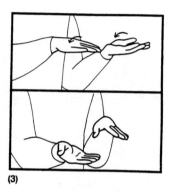

(3)

STILLBIRTH

A fetus that has died in the womb after seven months of pregnancy.

A pregnant woman's obstetrician can detect a stillbirth before it happens if the woman is coming in regularly for check-ups because he won't hear a fetal heartbeat and her abdomen will stop growing.

(1) Sign BABY — the right hand and forearm face up, resting on the left hand and forearm which also face up. Both are then rocked back and forth as if holding a baby. (MM)

(2) Sign BORN — the left "flat" hand faces in at chest level. The right "flat" hand also faces in behind the left hand. Move the right hand down under the left and out forward. (SM)

(3) Sign DEAD — the left "flat" hand faces up at chest level and the right "flat" hand faces down. Turn both hands over so that the left hand ends facing down and the right hand ends facing up. (SM)

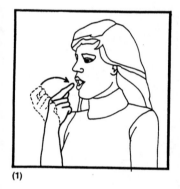

(1)

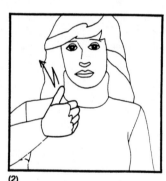

(2)

STIMULANT

Any drug which increases mental activity, increases the activity of a part of the body, or makes a person more alert. Examples of stimulants are caffeine, cocaine, amphetamine, dextroamphetamine and methamphetamine. "Uppers" is a slang name often used for a stimulant.

Most pain-relievers such as aspirin contain the stimulant caffeine because it makes the pain-relievers work better.

(1) Sign PILL — the right thumb and index finger touch, the palm faces in. Flick the index finger towards the mouth as if imitating popping a pill in the mouth. (SM)

(2) Sign UPPER — the right "A" hand with the thumb extended, faces in at shoulder level and moves up twice. (DM)

* This is a general sign for stimulants ("uppers"). The specific type of drug should also be fingerspelled and all side effects explained.

STIMULUS

Anything causing a change in a condition.

A thermal stimulus is one that changes the temperature of a person's body.

STING
See INSECT STING or BITE

STIRRUP
The common name for the stapes, one of the three small bones in the middle ear which helps carry sound waves from the eardrum to the inner ear. In the inner ear, the movement is picked up and detected as sounds by the brain. *See Figure 20*

STITCHES
Pieces of thread, wire or gut which are sewn into the skin or tissue to hold two things together or to hold something in place and help healing; also called "sutures."

When a person gets stitches inside the body, special material is used which will dissolve and be absorbed by the body.

(1) The right "F" hand imitates stitching on the left arm. (MM)
* This could be signed at the area where stitches are being done.

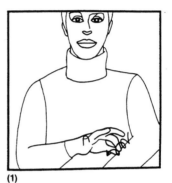
(1)

STOMA
An opening made by a surgeon between a space or passage in the body and the surface of the body.

A stoma may be made in a person's trachea or throat so he can breathe easier.

(1) Sign CUT — the thumb of the right "A" hand moves down the neck as if imitating cutting. (SM)
(2) The right "F" hand faces out at the neck. (SM)

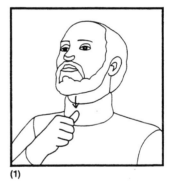
(1)

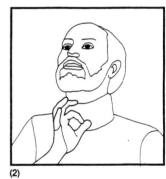
(2)

STOMACH
A sac-like organ connected to the lower end of the esophagus at one end and the upper end of the in-testines at the other end. The stomach is the part of the digestive tract found in the upper abdomen just below the chest. The stomach takes food from the esophagus which has been chewed and swallowed, holds it and lets it into the small intestine slowly. The stomach puts out digestive juices with acids and enzymes in it which help digest the food while it is in the stomach. The stomach does not absorb many foods but it does absorb aspirin and alcohol. *See Figure 9*

(Continued on next page)

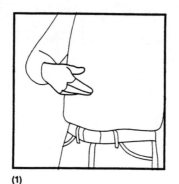

STOMACH, *continued*

(1) The fingertips of the right "cupped" hand tap the stomach. (MM)

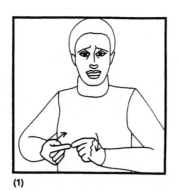

STOMACH ACHE

Pain in the abdomen area.

A stomach ache may also be called a "belly ache."
(1) Sign PAIN — both "one" hands face each other at the stomach and twist in opposite directions a few times. (MM)

* *The facial expression should reflect pain.*

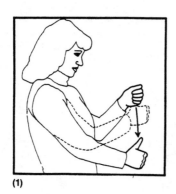

STOOL

Feces; the solid wastes released from the rectum in a bowel movement.

The bile secreted into the small intestine is what gives stools their brownish color but the color and consistency of the stools can be affected by what a person eats or by any disorder of the digestive tract.
(1) Sign DEFECATE — the left "A" hand faces right at chest level. The thumb of the right "A" hand is inside the left fist. Move the right hand down. (SM)

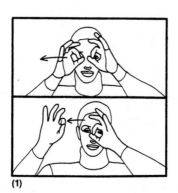

STRABISMUS

A disorder of the eyes in which both eyes do not look directly at the same thing at the same time, as they should. A person with strabismus will have one eye looking off at an angle when the other is looking at something.

One of the causes of strabismus is that the muscles that control movement of the eyeball do not work together as they should, and if this is the case, surgery may help correct the problem.
(1) Both "F" hands face out at the eyes. Move the right hand out forward. (SM)

STRAIN

An injury to a part of the body, usually a muscle; also a form of stress.

A strain may be caused by using or stretching a muscle too much.

(1) Both "S" hands face in at chest level, the left hand on top of the right. Move the right hand down. Grit the teeth while signing. (SM)

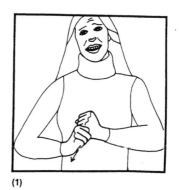
(1)

STRANGLE

To be choked or suffocated because of pressure on the trachea in the neck.

A person could die by being strangled because fresh air with oxygen in it can't be carried into the lungs and carbon dioxide can't be carried away from the lungs.

(1) Both hands grab the throat as if choking. (SM)

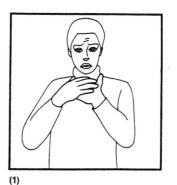
(1)

STRANGULATION

The closing down or shutting off of a passage, which stops the movement of material through them. Strangulation can occur in the throat and stop breathing, in a blood vessel and cut off the blood supply to an area, or in the intestines and stop the movement of food through it.

A loop of the intestine may push out of the abdomen through a hole causing a hernia and if it is a tight fit, strangulation of the part pushed out may occur; it is called a strangulated hernia.

(1) Sign STRANGLE — both hands grab the throat as if choking. (SM)

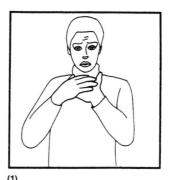
(1)

STREP THROAT

A serious throat infection caused by a certain kind of bacteria (streptococci); also called streptococcal sore throat. Strep throat can be very dangerous because the bacteria which causes the disease may spread to the ear or the meninges of the brain and make a poison which causes scarlet fever. These bacteria may also infect and damage the heart or cause rheumatic fever.

Symptoms of strep throat are a sore throat, swollen lymph nodes in the neck area and swelling and redness in the throat.

(Continued on next page)

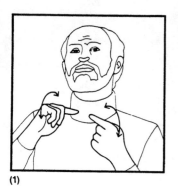

(1)

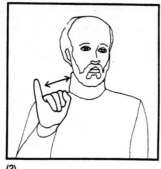

(2)

STREP THROAT, continued

(1) Sign PAIN — both "one" hands face each other at the throat and twist in opposite directions a few times. (MM)
* The facial expression should reflect pain.

(2) Sign INFECTION — the right "I" hand faces out at chest level. Shake the hand slightly a few times. (MM)
* Mouth the word "infection" while signing.

STREPTOCOCCAL SORE THROAT
See STREP THROAT

STREPTOMYCIN
An antibiotic made from a certain kind of bacteria which can be used to stop an infection caused by several other types of bacteria.

Streptomycin is usually given along with other antibiotics to treat plague, tuberculosis and heart infections.

STRESS
Physical or mental pressure, strain or tension caused by the surroundings.

It is believed that a certain amount of stress is needed for well being but too much stress cannot be handled by the body and may result in disease.

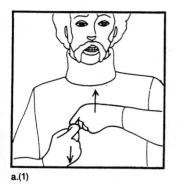

a.(1)

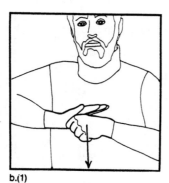

b.(1)

a. (1) Sign STRESS — both "modified-A" hands face in at chest level, the left hand above the right. Move both hands away from each other as if indicating putting stress on something. Grit the teeth while signing. (SM)

b. (1) Sign PRESSURE — the left "S" hand faces in at chest level. The right "flat" hand faces down on top of the left fist. Move both hands down as if indicating putting pressure on something. Grit the teeth while signing. (SM)

STRETCHER
A device just big enough for a sick or injured person to lie on, with wheels or handles on it.

A stretcher may also be called a "litter."

(Continued on next page)

STRETCHER, *continued*

(1) Sign LIE DOWN — the right "H" hand faces up in the palm of the left "flat" hand. (SM)
(2) Both "S" hands face each other at waist level with the arms slightly bent. Bounce both hands up and down slightly as if imitating carrying a stretcher. (MM)

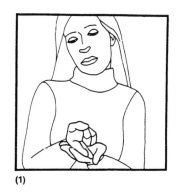
(1)
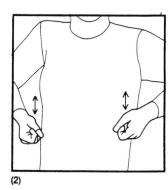
(2)

STROKE

A sudden, severe attack, especially one caused by the bursting of a blood vessel in the brain. Symptoms of a brain stroke are sudden unconsciousness, loud and difficult breathing, paralysis on one side of the body, a cold sweat on the body, a below-normal temperature, and speech problems.

A stroke may leave a person partly paralyzed, damage memory, affect speech, or even cause death depending on how bad it is.

STRYCHNINE

A poisonous substance made from plants, especially the seeds of a certain tree. Strychnine is not used much except experimentally with the nervous system. A person poisoned with strychnine will become nervous, have stiff muscles, have convulsions, the arms and face will twitch, the person's body may become arched because the muscles contract and don't relax and the skin may turn blue.

A person poisoned with strychnine, may die after one to three hours because the muscles which help us breathe, contract and don't relax, so air can't be moved in and out of the lungs, causing suffocation.

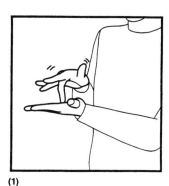
(1)
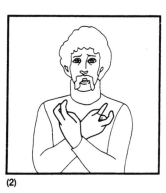
(2)

(1) Sign MEDICINE — the left "flat" hand faces up at chest level. The middle finger of the right "eight" hand touches the left palm and pivots slightly from side to side a few times. (MM)
(2) Sign POISON — both "bent-V" hands face in and cross at the chest. (SM)

STUPOR

A condition of unconsciousness; a decrease in sense or feeling.

Stupors can occur in infectious diseases, epileptic attacks, mental depression or poisoning.

(Continued on next page)

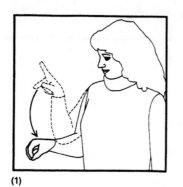

(1)

STUPOR, *continued*

(1) The right "K" hand faces out at chest level and drops slightly to an "O" hand. (SM)

STUTTER
See STAMMERING

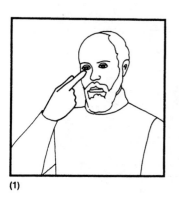

(1)

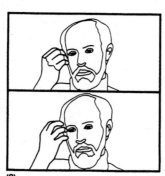

(2)

STY

An inflammation of an eyelid caused by bacteria infecting one of the glands of the eyelid. Symptoms of a sty are swelling, redness and pain in the eyelid and pus may form in the area.

If a sty is bad enough, hot packs should be put on it and the person may be given antibiotics to fight the infection.

(1) Sign EYE — the index finger of the right "one" hand points to the right eye. (SM)
(2) Sign SWELL — the right "O" hand faces in at the right eye. Open the hand slightly to a "claw" hand as if imitating swelling. (SM)

SUBCLAVIAN ARTERY

The large artery at the base of the neck which carries fresh blood to the arm and upper chest. The subclavian artery becomes the brachial artery when it leaves the chest region and enters the arm. *See Figure 6*

SUBCONSCIOUS

The mental activities which go on without a person knowing about them or being aware of them.

In psychoanalysis, a therapist tries to find and get out past emotions, feelings or occurrencs which are hidden in a person's subconscious and which are causing abnormal behavior.

SUBCUTANEOUS INJECTION

A shot in which the drug, released from a needle, is placed under the skin but not into a vein or muscle.

A person who is having surgery and who needs only a local anesthetic will usually be given a subcutaneous injection of a pain killing drug in the area.

(1) Sign INJECTION — the index finger of the right "L" hand touches the left inside arm. Bend the thumb in as if imitating injecting something into the arm. (SM)

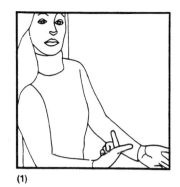

(1)

SUBSTANCE

The material that makes up something.

The hardest substance in the body is the enamel which forms the outer layer of a tooth.

SUCKING WOUND

A puncture wound of the chest which air flows in and out of because the wound has gone all the way through the chest wall to a lung. Instead of the air being brought into the chest through the mouth or nose, it is sucked in through the hole when a person inhales.

A sucking wound of the chest is very dangerous because the air getting inside the chest will collapse the lung, interfering with oxygen getting into the blood-stream.

(1) Sign LUNGS — the fingertips of both "cupped" hands rub up and down on the chest a few times. (MM)

(2) Sign PUNCTURE — the left "flat" hand faces up at chest level. The index finger of the right "one" hand moves down through the fingers of the left hand as if imitating puncturing something. (SM)

(1) The right "F" hand faces out at chest level.

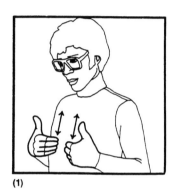

(1)

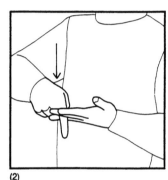

(2)

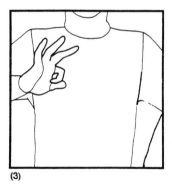

(3)

SUCROSE

A table sugar (cane, beet or maple sugar), made up of two other kinds of sugars, glucose and fructose. Sucrose is a carbohydrate.

When sucrose is eaten, it is broken down into glucose and fructose, absorbed in the intestines and then these two sugars are taken to the liver where they are changed and stored until they are needed for energy.

(Continued on next page)

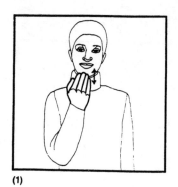
(1)

(1) Sign SUGAR — the fingertips of the right "flat" hand brush up and down on the chin a few times. (MM)

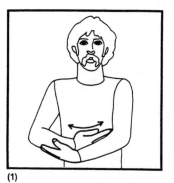
(1)

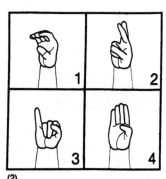

1   2

3   4

(2)

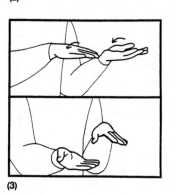
(3)

SUDDEN INFANT DEATH SYNDROME

The condition in which a baby, usually less than one year old, dies without apparent reason, usually while sleeping and with no warning; also called "crib death", cot death or SIDS. The exact cause of Sudden Infant Death Syndrome is unknown but researchers now think that it may be caused by a failure in the part of the brain that controls breathing during sleep.

About 10,000 children die each year of Sudden Infant Death Syndrome; it is more common in boys than girls, in the winter months, and in children of low birth weight.

(1) Sign BABY — the right hand and forearm face up, resting on the left hand and forearm which also face up. Both are then rocked back and forth as if holding a baby. (MM)

(2) Fingerspell "C-R-I-B".

(3) Sign DEAD — the left "flat" hand faces up at chest level and the right "flat" hand faces down. Turn both hands over so that the left hand ends facing down and the right hand ends facing up. (SM)

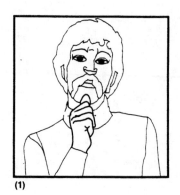
(1)

SUFFER

To feel pain, injury or harm.

*Lighter-skinned people may **suffer** from sunburn more than darker-skinned people because of lack of melanin in the skin.*

(1) The thumb of the right "A" hand touches the chin. Pivot the hand slightly from side to side a few times. (MM)

* *The facial expression should reflect pain.*

594

SUFFOCATION

Inability to breathe because the airways are blocked so that oxygen can't get into the lungs. Some causes of suffocation are drowning (the mouth and nose being covered so air can't pass through them), strangling (in which the trachea is flattened and air can't get through), and inhaling dangerous gases. Symptoms of suffocation may be loss of alertness, a purple and swollen face, convulsions, unconsciousness and death.

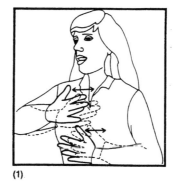 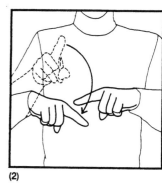

(1)   (2)

A victim of suffocation should always be given CPR or mouth-to-mouth resuscitation because he may be revived and survive if he doesn't go more than a few minutes without breathing.

(1) Sign BREATHE — both "flat" hands move in and out from the chest as if imitating breathing. (MM)
(2) Sign CAN'T — the left "one" hand faces down at chest level. The right "one" hand moves down to strike the left index finger. (SM)

SUICIDE

Killing oneself on purpose. Attacks of insanity or depression sometimes lead to suicide.

It is very important for someone to find out side-effects of drugs he is taking because some drugs can cause severe enough depression to lead to suicide.

a. (1) Sign KILL — the left "five" hand faces right at chest level. The right "one" hand moves down past the left hand. (SM)
(2) Sign MYSELF — the thumb of the right "A" hand taps the chest. (DM)
* *Use these signs if talking about killing yourself.*

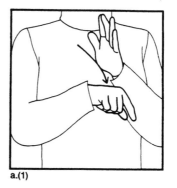 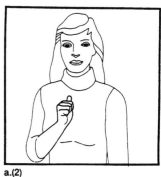

a.(1)   a.(2)

b. (1) Sign KILL — the left "five" hand faces right at chest level. The right "one" hand moves down past the left hand. (SM)
(2) Sign HIMSELF or HERSELF — the right "A" hand faces left and pivots forward from the wrist. (DM)
* *Use these signs if referring to someone else killing himself.*

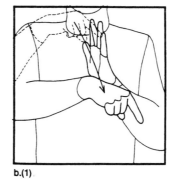 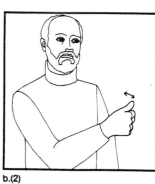

b.(1)   b.(2)

SULFA DRUGS

A group of antibiotic drugs, made from the same basic substance, which will stop infections caused by several different kinds of bacteria; the sulfonamides. Sulfa drugs may be injected into the body or taken through the mouth.

The most common use of sulfa drugs is to fight infections of the bladder or kidneys, the intestines and some kinds of pneumonia.

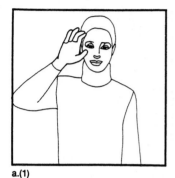

a.(1)

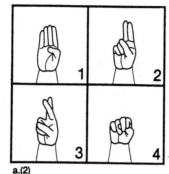

a.(2)

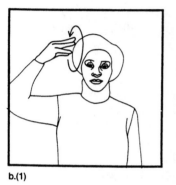

b.(1)

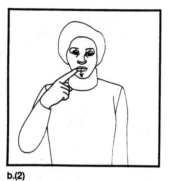

b.(2)

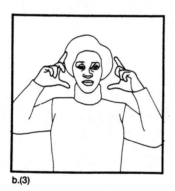

b.(3)

SULFONAMIDES

See SULFA DRUGS

SUNBURN

Redness and inflammation of the skin caused by being in the sun too long. Sunburn is a kind of burn caused by ultraviolet radiation, and may even cause blistering of the skin if it is bad enough.

People who are light-skinned, like blonds and redheads, will sunburn more easily because they don't have as much melanin in the skin which prevents the sun rays from harming the skin.

a. (1) Sign SUN — the right "C" hand faces out at the right side of the head. Move the hand up. (SM)

(2) Fingerspell "B-U-R-N-".

b. (1) The right "five" hand faces in at the right side of the head and moves in a circular movement a few times. (MM)

(2) Sign RED — the index finger of the right "one" hand brushes down the chin a few times. (MM)

(3) Both "L" hands face out at the sides of the head. (SM)

SUNSTROKE

An illness caused by being out in the sun or in hot weather too long; also called heatstroke. A person with sunstroke will have a high temperature, dry skin, be confused, have a headache, convulsions and perhaps go into a coma and die.

A person with sunstroke needs to be put in ice water quickly because the part of the brain which controls body temperature has been affected and the body can't cool itself off.

(Continued on next page)

SUNSTROKE, *continued*

(1) Sign SUN — the right "one" hand faces in at head level and makes a circle in the air, indicating the sun. (SM)
(2) The right "five" hand faces in at head level and moves down towards the face, indicating the sun's rays. (SM)
(3) Sign ATTACK — the left "one" hand points up and faces out at chest level. The right "S" hand faces in and sharply hits the left index finger. (SM)
(4) Sign SICK — the middle finger of the right "eight" hand touches the forehead and the middle finger of the left "eight" hand touches the stomach. Twist both hands slightly. (SM)

* *The facial expression should reflect illness.*

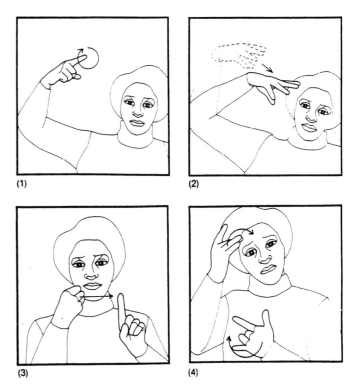

(1)　　(2)

(3)　　(4)

SUPEREGO

According to some branches of psychology, the part of a person's personality that is responsible for their morals, acting as their conscience. The superego, along with the ego and id, make up the parts of the personality, according to psychoanalysts.

> The **superego** is what makes us feel good when we behave well and what makes us feel guilty when we do wrong things.

SUPERFICIAL TEMPORAL ARTERY

The large artery which carries fresh blood to the scalp region. *See Figure 6*

SUPERFICIAL

On or near the surface.

> In a first degree burn, the damage done is *superficial* and the higher the degree, the deeper and more severe the damage.

(1) The right "flat" hand rubs in small circular movements on the top of the left "flat" hand. (MM)

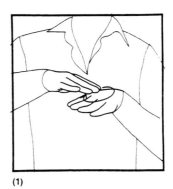

(1)

SUPERIOR

Higher or above something else. The superior limbs of the body are the arms.

SUPINE

Lying flat on the back with the face upward. Supine is the opposite of prone.

It is better for a person's back and neck to sleep in a supine position rather than a prone position.

(1) Sign LIE DOWN — the right "H" hand faces up in the palm of the left "flat" hand. (SM)

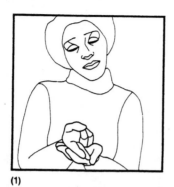

(1)

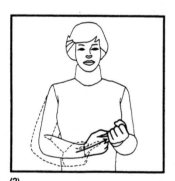

a.(1)

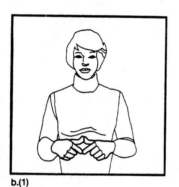

b.(1)

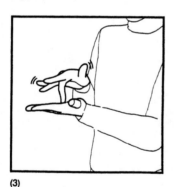

(2)

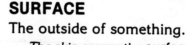

(3)

SUPPOSITORY

A small solid piece of medicine, usually shaped like a cone, which is placed in the rectum, vagina or urethra, where it melts. A suppository is a solid at room temperature but melts at body temperature, like cocoa butter or gelatin.

A suppository is used to concentrate a medicine in a certain part of the body or to get a medicine into the body quickly.

a. (1) Sign BUTTOCKS — the index finger of the right "one" hand points to the buttocks. (SM)

b. (1) Sign VAGINA — both "L" hands face in with the thumbs and index fingers touching. (SM)

(2) Sign INSERT — the left "S" hand faces up at chest level. The index finger of the right "one" hand moves into the left fist. (SM)

(3) Sign MEDICINE — the left "flat" hand faces up at chest level. The middle finger of the right "eight" hand touches the left palm and pivots slightly from side to side a few times. (MM)

* *Sign BUTTOCKS or VAGINA, whichever applies, then sign INSERT and MEDICINE.*

SURFACE

The outside of something.

The skin covers the surface of the body and helps protect it.

(1) The right "flat" hand rubs in small circular movements on top of the left "flat" hand. (MM)

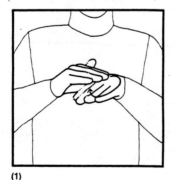

(1)

SURGEON

A doctor who specializes in surgery or doing operations.

Usually a team of people work on a person having an operation: the surgeon who does the operating, a nurse who helps the surgeon, and an anesthesiologist who gives the person drugs or gases to make him unconscious.

(1) Sign DOCTOR — the right "M" hand taps the left inside wrist. (DM)

(2) Sign SPECIALIZE — the left "B" hand faces right at chest level. The right "B" hand faces left and moves out along the left index finger. (SM)

(3) Sign OPERATE — the left "flat" hand faces right at chest level. The thumb of the right "A" hand moves down the left palm as if imitating cutting. (SM)

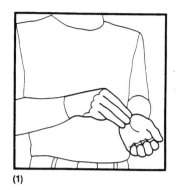
(1)

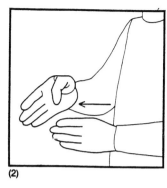
(2)

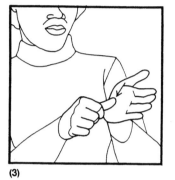
(3)

SURGERY

The area of medicine which treats and cures some diseases, deformities and injuries by doing operations on the patient; also, the area where the surgeon works and the actual operation.

There are different areas of surgery a doctor can specialize in such as plastic surgery, orthopedic surgery, cosmetic surgery and oral surgery.

(1) Sign OPERATE — the left "flat" hand faces right at chest level. The thumb of the right "A" hand moves down the left palm as if imitating cutting. (SM)

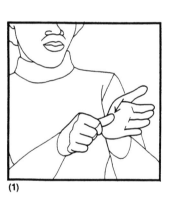
(1)

SURVIVE

To stay alive or to exist.

People who do outdoor activities, such as hiking or camping, should learn how to survive in the woods in case of an emergency when medical assistance is not available right away.

(1) Sign LIVE — both "A" hands, with the thumbs extended, face in and move up the body from waist to chest level. (SM)

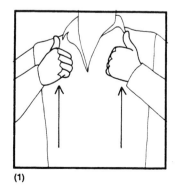
(1)

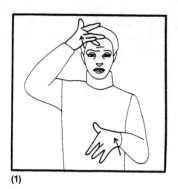
(1)

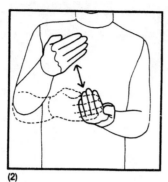
(2)

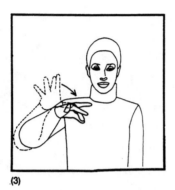
(3)

SUSCEPTIBLE

In medicine, it means being unable or less likely to fight off an infectious disease, so the person is more likely to get that disease.

An older person with a bad cold is more susceptible to developing pneumonia than a younger person.

(1) Sign SICK — the middle finger of the right "eight" hand touches the forehead and the middle finger of the left "eight" hand touches the stomach. Twist both hands slightly. (SM)
* *The facial expression should reflect illness.*

(2) Sign EASY — the fingers of the right "cupped" hand brush up the back of the fingers of the left "cupped" hand twice. (DM)

(3) Sign ACCEPT — the thumb of the right "five" hand touches the chest, the hand faces out. Close the hand to an "eight" hand with the middle finger and thumb touching. (SM)

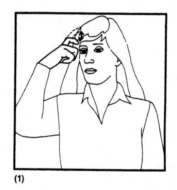
(1)

SUSPICIOUS

Being questionable or distrustful.

When a child is taken to the hospital for treatment of suspicious injuries, such as cuts or bruises, the doctor may question the parents as to the cause of the injuries in case there is a chance of child abuse.

(1) The right "one" hand faces in at the forehead. Bend and straighten the index finger a few times. (MM)
* *The facial expression should reflect suspicion.*

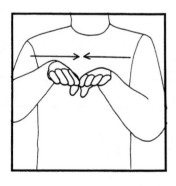

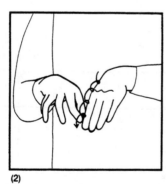
(2)

SUTURE

The sewing together of two parts to hold them together and help them heal; also the thread, wire or other material used to sew two parts together; a stitch.

A doctor will sometimes want to suture deep or bad cuts which he doesn't think will close normally or quickly if left to heal naturally.

(1) Both "four" hands face down at chest level and move towards each other. (SM)
(2) The right "F" hand imitates stitching on the left index finger ..(MM)

* *This could be signed at the area where sutures are being done.*

SWAB

A slender stick with cotton or gauze on the end used to clean an area or to apply medicine; also to wipe away something.

Sometimes a swab will be used to collect tissue or secretions for examination of bacteria.

SWALLOW

To move food or drink from the mouth through the throat into the esophagus and stomach.

Once a swallow has begun, a person cannot stop it from happening because, beyond a certain point, it is a reflex.

(1) The left "cupped" hand faces in at chest level. The right "one" hand points up and faces in above the left hand. Move the right hand down to waist level.

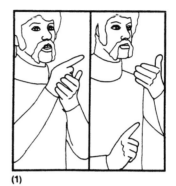

(1)

SWALLOWING

The action in which food is moved from the mouth through the throat and into the esophagus and stomach. The action of swallowing is started by us but beyond a certain point, it is a reflex and we have no control over it. Swallowing involves putting the food on the tongue, tipping the tongue up and forcing the food into the very back of the mouth. The food is then forced through the pharynx and directed into the esophagus.

Even though swallowing is mostly a reflex and goes on automatically, trying to talk, breathe or laugh while doing it may cause food to get into the larynx, which makes us cough.

(1) The left "cupped" hand faces in at chest level. The right "one" hand points up and faces in above the left hand. Move the right hand down to waist level. (SM)

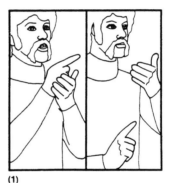

(1)

SWEAT

A colorless, salty-tasting fluid given off through the skin; to perspire. Sweat comes from special glands in the skin; the places where these glands open into the skin are called pores.

Sweat cools the body by evaporating off it and also acts to get rid of wastes.

(1) The left "five" hand points down at chest level. The right "S" hand faces down at the forehead. Drop the right hand down into a "five" hand as if imitating sweating. (SM)

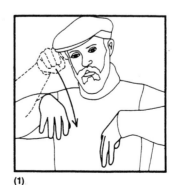

(1)

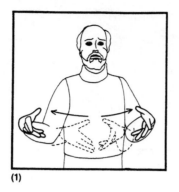
(1)

SWELLING

An abnormal increase in the size of a part of the body, usually on the surface. Swelling may be caused by an injury, inflammation or edema.

Swelling is not caused by an increase in the size or number of cells but by an increase in the amount of blood and fluid in the area.

(1) Both "five" hands face each other at waist level. Move both hands out to the sides as if imitating something swelling and at the same time, the cheeks should puff out. (SM)

SWIMMER'S ITCH

Small bumps which look like insect bites that show up on a person's skin three to fourteen days after swimming in water.

Swimmer's itch is caused when a parasite of birds, such as ducks, by mistake enters human skin and causes irritation.

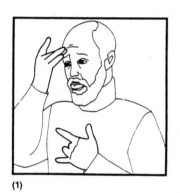
(1)

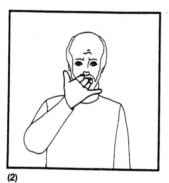
(2)

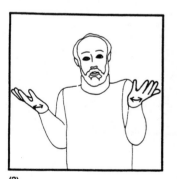
(3)

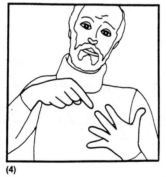
(4)

SYMPTOM

Any change in the body or the way it works that is caused by a disease or disorder. A symptom of a disease is usually an uncomfortable or painful feeling or a part of the body not working normally. Depending on the disease a person has, there can be many different symptoms. Examples of some possible symptoms are a headache, pain, weakness, coughing, itching, vomiting, sweating or a fever.

A person who isn't feeling well and has gone to see a doctor will be examined and asked questions so the doctor can find out all of the person's symptoms and then come up with a diagnosis.

(1) Sign SICK — the middle finger of the right "eight" hand touches the forehead and the middle finger of the left "eight" hand touches the stomach. (SM)
* The facial expression should reflect illness.

(2) Sign WRONG — the right "Y" hand faces in and taps the chin. (SM)

(3) Sign WHAT — both "five" hands face up at chest level and shake slightly from side to side a few times. (MM)
* The facial expression should reflect questioning.

(4) The left "five" hand faces in at chest level. The right "one" hand points to each finger. (SM)

SYNDROME

A group of signs and symptoms which regularly occur together when a person has a certain disease or disorder. Syndrome is often used with another word to tell which syndrome it is.

Down's syndrome is the preferred word for mongolism, a kind of mental retardation caused by an abnormal number of chromosomes.

SYNTHETIC

Something made artificially by man; not natural.

There are several different kinds of synthetic penicillin and new ones have to be made all the time because this antibiotic is used so often that, after a while, bacteria develop a tolerence to one type and a new type must be used to kill them.

(1) Sign FALSE — the right "L" hand faces left and brushes past the nose. (SM)

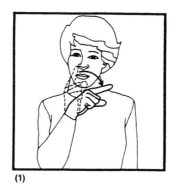

(1)

SYPHILIS

A severe contagious venereal disease caused by bacteria (Treponemataceae), spread mostly by sexual contact or through the transfusion of infected blood or plasma. Symptoms of syphilis include a sore usually appearing on the genitals two to four weeks after sexual intercourse with an infected person, healing and then (a couple weeks later) the lymph nodes swell. The disease then seems to go away for several weeks but a red rash will appear along with moist bumps around the genitals, armpits or mouth. Both kinds of open sores have bacteria in them which can infect other people. About a third of all infected people will have the disease cure itself and go away, another third will still have the disease but not show any more sign of it, and the rest will be affected by the disease many years later. The person may have the heart, blood vessels or nervous system affected. If this happens, the person will have sores develop on the skin, bones and liver and may have heart damage, paralysis or insanity.

Penicillin is the drug used to treat syphilis.

603

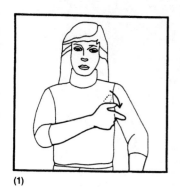
(1)

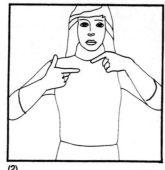
(2)

SYRINGE

An instrument used to give shots or inject something into the body or, to take fluids such as blood out of the body.

Syringes are different sizes and designs depending on what they are to be used for.

(1) Sign INJECTION — the index finger of the right "L" hand touches the left upper arm. Bend the thumb in as if imitating injecting something in the left arm. (SM)

(2) The left "one" hand points to the right "L" hand. (SM)

SYSTEM

In medicine, a group of organs or structures which work together to perform an activity. The body is divided into several major systems, each of which has a job that it does to keep us alive.

The body systems are the circulatory system, digestive system, endocrine system, muscular system, nervous system, reproductive system, skeletal system, excretory system and respiratory system.

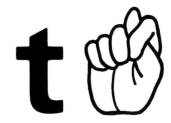

TABLET

In medicine, referring to a small disk-like pill containing powdered medicine.

Tablets are taken orally and are sometimes coated with sugar or chocolate.

(1) The right "F" hand faces in at chest level.
(2) Sign PILL — the thumb and index finger of the right hand touch, the palm faces the mouth. Flick the index finger towards the mouth as if popping a pill into the mouth. (SM)

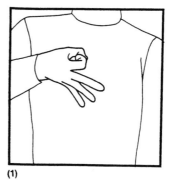
(1)

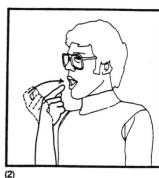
(2)

TAILBONE

The last small bone at the bottom of the human spinal column; the coccyx. The tailbone is usually made up of four vertebrae attached to each other to form one bone. *See Figure 26*

TALUS

The bone in the ankle just below the tibia and fibula of the lower leg. The weight of the whole body is carried by the talus, which then transfers the weight to the other bones of the ankle. *See Figure 26*

TAMPON

In medicine, a roll or piece of material like cotton or gauze, used to absorb blood or fluids from a wound or space in the body. Tampon usually refers to a small round piece of material which is placed by a woman in her vagina while she is menstruating to absorb the blood and secretions. Tampons have a string attached to them so they can be easily removed and depending on the brand, they may have a stick or tube which is used to place them in the vagina.

(Continued on next page)

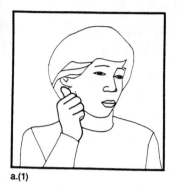
a.(1)

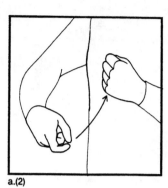
a.(2)

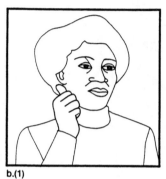
b.(1)

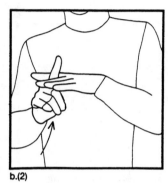
b.(2)

TAMPON, *continued*

Recent research has found that the use of tampons can increase the risk of a woman getting Toxic Shock Syndrome and that the use of sanitary napkins instead of tampons will prevent the disease in almost all cases.

a. (1) Sign MENSTRUATE — the right "A" hand taps the right cheek a few times. (MM)
(2) The left "S" hand faces in at chest level. The right "modified-A" hand faces in and moves up to the left hand. (SM)

b. (1) Sign MENSTRUATE — the right "A" hand taps the right cheek a few times. (MM)
(2) The left "flat" hand faces down at chest level. The right "one" hand points up and moves up through the left index and middle fingers. (SM)

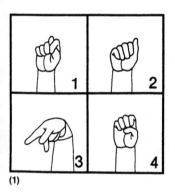
(1)

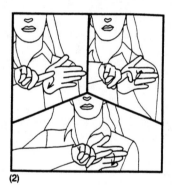
(2)

TAPEWORM

A type of flat, white worm which is a parasite of man and other meat eating animals. Tapeworms live in the intestines and people can get them by eating poorly cooked beef, pork or fish which are infected. A tapeworm will attach to the walls of the intestine and grow on the food we are digesting. Some tapeworms can live a long time and grow to be very long. There are often no symptoms when someone has a tapeworm but the person may feel tired, have nausea and diarrhea, lose appetite, be dizzy and weak. If there are many tapeworms, they may block the intestines.

A tapeworm is actually a string of segments which produce millions of eggs; the segments break off and may appear in the feces looking like pieces of rice.

(1) Fingerspell "T-A-P-E".
(2) Sign WORM — the left "flat" hand faces right at chest level. The right "one" hand faces down on the left palm. Move the right hand out on the left palm and at the same time, bend and straighten the index finger a few times. (MM)

TARSAL BONES

The seven bones that make up the ankles. *See Figure 26*

TARTAR

The hard substance made up of minerals and bacteria which is deposited on teeth and can cause cavities. Plaque on teeth helps in the formation of tartar.

*A dentist or dental hygienist will scrape and polish the teeth to remove **tartar** which has built up.*

TASTE

The sense which allows us to pick up the flavor of something placed on the tongue.

*Taste buds on the tongue allow us to **taste** different foods.*

(1) The middle finger of the right "eight" hand touches the chin or lip. (SM)

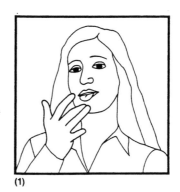

(1)

TASTE BUDS

Special groups of cells found mostly on the tongue which can sense chemicals from foods in the mouth. Taste buds can detect four tastes: salt, sweet, sour and bitter. Each individual taste bud can detect one taste better than the others. *See Figure 23*

TB

See TUBERCULOSIS

TEAR

See AVULSION

TEAR GAS

A gas which irritates the conjunctiva of the eye causing tears.

*There is no special treatment for the irritation of **tear gas** but sometimes washing out the eyes with large amounts of water will help.*

(Continued on next page)

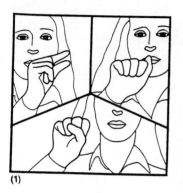
(1)

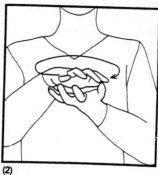
(2)

TEAR GAS, *continued*

(1) Fingerspell "G-A-S".

(2) Sign MIX — both "claw" hands face each other at chest level. Move both hands in alternating circular movements a few times. (MM)

(3) Sign TEARS — the index fingers of both "five" hands touch the cheeks. Move both hands down slightly and at the same time, wiggle the fingers. (SM)

* The facial expression should reflect tearing. This term may need a more detailed explanation.

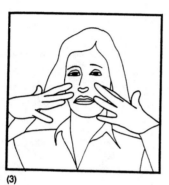
(3)

TECHNICIAN

A person who is highly trained in a certain activity or science.

An X-ray technician is one who specializes in X-rays.

TECHNOLOGIST

See TECHNICIAN

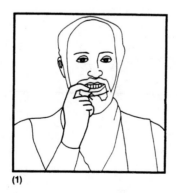
(1)

TEETH

The hard, white, bony structures in the jaws of the mouth which help us chew our food. There are four kinds of teeth in a person's mouth: the incisors, canines or cuspids, premolars or bicuspids, and molars.

We have two sets of teeth during our life: 20 temporary or deciduous teeth, which start to fall out around age six, and 32 permanent teeth.

(1) The index finger of the right "one" hand moves across the teeth from left to right. (SM)

TEETHING

The process of a tooth growing out and piercing the gum, also called cutting of the teeth.

*When a baby is **teething**, it often becomes irritable and cries because the process hurts.*

(1) Sign BABY — the right hand and forearm face up, resting on the left hand and forearm which also face up. Both are then rocked back and forth as if holding a baby. (MM)
(2) The left "flat" hand faces down at chest level. The right "V" hand faces in and moves up through the fingers of the left hand. (SM)
(3) The index finger of the right "one" hand moves across the teeth from left to right. (SM)

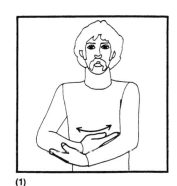
(1)

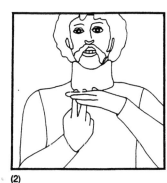
(2)

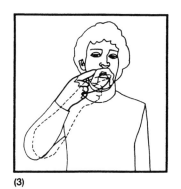
(3)

TEMPERATURE

In medicine, the amount of heat in a body, measured with a thermometer; also, a fever (an abnormally high temperature). Body temperature varies with the area of the body and with the time of day. The normal temperature of the body is 98.6° F or 37° C.

*When we are cold, shivering will raise the body's **temperature** and when we are warm, sweating will lower the body's **temperature**.*

a. (1) The left "flat" hand faces right at chest level. The right "flat" hand faces down and moves up and down on the index finger of the left hand a few times. (MM)
b. (1) The left "one" hand faces right at chest level. The right "one" hand faces down and moves up and down on the index finger of the left hand a few times. (MM)

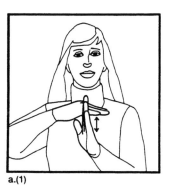
a.(1)

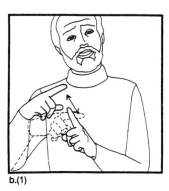
b.(1)

TEMPLE

The part of the head in front of the ear and above the cheek. *See Figure 2*

(Continued on next page)

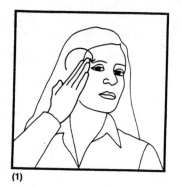
(1)

(1) The fingertips of the right "flat" hand make a circular movement on the right temple. (SM)

TEMPORAL

In medicine, referring to the temples.

The temporal artery is an artery which carries blood to the temple region.

TEMPORAL ARTERY

A large blood vessel which carries fresh blood to the scalp. The temporal artery branches off of the carotid artery. *See Figure 6*

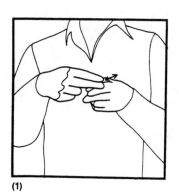
(1)

TEMPORARY

Something which lasts or is used for a short time.

The deciduous teeth are temporary teeth which a baby starts to get around six months of age and which begin to be replaced at six years of age.

(1) Sign SHORT — the left "H" hand faces in at chest level. The fingers of the right "H" hand move back and forth on the left fingers a few times. (MM)

* *This sign means "short time period" and should not be used to mean height.*

TEMPOROMANDIBULAR JOINT SYNDROME

A disorder affecting the muscles in the jaw joint in which the person can't close their teeth together normally, there is pain in the joint, the mouth can't be opened wide and clicking or popping noises are made when moving the joint.

Temporomandibular joint syndrome may be caused by hormonal dysfunction or disease and it may be treated by changing the occlusion.

TENDERNESS

In medicine, sensitive or painful, especially when touched.

There will be tenderness in an injured or inflamed area of the body because of irritation to nerves.

(1) Sign PAIN — both "one" hands point to each other at chest level and twist in opposite directions a few times. (MM)

* The facial expression should reflect pain. This could be signed at the area of tenderness.

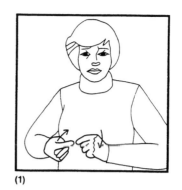

(1)

TENDON

A strong tissue of fibers which connects muscles to bones and other structures.

To test our reflexes and to see that our nervous system is working normally, a doctor will tap some tendons with a small hammer.

TENSION

Physical, mental or emotional stretching or straining.

When too much tension is placed on a bone in one place, it may break or snap and the person may end up with a fractured bone.

a. (1) Sign EMOTION — both "E" hands face each other at chest level and move alternately in inward circular movements a few times. (MM)

* The facial expression should reflect emotional tension.

b. (1) Both "S" hands face in, the right above the left. Move both hands away from each other as if imitating stretching something. (SM)

* The facial expression should reflect tension.

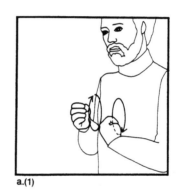

a.(1)

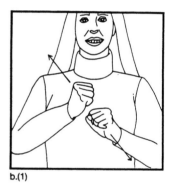

b.(1)

TERMINAL

In medicine, ending in death; fatal.

Patients who are dying from a disease such as cancer, are called terminal or terminally ill.

(1) Sign WILL — the right "flat" hand faces left and moves forward slightly. (SM)

(2) Sign DIE — the left "flat" hand faces up at chest level and the right "flat" hand faces down. Turn both hands over so that the left hand ends facing down and the right hand ends facing up. (SM)

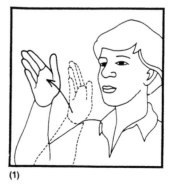

(1)

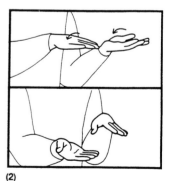

(2)

TESTES

See TESTICLE

611

TESTICLE

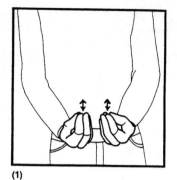

One of the two male reproductive glands found in a sac below and behind the penis called the scrotum; a testis. The testicles (testes) make sperm and the male sex hormone testosterone. Each testicle is a small oval structure with coiled tubes in it which make the sperm. Between the tubes are special cells which make the male sex hormones. When sperm have grown to a certain point in the testicles, they move to the epididymis, a mass of coiled tubes sitting on top of each testicle, where they are stored. *See Figure 13*

(1) Both "flat-O" hands face up at waist level and bounce a few times. (MM)

(1)

TESTIS

See TESTICLE

TESTOSTERONE

A hormone made in the adrenal glands and testes of a male that controls the development of male characteristics such as a deep voice, larger muscles, the growth of body, facial and pubic hair, and the development of the penis. Testosterone is also needed for normal sexual behavior and erections to occur in men. Testosterone is also normally made in women by the adrenal glands.

When a boy reaches puberty, the testicles start to make testosterone which begins the development of male characteristics.

TETANUS

A disease caused by poison made by a bacteria (Clostridium tetani) getting into the body through a wound. The bacteria, widely found in dirt and manure, usually gets into the body through a puncture wound. The bacteria stays in the wound but the poison gets into the bloodstream and affects the nervous system. Symptoms of the disease include painful contractions of muscles, especially in the face and neck. About half of the people getting tetanus will die because of contractions of the muscles which help us breathe.

Once a person has tetanus, it is very hard to treat, so it should be prevented by immunization with tetanus toxoid, cleaning wounds well and, if someone gets a very bad wound or shows signs of tetanus, having shots of penicillin and tetanus antitoxin.

TETANUS ANTITOXIN

An antitoxin made from the blood of horses and cattle for treating tetanus toxin.

*If a person shows signs of tetanus, they should have shots of penicillin and **tetanus antitoxin**.*

TETRACYCLINES

A group of antibiotics which stop infections caused by several different kinds of bacteria. Tetracyclines are used to treat plague, cholera, gonorrhea, gangrene and severe acne. Tetracycline may cause nausea, diarrhea, rashes or a fever if it is taken for a long time.

*Because **tetracycline** can cause yellowing of teeth if taken while they are forming, it shouldn't be taken by pregnant women or children under twelve years of age.*

THALAMUS

A large gray structure in the brain that has to do with many body functions and sending sense impulses to the brain (cerebral cortex). *See Figure 18*

THAW

To warm or melt something.

*When a part of the body has become frozen or frost bitten, it should be **thawed** quickly by placing it in warm but not hot water (102°F - 105°F).*

(1) Sign FREEZE — both "five" hands face down at waist level. Move both hands up slightly into "claw" hands. (SM)
(2) Sign MELT — both "flat-O" hands face up at chest level. Move both hands slightly to the sides and at the same time, the thumbs rub across the fingertips. (SM)

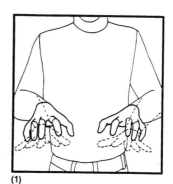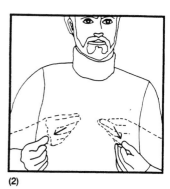

(1)   (2)

THERAPEUTIC

Having to do with treating or curing a disease.

*The **therapeutic** dose of medicine needed to cure a disease varies from person to person and may depend on how bad the disease or infection is, how healthy the person is, how the person's body handles the medicine, and the size of the person.*

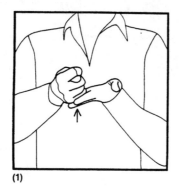
(1)

THERAPY

The treatment that someone goes through to cure a disease or disorder. The word therapy is often used with another word to tell exactly what kind of therapy it is, such as drug therapy, physical therapy, occupational therapy or group therapy.

A severely injured or ill person will often need months or years of different kinds of therapy to help the recovery and return to normal life.

(1) The left "flat" hand faces up at chest level. The right "T" hand faces left on the left palm. Move both hands up. (SM)

* *This is a newer English version and may need further explanation.*

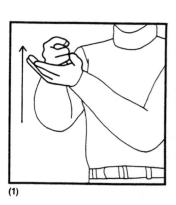
(1)

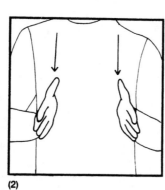
(2)

THERAPIST

A person who specializes in giving treatment to people with a disease or disorder.

A physical therapist may use exercise, heat, light or massage for treatments.

(1) Sign THERAPY — the left "flat" hand faces up at chest level. The right "T" hand faces left on the left palm. Move both hands up. (SM)

* *This is a newer English version and may need further explanation.*

(2) Sign PERSON — both "flat" hands face each other at chest level and move down to waist level. (SM)

THERMAL BURNS

Burns or injury to the skin or other tissue caused by heat. A thermal burn should be placed in cool water quickly or covered with cold packs and kept as clean as possible.

Depending on how deep a thermal burn is, how much damage was done, and what the burn looks like, it may be classified as a first, second, or third degree burn.

THERMOMETER

An instrument used to measure how hot or cold something is. In medicine, a clinical thermometer is used to measure the temperature of the body. It is a thin glass tube with a bulb filled with mercury on one end. The mercury will move into the tube and go up to a certain point in the tube, depending on how warm something is. The two kinds of thermometers used to measure body temperature are the rectal thermometer and the oral thermometer.

(Continued on next page)

THERMOMETER, *continued*

Before and after use, a **thermometer** *should be cleaned well and, because the mercury used to fill the thermometer will stay at the same level, it should be shaken down before it is used.*

a. (1) The index finger of the right "one" hand is in the mouth. Pull the hand out then shake it as if shaking a thermometer down. (MM)

' *Use this sign if referring to an oral thermometer.*

b. (1) The right "one" hand points to the buttocks. (SM)

(2) The index finger of the right "one" hand is in the left "S" hand. Pull the the hand out then shake it as if shaking a thermometer down. (MM)

* *Use this sign if referring to a rectal thermometer.*

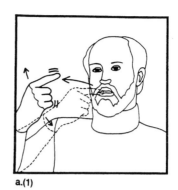

a.(1)

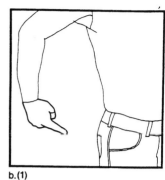

b.(1)

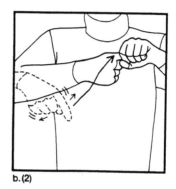

b.(2)

THIAMINE
See VITAMIN B COMPLEX

THIGH
The part of the leg between the hip joint and knee.
See Figure 1

THIGH BONE
See FEMUR

THIN
Light, slender or underweight.

Skinny is another word for **thin** *when referring to a person's weight.*

a. (1) The thumb and index finger of the right "F" hand touch the chin. Move the hand down slightly. (SM)

b. (1) Both "I" hands are at chest level with the little fingers touching. Move both hands in opposite directions. (SM)

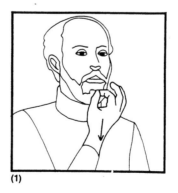

(1)

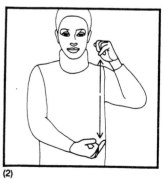

(2)

THIRD DEGREE BURN

Burns which damage both layers of skin, the epidermis and dermis. Third degree burns may damage tissues beneath the skin.

*Because of the severe damage to the skin, skin grafts are often used to help **third degree burns** to heal; otherwise, they would have to heal from the edges, causing much scarring.*

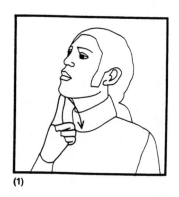
(1)

THIRST

A feeling of wanting to drink fluids, especially water.

Drying out of the lining of the mouth and throat, a fever, or dehydration caused by bleeding, sweating or vomiting may cause thirst.

(1) The index finger of the right "one" hand moves down the throat. (SM)

THORACIC

Having to do with the chest or thorax.

The thoracic cavity is a space in the chest made up by the diaphragm and ribs, containing the heart and lungs.

THORACIC VERTEBRAE

The 12 vertebrae which make up the spinal column in the chest region. Each of the 12 thoracic vertebrae has two ribs attached to it. *See Figure 26*

THORAX

The part of the body between the neck and abdomen; the chest. *See Figure 2*

THORAZINE®

The name under which the drug chlorpromazine is sold. Thorazine is a strong tranquilizer used to treat people with mental diseases, to calm people with severe diseases and those about to have surgery, to lessen the symptoms of withdrawal from alcohol and to treat severe nausea.

There are many side effects which may be caused by thorazine that someone taking the drug should know about.

616

THROAT

The front part of the neck; the pharynx. The throat runs from the back of the mouth down to the top of the esophagus and trachea. *See Figure 1*

(1) The right "G" hand moves down the throat. (SM)

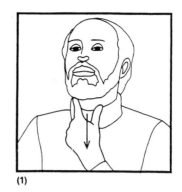

(1)

THROB

To beat or pound rapidly.

If a person hits his thumb with a hammer, it will throb and be painful.

(1) The left "S" hand faces in at chest level. The right "claw" hand faces the left hand slightly above and moves out slightly as if imitating throbbing. (SM)

* *This could be signed at the area that is throbbing.*

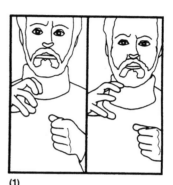

(1)

THROMBOSIS

The formation of a thrombus or blood clot inside a blood vessel. Thrombosis is most often caused by an injury of some sort, an operation, or childbirth. A thrombosis may interfere with blood flow to a part of the body.

Thrombosis is more likely to occur in people who have heart trouble, blood vessel disorders, are overweight, are older or who have a bacterial infection of the blood.

THROMBUS

A blood clot which interferes with or blocks the flow of blood through a blood vessel or through the heart. Symptoms of a thrombus may be pain in the area which is having its blood supply interferred with, coldness, paleness, and blueness or swelling of the part. The pulse may not be felt and gangrene may result. A thrombus which breaks loose and moves through a blood vessel with the blood is called an embolus.

Surgical removal or drugs called anticoagulants are used to treat or prevent a thrombus.

(Continued on next page)

617

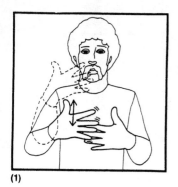
(1)

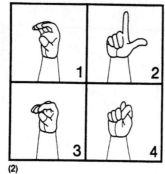
(2)

THROMBUS, *continued*

(1) Sign BLOOD — the left "five" hand is at chest level with the palm toward the body. The palm of the right "five" hand is toward the body with the middle fingertips touching the mouth. Move the right hand down the back of the left hand. Wiggle the fingers of the right hand as it moves. (MM)

* *This movement should be short, repeated and somewhat restrained.*

(2) Fingerspell "C-L-O-T".

THRUSH

An infection of the mouth or throat caused by a fungus. Symptoms of thrush are white spots in the lining of the mouth which become open sores, and often a fever and upset stomach. Thrush occurs most often in children.

*Infants and people taking certain kinds of antibiotics are more likely to get **thrush** than others.*

THUMB

The short, first finger on the inside of the hand. The thumb opposes the other four fingers and allows us to grasp things. *See Figure 1*

(1) The index finger of the right "one" hand points to the left thumb. (SM)

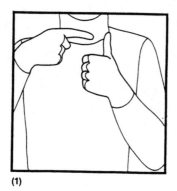
(1)

THYMUS

A gland-like organ behind the sternum (breastbone) and above the heart. The thymus is large in babies and continues to grow until puberty, when it starts to shrink.

*The **thymus** is important in helping develop immunity or resistance against disease.*

THYROID GLAND

The gland found at the base of the neck around the upper end of the trachea. The thyroid gland makes, stores, and puts out a hormone which controls body growth and metabolism. The thyroid gland becomes enlarged in a disease called goiter. The reason iodine is needed by the body is that it helps make up the hormone made by the thyroid gland.

See Figure 10

TIBIA

The inner, larger bone of the lower leg, connected to the femur above and the talus below; the shinbone. *See Figure 26*

TIC

See TWITCH

TICK

An eight legged insect related to spiders which feeds on the blood of animals and man. A tick will attach to the skin with its mouth and suck blood anywhere from several minutes to a few days. Usually tick bites aren't painful and the animal may not even know the tick is there. Ticks can be very dangerous because they can spread diseases like Rocky Mountain Spotted Fever, typhus and tularemia.

Ticks are most often found on uncleared land and paths in the woods, where they are attached to bushes which they will drop from when they detect the sweat of an animal passing by.

(1) Sign INSECT — the thumb of the right "three" hand touches the nose. Bend and straighten the index and middle fingers a few times. (MM)
(2) Fingerspell "T-I-C-K".

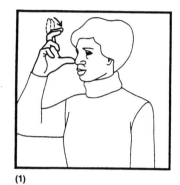

(1)

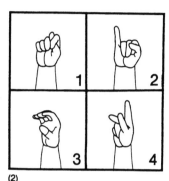

(2)

TICK FEVER

A general term for a group of diseases spread to people by tick bites, especially the diseases which have symptoms like those of Rocky Mountain Spotted Fever. The symptoms start about a week after the bite and include weakness, chills, vomiting, a headache, sore eyes, general body pain and the appearance later of spots on the body.

Tick fever can be prevented by staying out of tick infested areas, by wearing insect repellents and by removing ticks carefully as soon as they are noticed and cleaning the area well.

(1) Sign INSECT — the thumb of the right "three" hand touches the nose. Bend and straighten the index and middle figners a few times. (MM)
(2) Fingerspell "T-I-C-K".

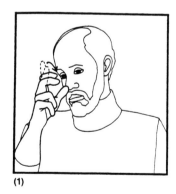

(1)

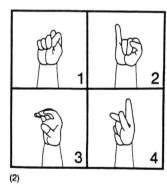

(2)

(Continued on next page)

619

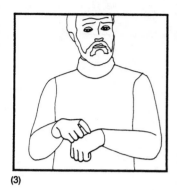

(3)

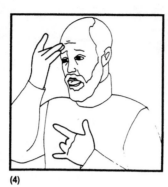

(4)

TICK FEVER, *continued*

(3) Sign BITE — the left "S" hand faces down at chest level. The index finger of the right "one" hand touches the back of the left hand. (SM)

(4) Sign DISEASE — the middle finger of the right "eight" hand touches the forehead and the middle finger of the left "eight" hand touches the stomach. (SM)

* *The facial expression should reflect sickness.*

TINE TEST

A skin test done to see if a person has or has had tuberculosis. To do the tine test, several prongs with materials made by the tuberculosis bacteria on them are pressed just beneath the skin, usually some place on the inside of the forearm. If a person has or has had tuberculosis at some time, he will have antibodies against tuberculosis. When these materials made by the tuberculosis bacteria are put in the body, the antibodies will go to the area, attack and destroy these materials, causing a red, inflamed bump to appear. This is a positive reaction to the tine test, showing the person has had tuberculosis at some time. If the person has never had tuberculosis, he won't have any antibodies against the disease so the materials placed under the skin won't cause a bump to form. This is a negative reaction to the tine test.

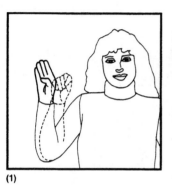

(1)

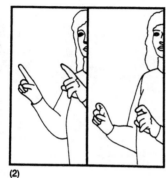

(2)

> *During a routine physical examination, a tine test is often done and should be checked 48-72 hours later for the formation of a hard, red bump.*

(1) Fingerspell "T-B".

(2) Sign TEST — both "one" hands face out and point up at chest level. Move both hands down slightly and at the same time, bend and straighten the index fingers. Repeat this movement three times until the hands end at waist level. (MM)

TINNITUS

A ringing, buzzing, humming or tinkling sound heard by a person in the ears.

> *Tinnitus is usually found along with a disorder or disease of the ear.*

(1) The index finger of the right "one" hand points to the ear. (SM)

(2) The right "five" hand faces down at the right ear and shakes slightly as if indicating ringing in the ear. (MM)

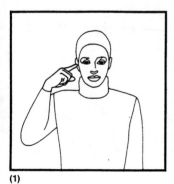

(1)

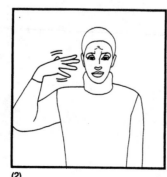

(2)

TIRED

Worn out, exhausted or fatigued.

> *If a person has a low level of glucose in the blood (hypoglycemia), he may become very **tired** and weak.*

a. (1) Sign EXHAUSTED — the right "H" hand faces up in the palm of the left "flat" hand. Move both hands back slightly. (SM)

* *The facial expression should reflect exhaustion.*

b. (1) The fingertips of both "cupped" hands touch the chest. Keeping the fingertips in place, drop both hands slightly. (SM)

* *The facial expression should reflect exhaustion.*

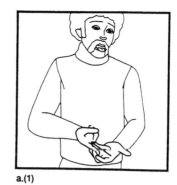
a.(1)

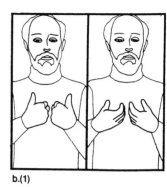
b.(1)

TISSUE

A group of cells in an area which are similar to each other and which work together to perform an activity. Examples of different kind of tissues are muscles, skin, nerves, fat and cartilage.

> *The body's connective **tissues** are those that support and hold the body together, such as cartilage, bone, tendons, and ligaments.*

TOE

One of the five digits on the foot. *See Figure 1*

TOLERANCE

The ability to stand or resist the effects of something like a drug, food or poison.

> *If a person takes a drug for a long time, he may develop a **tolerance** to it and then he will have to take a larger amount to get the same effect from the drug.*

(1) Sign MEDICINE — the left "flat" hand faces up at chest level. The middle finger of the right "eight" hand touches the left palm and pivots slightly from left to right a few times. (MM)

* *The sign for FOOD, POISON, or a specific drug could be used instead of MEDICINE.*

(2) The thumbs of both "five" hands touch the chest. Close both hands to "flat-O" hands. (SM)

(3) The left "flat" hand faces down at chest level. The right "flat" hand faces down at waist level and moves up to the left hand. (SM)

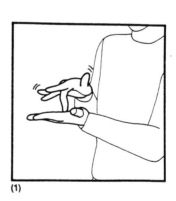
(1)

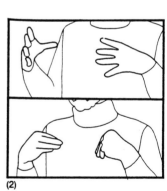
(2)

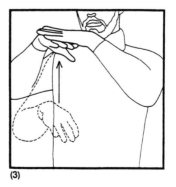
(3)

TONE DEAFNESS

The inability to tell the difference between specific musical sounds.

Tone deafness is also called amusia.

TONGUE

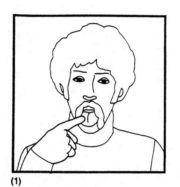
(1)

The flexible, muscular structure attached to the floor of the mouth. The tongue moves food around the mouth in chewing and swallowing and helps us to taste things and to talk. *See Figure 23*

(1) The index finger of the right "one" hand touches the tongue. (SM)

TONOMETER

An instrument used to measure pressure inside the eye.

A tonometer is used to check for glaucoma.

TONSIL

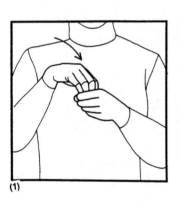
(1)

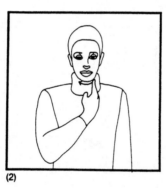
(2)

A small mass of tissue found on either side of the back part of the mouth or upper throat. The tonsils are a collection of lymphatic tissues which filter out and protect the body from bacteria and also make white blood cells. *See Figure 23*

(1) Sign IN — the right "flat-O" hand faces down and moves into the left "O" hand. (SM)

(2) The index finger of the right "one" hand touches the left then the right sides of the throat. (SM)

TONSILLECTOMY

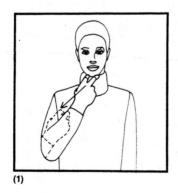
(1)

An operation removing the tonsils.

A tonsillectomy is usually not done unless a person's tonsils are inflamed and infected.

(1) The right "bent-V" hand faces in and moves from the throat out forward. (SM)

TONSILLITIS

Inflammation of the tonsils, usually caused by a bacterial infection. Symptoms of tonsillitis are a sore throat, fever, headache, chills, swollen lymph nodes in the neck area and swollen and inflamed tonsils.

Depending on the cause of a person's tonsillitis, the disease may be treated with rest, gargles or antibiotics.

(1) Sign IN — the right "flat-O" hand faces down and moves into the left "O" hand. (SM)
(2) The index finger of the right "one" hand touches the left then the right sides of the throat. (SM)
(3) Sign INFECTION — the right "I" hand faces out at chest level. Shake the hand slightly from side to side a few times. (MM)
* Mouth the word "infection" while signing.

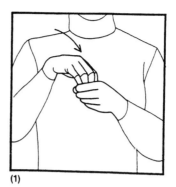
(1)

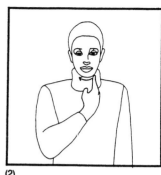
(2)

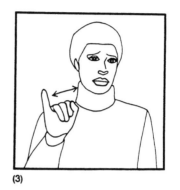
(3)

TOOTH

One of the whitish, bone-like structures in the upper and lower jaws used for chewing food. A tooth has a crown (the part above the gum that can be seen), a root (the part in the socket holding the tooth in place), and a neck (the narrower area between the two). A tooth is made up mostly of a material called dentin, covered by enamel. *See Figure 25*

(1) The index finger of the right "one" hand touches a tooth. (SM)

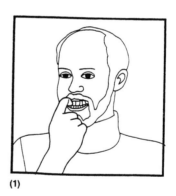
(1)

TOOTHACHE

Pain in or around the tooth.

There are many causes for a toothache but a deep cavity or an infection in the root are the most common.

(1) Sign PAIN — both "one" hands point to each other at the mouth and twist in opposite directions a few times. (MM)
* This could be signed at the area of the toothache. The facial expression should reflect pain.

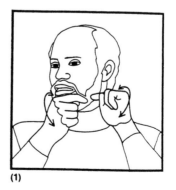
(1)

623

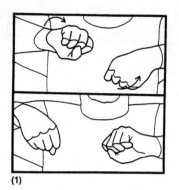
(1)

TORSION
Twisting something or being twisted.

(1) The right "S" hand faces out at chest level and the left "S" hand faces in. Twist both hands so that the right hand ends facing in and the left hand ends facing out. (SM)

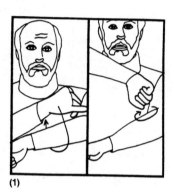
(1)

TOURNIQUET
Any device which can be tightened around an arm or leg to stop bleeding by shutting off blood flow through an artery. A tourniquet is also used to make a vein larger so a needle can be put into it more easily. To stop bleeding, a tourniquet is placed between the heart and the wound, as close to the wound as possible. A tourniquet should not be used if direct pressure over the wound will stop the bleeding.

After being in place about 15 minutes, a tourniquet should be loosened to see if bleeding has stopped because if it is left on too long, tissues will die.

(1) The right "A" hand moves around the left bent arm as if imitating wrapping something, then makes a quick twist. (SM)

* This could be signed at the area where the tourniquet is being applied.

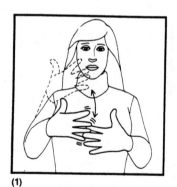
(1)

TOXEMIA
A general infection or poisoning of the body caused by poisonous substances getting into the blood. Toxemia is usually caused by toxins made by bacteria getting into the bloodstream from an infected area. Depending on the poison, symptoms of toxemia may be a fever, muscle pain, diarrhea, vomiting, paralysis, a rash, low blood pressure or shock.

After giving birth to a baby or after an abortion, there is a slight chance of getting a kind of toxemia caused by bacteria infecting the uterus.

(1) Sign BLOOD — the left "five" hand is at chest level with the palm toward the body. The palm of the right "five" hand is toward the body with the middle fingertips touching the mouth. Move the right hand down the back of the left hand. Wiggle the fingers of the right hand as it moves. (MM)

* This movement should be short, repeated and somewhat restrained.

(Continued on next page)

(2) Sign SICK — the middle finger of the right "eight" hand taps the forehead and the middle finger of the left "eight" hand taps the stomach. (MM)

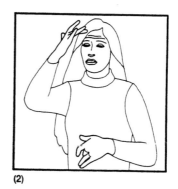

(2)

TOXIC

Poisonous, like a poison, or having to do with a poison.

> *Too much of almost anything can have a toxic effect on the body.*

(1) Sign MEDICINE — the left "flat" hand faces up at chest level. The middle finger of the right "eight" hand touches the left palm and pivots slightly from left to right a few times. (MM)
(2) Sign POISON — both "bent-V" hands cross at the wrists at chest level. (SM)

* The facial expression should reflect something bad.

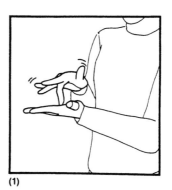

(1)

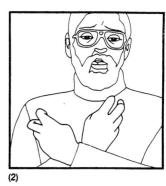

(2)

TOXIC SHOCK SYNDROME

A disease normally affecting women using tampons during the menstrual period; also called T.S.S. The cause of T.S.S. is unknown, but it is believed it may be a form of staph organism first affecting the vagina and moving into the uterus. Symptoms of Toxic Shock Syndrome are an overall body reaction; drop in blood pressure, vomiting, nausea, rash or scaly hands and feet, and dehydration. A person with T.S.S. should be hospitalized and treated with antibiotics and fluids. T.S.S. can cause death if not treated **immediately.**

> *A woman can prevent getting Toxic Shock Syndrome by not using tampons at all, or if used, they should be changed a lot or used between using sanitary napkins.*

(1) Fingerspell "T-S-S".

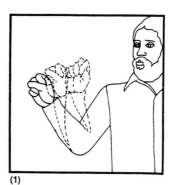

(1)

TOXIN

A poison or poisonous substance.

> *Many bacteria make a person sick by making a toxin which is spread to other parts of the body.*

(Continued on next page)

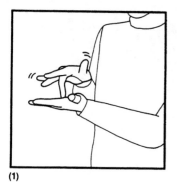
(1)

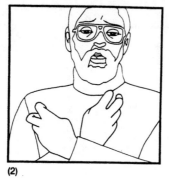
(2)

TOXIN, *continued*

(1) Sign MEDICINE — the left "flat" hand faces up at chest level. The middle finger of the right "eight" hand touches the left palm and pivots slightly from left to right a few times. (MM)

(2) Sign POISON — both "bent-V" hands cross at the wrists at chest level. (SM)

* The facial expression should reflect something bad.

TOXOID

A toxin which has been treated to change its structure and cause it to lose its ability to make someone sick. When a certain kind of toxoid is injected into someone, it will make the person immune to a disease because the toxoid is similar to the poison (toxin) made by the bacteria causing the disease. It will cause antibodies to be made that will work against the real poison (toxin).

To prevent tetanus, a person is given a toxoid which will cause antibodies to be made that will work against the real toxin in case of a tetanus infection.

TRACHEA

The tube running from the lower part of the throat through the neck and into the chest region, where it branches and forms the bronchi; commonly called the windpipe. The trachea carries air from the mouth or nose to the lungs. The trachea is about one inch across and four and a half inches long and is held open by rings of cartilage. *See Figure 10*

TRACHEOTOMY

A cut made into the trachea through the neck to allow a person to breathe or to remove something from the trachea.

A tracheotomy is also called a tracheostomy.

(1) The thumb of the right "A" hand moves down the throat as if imitating cutting. (SM)

(2) Sign BREATHE — both "flat" hands move in and out a few times from the chest as if imitating breathing. (MM)

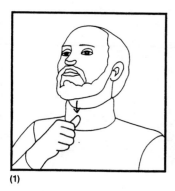
(1)

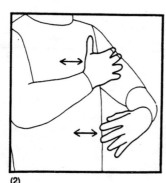
(2)

TRACHOMA

A contagious disease of the conjunctiva of the eye causing inflammation, abnormal growth (hypertrophy), the formation of follicles and possible blindness. Trachoma is especially contagious during the early stages and can be passed on by having direct contact with the infected area or by using contaminated objects such as towels or handkerchiefs.

Trachoma may be treated by taking tetracycline or sulfonamides orally.

TRACTION

A steady pulling used to hold broken bones in the correct position while healing, to correct or straighten deformities or to lengthen muscles that won't relax.

Devices used for traction often include pulleys and weights to produce the steady pulling.

(1) The right "flat" hand brushes down the left arm. (SM)

* This is just an example, the area where the traction is being applied should be signed or fingerspelled first.

(2) The right "S" hand faces out and the left "S" hand faces in, both at chest level. Move both hands out in opposite directions as if indicating pulling something. (SM)

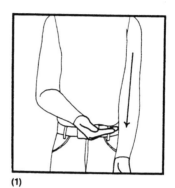
(1)

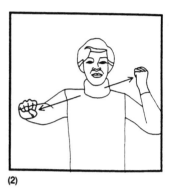
(2)

TRACTION SPLINT

A splint which is put on an injured limb, usually the leg, to hold the part still and to stretch the limb out so the broken ends don't overlap.

Putting a traction splint on a broken femur will prevent damage to the muscles, nerves and blood vessels around the break which may be caused by sharp bone ends.

(1) The right "flat" hand brushes down the left arm. (SM)

* This is just an example, the area where the traction splint is being applied should be signed first.

(2) The left "flat" hand faces down at chest level, the arm bent at the elbow. The right "flat" hand touches the top of the left arm then turns over to touch the bottom of the arm. (SM)

(3) The right "S" hand faces out and the left "S" hand faces in, both at chest level. Move both hands out in opposite directions as if imitating pulling something. (SM)

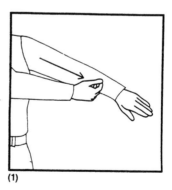
(1)

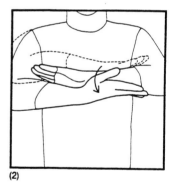
(2)

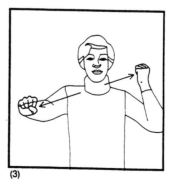
(3)

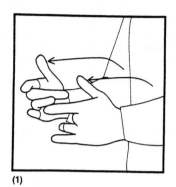
(1)

TRAIT

The qualities or features of a person or thing which makes it different from others.

Chromosomes are made up of genes, each of which will direct, control or be responsible for a certain trait.

(1) Sign TENDENCY — the middle fingers of both "eight" hands touch the chest then move slightly up and out forward. (SM)

* *The lips should mouth "PA".*

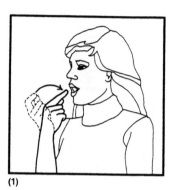
(1)

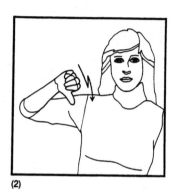
(2)

TRANQUILIZER

A drug which will lessen tension and anxiety without causing depression, drowsiness or lowered mental activity. Tranquilizers may be used to treat some kinds of mental problems. Examples of tranquilizers are chlorpromazine, meprobamate, reserpine and diazepam (Valium).

Tranquilizers increase the effect of alcohol and some can damage a developing fetus so they should always be used carefully.

(1) Sign PILL — the thumb and index finger of the right hand touch, the palm faces the mouth. Flick the index finger towards the mouth as if popping a pill into the mouth. (SM)

(2) Sign DOWNER — the right "A" hand with the thumb pointing down, moves down at shoulder level twice. (DM)

* *This is a general sign for depressants ("downers"). The specific type of drug should also be fingerspelled and all side effects explained.*

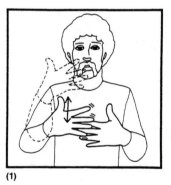
(1)

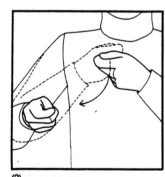
(2)

TRANSFUSION

Putting blood taken from one person into the blood vessels of another person. A transfusion is used to quickly replace blood lost through bleeding, to treat anemia, and to treat shock.

A person having a transfusion must get blood that is of the same blood group or of a special blood group to avoid having a reaction.

(1) Sign BLOOD — the left "five" hand is at chest level with the palm toward the body. The palm of the right "five" hand is toward the body with the middle fingertips touching the mouth. Move the right hand down the back of the left hand. Wiggle the fingers of the right hand as if moves. (MM)

* *This movement should be short, repeated and somewhat restrained.*

(2) Sign EXCHANGE — the left "A" hand faces in at chest level. The right "A" hand faces in behind the left hand. Move the right hand down under the left hand, then out forward. (SM)

628

TRANSMISSIBLE

Having the ability to carry on or pass on from one person to another, such as an infectious disease.

Communicable is another word for transmissible.

(1) Sign DISEASE — the middle finger of the right "eight" hand touches the forehead and the middle finger of the left "eight" hand touches the stomach. (SM)

(2) Sign EASY — the left "cupped" hand faces up at chest level. The right "cupped" hand faces in and brushes up the back of the left hand twice. (DM)

(3) Sign SPREAD — both "flat-O" hands face down at chest level. Move both hands out forward into "five" hands. (SM)

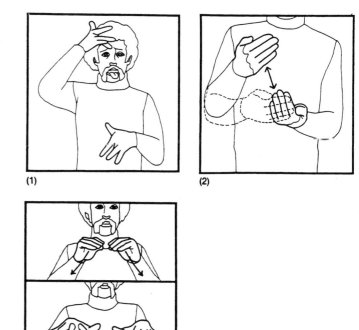

(1)

(2)

(3)

TRANSPLANT

Taking a tissue or organ from its normal place in someone's body and moving it to another part of that person's or another person's body.

A tissue or organ transplant is usually done to correct a defect or fix damage caused by an injury.

a. (1) Sign HEART — the middle finger of the right "eight" hand taps the chest a few times. (MM)

(2) Sign EXCHANGE — the left "A" hand faces in at chest level. The right "A" hand faces in behind the left hand. Move the right hand down under the left hand, then out forward. (SM)

* This is just an example and the specific thing should be signed or finger-spelled.

b. (1) Fingerspell "L-I-V-E-R".

(2) Sign EXCHANGE — the left "A" hand faces in at chest level. The right "A" hand faces in behind the left hand. Move the right hand down under the left hand, then out forward. (SM)

* This is just an example and the specific thing should be signed or finger-spelled.

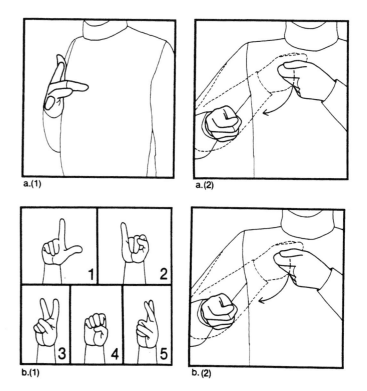

a.(1)

a.(2)

b.(1)

b.(2)

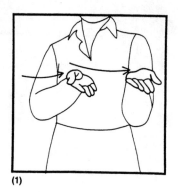
(1)

TRANSPORT

To move someone or something from one place to another.

Chemicals and liquids are carefully transported in and out of the cells.

(1) Sign MOVE — both "flat" hands face up at the right side. Move both hands to the left side. (SM)

TRAPEZIUS

A flat, triangle-shaped muscle on either side of the back part of the neck and shoulder. The trapezius helps us to tip our head back, to the sides and to move the shoulder blades. *See Figure 5*

TRAUMA

An injury or wound caused by something outside the body; also an emotional or mental shock.

A third degree burn causes much more trauma than a second or first degree burn.

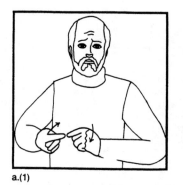
a.(1)

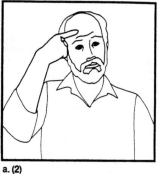
a. (2)

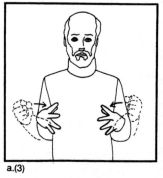
a.(3)

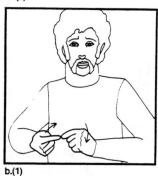
b.(1)

a. (1) Sign HURT — both "one" hands point to each other at chest level and twist in opposite directions a few times. (MM)
* The facial expression should reflect pain.

(2) Sign MIND — the index finger of the right "one" hand touches the forehead. (SM)

(3) Sign SHOCK — both "S" hands face each other at the sides of the body. Move both hands in towards the center, ending in "five" hands. (SM)
* These should be signed if referring to emotional or mental trauma.

b. (1) Sign HURT — both "one" hands point to each other at chest level and twist in opposite directions a few times. (MM)
* The facial expression should reflect pain.

(2) Sign BODY — both "flat" hands face in and touch the chest, then the stomach. (SM)

(3) Sign SHOCK — both "S" hands face each other at the sides of the body. Move both hands in towards the center, ending in "five" hands. (SM)
* These should be signed if referring to physical trauma.

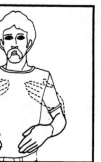
b.(2)

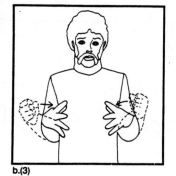
b.(3)

TREATMENT

The care, therapy or procedure used to help cure a disease or injury.

> Antibiotics are used in the *treatment* of infections or diseases caused by a virus.

(1) Sign CARE — both "K" hands tap a few times. (MM)

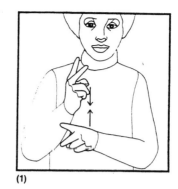
(1)

TREMBLE

An uncontrollable shivering or shaking.

> A person may *tremble* because of cold, disease, or strong emotions.

(1) Both "five" hands face in at chest level and shake slightly. (MM)

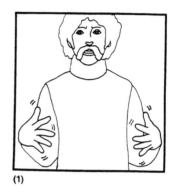
(1)

TREMOR

An uncontrollable shaking or quivering of a part of the body.

> *Tremors* may occur due to alcoholism, disease, mental disorders, excessive exercise, hunger or fatigue.

(1) The left hand grabs the right wrist. Shake the right hand a few times. (MM)

* In this example, the hand is shaken, you should use this motion and then point to the affected area.

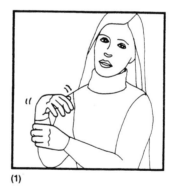
(1)

TRENCH MOUTH

An inflammation of the gums around the teeth caused by a bacteria, poor diet, severe diseases, poor mouth care or stress; also called Vincent's Disease or gingivitis. Symptoms of trench mouth are pain in the mouth, death of the tissue making up the gum, a bad odor to the breath, redness of the gums, thick saliva and also sores on the gums around the mouth and perhaps the throat.

> If *trench mouth* is caused by bacteria, it can be treated with antibiotics.

(1) Fingerspell "G-U-M".

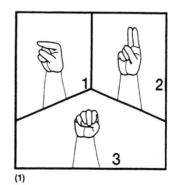
(1)

(Continued on next page)

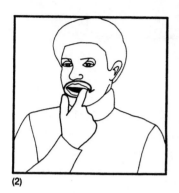

(2)

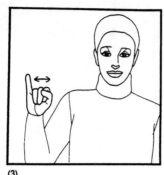

(3)

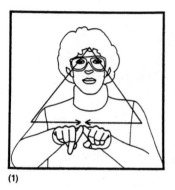

(1)

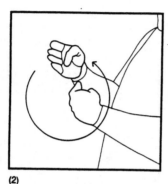

(2)

TRENCH MOUTH, *continued*

(2) The index finger of the right "one" hand circles around the gums. (SM)
(3) Sign INFECTION — the right "I" hand faces out at chest level and shakes slightly a few times. (MM)
* *Mouth the word "infection" while signing.*

TRIANGULAR BANDAGE

A square piece of cloth folded or cut to make a triangle-shaped bandage.

Triangular bandages are often used in first aid to cover large injured areas, make cravat bandages, make slings and, when folded, they can be used to provide pressure and stop bleeding.

(1) Both "one" hands draw a triangle in the air. (SM)
(2) Sign BANDAGE — the left "B" hand faces in at chest level. The right "B" hand also faces in and circles out and around the left hand as if imitating wrapping a bandage. (MM)
* *This could be signed at the area where the bandage is being applied.*

TRICEPS

The muscle found on the back of the upper arm that straightens the arm. *See Figure 5*

TRICHINOSIS

A disease caused by eating raw pork or poorly cooked meat which is infected by a certain kind of parasite (Trichinella spiralis). The parasite is a very small worm found in the muscles of animals like pigs, bears, rats, cats and dogs. If this meat is not well cooked, small worms may get into our bodies through the intestine and infect our muscles. If enough infected meat is eaten, symptoms may be abdominal pain, diarrhea and nausea starting about one day after eating the meat. Then the person may have a fever, edema, severe muscle pain, difficulty in breathing or swallowing, and heart damage; in bad infections, the person may die.

There is no reliable cure for trichinosis, a wide spread disease which can affect anyone, anywhere, if a person is not careful about eating well-cooked meat.

(Continued on next page)

TRICHINOSIS, *continued*

(1) Sign EAT — the right "flat-O" hand taps the mouth a few times. (MM)

(2) Sign DISEASE — the middle finger of the right "eight" hand touches the forehead and the middle finger of the left "eight" hand touches the stomach. (SM)

(3) Sign WHY — the fingertips of the right "flat" hand touch the forehead. Move the hand out slightly, ending in a "Y" hand. (SM)

* The facial expression should reflect questioning.

(4) Sign MEAT — the index finger and thumb of the right "F" hand grab the left hand between the thumb and index finger, then shakes slightly. (MM)

(5) Sign NOT — the right "A" hand, with the thumb extended, faces left and brushes out forward from the chin. (SM)

(6) Sign ENOUGH — the left "S" hand faces in at chest level. The right "flat" hand faces down and brushes out over the left fist. (SM)

(7) Sign COOK — the left "flat" hand faces down at chest level. The right "five" hand faces in under the left hand. Wiggle the fingers of the right hand. (MM)

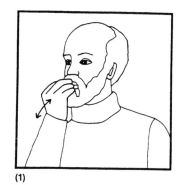

(1)

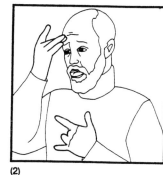

(2)

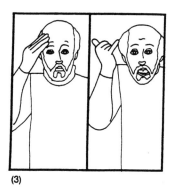

(3)

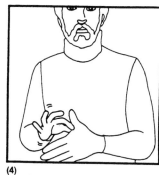

(4)

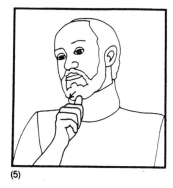

(5)

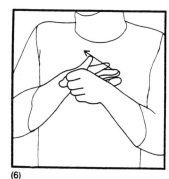

(6)

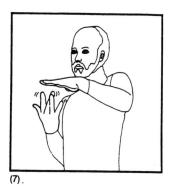

(7).

TRICHOMONIASIS

A disease caused by a very small parasite (Trichomonas) which infects the vagina and uretha of women and the prostate and uretha of man. The disease is usually passed by sexual intercourse or by infected clothing or towels. There are usually no symptoms in men but there may be some inflammation of the prostate or urethra. In women, there is inflammation of the vagina, bubbly yellow or white discharge and itching and burning of the vulva.

Flagyl (metronidazole) will clear up trichomoniasis in about five days; the infected person's sex partner should be treated at the same time.

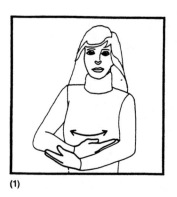
(1)

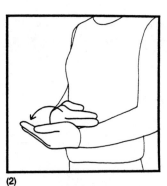
(2)

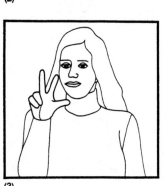
(3)

TRIPLETS

Three children given birth to by the same mother in the same pregnancy.

Sometimes women taking fertility pills will have multiple births such as triplets or quadruplets.

(1) Sign BABY — the right hand and forearm face up, resting on the left hand and forearm which also face up. Both are then rocked back and forth as if holding a baby. (MM)
(2) Sign BORN — the left "flat" hand faces in at waist level. The right "flat" hand faces in and moves down to rest in the left palm. (SM)
(3) Sign THREE — the right "three" hand faces out at chest level. (SM)

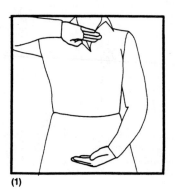
(1)

TRUNK

The main part of the body not including the head, arms or legs. *See Figure 2*
(1) The right "flat" hand faces down at the neck and the left "flat" hand faces up at the stomach.

TUBAL PREGNANCY

A pregnancy in which the fertilized egg has abnormally attached to the inside of one of the fallopian tubes; an ectopic pregnancy. As the fetus grows, there is usually pain and bleeding into the abdomen, which becomes severe if the tube bursts because of the pregnancy.

Surgery is needed to treat a tubal pregnancy or death may result.

TUBERCULIN TINE TEST

See TINE TEST

TUBERCULOSIS

An infectious disease caused by a bacteria (Mycobacterium tuberculosis) which usually affects the lungs but can also effect the intestines, bones, joints, skin, lymph nodes, urinary tract and genitals; also called consumption. Symptoms of tuberculosis vary, depending on the type. Small bumps usually form in the infected area, and there is fever, sweating, tissue death, scarring, weight loss and weakness. If it is affecting the lungs, the person will usually have a cough, chest pain and blood in the sputum. Tuberculosis can be treated more effectively now with antibiotics, rest, a good diet and sometimes surgery.

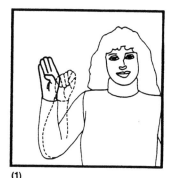

(1)

Because cattle can get tuberculosis and pass it to man, young children should drink only pasteurized milk instead of raw milk.

(1) Fingerspell "T-B".

* This may need some explanation before fingerspelling.

TULAREMIA

A severe infectious disease caused by the bite of an infected tick or other blood-sucking insect, contact with infected animals, by eating undercooked meat or by drinking water that has the organism in it. Symptoms of tularemia may include headache, chills, vomiting, pain and a fever. If the infected area develops into an abscess, a person may have sweating, loss of weight and weakness.

Tularemia can effectively be treated with streptomycin and tetracyclines.

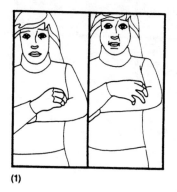
(1)

TUMOR

A swelling or abnormal growth of cells in an area. The cells in a tumor are not normal, do not work, and often grow out of control.

The cause of tumor growth is often unknown and there is usually no inflammation.

(1) The right "O" hand faces down on the left bent arm. Open the right hand slightly into a "claw" hand and at the same time, the cheeks should puff out. (SM)

* *This could be signed at the area of the tumor.*

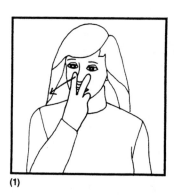
(1)

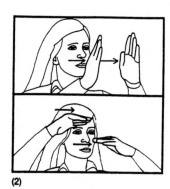
(2)

TUNNEL VISION

A vision problem in which a person can see only a small area, as if he were looking through a tunnel.

Glaucoma and emotional problems may cause tunnel vision.

(1) Sign SEE — the right "V" hand faces in and moves out from the eyes. (SM)

(2) Both "flat" hands face each other at eye level and move out forward slightly. Both "flat" hands then face down at eye level and move out forward slightly. (SM)

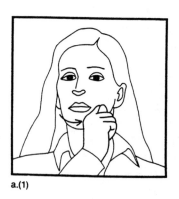
a.(1)

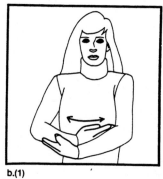
b.(1)

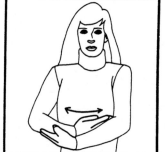
b.(2)

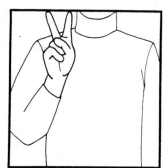
b.(3)

TWINS

Two children given birth to by a woman in the same pregnancy.

Twins are identical if a fertilized egg splits and then develops into two babies and they are fraternal if two eggs were released and fertilized at the same time.

a. (1) The right "T" hand touches both cheeks. (SM) cheeks. (SM)

b. (1) Sign BABY — the right hand and forearm face up, resting on the left hand and forearm which also face up. Both are then rocked back and forth as if holding a baby. (MM)

(2) Sign BORN — the left "flat" hand faces in at waist level. The right "flat" hand faces in and moves down to rest in the left palm. (SM)

(3) Sign TWO — the right "V" hand faces out at chest level.

636

TWITCH

A small, uncontrollable muscle contraction or tic of a face, head, neck or shoulder muscle, often repeated.

The cause of a twitch may be psychological or it may be a movement which has become a habit.

* This could be mimed.

TYMPANIC MEMBRANE

See EARDRUM

TYPHOID FEVER

A severe, infectious disease caused by a bacteria (Salmonella typhosa) which gets into the body through the digestive system and then spreads to the blood and entire body. The disease is usually caught by eating food, water or milk which has the germ in it. The bacteria can also be spread to others by contact with the feces or hands of an infected person. Early symptoms are a headache, weakness, general pain and nosebleeds. The person will then have a high fever, red spots on the abdomen and back, an enlarged abdomen and spleen, either constipation or diarrhea and perhaps vomiting and delirium. Typhoid can be prevented by a vaccine and if a person does get it, then antibiotics like ampicillin and chloramphenicol are used to treat it.

The use of good, clean water, sewage treatment, pasteurization of milk, control of people who carry the bacteria that causes typhoid and education of the public in cleanliness have all made typhoid fever an uncommon illness in the United States today.

TYPHUS

A severe infectious disease caused by a rickettsial organism. Typhus is spread by lice, fleas and ticks and occurs when large groups of people must live together in unclean conditions, as during wars or emergencies. Symptoms are a bad headache, pain in the back and limbs, severe weakness, a high fever, delirium, twitching, bluish spots on the body and constipation. A person with typhus is treated with rest, a liquid diet and antibiotics like tetracyclines and chloramphenicol.

If people must be kept in close contact for long periods of time, the spread of typhus can be prevented by vaccination, cleanliness, and control of rats and body lice.

637

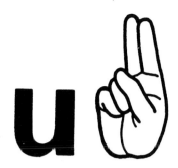

u

ULCER

An open sore on the skin or on an internal organ. Ulcers are areas of dead tissues which heal slowly and sometimes bleed and make pus. They are caused by the tissue in an area being killed by something like strong chemicals, by an injury or by bacteria, viruses or parasites. The most common kind of ulcers are those in the digestive system caused by the digestive enzymes and acids attacking and digesting the lining of the esophagus, stomach or small intestine.

An ulcer in the digestive tract is dangerous because it may bleed a lot or it may eat all the way through the lining, allowing food and other materials into the abdomen, which will cause an infection.

ULNA

The larger of the two bones in the forearm running between the elbow and wrist. The ulna is the inner bone on the side opposite the thumb. *See Figure 26*

ULNAR ARTERY

A large blood vessel in the forearm which carries fresh blood to the lower arm, wrist and hand. Below the elbow, the brachial artery branches to form the radial artery and ulnar artery. *See Figure 6*

ULTRASOUND

A sound wave of very high energy. We cannot hear this kind of sound wave but it is able to go through a person's body. Because ultrasound has different speeds in different types of tissues and structures in the body, it can be used to take a kind of picture of internal structures. Also, some of the energy in ultrasound is turned into heat in the body, so it is used to apply heat to deep tissues.

A common use of ultrasound is to form an image of a fetus while it is growing in a woman to make sure it is normal and healthy.

ULTRAVIOLET RAYS

An invisible light ray of a very high energy. These rays, a natural part of sunlight, can be made by a special kind of lamp. Because they have so much energy, these rays can pass through the surface layers of the skin and may damage lower layers if a person is exposed to them for a long time. Ultraviolet light is important in helping to make vitamin D in the skin and in killing bacteria in certain areas.

*A substance called melanin gives the skin its color and when we are in the sun a lot, more of it is made, causing a tan which protects us from **ultraviolet rays** in the sun's light.*

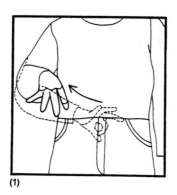

(1)

UMBILICAL CORD

A rope-like structure about 2 feet long and one half inch wide which connects the fetus to the placenta while it is in the uterus. The umbilical cord contains two arteries and one vein which carries oxygen and nutrients to and wastes from the baby.

*The **umbilical cord**, which is still attached to a baby when it is born, is cut shortly after birth, leaving a scar on a person's abdomen called the navel or bellybutton.*

(1) The right "F" hand faces out at the navel. Move the hand out forward slightly. (SM)

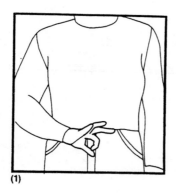

(1)

UMBILICUS

The navel or scar left on the abdomen where the umbilical cord was once attached to us.

*The **umbilicus** is also commonly called the bellybutton.*

(1) The right "F" hand faces out at the navel. (SM)

UNCONSCIOUS

Unable to sense things and unaware of what is going on around a person. Being unconscious is somewhat like sleeping but the person cannot be brought back to full alertness as a sleeping person can. A person can become unconscious from lack of oxygen, too much alcohol, a brain or head injury, poisoning, an overdose of certain drugs, epilepsy, fear, a stroke or severe shock. Unconscious is also used in psychology for the part of our mind or personality made up of feelings and drives that we aren't aware of but which can still affect our behavior.

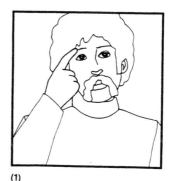
(1)

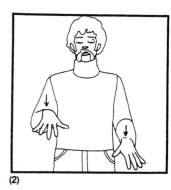
(2)

A person who is unconscious for any reason should have the head turned to the side so any saliva or vomit will drain out instead of being inhaled.

(1) Sign MIND — the index finger of the right "one" hand touches the forehead. (SM)
(2) Both "five" hands face down and move down slightly, the eyes should be closed. (SM)

UNCONTROLLABLE

Unable to be controlled.

Someone having a grand mal seizure will experience uncontrollable movements for a short time.

(1) Sign CAN'T — the left "one" hand faces down at chest level. The right "one" hand moves down to strike the left index finger. (SM)
(2) Sign CONTROL — both "modified-A" hands face each other at chest level. Move both hands alternately forward and back a few times. (MM)

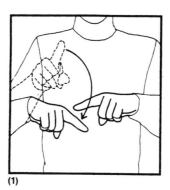
(1)

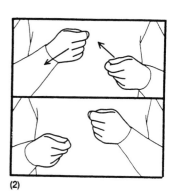
(2)

UNILATERAL

Happening on or affecting only one side of the body.

A person who has lived through a stroke will usually have unilateral paralysis because of damage to one side of the brain.

(1) The right "cupped" hand moves down the body from the center of the head to waist level. (SM)
(2) The left "flat" hand moves across the body from right to left. (SM)

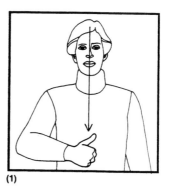
(1)

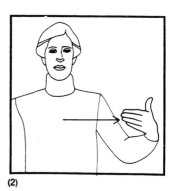
(2)

UNIT TYPE KIT

One of two common types of first aid kits. This type of kit has a wide range of bandages, compresses, gauze pads and rolls of gauze wrapped individually. Because there is just enough dressing in each package to treat one injury, there is no waste and the other things stay sterile.

In a unit type kit, all medications are put in one-dose containers so they aren't wasted or contaminated.

UNIVERSAL DONOR

A person who belongs to the O blood group. This person's blood may be given to people who belong to another group such as the A, B or AB groups, without causing them to have an allergic reaction. A person who belongs to the O blood group has no proteins called antigens on the surface of their blood cells so when their blood is given to someone else, the new blood won't be recognized as not belonging in that person's body and there will be no allergic reaction.

Because there are other blood grouping systems than A, B, AB, and O group, like the Rh group, a universal donor's blood cannot be given to just anyone without further tests.

UNIVERSAL RECIPIENT

A person who belongs to the AB blood group. This person may get blood from people whose blood is not of the same blood group as theirs, such as A, B, or O blood without causing an allergic reaction. A person who belongs to the AB blood group has two kinds of proteins, called the A-antigens and B-antigens, on the surface of the blood cells so that he could get blood from the A blood group, B blood group or O blood group (which has no proteins on the cells) and the body would not recognize the new blood as not belonging in the body and there would be no reaction.

There are other blood grouping systems besides the A, B, AB and O systems like Rh system, so blood given to a universal recipient is tested in other ways to prevent a reaction.

UNSTERILE

Dirty or not clean. Unsterile is used in medicine for something which has very small living things on it such as viruses, bacteria or fungi, which could cause an infection.

Hepatitis and other infections are more common among people who inject themselves with illegal drugs because unsterile needles and syringes are often used.

(1) Sign NOT — the thumb of the right "A" hand touches under the chin. Move the hand out forward. (SM)

(2) Sign CLEAN — the left "flat" hand faces up at chest level. The right "flat" hand faces down and rubs out across the left palm. (SM)

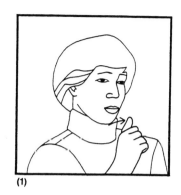 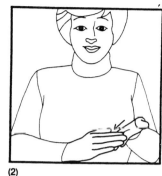

(1)　　　　　　(2)

UPPER ARM

See BICEPS

UPPERS

The slang name for a stimulant drug that will increase activity and make a person less tired and more alert.

Drugs like amphetamine, dextroamphetamine and methamphetamine are often called "uppers."

(1) Sign PILL — the right thumb and index finger touch, the palm faces in. Flick the index finger towards the mouth as if imitating popping a pill in the mouth. (SM)

(2) Sign UPPERS — the right "A" hand, with the thumb extended, faces in at shoulder level and moves up twice. (DM)

* This is a general sign for stimulants ("uppers"). The specific type of drug should also be fingerspelled and all side effects explained.

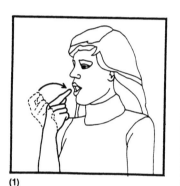 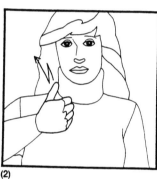

(1)　　　　　　(2)

URETER

One of the two tubes connected to the kidneys and bladder that carries urine from the kidneys, where it is made, to the bladder, where it is held until it is released from the body. The ureters are muscular tubes which can contract and help move the drops of urine to the bladder. *See Figure 12 or 13*

URETHRA

A muscular tube which goes from a person's bladder to the outside of the body. The urethra carries urine from the bladder to the outside of the body. In a woman, the urethra is a short straight tube which opens between the vagina and clitoris. In a man, the urethra is longer and more complicated because it goes through the length of the penis and also is a part of the reproductive system. *See Figure 12 or 13*

643

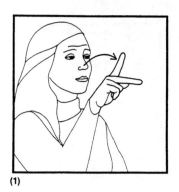
(1)

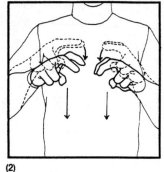
(2)

URINALYSIS

The chemical examination of urine for the color and presence of cells, chemicals or other substances.

A doctor might want a urinalysis done when diagnosing a disease because urine can tell a lot about how the body is working.

(1) Sign URINATE — the right "P" hand faces out and moves from the nose forward. (SM)
(2) Sign ANALYZE — both "bent-V" hands face down at chest level. Drop both hands down slightly and at the same time, move both hands down to waist level. (MM)

URINARY SYSTEM

The system made up of the kidneys, ureter, bladder and urethra which helps get wastes out of the body. The urinary system is a part of the excretory system. *See Figure 12 'or 13*

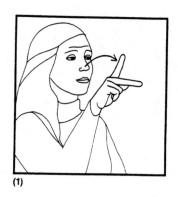
(1)

URINATE

To release urine from the bladder to the outside of the body through the urethra.

To urinate, two muscles around the urethra must be relaxed so the urine can flow through it.

(1) The right "P" hand faces out and moves from the nose forward. (SM)

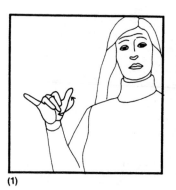
(1)

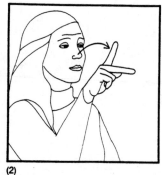
(2)

URINE

The yellowish fluid made from the blood by the kidneys and stored in the bladder until it is released from the body through the urethra. The urine is carried to the bladder from the kidneys by the urethers.

Healthy people produce around one to one and a half quarts of urine a day.

(1) Sign YELLOW — the right "Y" hand faces out at chest level and shakes slightly from side to side a few times. (MM)
(2) Sign URINATE — the right "P" hand faces out and moves from the nose forward. (SM)

UROLOGIST

A doctor who specializes in treating diseases and disorders of the kidney, ureters, bladder and urethra of both men and women and the reproductive system in men.

A person who has painful or difficult urination should see a **urologist.**

UROLOGY

The area of medicine which deals with diseases and disorders of the kidneys, ureter, bladder and urethra of both men and women and the reproductive system in men.

Ureteralgia, pain in the ureter, is a disorder that is studied in **urology.**

UTERUS

A muscular, hollow, pear-shaped organ found in a female's abdomen; also called the womb. The uterus is about three inches long and two inches wide. The two fallopian tubes open into it at the top; the lower end, called the cervix, opens into the vagina. The uterus holds a developing fetus and provides nutrients to it from the time the fertilized egg attaches to the wall of the uterus until the baby is born. The uterus expands during this time of development. *See Figure 12*

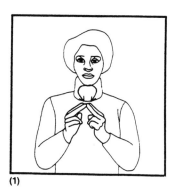
(1)

(1) Both "H" hands outline the shape of the uterus. (SM)

* *This may need to be fingerspelled first to clarify.*

UVULA

The small bag-shaped structure hanging from the back, top part of the mouth. The uvula is made up mostly of muscle. *See Figure 23*

(1) The index finger of the right "one" hand points to the mouth. (SM)
(2) With the mouth open, the right "one" hand points down and wiggles slightly as if imitating the uvula moving. (SM)

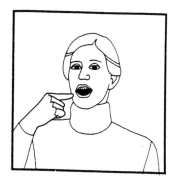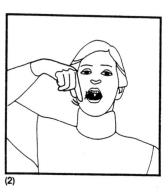
(2)

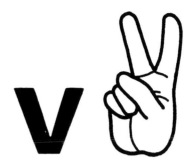

V

VACCINATE

To inject a weakened dose of a disease-causing virus or bacteria, a dead virus or bacteria or a certain part of the virus or bacteria into someone to make him immune to the strong or real form of the disease.

> It is very important to **vaccinate** all children against polio, diptheria, tetanus, whooping cough, measles, and German measles, and to make sure they get boosters when needed to keep them protected.

a. (1) The index finger of the right "L" hand touches the left upper arm. Bend the thumb in as if imitating injecting something into the arm. (SM)

* This could be signed at the area being vaccinated.

b. (1) The index finger of the right "X" hand taps the left upper arm a few times as if imitating vaccinating. (SM)

* This could be signed at the area being vaccinated.

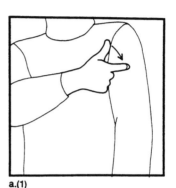

a.(1)

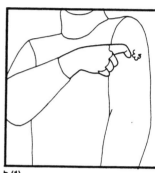

b.(1)

VACCINE

A solution containing a weakened form of a disease-causing organism, a dead disease-causing organism or certain parts of a disease-causing organism. The solution is swallowed, injected or even inhaled to cause the body to make special proteins called antibodies which will fight off the strong or real form of the disease if it gets into the body. (There are many vaccines that will safely prevent infections caused by dangerous viruses or bacteria but only if they are given at the right times and in the right amounts.)

> Some diseases that can be prevented by a **vaccine** are diphtheria, tetanus, whooping cough, influenza, measles, mumps, polio, rabies, German measles, smallpox, typhoid and typhus. (Continued on next page)

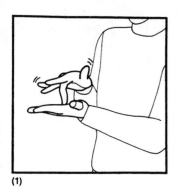
(1)

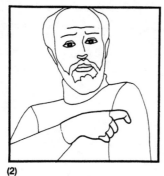
(2)

VACCINE, continued

(1) Sign MEDICINE — the left "flat" hand faces up at chest level. The middle finger of the right "eight" hand touches the left palm and pivots slightly from side to side a few times. (MM)

(2) The index finger of the right "X" hand taps the left upper arm a few times as if imitating vaccinating. (SM)

* *This could be signed at the area where the vaccination is being given. Sign IN-HALE or DRINK if referred specified.*

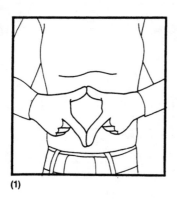
(1)

VAGINA

The structure in a woman which goes from the bottom of the uterus to the outside of the body. The vagina is about three and a half inches long and lies between the bladder and the rectum, with the opening between the urethra and the anus. The vagina is like a collapsed or flattened tube which can expand. The vagina receives the penis during sexual intercourse, is the place where semen is deposited, allows menstrual fluid from the uterus to leave the body and is the passage a baby moves through during birth. *See Figure 12*

(1) The thumb and index fingers of both "L" hands touch. (SM)

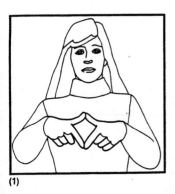
(1)

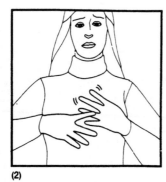
(2)

VAGINAL DISCHARGE

The flowing away of a secretion, usually pus, blood or urine, from the vagina.

> *Vaginal discharge may be a symptom of some disorders such as in candidiasis (yeast infection) or vaginitis (inflammation of the vagina).*

(1) Sign VAGINA — the thumb and index fingers of both "L" hands touch. (SM)

(2) The left "five" hand faces in at chest level. The right "five" hand faces in below the left hand. Move the right hand down slightly and at the same time, wiggle the fingers. (SM)

* *These signs could be followed by fingerspelling "P-U-S", by signing BLOOD or the colors YELLOW or WHITE, to specify.*

VAGINISMUS

Painful contractions of the muscles around the vagina which may be caused by vaginitis, menopause, abnormal formation or the person being afraid of sexual intercourse. The symptoms of vaginismus are tension of the tissues around the vagina and extreme sensitivity when touched.

Vaginismus may be treated with psychotherapy and by teaching the person not to be afraid of sexual intercourse.

VAGINITIS

Inflammation of the vagina. Vaginitis may be caused by uncleanliness, chemical irritation (which could be caused by douching with too strong chemicals), menopause, irritation by some foreign objects or an infection caused by a fungus, bacteria or other parasite. Symptoms of vaginitis are a pus-like and perhaps bloody discharge from the vagina, painful urination, redness in the area and perhaps sores.

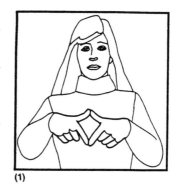 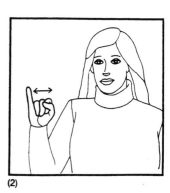
(1)   (2)

Most women experience vaginitis at some time in their lives and the treatment of it will depend on the cause.

(1) Sign VAGINA — the thumb and index fingers of both "L" hands touch. (SM)
(2) Sign INFECTION — the right "I" hand faces out at chest level and shakes slightly from side to side a few times. (MM)
* Mouth the word "infection" while signing.

VALIUM®

The brand name that the drug diazepam is sold under. Valium is used to lessen tension and anxiety caused by mental problems or surgery, to relax muscles and to lessen the symptoms caused by withdrawal from alcoholism. Valium is the most frequently prescribed drug in the country and has been since 1972. Even so, many people don't know of the possible side affects that may occur, such as tiredness, poor coordination, a rash, nausea, dizziness, headaches, confusion, depression, irritability, constipation and problems with the blood.

One of the greatest dangers of valium is that it can produce dependency so that if a person stops using the drug all of a sudden after taking it for several months, he may become upset, be unable to sleep, tremble, have cramps or even go into convulsions.

(Continued on next page)

649

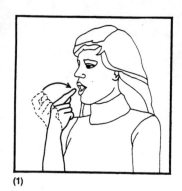
(1)

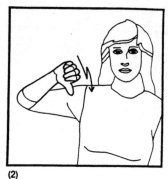
(2)

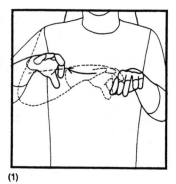
(1)

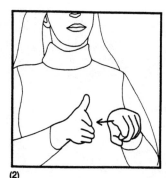
(2)

VALIUM ,*continued*

(1) Sign PILL — the right thumb and index finger touch, the palm faces in. Flick the index finger towards the mouth as if imitating popping a pill in the mouth. (SM)

(2) Sign DOWNER — the right "A" hand, with the thumb extended, faces down at shoulder level and moves down twice. (DM)

VALVE

A flap-like structure, often shaped like a cup and found in a hollow structure or tube, that will close at certain times in order to keep a fluid moving in one direction.

There are valves in the heart between the atrium and ventricle on each side to keep blood flowing in the correct direction when the heart muscle contracts.

(1) Both "modified-O" hands face down at chest level. Move the right hand out to the side. (SM)

(2) The left "O" hand faces down at chest level. The right "flat" hand faces left next to the left hand. Pivot the right hand out at the wrist as if imitating a valve opening and closing. (SM)

VARICELLA

See CHICKENPOX

VARICELLA ZOSTER

See SHINGLES

VARICOSE VEINS

Swollen, twisted and knotted veins. Varicose veins can occur anywhere on the body but are most common in the legs. Veins have little valves along their length that allow blood to move along them in only one direction and prevent it from returning. If a vein enlarges, the valves won't close together and blood can then flow back and pool in the vein causing varicose veins. Varicose veins may be caused by standing for long periods of time, being overweight, pregnant, or the valves being abnormal. Symptoms of varicose veins are pain in the lower legs, muscle cramps, swelling, the appearance of large, bluish veins just under the skin and perhaps the formation of sores.

(Continued on next page)

650

Bad cases of **varicose veins** may be treated by totally removing the damaged veins.

(1) Fingerspell "V-E-I-N".
(2) Both "S" hands face down at chest level. Open both hands slightly into "claw" hands, indicating the vein swelling. (SM)

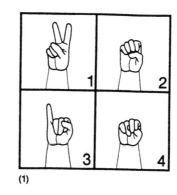
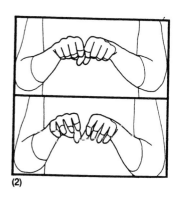

VARIOLA
See SMALLPOX

VAS DEFERENS
Coiled tubes, each about 18 inches or more in length, that go from each testicle to join the urethra in the region of the prostate gland. The vas deferens carry sperm from the testicles to the urethra during ejaculation. *See Figure 13*

VASECTOMY
An operation in which small sections of the vas deferens are removed, usually in the area between the testicles and where the vas deferens enter the body. A vasectomy is a form of contraception that makes a man sterile but not impotent. A vasectomy is minor surgery, does not require hospitalization, and can be done in a doctor's office. A small incision is made on each side of the scrotum under a local anesthetic and the doctor will remove a small section of the vas deferens and then tie the ends to prevent them from rejoining. A man who has had this operation will ejaculate in the normal manner but the semen will contain no sperm because it can no longer leave the testicles.

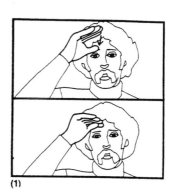
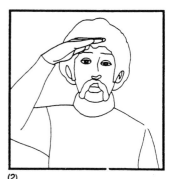

There is absolutely no physical reason for a **vasectomy** to affect a man's sex drive or performance.

(1) Sign MAN — the right open "flat-O" hand faces down at the forehead. Close the hand into a "flat-O" hand and move it out slightly. (SM)
(2) The right "flat" hand faces down at the forehead and moves out slightly. (SM)
(3) Both "A" hands face in at the lower stomach area and imitate tying. (DM)

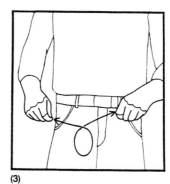

V.D.

See VENEREAL DISEASE

VEIN

The kind of blood vessel which carries blood from all parts of the body back to the heart. Both veins and arteries are blood vessels and together they make up an important part of the circulatory system.

A vein carries blood which is dark red, low in oxygen, high in carbon dioxide and high in wastes back from the cells and capillaries to the heart.

(1) Fingerspell "V-E-I-N".

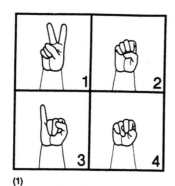

(1)

VENA CAVA

A large vein which enters the right atrium of the heart. The superior vena cava carries blood from the head, neck, chest and arms back to the heart and the inferior vena cava carries blood from the legs and abdomen back to the heart. *See Figure 15 or 16*

VENEREAL

Causing or having to do with sexual intercourse.

A venereologist is a doctor who treats venereal diseases.

(1) Sign CONNECT — the thumbs and index fingers of both "F" hands join together. (SM)
(2) Sign SEX — the right "X" hand faces out and touches the side of the head at eye level, then at the chin. (SM)

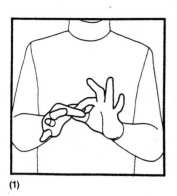

(1)

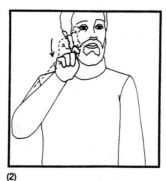

(2)

VENEREAL DISEASE

A disease which a person gets by having sexual intercourse with a person who has or is infected with the disease. Examples of venereal diseases are gonorrhea, syphilis, a type of herpes which affects the genitals, venereal warts, and, in some cases, trichamoniasis. The symptoms of venereal diseases vary depending on which one a person has but they usually start out with a sore or inflammation somewhere on the genitals, a pus-like discharge, swollen lymph nodes in the area, painful urination and perhaps other symptoms such as a fever and general pain.

(Continued on next page)

Several years ago, gonorrhea was the most common venereal disease but recently, the number of people with herpes may have passed those with all other venereal diseases combined.

(1) Fingerspell "V-D".

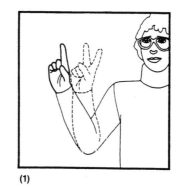

(1)

VENOM

A poison made by some animals and insects which can be injected into other animals by bites or stings. Venom is used by these animals to get their food or to protect themselves. Most venoms contain proteins which are usually toxins and enzymes.

There is an antivenom available to work against any venom which has been injected into the body.

a. (1) Sign ANIMAL — the fingertips of both "cupped" hands touch the chest. Keeping the hands in place, bend and straighten the fingers at the knuckles a few times. (MM)

b. (1) Sign INSECT — the thumb of the right "three" hand touches the nose. Bend and straighten the fingers a few times. (MM)

(2) Sign POISON — both "bent-V" hands face in and cross on the chest. (SM)

* *Sign ANIMAL or INSECT, whichever applies, then sign POISON.*

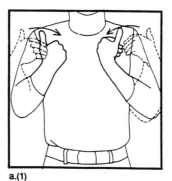

a.(1)

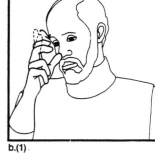

b.(1)

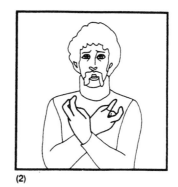

(2)

VENTRAL

Having to do with the belly or abdomen; the opposite of dorsal. In a four-legged animal, ventral refers to lower side or underside of the body. In man, ventral refers to the front side of the body. For example, the sternum or breastbone is attached to the ventral side of the rib cage.

VENTRICLES OF THE BRAIN

The spaces in the brain which are filled with a fluid called cerebrospinal fluid. There are four ventricles in the brain, connected to each other by narrow passageways. *See Figure 18*

VENTRICLES OF THE HEART

The two lower chambers in the heart. The right ventricle and the left ventricle are separated from each other but each ventricle is connected to the atrium above it. The right ventricle has blood forced into it by the right atrium. It contracts and forces the blood in it into the pulmonary artery, which takes the blood to the lungs. The left ventricle has blood forced into it by the left atrium and then contracts and forces the blood into the aorta, which takes blood to all parts of the body. *See Figure 16*

VENTRICULAR FIBRILLATION

The ventricles of the heart beating quickly, irregularly and abnormally. Ventricular fibrillation, unlike atrial fibrillation, can cause death in a few minutes and is a serious emergency because the ventricles are the parts of the heart that do most of the pumping of the blood. Ventricular fibrillation can be caused by severe heart damage or poisoning by certain drugs such as digitalis.

*Because **ventricular fibrillation** can quickly cause death, it must be treated immediately by specially trained doctors and nurses with drugs and defibrillation.*

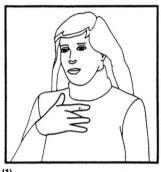

(1)

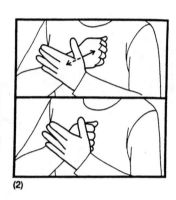

(2)

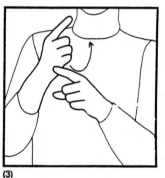

(3)

(1) Sign HEART — the middle finger of the right "eight" hand taps the chest a few times. (MM)
(2) The left "flat" hand faces in at chest level. The right "S" hand faces in behind the left hand. The right hand sharply hits the palm of the left hand a few times. (MM)
(3) Sign IRREGULAR — the left "one" hand faces right and the right "one" hand faces left on top of the left hand. Tap the hands together a few times, and at the same time, shake the head "no". (SM)

VERMIN

Small animals or insects like lice, fleas, bedbugs and mice which are hard to control and which may cause disease. Vermin may be parasites which live outside of a person on the surface of the body.

*When people are crowded together under unhealthy conditions such as emergencies or disasters, **vermin** should be controlled to prevent the spread of disease.*

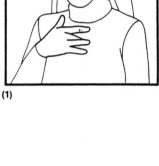

a.(1)

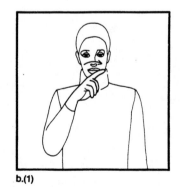

b.(1)

a. (1) Sign INSECT — the thumb of the right "three" hand touches the nose. Bend and straighten the fingers a few times. (MM)
b. (1) Sign RODENT — the right "R" hand faces left and brushes past the nose. (SM)

(Continued on next page)

VERMIN, *continued*

(2) Sign EASY — the fingers of the right "cupped" hand brush up the back of the fingers of the left "cupped" hand twice. (DM)
(3) Sign SPREAD — both "flat-O" hands face down at chest level. Move both hands out forward into "five" hands. (SM)
(4) Sign DISEASE — the middle finger of the right "eight" hand touches the forehead and the middle finger of the left "eight" hand touches the stomach. (SM)

* Sign INSECT or RODENT, whichever applies, then sign EASY, SPREAD, and DISEASE.

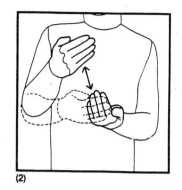
(2)

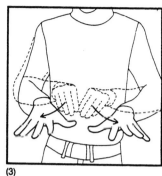
(3)

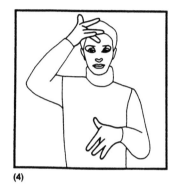
(4)

VERTEBRA

One of the 33 small bones that makes up the vertebral column or backbone. The vertebrae are separated into 5 groups: 7 cervical vertebrae, 12 thoracic vertebrae, 5 lumbar vertebrae, 5 sacral vertebrae and the coccyx, made up of 4 vertebrae. The five sacral vertebrae are joined together to form one bone called the sacrum and the four vertebrae in the coccyx are also joined together to form one bone. The vertebrae are separated from each other by an intervertebral disk. There is a hole in each vertebrae and when they are stacked on top of each other, they form a canal that the spinal cord runs through. *See Figure 26*

(1) Sign BACK — the right "flat" hand pats the back a few times. (MM)
(2) Fingerspell "B-O-N-E".
(3) The right "G" hand faces out at head level indicating one vertebra. (SM)

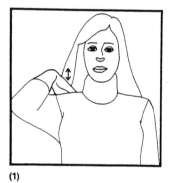
(1)

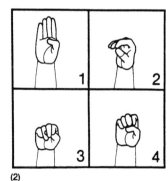
(2)

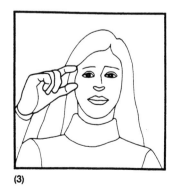
(3)

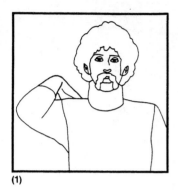
(1)

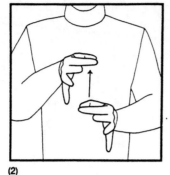
(2)

VERTEBRAL COLUMN

The series of bones which runs up and down a person's back; also called the spinal column, spine and backbone. The vertebral column is made up of 33 bones called vertebrae which are stacked one on top of the other. The vertebrae have a hole in them which makes a canal for the spinal cord to run through. The most important functions of the vertebral column are to support the head, neck, trunk and arms and to protect the spinal cord. *See Figure 26*

(1) Sign BACK — the right "flat" hand pats the back a few times. (MM)
(2) Both "F" hands face down at waist level. Move the right hand up to chest level as if imitating the shape of the backbone. (SM)

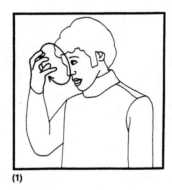
(1)

VERTIGO

A feeling of whirling around or of having things circle around a person; dizziness. Vertigo results when something irritates or upsets the parts of the ear or brain which help us keep our balance. Some causes of vertigo are disease of the inner ear, eye disease, brain disease, alcohol, some drugs, food poisoning, some infectious diseases or the start of an epileptic attack.

*Carsickness, airsickness and seasickness often have symptoms of **vertigo**, nausea and vomiting.*

(1) Sign DIZZY — the right "claw" hand faces in at the head and moves in counterclockwise circles a few times. (MM)

VESICLE

A small sac or bladder-like structure containing fluid; also a blister-like formation on the skin. Vesicles may vary in size and may be flat, round, clear or dark in appearance.

Vesicles may form in certain types of eczema or herpes, chickenpox, smallpox or scabies.

VESSEL

A tube, canal or duct in the body that carries a fluid.

The vessels that transport blood in the body are called arteries, veins and capillaries.

(1) Both "F" hands face out at chest level. Move both hands out slightly to the sides. (SM)
(2) Sign IN — the fingers of the right "flat-O" hand move into the left fist. (SM)
(3) Sign BODY — the fingers of both "flat" hands touch the chest, then the stomach. (SM)

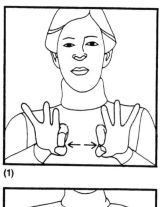

(1)

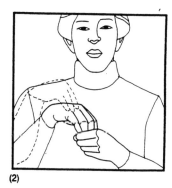

(2)

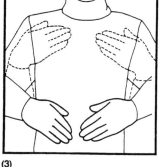

(3)

VESTIBULE

A small cavity, chamber or space at the beginning of a canal.

The vestibule of the ear is the middle part of the inner ear, behind the cochlea and in front of the semicircular canals.

VETERINARIAN

A doctor who specializes in the diseases of animals and their treatment. A veterinarian has gone to a special school for at least four years after finishing college.

Physicians and health officals often work closely with veterinarians to prevent the spread of diseases from animals to people.

a. (1) Sign ANIMAL — the fingertips of both "cupped" hands touch the chest. Keeping the hands in place, bend and straighten the fingers at the knuckles a few times. (MM)
(2) Sign DOCTOR — the right "M" hand taps the left inside wrist. (DM)
b. (1) Fingerspell "V-E-T."

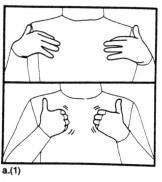

a.(1)

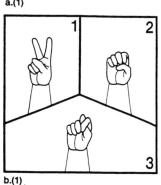

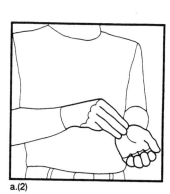

a.(2)

b.(1)

657

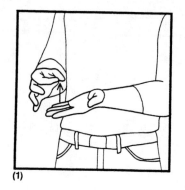
(1)

VIAL

A small glass or plastic bottle used to hold a medicine or chemical.

A vial usually has a tight-fitting lid and the material used to make the vial is usually dark to protect the medicine from sunlight which might damage or weaken it.

(1) The left "flat" hand faces up at chest level. The right "F" hand faces down and moves up from the left palm. (SM)

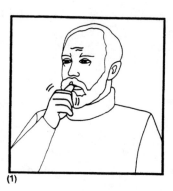
(1)

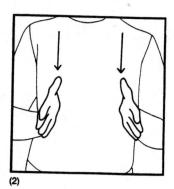
(2)

VICTIM

A person who suffers harm, injury or death from a certain condition.

During disasters, such as floods or fire, a person injured or killed is called a victim.

(1) Sign SUFFER — the thumb of the right "A" hand touches the chin. Pivot the hand slightly from side to side a few times. (MM)
* The facial expression should reflect pain or suffering.

(2) Sign PERSON — both "flat" hands face each other at chest level and move down to waist level. (SM)

VILLUS

A tiny hair-like structure that sticks out of membranes.

The chorionic villus help form the placenta.

VINCENT'S DISEASE

See TRENCH MOUTH

VIRULENT

Infectious; able to get into the body and cause a disease.

A vaccine is made by injecting a virus or bacteria that is changed, dead and not virulent into someone's body so antibodies can be made to protect against the virulent virus or bacteria.

(Continued on next page)

VIRULENT, *continued*

(1) Sign CAN — both "A" hands face out at chest level. Drop both hands down so that the palms face down. (SM)
(2) Sign CAUSE — both "S" hands face up at chest level. Drop both hands down to the left side, ending in "five" hands facing up. (SM)
(3) Sign INFECTION — the right "I" hand faces out at chest level and shakes slightly from side to side a few times. (MM)

* Mouth the word "infection" while signing.

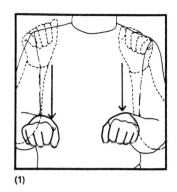
(1)

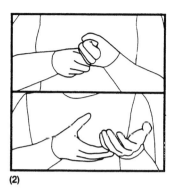
(2)

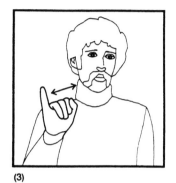
(3)

VIRUS

A very small structure which must get inside living cells to reproduce. Viruses are much smaller than bacteria, they are much simpler than bacteria, and some even infect bacteria. A virus is just a tiny pocket containing a chromosome and perhaps some enzymes. To reproduce, the virus needs the chemicals and other materials found in living cells. A virus will get into a cell and turn it into a virus factory, making the cell unable to do its normal job and even causing it to die. This is what makes a person sick when he has a disease caused by a virus. There are hundreds of different kinds of viruses causing diseases in bacteria, plants, animals and humans.

> *Some diseases of humans caused by a virus are the common cold, smallpox, chickenpox, measles, rabies, polio, mumps, cold sores, genital herpes and warts.*

(1) Fingerspell "V-I-R-U-S".

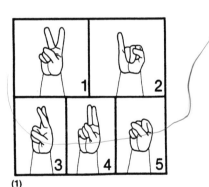
(1)

VISCERA

The organs found in the chest or abdomen, such as the stomach, intestines, spleen, liver, bladder, kidneys, lungs or heart.

> *A hernia is often caused by a part of the viscera pushing through a weakened muscle wall.*

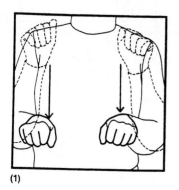
(1)

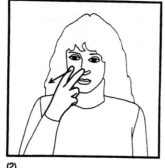
(2)

VISIBLE

Something which can be seen.

Visible signs of a disorder or disease may be a rash or boil on the skin.

(1) Sign CAN — both "A" hands face out at chest level. Drop both hands down so that the palms face down. (SM)
(2) Sign SEE — the right "V" hand faces in at eye level. Move the hand out forward slightly. (SM)

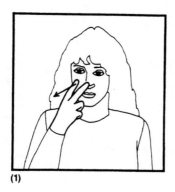
(1)

VISION

Sight, the sense which allows us to detect light and color.

The eyes are the organs of vision.

(1) Sign SEE — the right "V" hand faces in at eye level. Move the hand out forward slightly. (SM)

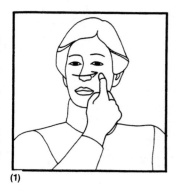
(1)

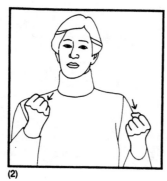
(2)

VISUAL ACUITY

A measure of how well a person sees. Visual acuity is measured with a Snellen chart and the results of the test are written as a fraction. Visual acuity of 20/20 (normal vision) means that a person can see at 20 feet what the normal person can see at 20 feet. 20/40 means that a person can see at 20 feet what a normal person could see at 40 feet.

A check of a person's visual acuity should be a part of every complete physical examination and every eye examination.

(1) Sign EYES — the index finger of the right "one" hand points to both eyes. (SM)
(2) Sign STRONG — both "S" hands face in at chest level and move out slightly. (SM)

VISUAL FIELD

The area in which objects can be seen when the eyes are focused.

The visual field may also be called the "field of vision."

(1) Sign EYES — the index finger of the right "one" hand points to both eyes. (SM)

(2) Sign SEE — both "V" hands face out at left chest level and move to the right. (SM)

(3) Both "flat" hands face each other at eye level and move out towards the sides. (SM)

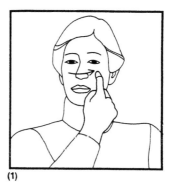
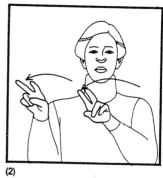

(1)

(2)

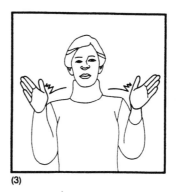

(3)

VITAL SIGNS

The respiration, heartbeat, and temperature of a person.

Hospitals have special devices which constantly check the vital signs of a very sick person and sound an alarm if there is an emergency with the person.

(1) Sign CHECK — the index finger of the right "one" hand makes a check movement in the palm of the left "flat" hand. (SM)

(2) Sign HEART — the middle finger of the right "eight" hand taps the chest a few times. (MM)

(3) Sign PULSE — the fingertips of the right "cupped" hand touch the left inside wrist as if feeling for a pulse. (SM)

(4) Sign TEMPERATURE — the index finger of the right "one" hand touches the mouth. Move the hand to the right, then shake it slightly as if shaking down a thermometer. (SM)

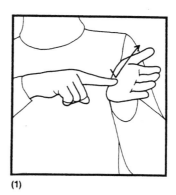
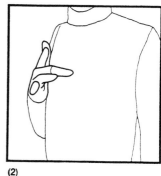

(1)

(2)

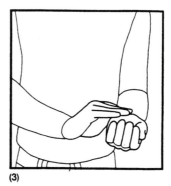
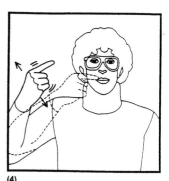

(3)

(4)

661

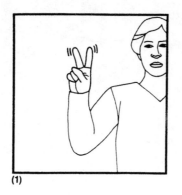
(1)

VITAMIN

Organic substances found in natural foods which the body needs for normal growth, health and life. Most vitamins are not made by the human body, so they must be gotten from other animals or plants. They work in very small amounts and each has an activity that it allows to happen normally or helps to direct.

Some vitamins, like the B vitamins and vitamin C, can be dissolved in water and these vitamins will be lost from the body more quickly than vitamins A, D, E and K, which can dissolve in fats and will stay in the body longer.

(1) The right "V" hand faces out at chest level and shakes slightly from side to side a few times. (MM)

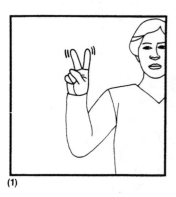
(1)
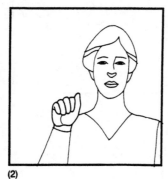
(2)

VITAMIN A

A vitamin found in fish, livers, some yellow and dark green vegetables, and dairy products. Vitamin A is important in helping the rods in the retina of the eye work properly so we can see in the dark. Vitamin A also helps keep the skin in good health.

(1) Sign VITAMIN — the right "V" hand faces out at chest level and shakes slightly from side to side a few times. (MM)
(2) Sign "A" — the right "A" hand faces out at chest level. (SM)

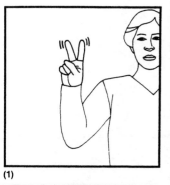
(1)
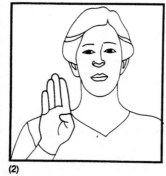
(2)

VITAMIN B COMPLEX

Several different B vitamins; thiamine (B1), riboflavin (B2), niacin, biotin, pyridoxine (B6), inositol, para-aminobenzoic acid (PABA), cyanocobalamine (B12) and folic acid. Because of their chemical make-up, B vitamins are easily lost from the body and if a person has less than needed of one, he is more likely to have less of another.

(1) Sign VITAMIN — the right "V" hand faces out at chest level and shakes slightly from side to side a few times. (MM)
(2) Sign "B" — the right "B" hand faces out at chest level. (SM)
(3) Sign DIFFERENT — both "one" hands point up and face out at chest level with the index fingers crossing. Move both hands to the sides. (SM)
(4) Sign COMBINE — both "claw" hands face each other at chest level. The right hand moves in counterclockwise circles a few times. (MM)

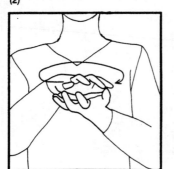

(3)
(4)

VITAMIN B1

A vitamin found in grains, Brewer's yeast, nuts, wheat germ, most vegetables and some meats (pork, liver, heart and kidneys); also called thiamine. Vitamin B1 is needed for normal use of carbohydrates and proper working of the nervous, circulatory and digestive systems.

(1) Sign VITAMIN — the right "V" hand faces out at chest level and shakes slightly from side to side a few times. (MM)
(2) Sign "B-1" — the right "B" hand faces out at chest level and moves slightly to the side to a "one" hand. (SM)

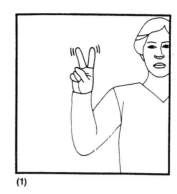
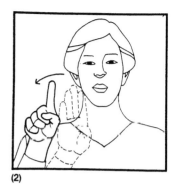

(1)   (2)

VITAMIN B2

A vitamin found in milk, liver, yeast, green leafy vegetables and eggs; also called riboflavin. It is important in normal growth and cell metabolism.

(1) Sign VITAMIN — the right "V" hand faces out at chest level and shakes slightly from side to side a few times. (MM)
(2) Sign "B-2" — the right "B" hand faces out at chest level and moves slightly to the side to a "two" hand. (SM)

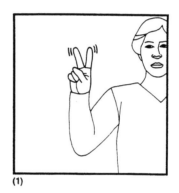
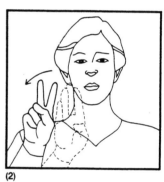

(1)   (2)

VITAMIN B6

A vitamin found in meats, grains, wheat germ and blackstrap molasses; also called pyridoxine. It is important in using certain kinds of fats and some amino acids.

(1) Sign VITAMIN — the right "V" hand faces out at chest level and shakes slightly from side to side a few times. (MM)
(2) Sign "B-6" — the right "B" hand faces out at chest level and moves slightly to the side to a "six" hand. (SM)

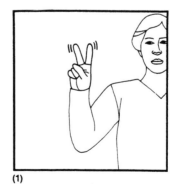
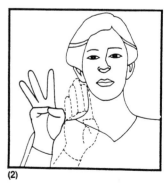

(1)   (2)

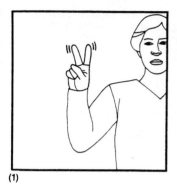
(1)

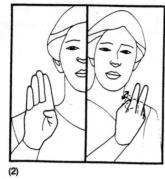
(2)

VITAMIN B12

A vitamin found in liver, kidney and dairy products: also called cyanocobalamine. It is also made by bacteria living in our intestines. Vitamin B12 is needed for making red blood cells.

(1) Sign VITAMIN — the right "V" hand faces out at chest level and shakes slightly from side to side a few times. (MM)
(2) Sign "B-12" — the right "B" hand faces out at chest level. Turn the hand around to a "V" hand facing in and bend and straighten the index and middle fingers. (SM)

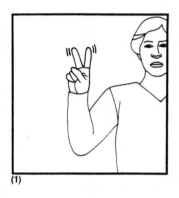
(1)

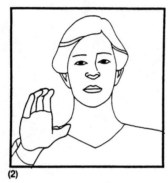
(2)

VITAMIN C

A vitamin found mostly in fresh fruits and vegetables; also called ascorbic acid. It helps form the substances holding cells together, in healing wounds and fractures and prevents scurvy. Vitamin C also helps in absorbing iron.

(1) Sign VITAMIN — the right "V" hand faces out at chest level and shakes slightly from side to side a few times. (MM)
(2) Sign "C" — the right "C" hand faces out at chest level. (SM)

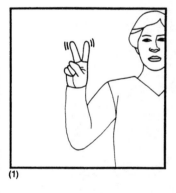
(1)

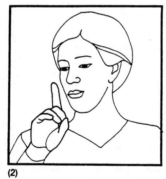
(2)

VITAMIN D

A vitamin found in butter, egg yolks, liver, fish and oysters. It is also formed in the skin by sunlight. Vitamin D helps absorb calcium into the body to be used in bones and teeth.

(1) Sign VITAMIN — the right "V" hand faces out at chest level and shakes slightly from side to side a few times. (MM)
(2) Sign "D" — the right "D" hand faces out at chest level. (SM)

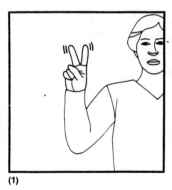
(1)

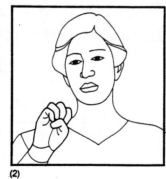
(2)

VITAMIN E

A vitamin found in rice, wheat germ oil and green leafy vegetables.

(1) Sign VITAMIN — the right "V" hand faces out at chest level and shakes slightly from side to side a few times. (MM)
(2) Sign "E" — the right "E" hand faces out at chest level. (SM)

664

VITAMIN K

A vitamin found in fats, oats, wheat, rye and alfalfa. Vitamin K is needed to help blood clot.

(1) Sign VITAMIN — the right "V" hand faces out at chest level and shakes slightly from side to side a few times. (MM)
(2) Sign "K" — the right "K" hand faces out at chest level. (SM)

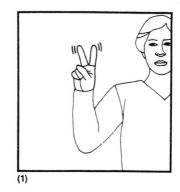
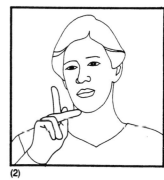

(1)   (2)

VITREOUS BODY

The clear, jelly-like material that fills the eyeball. *See Figure 22*

VOCAL CORDS

Bands of elastic tissue stretched across the opening of the trachea in the throat. Sounds are made by the vocal cords' vibrating back and forth as air moves past them out of the trachea. Words are not actually formed in the throat but the sounds produced there are shaped into speech by the mouth, tongue, teeth and lips. *See Figure 10*

(1) The right "V" hand faces in at the throat and makes a small circular movement. (SM)
(2) The right "G" hand faces in and moves up and down the throat a few times. (MM)

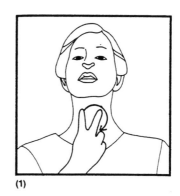
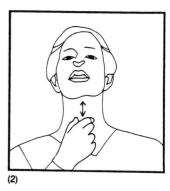

(1)   (2)

VOLATILE

Able to evaporate quickly or change quickly from a liquid to a gas. Examples of volatile substances are ether, gasoline and alcohols.

> *Many volatile liquids are also flammable or explosive so no matches should be lit around them and no sparks should be produced.*

(1) The left "C" hand faces right at chest level. The right "claw" hand faces down on top of the left fist. Move the right hand up and out as if imitating taking the lid off of a jar. (SM)
(2) The middle finger of the right "eight" hand is inside the left "C" hand. Move the right hand up to a "S" hand. At the same time, the mouth should indicate sucking in. (SM)

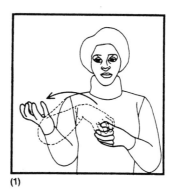
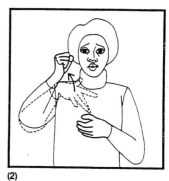

(1)   (2)

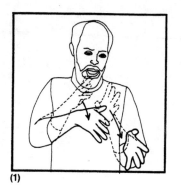
(1)

VOMIT

Materials or food which are in the stomach passing back up through the esophagus and mouth; often called "throwing up." Vomiting is a reflex action that is controlled by the brain. Many things may cause a person to vomit such as some poisons, early pregnancy, brain tumors or infections, motion sickness, ulcers, blocking of the intestines, worms in the intestines or an infection of the intestines such as the flu.

A person who is going to have an operation is not allowed to eat before surgery because the anesthetics used to make a person unconscious may also make him vomit.

(1) Both "five" hands face each other at the mouth. Drop both hands down forward. (SM)

VULNERABLE

Easily injured or wounded; not protected from danger.

People who are not immunized against certain diseases are more vulnerable to illnesses.

a. (1) Sign EASY — the fingers of the right "cupped" hand brush up the back of the fingers of the left "cupped" hand twice. (DM)
(2) The thumbs of both "five" hands touch the chest, the hands face each other. Close both hands to "eight" hands. (SM)

b. (1) Sign TENDENCY — the middle fingers of both "eight" hands touch the chest. Move both hands out forward. (SM)
(2) Sign EASY — the fingers of the right "cupped" hand brush up the back of the fingers of the left "cupped" hand twice. (DM)
(3) Sign HURT — both "one" hands point to each other at chest level and twist in opposite directions a few times. (MM)

* The facial expression should reflect pain.

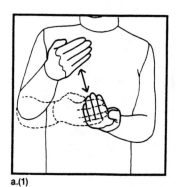
a.(1)

a.(2)

b.(1)

b.(2)

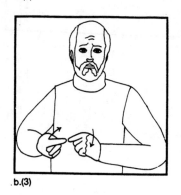
. b.(3)

VULVA

The female genitals; the structures around the opening of the vagina. The vulva includes the clitoris, the opening of the vagina, the perineum and the lips around the clitoris, urethra opening and vagina opening. *See Figure 12*

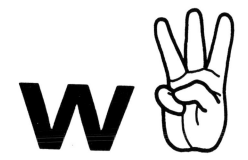

WAKEFUL

Not able to sleep.

Most teas, soft drinks, coffee and hot chocolate contain caffeine, so drinking them before bed will make the person feel wakeful instead of sleepy.

(1) Sign AWAKE — both "C" hands face out at the sides of the face. Open the eyes wide. (SM)

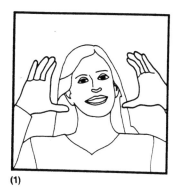

(1)

WALKER

A device used to help a person walk. It is a stable platform made of light metal tubing which will stand alone. A person can hold onto it for support while taking a step and then it can be moved forward and another step taken.

People who are unsteady on their feet, such as older people or people who have had leg injuries, may be able to move about more safely by using a walker.

a. (1) Sign METAL — the index finger of the right "X" hand brushes down the chin a few times. (MM)

(2) Both "F" hands face down at waist level. Move both hands to the sides, then down slightly. (SM)

b. (1) Sign METAL — the index finger of the right "X" hand brushes down the chin a few times. (MM)

(2) Both "F" hands face down at chest level, the right hand under the left. Move the right hand down slightly to a "claw" hand facing down. (SM)

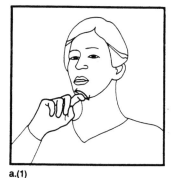

a.(1)

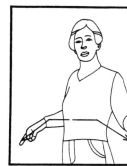

a.(2)

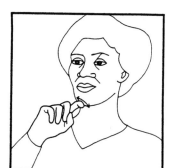

b.(1)

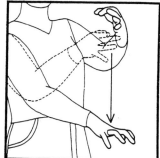

b.(2)

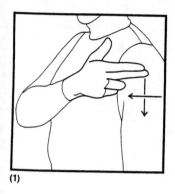

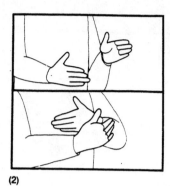

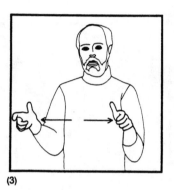

WARD

A large room or area in a hospital where several patients stay and are treated.

The word ward is usually used with another word to tell what kind of patient stays there, such as post-operative ward, maternity ward, or isolation ward.

(1) Sign HOSPITAL — the fingers of the right "H" hand make a cross on the left upper arm. (SM)
(2) Sign ROOM — both "flat" hands face each other at chest level. Turn both hands to the center so that both hands face in, the right hand in front of the left. (SM)
(3) Sign LARGE — both "modified-L" hands face each other at chest level and move out to the sides. (SM)

WARFARIN

A drug which prevents blood from clotting, used to treat blood clots which have formed in the blood vessels and may plug veins or arteries. Poisoning or an overdose of warfarin occurs after taking it in smaller amounts. Symptoms are nosebleeds, bleeding gums, paleness, blood in the urine or feces and bleeding under the skin, especially around the knees and buttocks. Warfarin, like any other poison, should be handled carefully and kept away from children.

Rat or mouse poisons often contain warfarin to cause the animal to bleed to death.

WART

A bump on the skin caused by a virus (verruca) infecting cells in the skin. The virus gets into the cells and causes them to divide more rapidly than normal, producing a raised area of skin. Because warts are caused by a virus, they can be spread from person to person or from one part of the body to another. Different kinds of warts appear on different parts of the body, such as plantar warts, which usually occur on the soles of the feet, and venereal warts which occur on the genitals.

(Continued on next page)

*A **wart** should not be picked at or irritated but can be removed by freezing with very cold substances, such as liquid nitrogen, or by putting chemicals on it which will dissolve it.*

(1) The left "S" hand faces down at chest level. The index finger of the right "one" hand makes a small bump on top of the left hand and at the same time, the cheeks should puff out. (SM)

(2) The fingertips of the right "claw" hand touch the cheek. Open the hand slightly and at the same time, the cheeks should puff out. (SM)

* This could be signed at the area of the wart.

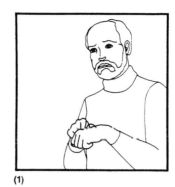
(1)

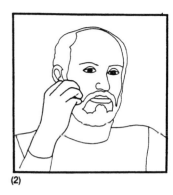
(2)

WASTE

Materials or products which are useless or present in too large amounts.

*Some of the **wastes** made by the body are urine, carbon dioxide, water and feces or undigested food.*

a. (1) Sign URINATE — the right "P" hand faces out and moves from the nose forward. (SM)

b. (1) Sign DEFECATE — the left "A" hand faces right at chest level. The thumb of the right "A" hand is inside the left fist. Drop the right hand down. (SM)

* These are just examples, the specific should be fingerspelled or signed if known.

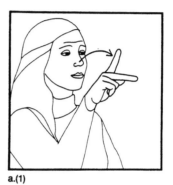
a.(1)

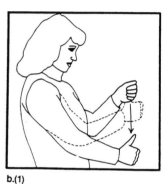
b.(1)

WASTING ALONE

Shrinking in size or lessening in strength; also called wasting away.

*There are many causes of **wasting alone** such as paralysis, not getting enough food, food not being digested or absorbed correctly, hormone problems, cancer and being sick for a long time.*

(1) Sign DECLINE — the right "flat" hand faces in and moves down the left arm, touching it several times. (MM)

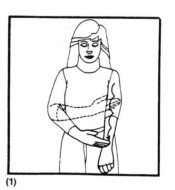
(1)

WATER

A clear fluid which cannot be tasted or smelled. Water is made up of a combination of hydrogen and oxygen. Water makes up 75% of the body and is necessary for life. It is important because all chemical reactions that go on in and around cells in the body happen in water. Water is used to dissolve and transport materials in the body and it helps control body temperature by evaporation.

(Continued on next page)

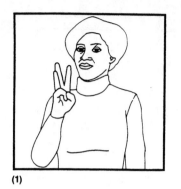
(1)

WATER, *continued*

All body fluids and secretions, such as blood, lymph, saliva, sweat, gastric juices and urine, are made up mostly of water.

(1) The index finger of the right "W" hand taps the mouth a few times. (MM)

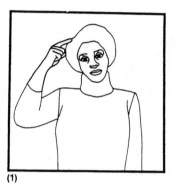
(1)

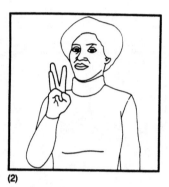
(2)

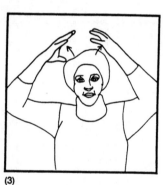
(3)

WATER ON THE BRAIN

A disease where there is an increase of cerebrospinal fluid in the ventricles of the brain; also called hydrocephalus or hydrencephalus. It can be caused by infection, brain injury or tumors, or abnormal development.

In older people water on the brain may cause headaches, vomiting, problems with the optic nerve and mental disorders.

(1) The index finger of the right "one" hand touches the head.
(2) Sign WATER — the index finger of the right "W" hand taps the mouth a few times. (MM)
(3) Both "claw" hands face in at the head and move up slightly as if imitating the head swelling. (SM)

WATERS

See AMNIONIC FLUID

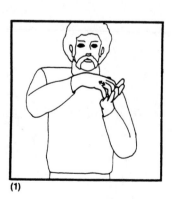
(1)

WEAK

Not having much strength or activity.

An injury or disease will usually make a person weak because the body's energy is being used to fight the infection or repair damage which has been done.

(1) The fingertips of the right "claw" hand touch the left "flat" palm. Keeping the right hand in place, bend and straighten the fingers at the knuckles a few times. (MM)

WEIGHT

A measure of how heavy something is.

*By keeping his **weight** in a normal range, a person will be healthier and less likely to have high blood pressure, heart disease, joint problems, diabetes or gallbladder problems.*

(1) The fingers of the right "H" hand pivot slightly on the fingers of the left "H" hand. (MM)

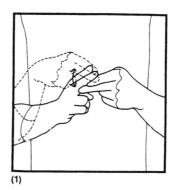

(1)

WEIGHT GAIN

See GAIN WEIGHT

WEIGHT LOSS

See LOSE WEIGHT

WELL

Healthy.

*If a person is **well** he is in good condition.*

(1) Sign HEALTHY — the fingers of both "claw" hands touch the chest. Move both hands up to "S" hands. (SM)

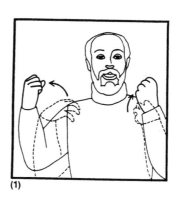

(1)

WEN

A bump on the skin caused by the plugging of a skin gland and the material made by glands building up; a kind of cyst.

*A **wen**, which usually forms slowly on the head, face or back, should be removed by a doctor to keep it from coming back.*

(1) The left "S" hand faces down at chest level. The index finger of the right "one" hand makes a small bump on the top of the left hand. At the same time, the cheeks should puff out. (SM)

(2) The fingertips of the right "claw" hand touch the head. Move the hand up slightly, and at the same time, the cheeks should puff out. (SM)

* *This could be signed at the area of the wen.*

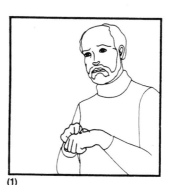

(1)

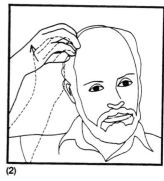

(2)

WET DREAM

See NOCTURNAL EMISSION

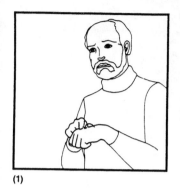

(1)

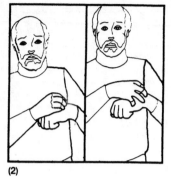

(2)

WHEAL

A general term for a raised area of skin which may be a round bump or a long ridge. A wheal is usually white with a red area around it.

An insect bite or sting often leaves a wheal caused by an allergic reaction to the things the insect injected under the skin.

(1) The left "S" hand faces down at chest level. The index finger of the right "one" hand makes a small bump on the back of the left hand. At the same time, the cheeks should puff out. (SM)

* This could be signed at the area of the wheal.

(2) The fingertips of the right "claw" hand touch the back of the left hand. Move the right hand up slightly as if imitating swelling. (SM)

* This could be signed at the area of the wheal.

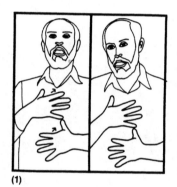

(1)

WHEEZE

A whistling sound made by someone who is having difficulty breathing.

A wheeze is caused by narrowing of the airways because of a tumor, something being inhaled, asthma, or inflammation caused by an infection.

(1) Sign BREATHE — both "five" hands touch the chest. Move both hands up slightly. (SM)

* The facial expression should reflect wheezing.

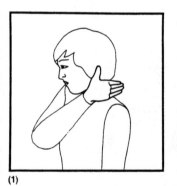

(1)

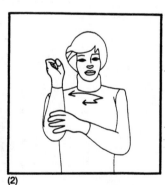

(2)

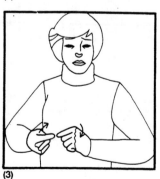

(3)

WHIPLASH INJURY

A general name for an injury to the vertebrae in the neck and the ligaments and muscles around them caused by a quick forward and backward movement of the head. Symptoms of whiplash are pain and swelling in the neck area and being unable to move the head easily.

A common cause of whiplash injury is being in a car which is hit from behind by another car.

(1) The fingers of the right "flat" hand rub the back of the neck. (SM)

(2) The right "S" hand faces left, the arm is bent. The left hand grabs the right arm. The right hand moves in a whipping movement from the left to the right. (SM)

(3) Sign HURT — both "one" hands point to each other at chest level and twist in opposite directions a few times. (MM)

* The facial expression should reflect pain.

674

WHIPWORM

Small, white, whip-shaped worms which live in the end of the small intestine. Whipworms burrow into the lining of the intestine and suck blood out, causing irritation and bleeding. Symptoms of whipworm infection are anemia, loss of appetite, vomiting, diarrhea, nervousness and perhaps an infection of the intestines. People usually get whipworms in areas with poor sanitation, by drinking water with the worm in it or by accidently eating dirt with the worm in it.

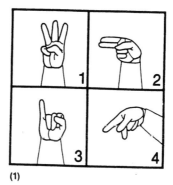
(1)

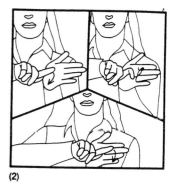
(2)

A whipworm infection can be treated with drugs by mouth and also by medicated enemas.

(1) Fingerspell "W-H-I-P".
(2) Sign WORM — the left "flat" hand faces right at chest level. The right "one" hand points out on the left palm. While moving the right hand out along the left palm, bend and straighten the index finger a few times. (MM)

WHITE BLOOD CELLS

A kind of cell found in the blood and also in the tissues; also called leukocytes. These cells, not actually white but colorless, are very different from the red blood cells. There are a lot fewer white blood cells than red blood cells and the number of them in the body can change quickly. White blood cells are able to change their shape and move through small spaces. This is how they get out of the blood stream into the tissues. There are five different kinds of white blood cells and the most important job they have is fighting infections. Some white blood cells go to injured or infected areas of the body and swallow up bacteria, damaged or dead cells and other materials. Some make antibodies and others help stop blood from clotting.

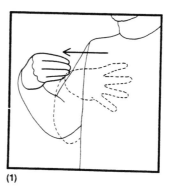
(1)

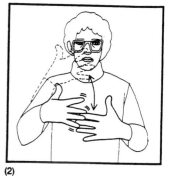
(2)

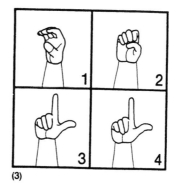
(3)

In some infections, many white blood cells will collect in an area to fight an infection and when a lot of them are killed and not carried away, they form pus.

(1) Sign WHITE — the fingertips of the right "five" hand touch the chest. Move the hand out slightly into a "flat-O" hand. (SM)
(2) Sign BLOOD — the left "five" hand is at chest level with the palm toward the body. The palm of the right "five" hand is toward the body with the middle fingertips touching the mouth. Move the right hand down the back of the left hand. Wiggle the fingers of the right hand as it moves. (MM)

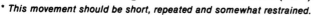
* This movement should be short, repeated and somewhat restrained.

(3) Fingerspell "C-E-L-L".

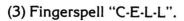

675

WHOOPING COUGH

A contagious disease caused by a bacteria (Hemophilus pertussis) which attacks the lining of the respiratory tract; also called pertussis. The disease starts out with cold-like symptoms, with a fever, sneezing, runny nose and cough. Later, the cough becomes severe; the person coughs hard several times and then inhales loudly, causing the "whoop" the disease gets its name from. This cough tires the person out very quickly and it often makes him turn blue from lack of oxygen. After coughing, the person often vomits. It often takes several months to recover from whooping cough.

*Antibiotics can be given to help fight off a **whooping cough** infection but every baby should be vaccinated against it in the first year of life, along with tetanus and diphtheria vaccinations.*

WINDCHILL FACTOR

The amount of cooling of the skin or the loss of heat from the skin caused by wind blowing over it. The amount of heat lost depends on the speed of the wind. For example, if the wind is blowing at 20 miles per hour and the temperature is 0°F, the effect on the skin would be the same as in still air at 46°F. Or, if the temperature is 20°F and the wind is blowing at 10 miles per hour, the effect on the skin would be the same as −46°F in still air.

*Besides checking the temperature, a person should also remember the **windchill factor** when dressing to go out of doors or else hypothermia or frostbite could occur.*

WINDPIPE

See TRACHEA

WISDOM TOOTH

The last tooth, which may or may not appear behind the two molars in each jaw. The four wisdom teeth usually come in between 17 and 25 years of age. Because the wisdom teeth are so far back in the mouth and hard to clean and because they often crowd the other teeth out of position, they are usually removed. *See Figure 24*

WITHDRAWAL

Pulling back or away from something. In medicine, it is usually used for no longer giving a person a drug or medicine they have become addicted to. The symptoms of withdrawal depend on the type of drug used but they usually include nervousness, loss of appetite, vomiting, diarrhea, shaking, being unable to sleep, and extreme weakness.

Many people who go through withdrawal from a drug are kept in a hospital or special treatment center so they can get all the help they need to lessen the symptoms and make themselves more comfortable.

WOMB

See UTERUS

WORM

In medicine, usually a kind of small, legless parasite that is harmful and lives in a person or other animal's body.

Depending on the kind of worm, the damage to the person may include eating the tissues, poisoning the person with wastes, and taking in nutrients before the person can absorb them.

(1) The left "flat" hand faces right at chest level. The right "one" hand points out on the left palm. While moving the right hand out along the left palm, bend and straighten the index finger a few times. (MM)

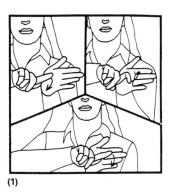

(1)

WORSE

A bad change in a condition; the opposite of better.

Most diseases will become worse if not treated.

(1) Both "K" hands cross at the wrists at waist level. While tapping the hands together in circular movements, move both hands up to chest level. (MM)

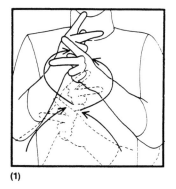

(1)

WOUND

An injury or damage to a part of the body, either on the inside or outside.

If a wound is deep or bad enough, the person should be given a tetanus shot.

(Continued on next page)

677

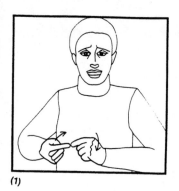
(1)

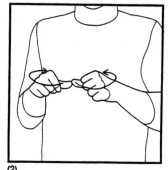
(2)

WOUND, *continued*

(1) Sign HURT — both "one" hands point to each other at chest level and twist in opposite directions a few times. (MM)
* The facial expression should reflect pain.

(2) Sign AREA — the thumbs of both "A" hands touch at chest level. Move both hands out forward and around back to the starting position. (SM)

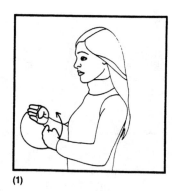
(1)

WRAP

To fold or cover something for protection.
> A person should be careful not to **wrap** a wound too tightly so as not to cut off circulation or nerve function.

(1) Sign BANDAGE — the left "B" hand faces in at chest level. The right "B" hand moves out and around the left hand as if imitating wrapping something. (SM)
* This could be signed where something is being wrapped.

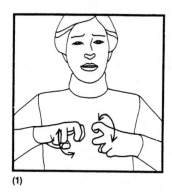
(1)

WRENCH

In medicine, a sudden, painful twisting of a part of the body.
> The ankle or wrist are joints that are often **wrenched**.

(1) The right "bent-V" hand faces out and the left "bent-V" hand faces in, both at chest level. Twist both hands slightly. (SM)
* This could be signed at the area of the body that is wrenched.

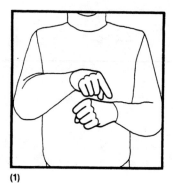
(1)

WRIST

The joint or area between the hand and lower arm. *See Figure 1*

(1) The index finger of the right "one" hand points to the left wrist. (SM)

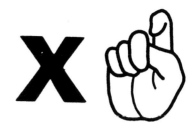
X

X CHROMOSOME

One of two sex chromosomes (X and Y) in the fetus.

The X chromosome determines that the fetus will have female characteristics.

X RAY

A strong, wave-like kind of energy made up of small particles which can pass through solid things. These particles can also cause changes on photographic film. Because of this, these rays can be passed through the body and used to take pictures of (internal) organs and other structures to diagnose a disease or disorder. X rays are a kind of controlled radiation.

Whenever X rays are used to take a picture, the ovaries or testicles should be covered with a lead shield to protect the ova and sperm from damage.

(1) Fingerspell "X-R-A-Y".

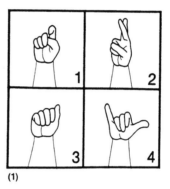

(1)

X-RAY

The photograph or picture made by X rays.

A person should not have any unnecessary X-rays taken because they can damage the body and a person should keep an accurate record of any X-rays he had taken.

(1) Fingerspell "X-R-A-Y".
(2) Sign PICTURE — the right "C" hand faces out at the head. Move the right hand down to the left "flat" hand. (SM)

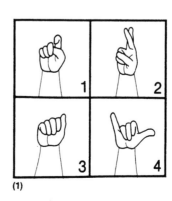

(1)

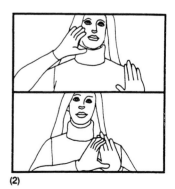

(2)

679

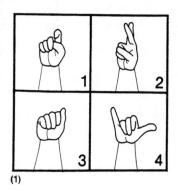
(1)

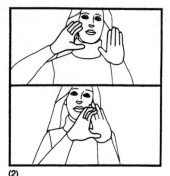
(2)

X-RAY (Dental)

A photograph taken of the head, jaws or teeth using X-rays that will help a dentist treat a problem with the teeth. Dental X-rays are usually taken with a special machine that can be moved around a person easily. A common kind of X-ray is the **Bitewing X-ray** which is a X-ray taken in a way that will show several upper and lower teeth all at once. A piece of cardboard in the shape of a "T" is placed between the teeth and bitten down on, leaving the crossbar of the "T" with the film in it on the inside of the teeth. The X-ray machine is placed against the cheek and the picture is taken from the outside in. Another common kind of X-ray is the **full mouth X-ray,** in which many pictures, usually more than 16, are taken of the teeth to get a complete set of all the teeth and their roots. Full mouth X-rays are usually taken before any major treatment is done on the mouth or teeth, such as orthodontic work. A **Panoramix X-ray** is a X-ray taken in a way that shows a large area of the mouth all at once. To take a Panoramix X-ray, the film is placed outside the mouth and the source of the X-rays is placed inside the mouth so the picture is taken from the inside of the mouth outwards.

(1) Fingerspell "X-R-A-Y".
(2) Sign PICTURE — the right "C" hand faces out at the mouth. Move the right hand down to the left "flat" hand. (SM)

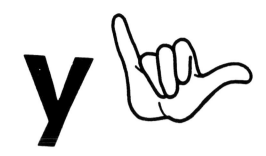

YAWN

To open the mouth wide with a deep inhalation.

When a person is tired or drowsy, he will usually yawn.
(1) The left "bent-V" hand faces up at chest level. The right "bent-V" hand faces out on the left palm. Move the right hand down to the left as if imitating the mouth yawning and, at the same time, the mouth should imitate yawning. (SM)

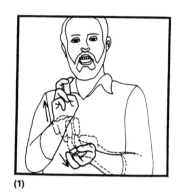

(1)

Y CHROMOSOME

One of two sex chromosomes (X and Y) in the fetus.

The Y chromosome determines that the fetus will have male sexual characteristics.

YEAST

A kind of one-celled fungus(saccharomyces). Yeasts are used to make alcohol, to make bread rise, and some kinds can cause diseases in people.

A common disease caused by yeast is "candidiasis."

YEAST INFECTION

See CANDIDIASIS

YELLOW FEVER

An acute infectious disease caused by a virus and spread by the bite of a mosquito. Symptoms of yellow fever include fever, jaundice (skin becomes yellow) and vomiting, containing dark blood.

There are preventive vaccines available for a person traveling or living in an area where yellow fever is common.

681

YELLOW JACKET
See PENTOBARBITAL

YOLK
The inside of the ovum and sometimes the part containing nutrients, especially proteins and fats.
The yolk sac surrounds the embryo, giving it necessary nutrients and also acting as the circulatory system.

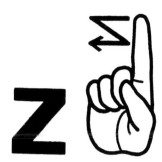

ZOONOSIS

A disease or parasite which is spread from animals to people. Examples of zoonosis are trichinosis, anthrax, tuberculosis, ringworm, fleas, mange and rabies.

People who live closely with animals, work with animals, or who live in unclean conditions are more likely to get a zoonosis.

ZOSTER

See HERPES-ZOSTER or SHINGLES

FIGURE 1 — Anterior (front) View of the Body

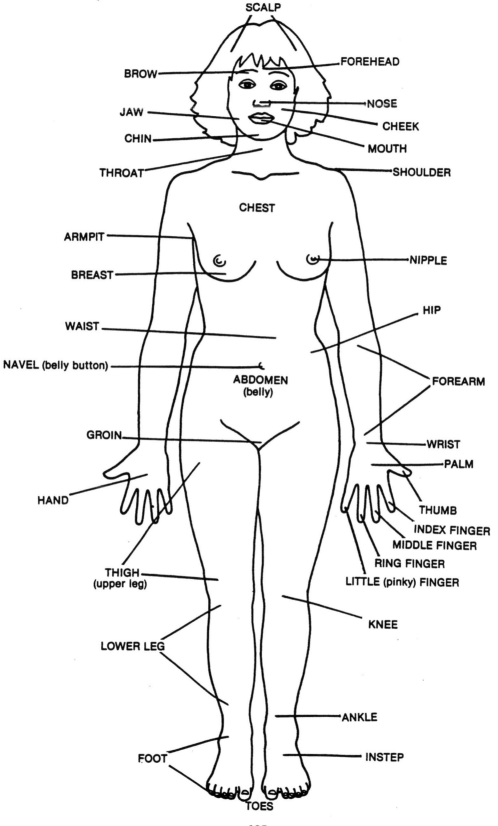

SCALP

BROW

FOREHEAD

JAW

NOSE

CHIN

CHEEK

THROAT

MOUTH

SHOULDER

CHEST

ARMPIT

NIPPLE

BREAST

WAIST

HIP

NAVEL (belly button)

ABDOMEN
(belly)

FOREARM

GROIN

WRIST

PALM

HAND

THUMB

INDEX FINGER

MIDDLE FINGER

THIGH
(upper leg)

RING FINGER

LITTLE (pinky) FINGER

KNEE

LOWER LEG

ANKLE

FOOT

INSTEP

TOES

FIGURE 2 — Lateral (side) View of the Body

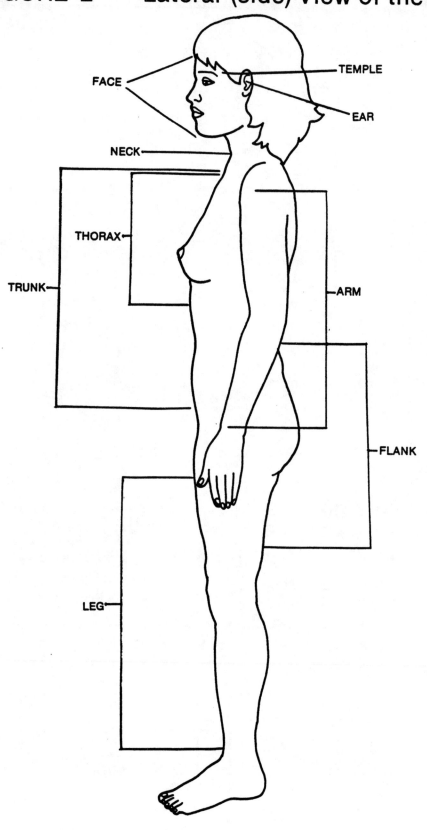

FACE

TEMPLE

EAR

NECK

THORAX

TRUNK

ARM

FLANK

LEG

FIGURE 3 — Posterior (back) View of the Body

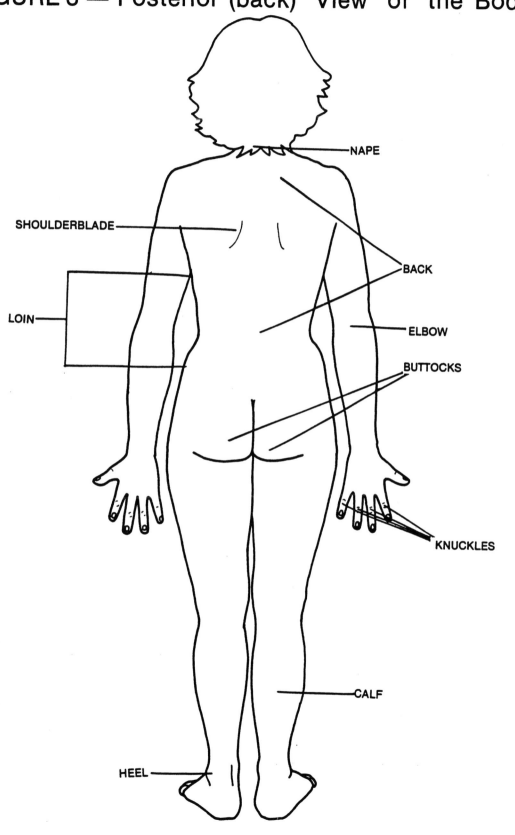

NAPE

SHOULDERBLADE

BACK

LOIN

ELBOW

BUTTOCKS

KNUCKLES

CALF

HEEL

FIGURE 4 — Anterior (front) View of Muscular System

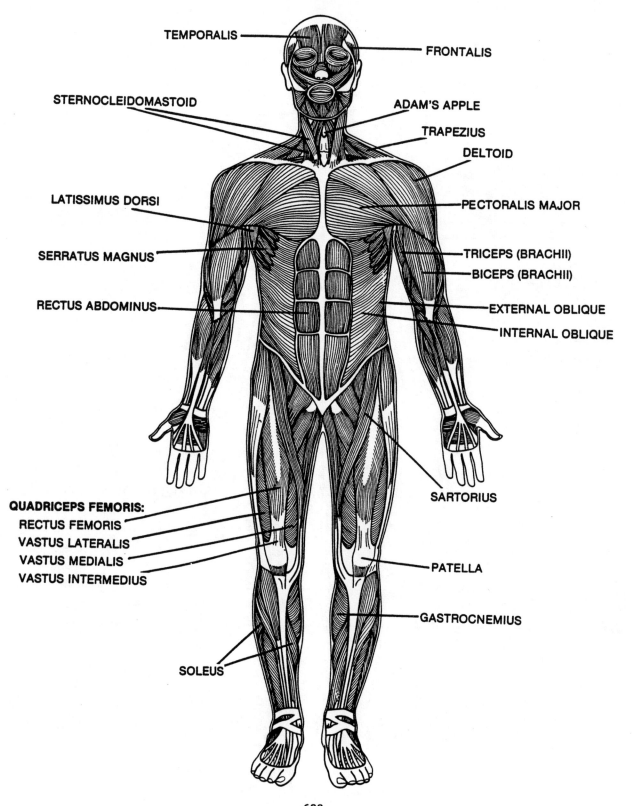

TEMPORALIS

FRONTALIS

STERNOCLEIDOMASTOID

ADAM'S APPLE

TRAPEZIUS

DELTOID

LATISSIMUS DORSI

PECTORALIS MAJOR

SERRATUS MAGNUS

TRICEPS (BRACHII)

BICEPS (BRACHII)

RECTUS ABDOMINUS

EXTERNAL OBLIQUE

INTERNAL OBLIQUE

SARTORIUS

QUADRICEPS FEMORIS:
RECTUS FEMORIS
VASTUS LATERALIS
VASTUS MEDIALIS
VASTUS INTERMEDIUS

PATELLA

GASTROCNEMIUS

SOLEUS

FIGURE 5 — Posterior (back) View of Muscular System

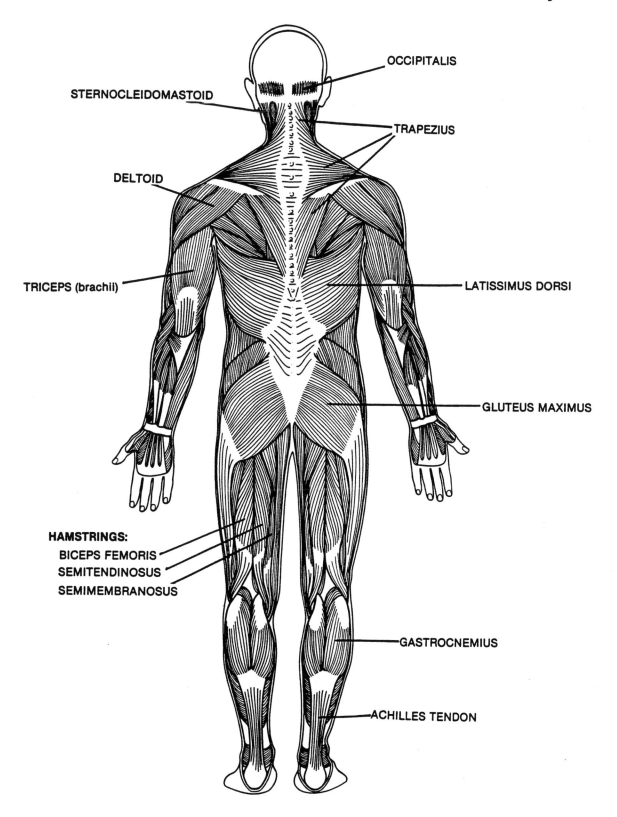

OCCIPITALIS

STERNOCLEIDOMASTOID

TRAPEZIUS

DELTOID

TRICEPS (brachii)

LATISSIMUS DORSI

GLUTEUS MAXIMUS

HAMSTRINGS:
  BICEPS FEMORIS
  SEMITENDINOSUS
  SEMIMEMBRANOSUS

GASTROCNEMIUS

ACHILLES TENDON

FIGURE 6 — Arteries (Circulatory System)

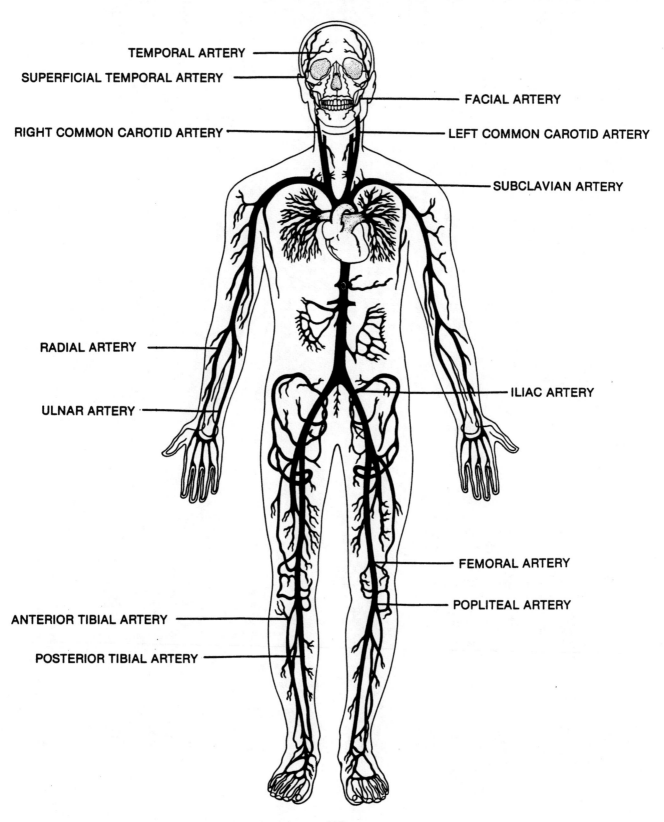

TEMPORAL ARTERY

SUPERFICIAL TEMPORAL ARTERY

FACIAL ARTERY

RIGHT COMMON CAROTID ARTERY

LEFT COMMON CAROTID ARTERY

SUBCLAVIAN ARTERY

RADIAL ARTERY

ULNAR ARTERY

ILIAC ARTERY

FEMORAL ARTERY

POPLITEAL ARTERY

ANTERIOR TIBIAL ARTERY

POSTERIOR TIBIAL ARTERY

FIGURE 7 — Veins (Circulatory System)

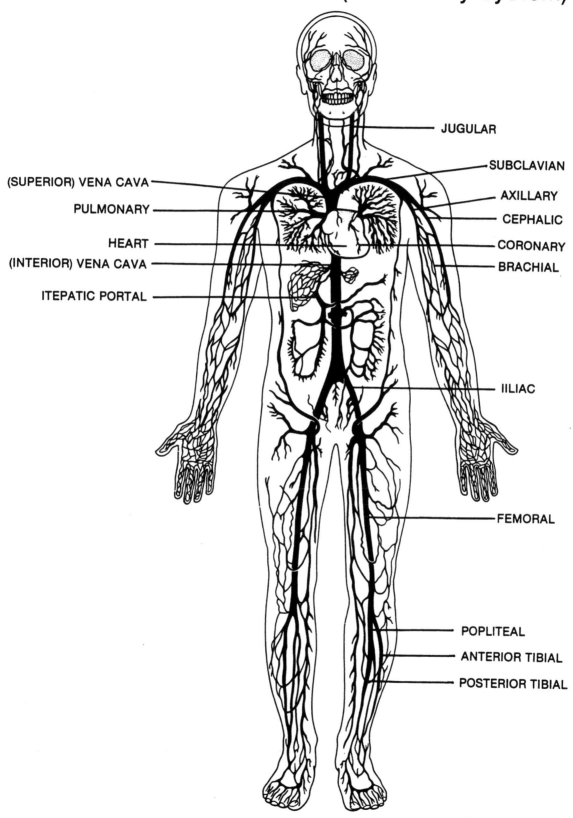

JUGULAR

SUBCLAVIAN

(SUPERIOR) VENA CAVA

AXILLARY

PULMONARY

CEPHALIC

HEART

CORONARY

(INTERIOR) VENA CAVA

BRACHIAL

ITEPATIC PORTAL

IILIAC

FEMORAL

POPLITEAL

ANTERIOR TIBIAL

POSTERIOR TIBIAL

FIGURE 8 — Nervous System

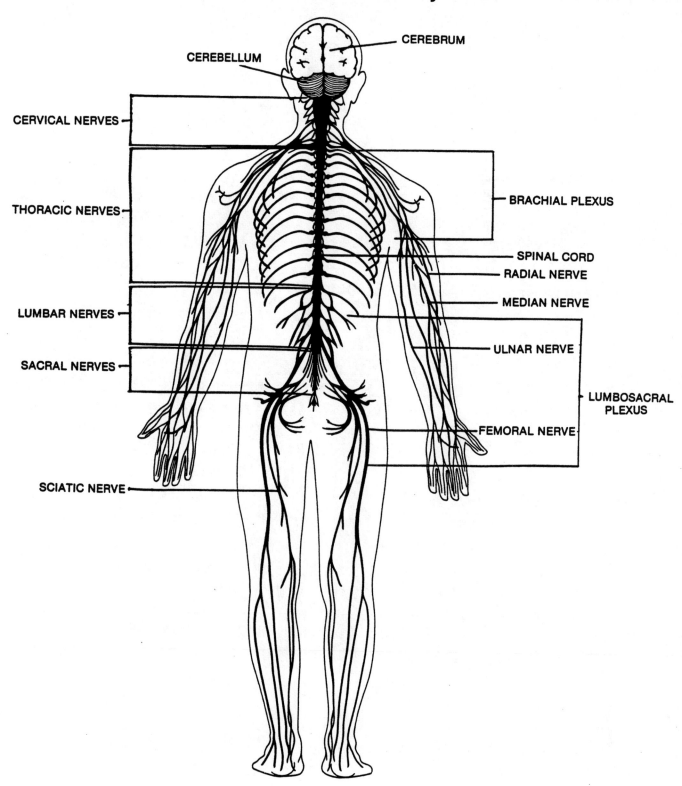

CEREBRUM

CEREBELLUM

CERVICAL NERVES

THORACIC NERVES

LUMBAR NERVES

SACRAL NERVES

SCIATIC NERVE

BRACHIAL PLEXUS

SPINAL CORD

RADIAL NERVE

MEDIAN NERVE

ULNAR NERVE

LUMBOSACRAL PLEXUS

FEMORAL NERVE

FIGURE 9 — Body Inside View

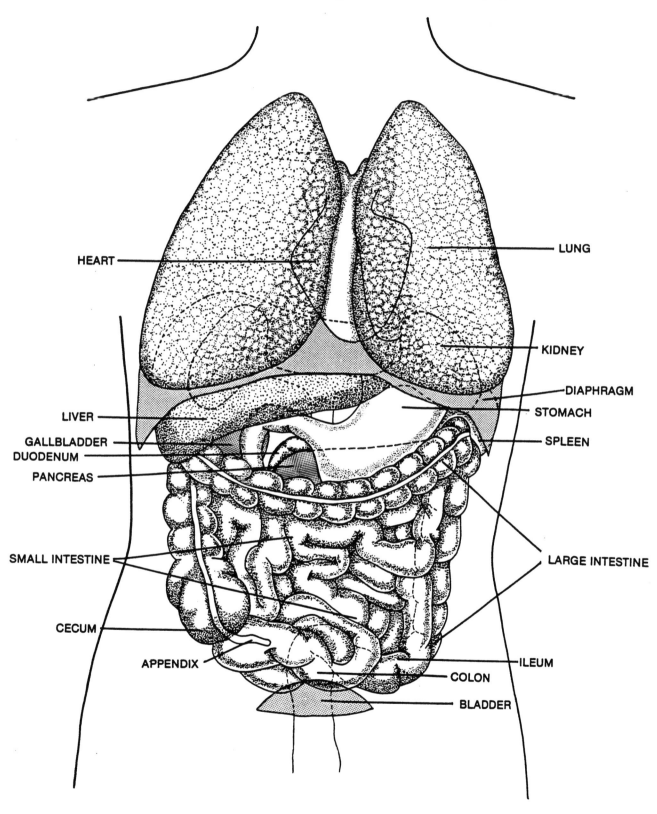

HEART

LUNG

KIDNEY

DIAPHRAGM

STOMACH

LIVER

SPLEEN

GALLBLADDER

DUODENUM

PANCREAS

SMALL INTESTINE

LARGE INTESTINE

CECUM

APPENDIX

ILEUM

COLON

BLADDER

FIGURE 10 — Respiratory System

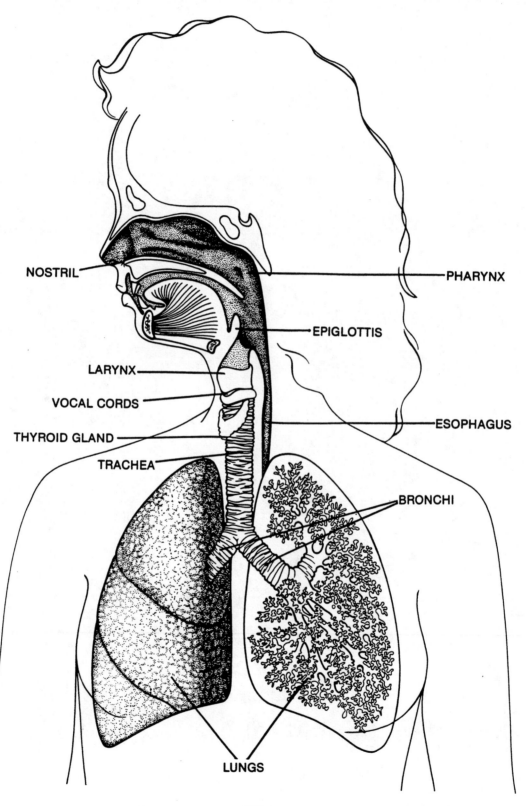

NOSTRIL

PHARYNX

EPIGLOTTIS

LARYNX

VOCAL CORDS

ESOPHAGUS

THYROID GLAND

TRACHEA

BRONCHI

LUNGS

FIGURE 11 — Urinary System

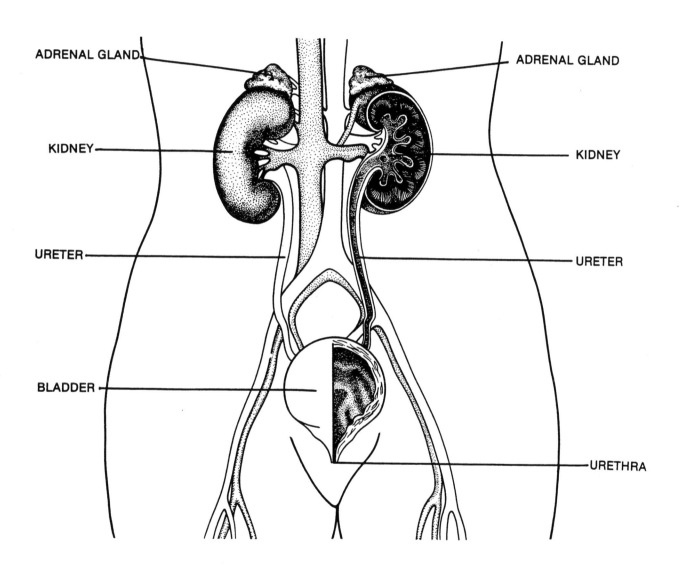

ADRENAL GLAND

ADRENAL GLAND

KIDNEY

KIDNEY

URETER

URETER

BLADDER

URETHRA

FIGURE 12 — Female Reproductive System

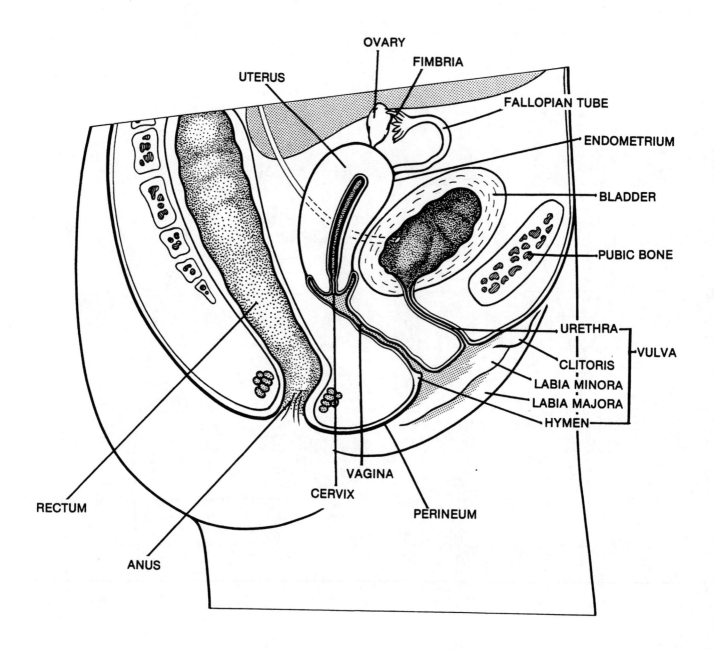

OVARY

FIMBRIA

UTERUS

FALLOPIAN TUBE

ENDOMETRIUM

BLADDER

PUBIC BONE

URETHRA

VULVA

CLITORIS

LABIA MINORA

LABIA MAJORA

HYMEN

VAGINA

CERVIX

PERINEUM

RECTUM

ANUS

FIGURE 13 — Male Reproductive System

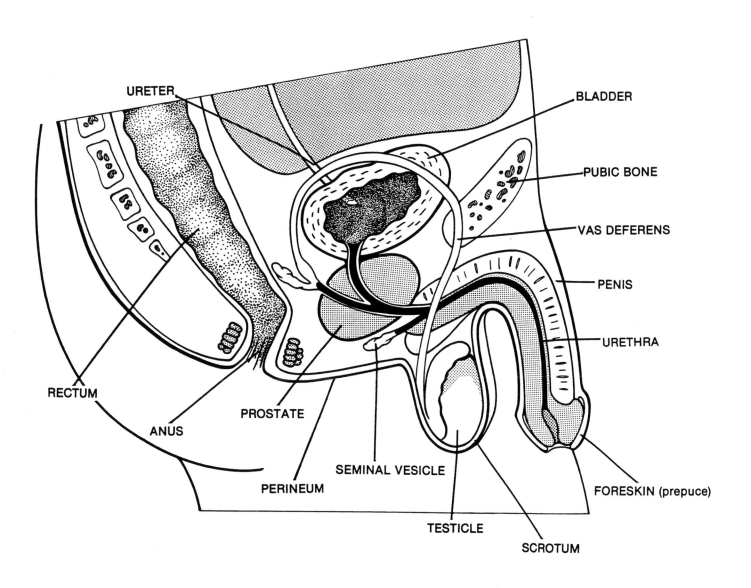

URETER

BLADDER

PUBIC BONE

VAS DEFERENS

PENIS

URETHRA

RECTUM

PROSTATE

ANUS

SEMINAL VESICLE

FORESKIN (prepuce)

PERINEUM

TESTICLE

SCROTUM

FIGURE 14 — Fetus

THREE MONTHS

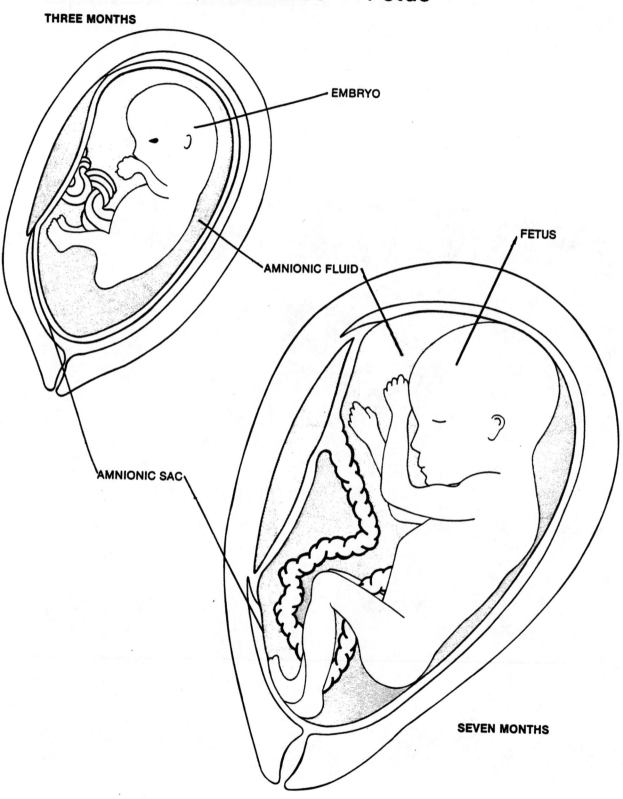

EMBRYO

AMNIONIC FLUID

FETUS

AMNIONIC SAC

SEVEN MONTHS

FIGURE 15 — Heart

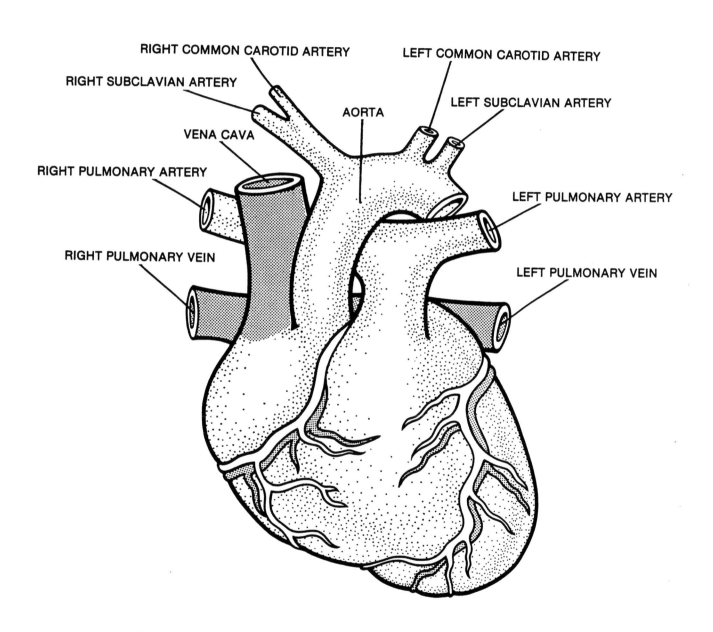

RIGHT COMMON CAROTID ARTERY

LEFT COMMON CAROTID ARTERY

RIGHT SUBCLAVIAN ARTERY

LEFT SUBCLAVIAN ARTERY

AORTA

VENA CAVA

RIGHT PULMONARY ARTERY

LEFT PULMONARY ARTERY

RIGHT PULMONARY VEIN

LEFT PULMONARY VEIN

FIGURE 16 — Heart Cross Section View

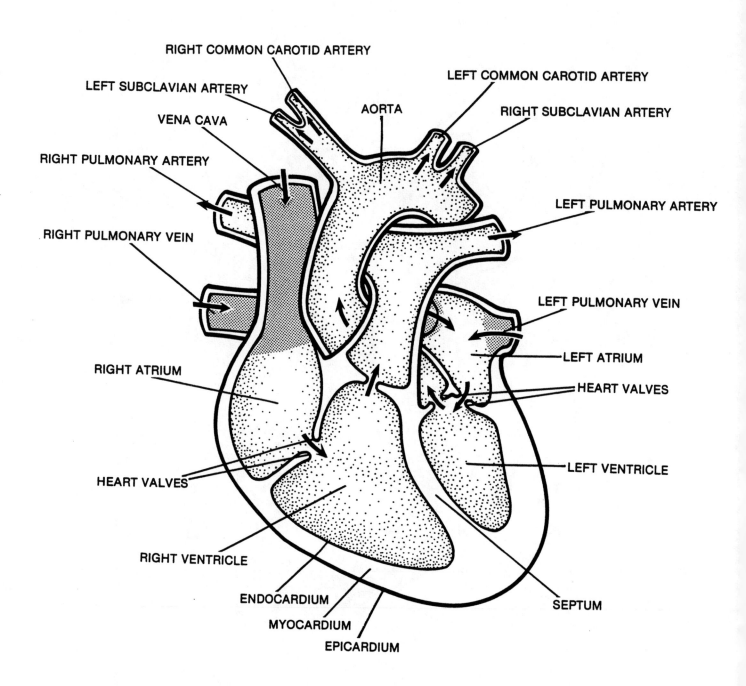

RIGHT COMMON CAROTID ARTERY

LEFT SUBCLAVIAN ARTERY

VENA CAVA

RIGHT PULMONARY ARTERY

RIGHT PULMONARY VEIN

RIGHT ATRIUM

HEART VALVES

RIGHT VENTRICLE

ENDOCARDIUM

MYOCARDIUM

EPICARDIUM

LEFT COMMON CAROTID ARTERY

AORTA

RIGHT SUBCLAVIAN ARTERY

LEFT PULMONARY ARTERY

LEFT PULMONARY VEIN

LEFT ATRIUM

HEART VALVES

LEFT VENTRICLE

SEPTUM

FIGURES 17 & 18 — Brain and Brain Cross Section View

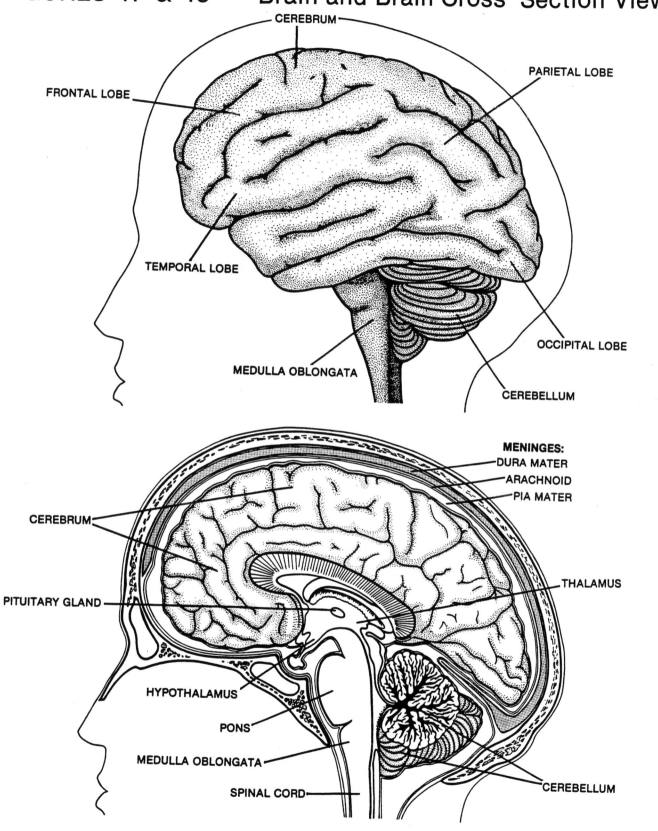

CEREBRUM

FRONTAL LOBE

PARIETAL LOBE

TEMPORAL LOBE

OCCIPITAL LOBE

MEDULLA OBLONGATA

CEREBELLUM

MENINGES:
DURA MATER
ARACHNOID
PIA MATER

CEREBRUM

THALAMUS

PITUITARY GLAND

HYPOTHALAMUS

PONS

MEDULLA OBLONGATA

SPINAL CORD

CEREBELLUM

FIGURE 20 — Ear

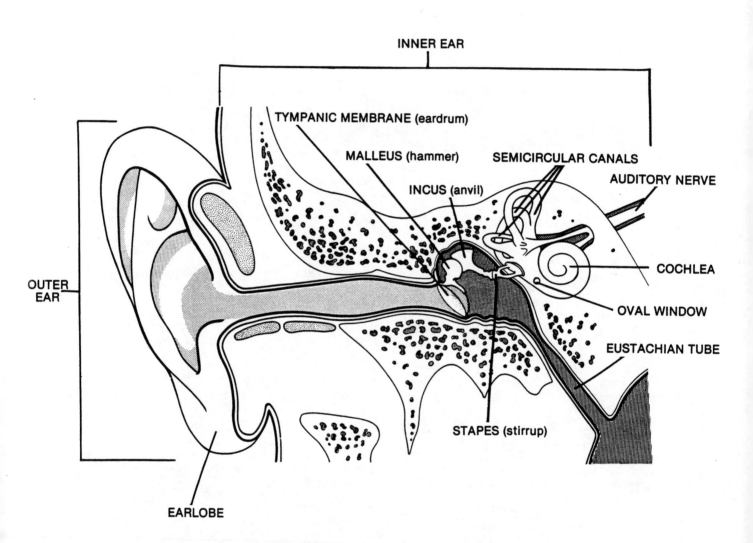

INNER EAR

TYMPANIC MEMBRANE (eardrum)

MALLEUS (hammer)

SEMICIRCULAR CANALS

INCUS (anvil)

AUDITORY NERVE

COCHLEA

OVAL WINDOW

EUSTACHIAN TUBE

STAPES (stirrup)

OUTER EAR

EARLOBE

702

FIGURES 21 & 22 — Eye and Eye Cross Section View

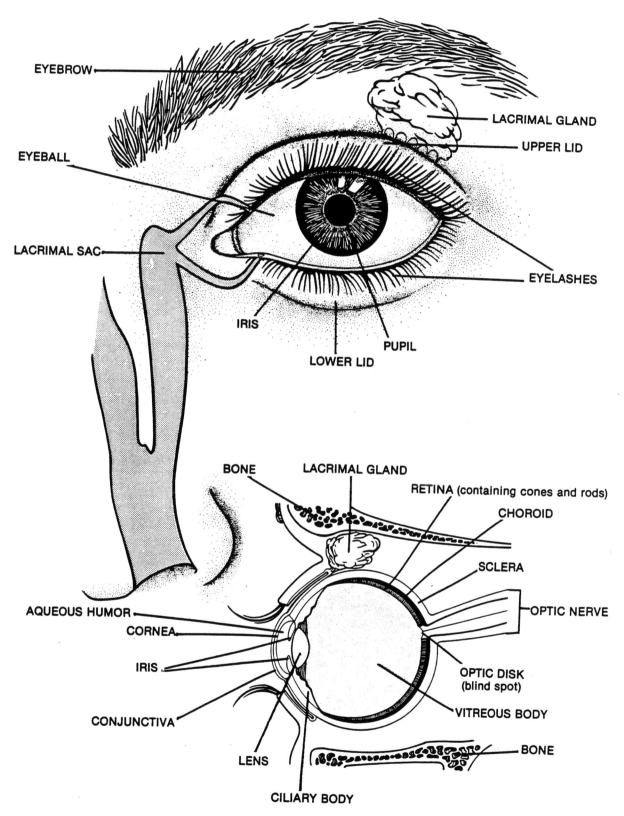

EYEBROW

LACRIMAL GLAND

UPPER LID

EYEBALL

EYELASHES

LACRIMAL SAC

IRIS

PUPIL

LOWER LID

BONE

LACRIMAL GLAND

RETINA (containing cones and rods)

CHOROID

SCLERA

AQUEOUS HUMOR

OPTIC NERVE

CORNEA

IRIS

OPTIC DISK
(blind spot)

CONJUNCTIVA

VITREOUS BODY

LENS

BONE

CILIARY BODY

FIGURE 23 — Mouth

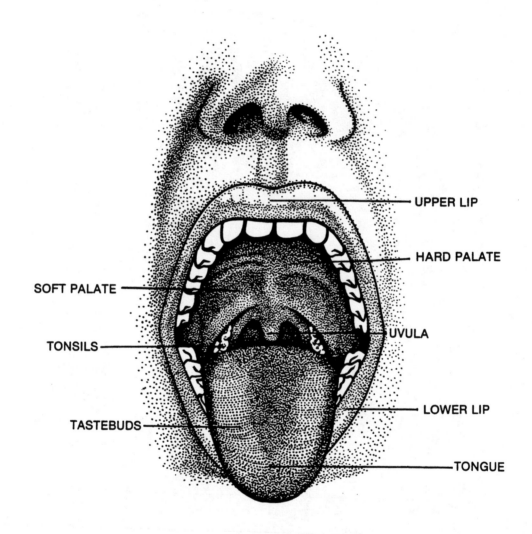

UPPER LIP

HARD PALATE

SOFT PALATE

UVULA

TONSILS

LOWER LIP

TASTEBUDS

TONGUE

FIGURE 24 — Teeth

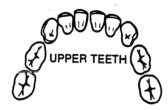

UPPER TEETH

LOWER TEETH

PERMANENT (adult) TEETH

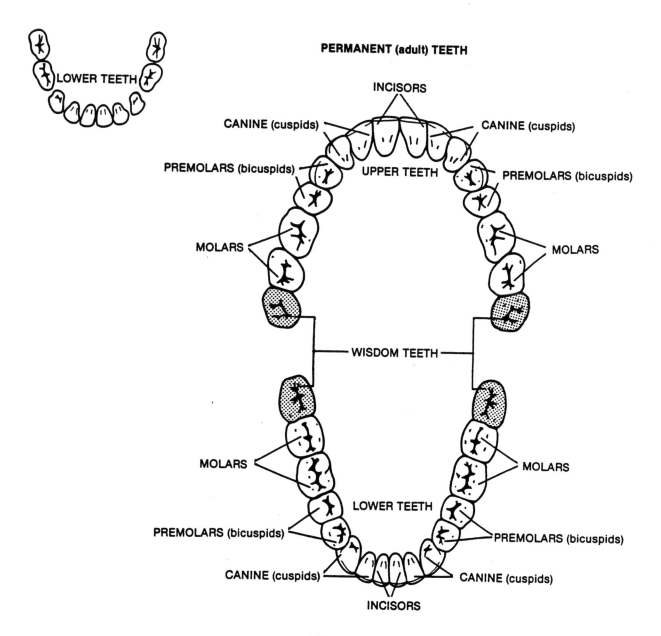

INCISORS

CANINE (cuspids)

CANINE (cuspids)

PREMOLARS (bicuspids)

UPPER TEETH

PREMOLARS (bicuspids)

MOLARS

MOLARS

WISDOM TEETH

MOLARS

MOLARS

LOWER TEETH

PREMOLARS (bicuspids)

PREMOLARS (bicuspids)

CANINE (cuspids)

CANINE (cuspids)

INCISORS

FIGURE 25 — Tooth Cross Section View

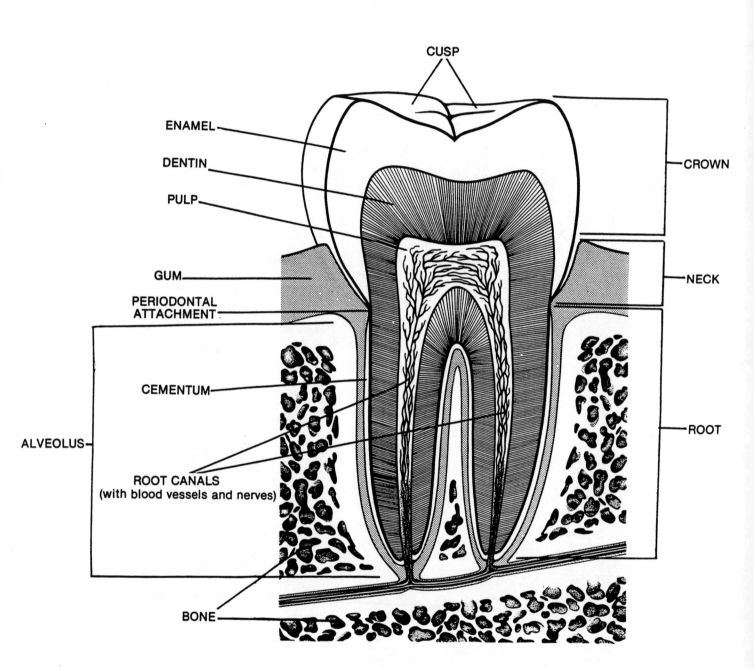

CUSP

ENAMEL

DENTIN

PULP

GUM

PERIODONTAL ATTACHMENT

CEMENTUM

ALVEOLUS

ROOT CANALS
(with blood vessels and nerves)

BONE

CROWN

NECK

ROOT

FIGURE 26 — Skeletal System

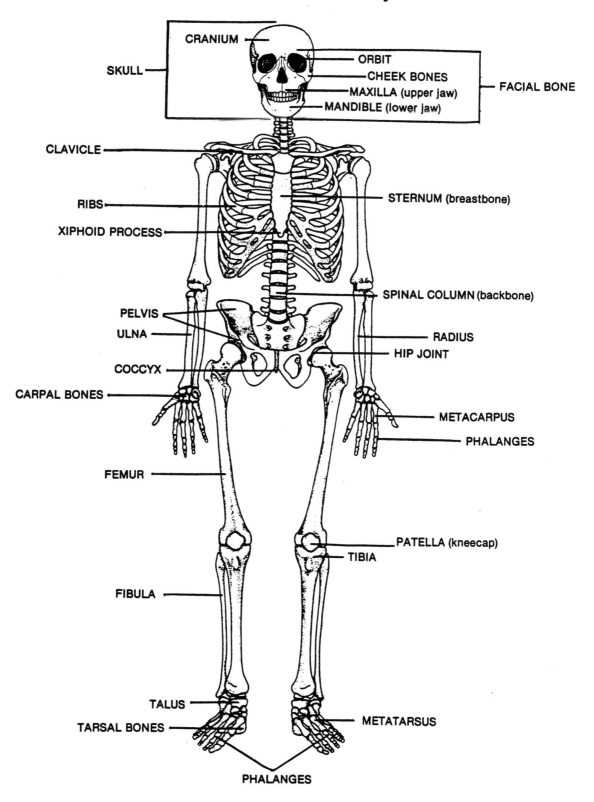

SKULL

CRANIUM

ORBIT

CHEEK BONES

MAXILLA (upper jaw)

MANDIBLE (lower jaw)

FACIAL BONE

CLAVICLE

RIBS

XIPHOID PROCESS

STERNUM (breastbone)

SPINAL COLUMN (backbone)

PELVIS

ULNA

COCCYX

RADIUS

HIP JOINT

CARPAL BONES

METACARPUS

PHALANGES

FEMUR

PATELLA (kneecap)

TIBIA

FIBULA

TALUS

TARSAL BONES

METATARSUS

PHALANGES

FIGURE 26 — Spinal Column (Vertebral Column)

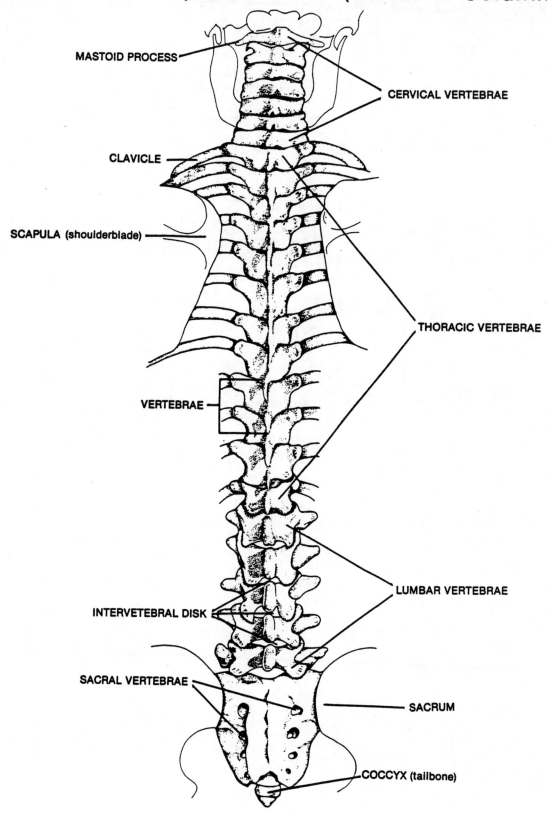

MASTOID PROCESS

CERVICAL VERTEBRAE

CLAVICLE

SCAPULA (shoulderblade)

THORACIC VERTEBRAE

VERTEBRAE

LUMBAR VERTEBRAE

INTERVETEBRAL DISK

SACRAL VERTEBRAE

SACRUM

COCCYX (tailbone)

BIBLIOGRAPHY

Boucher, Carl O., 1974. *Current Clinical Dental Terminology*, St. Louis: C.V. Mosby Company.

Doughten, Minkin, Rosen, 1978. *Signs for Sexuality*, Seattle Wa.: Planned Parenthood of Seattle/King County.

Duncan, Helen A., 1971. *Duncan's Dictionary for Nurses*, New York: Springer Publishing Co. Inc.

Elson, Lawrence M., Kapit, Wynn, 1977. *The Anatomy Coloring Book*, New York: Harper & Row.

Graedon, Joe, 1980. *Peoples Pharmacy*, New York: Avon Publishers of Bard, Camellot and Discus.

Gray, Henery, 1974. *Anatomy Descriptive and Surgical*, Philadelphia Pa.: Running Press.

Masters, R.E.L. and Huston Jean, 1977. *The Varieties of Psychodelic Experiences*, Holt, Rinehart & Winston.

Nourse, Alan E. 1964. *The Body*, New York: Rhett Austell.

Taber, Clarence Wilber, 1980. *Cyclopedic Medical Dictionary*, Philadelphia Pa.: F.A. Davis Company.

Woodward, James, 1980. *Signs of Drug Use*, Silver Spring Md.: T.J. Publishers.

Woodward, James, 1970. *Signs of Sexual Behavior*, Silver Spring Md.: T.J. Publishers.

TO OUR READERS

We would like your help in making this a better book. If there are dental, first-aid, or medical-related terms you feel should be added, please list them here and mail this page. If there are signs or a combination of six or less signs for a medical-related term you feel is commonly used, please let us know and we will include it in future revisions.

We would also like your comments on the text itself. Please circle numbers 1 to 6 according to your feelings concerning the following statements with the numbers corresponding as follows:

1 – of no help
2 – of little help
3 – average
4 – good
5 – very good
6 – excellent

1. I found this book useful when communicating with the deaf.

    1   2   3   4   5   6

2. As an interpreter, I found the suggested signs useful when interpreting.

    1   2   3   4   5   6

3. As a deaf person, I found the book's definitions easy to read and understand.

    1   2   3   4   5   6

NAME _____

ADDRESS _____

_____

COMMENTS:

RETURN TO: SILENT ENVIRONMENT EDUCATIONAL KAMP
              P.O. BOX 1026
              ELLENSBURG, WA 98926

Cut along this line